BARRON'S

HOW TO PREPARE FOR THE

MCAT

MEDICAL COLLEGE ADMISSION TEST

9th EDITION

Hugo R. Seibel, Ph.D.
Professor of Anatomy
Associate Dean of Medicine for
  Student Activities
School of Medicine
Virginia Commonwealth University
Richmond, Virginia

Kenneth E. Guyer, Ph.D.
Associate Professor of Biochemistry
School of Medicine, Marshall University
Huntington, West Virginia

A. Bryant Mangum, Ph.D.
Professor of English
Virginia Commonwealth University

Carolyn M. Conway, Ph.D.
Assistant Professor of Biology
Virginia Commonwealth University

Arthur F. Conway, Ph.D.
Associate Professor of Biology
Randolph-Macon College
Ashland, Virginia

Wesley L. Shanholtzer, Ph.D.
Professor
Department of Physics and
  Physical Sciences
Marshall University

BARRON'S

All inquiries should be addressed to:
Barron's Educational Series, Inc.
250 Wireless Boulevard
Hauppauge, New York 11788
http://www.barronseduc.com

Library of Congress Catalog Card No. 00-058524

International Standard Book No. 0-7641-1379-8

Library of Congress Cataloging-in-Publication Data
How to prepare for the MCAT : medical college admission test / Hugo R. Seibel . . . [et al.]. – 9th ed.
     p. cm.
    Includes index.
    ISBN 0-7641-1379-8
    1. Medical colleges—United States—Entrance examinations—Study guides. I. Seibel, Hugo R.

R838.5.H67 2001
610'.76—dc21   00-058524

PRINTED IN THE UNITED STATES OF AMERICA
9 8 7 6 5 4 3

CONTENTS

PREFACE

Can you prepare for the Medical College Admission Test (MCAT)? Some students are hesitant to utilize a book of this sort to assist in preparation for the Medical College Admission Test, perhaps believing there is something dishonest about this method of preparation. Other students may believe that they can utilize this book or a similar one just before the test to prepare themselves.

In our estimation both of these viewpoints are incorrect. These practice materials should provide experience in timed tests of this type and point out areas of weakness for additional study in appropriate textbooks. By proper and careful preparation utilizing all possible modes, the individual is simply presenting his or her true potential for the study of medicine. For maximum benefit we would suggest that students begin their preparation two or three months before the examination. This will allow time to take some of the practice examinations, review the areas of weakness, and retake some of the practice examinations without having the pressure of time to produce undue frustration and a feeling of hopelessness.

Obtaining admission to medical school is a very difficult task today. We hope that, in preparing this volume, we have been able to offer you a greater chance of success. Good luck!

We wish to acknowledge the help we have received from many of our colleagues; a special thank you should be extended to H. Meetz; G. D. Meetz; J. Gregorek; J. D. Reynolds; W. M. Reams; C. Kirksey; R. J. Krieg; J. H. Johnson; S. S. Craig; J. D. Povlishock; W. Seibel; L. Crane; L. P. Gartner; L. M. Sawyer; G. J. Somori; W. J. McIntyre; J. Washburn; J. L. Poland; S. L. Quattropani; M. P. Golka; F. M. Bush; R. L. Salisbury; M. M. Sholley; G. Miller; C. H. Fowlkes; R. B. Brandt; P. L. Szabo; N. Whisner; J. Wood; J. P. Guyer; J. Kass; Lester Schlumpf; B. P. Dezzutti; S. Falzone; I. K. Schneider; L. S. Costanzo; S. C. Dudley; J. Pettit; W. M. Grogan; S. G. Bradley; A. N. Avakian; C. P. Ruch; S. M. Ayers; J. J. McGovern; W. J. Borowy; J. Astruc, Jr.; J. F. Snyder; J. I. Townsend; J. Perlin; W. L. Banks; W. E. Blake, Jr.; L. Padilla; S. E. Kennedy; J. M. Messmer; S. A. Messmer; J. A. Rosecrans; M. N. De Pillars; B. Owen; R. G. Bass; R. S. Vacca; J. Mundie; E. Pollard; D. James; P. F. H. Campbell; T. Fleet; H. Tuttle; M. Ripley; R. Perry; R. Dale; S. V. Doud; L. Graham; D. J. Vick; Robert Lehrman; N. Sharp; E. Hodges; L. Carleton; and A. Arnold. Particular gratitude is extended to Mrs. Marilyn P. Bertrand for her cheerful and spirited assistance and the typing of the manuscript. We are indebted to Dr. Edith E. Seibel for her contributions and the proofreading of the book. Dr. Erwin E. Seibel deserves a special commendation since he contributed the bulk of the physics review for the first edition.

In preparing the 9th edition of this book we received extraordinary help and wish to extend our special gratitude to Karl S. Roth, Charles H. O'Neil, David G. Simpson, J. Dennis Hoban, Donald G. Roebuck, Ruth L. Dennis-Phillips, John W. Bigbee, Caroline G. Jackson, Phyllis J. Jett, Thomas L. Tucker, Emily Mistr, and William L. Banks, Jr.

INTRODUCTION

The MCAT represents an attempt to evaluate (1) the student's knowledge and ability to solve problems in the areas of biology, chemistry, and physics, (2) the student's skill in analysis of paragraphs, tabular material, graphs, etc., and (3) the ability to write two first draft compositions in correct English. Separate scores will be reported for Verbal Reasoning, Physical Sciences, Writing Sample, and Biological Sciences.

It is expected that those taking the test will have the equivalent of one year of college study in each of the following scientific areas: biology, general and/or inorganic chemistry, organic chemistry, and physics. Although advanced study in one or more of these disciplines may give a better understanding of concepts, it is not intended that the questions will require a knowledge of concepts not taught in basic courses.

A mathematics background including one year of college mathematics should suffice for the science questions; calculus is not required. Indeed, it has been suggested that high school courses, which included the following, would represent adequate preparation in mathematics: two years of algebra; use of trigonometric functions; memorization of sine and cosine of 0°, 90°, and 180°; facility in use of metric and English units and conversion from one set of units to another (when conversion factors are given); experimental error; statistics to include the concepts of arithmetic mean, range, variability, and significant figures; and vector addition and subtraction.

It is our suggestion that you begin preparation by studying the review sections of this book. Areas that are particularly difficult for you may require some review of your college texts. When you begin taking the practice tests, try to pace yourself to allow completion of each section within the allotted time. (If it is necessary to omit some questions because of time limitations, you may wish to go back after you have scored the test and try to answer them without the pressure of time.)

After taking your first practice test and correcting the answers, you should score your test as it will be done after the actual test. First count the number of correct answers in (1) Verbal Reasoning, (2) Physical Sciences, and (3) Biological Sciences. In each case this will represent the number of correct answers in that discipline.

The number of correct answers is the raw score and must then be converted into a 15-point scaled score *approximated* by the following tables. The approximation exists because raw score to scaled score tables may vary from test to test due to slight differences in degree of difficulty.

Although individual medical schools will vary with respect to the scores they require, a standard score of 11 or greater will probably be considered to be quite competitive. A standard score of 7 or less would indicate an area requiring substantial additional preparation. Before taking the next practice test, you should concentrate on areas of low score.

The Science area may be remediated by additional study and working problems. The area of Verbal Reasoning, however, may require a slightly different approach. Try going back over this part of the examination, reading carefully, and answering the questions again without a time limit. Read the paragraph again and try to determine why you missed certain questions. Be sure to use only the information in the paragraph. Then go on to additional practice examinations. One additional suggestion: Read the questions carefully before answering. Sometimes students answer the question they *expected* rather than the question that was asked. Try to avoid this pitfall.

If you are unable to read at the required rate and comprehension level, then your problem may be more serious. After studying the Verbal Reasoning section of this book, you may want to review some reading selections from your Freshman English course. You may also want to practice by reading articles in magazines such as *Time, Newsweek,* or *The Atlantic Monthly,* consciously noting the central ideas and distinguishing major from minor points in each article as you read.

Verbal Reasoning		Physical Sciences		Biological Sciences	
Raw Score	Scaled Score	Raw Score	Scaled Score	Raw Score	Scaled Score
0–7	1	0–8	1	0–8	1
8–14	2	9–16	2	9–16	2
15–20	3	17–28	3	17–28	3
21–26	4	29–33	4	29–33	4
27–31	5	34–39	5	34–39	5
32–36	6	40–44	6	40–44	6
37–41	7	45–49	7	45–49	7
42–46	8	50–55	8	50–55	8
47–50	9	56–60	9	56–60	9
51–53	10	61–64	10	61–64	10
54–57	11	65–67	11	65–67	11
58–60	12	68–70	12	68–70	12
61–62	13	71–73	13	71–73	13
63–64	14	74–75	14	74–75	14
65	15	76–77	15	76–77	15

As you progress through the other practice tests, you should develop facility in working faster to allow completion of each section. Although wild guessing is of no value, it is to your advantage to guess among a select number of answers if you have ruled out some answers.

Remember that we cannot hope to present everything you should have learned in years of study. We can only help you to identify areas of weakness, give some review of important concepts, and provide experience and confidence in taking a test having the format of the Medical College Admission Test. We hope that this will allow you to reach your own potential on this test.

The following four sections comprise the MCAT examination: Biological Sciences, Physical Sciences, Verbal Reasoning, and Writing Sample.

The Biological Sciences test will concentrate on basic biology and biologically related chemistry, whereas the Physical Sciences examination will focus on physics and physically related chemistry areas. The Verbal Reasoning passages will be taken from the social sciences, from the humanities, and from areas of the natural sciences not tested in the Biological and Physical Sciences section of the MCAT. Topics for the Writing Sample are not taken from the content of physics, biology, or chemistry, nor will they ask for personal reasons why the student has chosen medicine as a career.

TIMETABLE FOR THE MCAT

TOTAL TIME: Approximately 5 hours and 45 minutes, plus 1 hour for lunch, 20 minutes for breaks

85 minutes	Verbal Reasoning (65 questions)	9 passages 6–10 questions/passage
10 minutes	REST PERIOD	
100 minutes	Physical Sciences (77 questions)	10 problem sets 5–10 questions/set 15 problems 1 question/set
60 minutes	LUNCH	
60 minutes	Writing Sample (2 essays)	2 topics 30 minutes/topic
10 minutes	REST PERIOD	
100 minutes	Biological Sciences (77 questions)	10 problem sets 5–10 questions/set 15 problems 1 question/set

Verbal Reasoning

Typically this section will be composed of 9 passages from the humanities, social sciences, and natural sciences; each passage will be followed by 6–10 questions. These questions will be based on, and can be answered from, the information presented.

Physical Sciences

Typically this section will be composed of a series of problems upon which the subsequent multiple-choice questions are based. There usually will be 10 problem sets that will be followed by 5–10 questions each and 15 problems to be followed by a single question.

Writing Sample

Typically this section will be composed of two topics; 30 minutes will be allowed for each. The student will be asked to develop a central thesis, synthesize material, separate major from minor issues, propose alternative solutions, present ideas in a logical and coherent manner, and write in standard English, which conforms to accepted practices regarding such mechanical matters as grammar and syntax.

Biological Sciences

Typically this section will be composed of a series of problems upon which the subsequent multiple-choice questions are based. There usually will be 10 problem sets that will be followed by 5–10 questions each and 15 problems to be followed by a single question.

ROLE OF THE MCAT

The MCAT, in combination with college grades (overall and science GPA), types and quality of courses, letters of recommendation, extracurricular activities, major undergraduate institution attended, the interview, SAT, etc., is a screening device. The test is an objective measure and high scores will help an individual with average grades. Average or slightly lower MCAT scores probably do not significantly affect a superior college record. The literature points to a positive correlation between high MCAT scores (especially science subtests) and future success in the basic medical sciences (preclinical phase) and National Board of Medical Examiners Part I examination scores.

TOOLS FOR LEARNING, TEST PREPARATION, AND TEST-TAKING STRATEGIES

> *Failure to prepare is preparation for failure.*

PRINCIPLES OF STUDYING

Introduction

The authors have been involved in the training of thousands of medical students and have explored and discussed with these students their test preparation and test-taking strategies. These students have developed into efficient, skillful test takers in order to cope with the volumes of detailed material on which they are tested. They learned to recognize key elements of course content and to train themselves to successfully answer thousands of test questions.

It is not just our observations of medical students, however, that we rely on to give you advice. There is a growing body of scientific literature emerging from psychology and the neurosciences that provides useful information about how to study for tests. These studies have identified the following very important test preparation topics.

- *Study time*: HOW much you use; HOW you use it
- *Study location*: WHERE and WHEN you study
- *Input*: HOW you ENTER knowledge into memory
- *Storage*: HOW you SAVE knowledge in memory
- *Retrieval*: HOW you GET knowledge from memory

All these topics offer something to help you study and prepare for any type of examination you could encounter in the future.

Study Time

Preparation time is a *necessary* element for successful performance on tests but is found to be insufficient when used alone. Students have told us that they must set aside *regular time* periods for studying which increases their efficiency. It is not just setting aside time, however, that allows learning to take place. Rather, it is what happens during the regular study periods. We all know people who spend large amounts of time looking at textbooks or notes but still have poor grades because they lack effective study strategies. The most important strategy is for you to *concentrate* on what you are learning and to have *learning* as your *sole purpose for studying*. The goal of every study period should be to learn something new or relearn something that you have partially forgotten.

Here is a hint to help you concentrate or *pay attention*: If you find that your eyes are crossing a page of text but nothing is registering in your mind, and you are having trouble paying attention, you need to read faster. So fast that you will finally pay attention but not so fast that you aren't actually reading. *Speed helps you concentrate.* Suppose you are driving along a winding, country road at 20 mph. What are you likely to be doing? Perhaps you are enjoying the scenery—taking in the trees, the horses in the pasture, or the ducks flying overhead. Now push down on the accelerator until you are going 55 mph. What will you do? You either are paying attention to your driving or are likely to find yourself in serious trouble. The point is that speed forces you to focus on what you are doing. Reading rapidly helps you pay attention to what you are reading.

Study Location

Research tells us *where and when* to study. If you learn something in a certain environment, you are more likely to remember this information when you are again in that environment; therefore, study in a place similar to that in which you will be tested.

Even your mood is thought to play a role in memory. While the effect is not thought to be a powerful one, researchers do believe it influences memory in two ways:

1. Recall is better for pleasant than for unpleasant material.
2. Recall is better when you are in the same mood at retrieval time as you were when you encoded the knowledge.

You will want to *study in spurts*. Spread out practice over time with rest intervals spaced between. This is called *distributed study or spaced practice*. The amount of study material and the distribution of practice sessions affects your ability to retrieve the things you have learned. *Massed practice* refers to long study periods and produces the poorest learning outcome. For most academic subjects it is best to work in a series of shorter study sessions distributed over several days. If, however, you are cramming for a test, then long study sessions are better. The problem with cramming is that you do all right on an exam but don't remember much two weeks later.

Putting Knowledge into Short-Term Memory

Putting information into memory involves the encoding of incoming sensory information into a form that the brain can understand. In other words, our senses take in information from the environment, and our brain makes sense of it. A key to storing information in long-term memory so that you can easily retrieve it is *organization*.

Short-term memory (STM), also known as *working memory*, has a capacity limited to 5 to 9 items. Unrehearsed material stays in STM for 15 to 20 seconds.

What is the usual length of a telephone number? Count the digits in 555-4567. Interestingly, most phone numbers have 7 digits (the ideal number of items to be remembered in working memory). Fortunately, there are ways that your brain can manipulate the limitation of remembering just 5 to 9 items. One way is called *chunking,* in which you arrange pieces of information into meaningful clusters and increase your capacity to remember. Take, for example, the following numbers: 76823318289190827103135466542594214. You can't even hold this 35-digit number in your working memory. Maybe you could remember the first 3 or 4 or last 3 or 4 numbers but you're not going to hold all 35 numbers in your working memory. Now look at the same number chunked into 5 telephone numbers.

768-2331
828-9190
827-1031
354-6654
259-4214

Interesting, isn't it? Do you think you could use chunking to learn material just as apparently overwhelming and meaningless as the 35-digit number you just chunked? What is the key to chunking? You're right—*organization*. It is a key to storing information in your long-term memory.

Storing Knowledge in Long-Term Memory

Strategies that encode information in a meaningful manner help you retrieve easily information from long-term memory (LTM). There are two ways to increase retention of what you are learning. Both require you to practice what you are learning. The first, *overlearning*, involves practicing with the material over and above what is needed to just learn it and is particularly good for learning basic facts and skills. When you learned the multiplication tables, you overlearned them by practicing them over and over again. Furnish yourself with opportunities for overlearning of key concepts and skills. Make up flash cards and use them over and over until you have the facts locked in memory. Repeat until you "know it cold." Most people don't have the time, patience, or determination for this approach, and it's not very efficient when you have a lot to learn in a short period of time.

Because of these deficiencies, an approach called *elaboration* is often recommended. When you elaborate, you reorganize information and make it meaningful by relating it to something already in your memory. In order for you to engage in elaborative activities, you need to connect new information to something you already know. An organizational plan that is useful for school subjects utilizes logical schemes: places, dates, hierarchies, etc. Semantic categories allow you to organize by any meaningful strategy that you prefer. For example, you can categorize alphabetically, by body part, by size, by function, or by structure. Still other ways of organizing information are sounds, pictures, and colors. You should use personally meaningful categories to organize the knowledge you are attempting to store in long-term memory.

Mnemonics are schemes designed to assist you in remembering. "Fall back, spring forward" is a way of remembering to set your clock forward in the spring and back in the fall. "Every good boy does fine" and "FACE" help us remember the lines and spaces of the musical staff. "Please Excuse My Dear Aunt Sally" stands for the order of the following mathematical operations: Parentheses, Exponents, Multiplication, Division, Addition, and Subtraction. You remember these mnemonics, don't you? They are unforgettable acronyms or sentences used to recall a set of already existing strong associations. Other mnemonic schemes include methods of associating things you are trying to remember with words (peg word method) and with locations (loci method).

Peg Word Method

With the peg word method, you begin by using the sequence of numbers 1 to 10 to memorize a word that is concrete and rhymes with the number beside it. For each number, you memorize the word that rhymes with it. Here are 10 numbers and words.

1. bun
2. shoe
3. tree
4. door
5. hive
6. stick
7. heaven
8. gate
9. line
10. hen

These words make up a peg list. You use it to memorize new, unrelated sets of items. Place each item to be remembered in an image with a peg word. For example, if you wanted to memorize a list of words that begins *muscle, tissue, cell, energy* . . ., you could imagine a muscle burger bulging through a bun, Mother Hubbard's shoe house covered with toilet tissue as a result of your high school's big victory, a tree growing through a jail cell, and a door swirling in the sky captured by the energy of a tornado. Try this method with lists that you need to memorize. It could be fun to use the peg word method.

Loci Method

The loci method lets you use knowledge of the spatial arrangement and contents of some familiar place, like your own home or neighborhood. When trying to remember a list of words, take an imagined walk through your location, placing each item in, on, or near some familiar, easily remembered object. To return to the sample words above, your muscles would be seen in the mirror in the bathroom, tissues would be on the nightstand in your bedroom, the cell phone would be on the kitchen table where you left it, and the energy would come from the furnace in the garage. To retrieve these items you recreate the stroll and retrieve each item as you come to it. To remember these words, you imagine driving into the garage and seeing that the furnace is aglow with energy. You open the door inside the garage and enter the kitchen, where you immediately notice your cell phone on the kitchen table. While picking up the phone, you knock over the pepper shaker and start sneezing. You run to your bedroom, where you pick up tissues from the nightstand so you can blow your nose. Then you decide to take a shower. While entering the bathroom, you can't help but stop and admire your muscles in the mirror on the bathroom door.

These methods may seem silly, but you really ought to try them.

Retrieving Knowledge

Retrieval is difficult if the information you are trying to remember is not encoded appropriately. Remember, organization is the key to storing information in long-term memory so that you can easily retrieve it. Also, do you remember the importance of studying in an environment similar to the one in which you will be tested? Retrieval tends to be best when the *context* in which it takes place matches the *context* present at encoding. Two things that you have control over and that affect your ability to retrieve knowledge from memory are the *amount of time* you spend practicing and how you *distribute your practice*. What is the best way to distribute practice? That's right—study in spurts, take breaks, and study over time.

There are two ways in which you are asked to remember on tests. One is to *recall* information without cues, as with fill-in-the-blank and essay questions. These are considered the hardest questions, because recall tasks provide few cues to the answers. The other way you are asked to remember is called *recognition*, which requires you to identify material previously learned. Multiple-choice and matching items are typically aimed at asking you to recognize word associations. Both recall and recognition require retrieval of data stored in long-term memory.

Forgetting

It appears that there is no practical limit to how much information we can put into long-term memory. Many psychologists believe that information is permanently stored in various places in our brain. For them, forgetting is failure in retrieval. Other psychologists theorize that aging, lack of use, and disease decay memory and cause our brain to forget. Still other psychologists think that the ability to remember is linked to the use of the same cues for encoding and retrieving items in long-term memory.

A basic problem with retrieving information from memory is that there are lots of things that interfere. So being forewarned may help you overcome some of the things that will interfere with your ability to remember for recall and recognition tasks.

There are two classic interference effects that we all face when trying to put new knowledge into memory: the recency/primacy effect and the retroactive and proactive interference effect. *Retroactive interference* refers to the new memories impairing the memory of something that you previously stored in memory. *Proactive interference* refers to the effect that old memories have on your ability to remember new material. For example, you memorized the names of the muscles and bones of the leg last week. This week you are trying to learn the names of the muscles and bones of the arm. What will happen? You will have a tendency to forget the parts of the leg as you learn the arm parts (retroactive interference), as well as a tendency to forget some of the arm parts because you learned the leg first (proactive interference). You should avoid studying similar things in consecutive time periods.

Remember that long list of 35 numbers you saw earlier? We told you that virtually no one would remember that list. But we did say that you might remember the first couple or the last couple of numbers, which is an example of the *recency/primacy effect*. You tend to remember the beginning and end of any list much more easily than you remember what is in the middle. When you go to a restaurant and the waitress names 8 or 10 salad dressings, you tend to ask for either the first or last one she mentioned. Or you ask her to repeat the list because you can't remember the fifth one she mentioned. The moral of this story is to make *short lists*.

Summary

Factors that enhance learning and memory are:

1. Study time and place.
2. Characteristics of what must be remembered.
3. Strategies for storing knowledge and remembering.
4. Context characteristics of practice and test situations.

Test Taking

Here are some common suggestions for taking tests. Note that most of them involve common sense, but we don't always think about or use many of these suggestions.

Before the Test

To prepare for tests, follow these guidelines:

1. Identify the subject matter that you need to prepare and prioritize it in terms of how much study time you need for difficult, moderate, and easy material.
2. Use review books but have comprehensive textbooks handy to fill in any gaps you discover in your reviewing.
3. Use old examinations. By going over old exams, you are relearning material in the context in which you will be tested and you begin to see how test makers think about a subject. The more old test questions you go over, the better.
4. Remember to use lots of short study periods.
5. It is not "old-fashioned" to use flashcards to help you memorize terms, processes, formulas, etc.
6. Seek help from professors when you hit a roadblock.
7. Reduce your stress through exercise, reading, music, etc.
8. Get plenty of rest.
9. Follow a nutritious diet.
10. The night before the examination, relax and get a good night's sleep.

During the Test

On the day of a test, keep in mind the following guidelines.

1. Read the directions carefully! Follow the directions!
2. Preview the test to see how much time you need to allot for each section.
3. Pace yourself during the examination so that you do not panic at the end.
4. Save time at the end of the exam to review your test and make sure you haven't left any questions unanswered.
5. Answer the question being asked. Do not change the question to fit your way of thinking.
6. You can change answers during the exam, but do so only if you are at least 90 percent sure that you are changing to the correct answer.
7. Stay calm. If you find yourself getting frustrated or annoyed, stop. Take a deep breath. Think of something pleasant and start again.
8. Stay focused on why it is important to do your best. Remind yourself that good performance on tests provides you with opportunities that otherwise will not be available to you.
9. Don't let your mind or eyes wander. Work efficiently and concentrate on speed and accuracy.
10. Remember that standardized tests are designed to be very difficult. Virtually no one gets all the questions correct, so don't worry when you see a bunch of questions for which you don't know the answer.

Strategies for Success

A. Time Management

1. Time management is an essential element and an effective tool for test preparation.
2. There are many time management strategies to help you effectively and productively use your time to study within an established time frame.
3. Become aware of the importance of time management, because time is an investment. It is unrelenting and irreplaceable. Once wasted, it is gone forever. If you lack the ability to control your time, you basically are not controlling your life. Experts feel that using time in a con-

trolled, deliberate fashion is far more beneficial than doing everything efficiently. Efficiency is important but time management is key. Of course, the ideal is a structured, solid balance.

4. Only you can determine how much return you want on your investment.

5. You must realistically allocate enough study hours daily to perform meaningful tasks yet balance all your other daily activities. You need not become an obsessed clock watcher.

6. Weigh the importance of each task to be accomplished, then make a decision on what to do. You must critically assess what you are doing; plan the activity but be flexible to change when necessary. Today's priority number one might become tomorrow's priority number three as the situation warrants.

7. When making conscious decisions, utilize the basic principle of time management:

Work smarter, not harder. One way to use this basic principle is a simple, yet effective time management formula:

$$PMS = W$$

Plan, Make a Molehill Out of a Mountain, and Safeguard (then you can) = Work Your "A" Off

Plan

- Plan an effective study schedule by prioritizing and concentrating on one task or subject at a time. Astute planning while focusing on the future puts the future in the present; you are doing something about the situation now, not when chance lets you.
- Prioritize what needs to be accomplished in your life. This is not an easy task unless you understand the broader picture and you have conceptualized established goals. Prioritizing is especially important when studying for an examination some time from now. Your daily school commitments have a certain definite priority, and therefore you must be able to adjust your schedule as necessary. Resolve your conflicts promptly and thoughtfully.
- Prioritize your tasks by establishing a to-do list. This is an extremely powerful tool because it is a method to organize yourself and reduce stress in your life. Write down tasks that need to be done within 24 hours or less (short-range goals, or your A list). Then, write down tasks that need to be done within one week (intermediate-range goals, or your B list). Now write down tasks that need to be accomplished within one month or more (long-range goals, or your C list). This is not a static world and goals can and should be revised periodically. In order to achieve your long-term goals, short-term planning is key. A priority list is essential, but above all realize it is subject to change.
- Determine which things are important to you and which things can be dropped from your list. You must eliminate low-priority items as they crop up.
- Your critical thinking skills will surface as you decide when to implement and how to execute tasks.
- Use the basic guidelines: *Be aware of all that needs to be done.*
- Never be too rigid in your planning. "Flexibility" is the key to a successful plan.
- You should revise and evaluate your plan weekly to analyze whether it is working or if it is taking too long to execute and complete tasks.
- Tailor the plan to fit your needs and know how you will spend your time.
- Allow sufficient time for studying each task by placing blocks of time in your schedule.

Do Not Make an Excuse for Planning

- Many of us fall into the time trap and use the excuse "I am too busy to take time out to plan." Think of it in these terms: If you feel that you have no spare time to plan, most certainly you need a plan.
- Every football team has a game plan, so do not look for a surprise victory.
- The best time to plan is open to debate. You are the best judge and determining factor—stay loose.
- Remember that a guide helps you operate more smoothly and less strenuously. It eliminates anxiety and fosters a positive self image.

Make a Molehill Out of a Mountain

- Make your plan work for you by reversing the cliché. "Make a molehill out of a mountain." You can break the mountain down for any major and difficult assignment if you have established a to-do list and have estimated the time it will take to complete each task.
- Estimate the amount of time you think it takes to complete each task on your to-do list. At first your guess may be wrong. Eventually, with practice, you will increase your accuracy regarding each task.
- If you spend 30 minutes each day on a major assignment, the assignment will become less intimidating as well as easier to complete by the end of one week. You will see instant results and be amazed at how much you have accomplished on this task.
- Always introduce a "safety net" with each task to be completed on your list. The safety net will assist you with the unexpected events in your plan such as sickness, surprise visitors, fatigue, interruptions, and family demands. You will need to use good judgment and be realistic about the length of time for these activities.
- Don't forget to include time for yourself. During this time you can relax and enjoy things you want to do for at least an hour—such as talk on the telephone, go shopping, or go to the gym.
- A break in the schedule creates a good balance and a healthier attitude.
- Sometimes you get more accomplished doing nothing. The moral is to work hard and play hard.
- Planned relaxing and having fun clears the way to more productivity. How you study is more relevant than how long you study. A clear, focused mind can process more information quickly.
- Utilize your commuting time. One of the authors usually had an hour's subway ride. This was his time to read a novel or magazine, and to set aside schoolwork. You might decide on the exact opposite.

Safeguard Your Time

- Safeguard your valuable time by placing it in a safety deposit box. (Isn't that where valuables are kept?) You are the safety deposit box!
- You must learn to say no to others who don't understand your purpose and goals.
- Strictly speaking in order to follow set priorities, you must learn when to say yes, and when to say no. Too many of us take the easy way out and rationalize; this method is not compatible with an effective plan. An effective plan has availability hours integrated into it. If your motivation waivers at times, do not be discouraged but give yourself credit for your accomplishments.
- Sometimes after succeeding in some very difficult tasks it is beneficial to slow down, refocus, and reward yourself. Whatever you do, do not use escape routes to justify procrastination.
- Do your best always; consider your successes and try and try again. If you do not, you will encounter problems.
- If you do your utmost you have a chance, even though you can never eliminate the possibility of failure. That is being honest and realistic.
- Avoid ploys that others use to break into your safety deposit box and steal your valuables (time and your to-do list.)
- When your open your safety deposit box, remove all external distractions (television and music) or distractions on your desk.
- Study difficult and boring information first.
- Be aware of when your energy and concentration level is high and plan your study periods around this time of the day. We all have our patterns.
- Find a better place to study when your productivity or level of energy decreases. Remember that your study area should provide the least distractions.
- Be critical of your study breaks; space them appropriately.
- Controlling your time gives you the luxury to adapt and to be spontaneous.

Work Your "A"

David Ellis, author of *Becoming a Master Student*, recommends a powerful technique to help students accomplish their goals and efficiently manage their time. To master this technique, stick with completing the "A," or the short-range goals that are on your to-do list.

- Start and finish one task at a time. Don't jump around to other items on the list.
- After each completed task, reward yourself.
- It is more efficient to work on one task no longer than three hours; at that point take an hour break.
- Take more breaks (10 minutes at a time) if you are under a lot of pressure, because you need time to digest and process the material. Also, more breaks will relieve your stress and sustain your motivation.

B. Memory and Association Techniques

1. Memory is the total storehouse of mentally retained impressions and knowledge.
2. You need total concentration (initial attention) to store information into your long-term memory.
3. There are three main strategies for aiding memory and giving a subject your initial attention. Try each one and see which idea or combination of ideas works for you.
   - **R** = repetition
   - **A** = association
   - **P** = pictures or symbols
4. Repetition is time-consuming to most students but it is an effective way to recall information. The more you see the information, the more you will recall it.
5. Association techniques are mnemonic devices—tricks to help you retain information for long-term use.
6. Mnemonic devices make learning faster and more efficient by linking the information to something familiar. Mnemonic devices are not a substitute for overall comprehension of the material. They provide a way to link difficult information to the main information learned.
7. There are limitations to mnemonic devices. The trick itself may be hard to remember and difficult to retain; the device can be forgotten if it is never stored into long-term memory; and no device can help you digest or understand the information.
8. Types of mnemonic devices are:
   - Acronyms, words formed from the initial letters of a series of words
   - Acrostics, series of words that form creative sentences
   - Songs and rhymes
   - Stories (created)
9. Create pictures and symbols as associations for difficult information you must remember.
10. Visualize the material by creating a story, and have fun with the material to be learned. The more unusual the story, the more likely the information will stick with you.
11. Make up a song with your favorite tune or create a rhyme to retain the information.
12. Take an active role in your learning by paying attention and using association techniques.

C. Memory Principles

1. Be interested in the material; show excitement at mastering the subject matter. There is pleasure in knowledge. As a physician, you will have to become a lifelong learner.
2. A positive attitude and approach will increase learning and remembering. It will add meaning to your work. Be cognizant of the fact that reasoning, analysis, and persistence will lead to positive conclusions.
3. Remember that the more solid your basic knowledge is, the easier new building blocks are mastered and added. Accept your strengths and weaknesses.
4. Develop associations between facts and concepts.
5. Visualize, conceptualize, and recite; be active on all fronts.

6. Give yourself a chance to consolidate your knowledge base; remember that everything takes time.

7. Set aside regular time periods for this specific task; do not squeeze it in here and there! Regular time periods increase efficiency and delineate purpose.

8. Skip superfluous material and adjust to repetitious material.

9. If you detect major gaps in your knowledge, fill these in. Otherwise, they will bother you and distract you from your effort. It's easier to remember a story than to remember isolated facts.

10. Study, if you can, in chronological order. You will feel more comfortable because of the sequence, and you will enhance your recall.

11. During your studying, vary your attack as required.
    - Read the material.
    - Speak out the material.
    - Write out the material.
    - Sketch some of the material.
    - Underline some of the material.
    - Outline some of the material.
    - Resort, if necessary, to mnemonic devices.

12. Understand the material before you commit it to memory.

13. Organize the material, and learn it in parts rather then in isolated, single details. Try to build a framework of facts.

14. Note and focus on similar ideas from different subject areas. Put them meaningfully together, and keep them in association. Integrate your material.

D. Review: General

Most students that we consulted did a thorough preliminary review of the material they expected to master before they undertook intensive, well-planned study. The purpose of a review is to create a sense of familiarity with the material to be studied so that when the period of intensive study begins, none of the material will appear new. It also points out areas that will need more attention for comprehension and understanding. The review helps students avoid the sense that they are cramming for the examination. Remember that the MCAT examination requires understanding, reasoning and deduction. Once the period of intensive study has begun, students will benefit from the guidelines below.

Guides to Success

1. In order to be successful and competitive, you must not only work harder but smarter. Facts and concepts must be organized and integrated; associations and differences must be looked for. You must develop the skill to draw inferences and utilize presented information effectively on standardized tests.

2. In reviewing, try to integrate and synthesize material that you have learned over the years in a course-by-course manner. Study as if you were preparing for an essay exam; it will help summarize and make your facts more coherent.

3. Despite the fact that the examination stresses reasoning, commit "the basics" to memory. They are the building blocks for reasoning.

4. Test-wise students think deductively; general principles applied wisely usually lead to specific conclusions. The integrated learner has the ability to make associations and to use information better.

5. Standardized tests require you to manipulate related concepts to reach the answer; this is a learned skill. Memorization of facts will serve you well, but thinking in an integrated fashion enhances understanding. What you know will never hurt you.

6. Question analysis requires you to identify the topic and to understand both the right and wrong answers. Understanding the wrong answers often leads to a better comprehension of the right answer.

7. Observe, note, and use all the relevant facts provided. Be systematic and do not jump to conclusions. Do not be sloppy; you cannot answer a question on the basis of superficial considerations or impressions.

8. Do not read too rapidly and skip words and facts. Reread difficult material.

9. Be consistent in your interpretation of words.

10. Break complex problems into parts and draw upon prior knowledge. Actively look for the main ideas; this helps understanding and reasoning.

11. Answer all questions in sequence, even if you have to guess sometimes (there is no penalty for guessing). If you skip here and there, you might inadvertently fill out your answer sheet inappropriately. An inordinate amount of time could be spent in correcting the mistake.

12. Fill in the areas on the bubble sheet as you proceed; do not leave that task to the end. You might not have time. A transcription error could be devastating.

13. Pace yourself and train yourself to answer one question per minute. Make a note of any question you were not sure of, since a subsequent question might provide you with the proper answer.

14. Be sure to read the entire question before your consider a quick answer. Circle or underline your key words and be cognizant of the fact that multiple-choice examinations quite often contain one answer that is ridiculous. The examination is not designed to mislead you. Most questions are quite straightforward. Just as you should rule out ridiculous options, so you should carefully examine options that are the same, since only one answer is the correct one. Always use your knowledge base before you eliminate a statement. Even partial familiarity and hunches are better than outright guessing.

15. Before you change an answer, you should have a very compelling reason.

E. Review: Specific Principles

Be Goal Directed

An old saying proposes: "If we have goals, we tend to do things that move us toward those goals."

1. Your goal is to transfer facts to your long-term memory, and the mechanism for accomplishing that is review. Memorization is a daily task, not just a cramming before an examination.

2. Reflect on what you want to accomplish and be. Stay in touch with your dreams. Frequently challenge yourself to live up to high standards academically and personally.

3. Acknowledge your accomplishments and be proud of yourself. Consistency and hard work got you this far and can help you realize your goals.

4. Remain motivated and realistic. There is no study system that is right for everyone. Find what works best for you and stick with it.

Plan

Planning is the unmistakable road map to success and has been proven to save hours and hours of misdirected, unproductive work.

1. Make a study plan and stick to it. Better students always have an effective study plan. Decide before you begin how many weeks and months you will require to review the material. If you have to deviate, immediately schedule when you will make up the work; compensatory study time is part of every plan.

2. Be cognizant of the fact that certain areas are more prone to be forgotten, so extra time to relearn material needs to be factored into your schedule.

3. Identify and allot more time to subject matter for which you feel the least prepared. There is no point in studying material you already know well.

4. Keep your efforts in proper perspective. You cannot know it all, but a well-rounded knowledge base and the intelligent use of that knowledge will serve you well both on the MCAT and in your future study. Keep the expression "Use it or lose it" in mind. You must focus on learning the material as you plan to use it and test yourself regularly to improve remembering.

5. As you lay out your study plan, take into account other responsibilities and commitments: present courses and exams, holidays, vacations, family occasions, sports commitments, etc.
6. Leaving things to the last minute is bad planning. It robs you of extended memory time and usually leads to quick forgetting. A systematic, orderly and properly paced and spaced procedure will "pay off in the end."

Strategies

Remember the adage "We forget much of what we learn over the long run." Forgetting is a normal and natural process, but the process can be slowed and lessened. The more organized your original study and review process, the more you will recall.

1. Utilize a regular work area and establish a routine; keep your workspace, books and notes organized.
2. Spend about 30 minutes each day reviewing the material you studied yesterday.
3. Review material you are least prepared for first; however, beware of the trap of studying material you already know. We sometimes have a subconscious tendency to gravitate to our comfort zones, and that can lead to a false sense of security.
4. You will remember more if both your material and review are organized.
   - Take advantage of summaries, tables, graphs, schematics, and review books. Draw out pathways and learn similarities and differences between them. Make flow charts for integration.
   - Be active in your review. Stop periodically and check your memory by jotting down abbreviated notes on what you just learned.
   - Remain alert and interactive. Guard against slipping into a passive mode. Underline, write, chart, draw—whatever. Be focused, ask questions, and utilize all your auditory and visual senses. Learn it so you can teach it.
5. Choose your sources carefully. Your own learning style should be a determining factor. Your previous class notes and summaries might greatly facilitate your recall and understanding again. Some books are just outlines, others are full-length prose, and most are a combination. Select what fits your needs and learning style.
6. Keep in mind that a review book cannot meet all your needs; therefore, you may have to refer to a comprehensive text with which you are familiar in order to fill in some of the gaps.
7. Divide your material into small units to sustain attention and a sense of accomplishment.
8. Actively tie what you learn or relearn to what you know already. The cornerstone of learning is linking new concepts (facts) to the familiar.
9. Memorization is critical to learning and must be done every day. Keep in mind that memorization requires repetition and that repetition is the mother of all learning.
10. Just because you have reviewed and memorized subject matter, you have no guarantee that you are in a position to solve problems. Use practice exams at least once a week to evaluate your proficiency and to identify your weaknesses.
11. Examine the detailed answers provided with practice questions. It will reinforce what you have learned, refresh your knowledge, and act as one more general guard against forgetting.
12. Vary your memorization methods. Mnemonic devices can get you through dry and boring material. "ACE" can add flavor and fun: Weave difficult lists into an Active, Colorful, Exaggerated story for recall later. Alliteration, flashcards, and acronyms can all be helpful.

F. Stress Management

1. One of the best stress management techniques is to take control of your life. Realize that you are responsible for your actions and destiny. Accept yourself—your strengths and weaknesses. Feel good about yourself as a person.
2. Do not shun activities that you enjoy. Include entertainment in your schedule so you remain charged and motivated. Treat yourself to anything that brings you pleasure.

3. Keep your study and living area clean and organized. Don't ignore other aspects of your daily responsibilities, such as paying bills. Feeling and being organized is a correlate motivation.
4. Don't study when you are overly tired. It adds to your frustration and translates to low productivity. Take a short nap but set an alarm clock.
5. Use exercise, a hot shower, music, or a chat with a friend to relax and regenerate.
6. Do not expect perfection. You cannot know it all and none of us is perfect.
7. Seek help when you hit roadblocks. Fellow students and professors are excellent resources for discussion. Asking for help is not a weakness but rather a symbol of strength.
8. Reward yourself for your weekly accomplishments. Catch a movie or a play or perhaps go to a sports event.
9. There is no magic formula. Accept that study is an ongoing challenge; remain persistent and you will be successful. Knowing that you know your material is a wonderful experience. Remember that success begets success!
10. Stay in touch with your dream! Visualize having completed the test successfully. Visualize being a medical student, becoming a physician, and having the kind of satisfying life you want for yourself.

G. Examination Day

1. Try to get a good night's rest before the examination. Be cautious about using sleep aids. They often leave you with residual dulling effects the next day.
2. Avoid changing daily habits. Eat foods that agree with you so that gastrointestinal discomfort is avoided. Follow your normal exercise routine but don't overdo it. A sore body is very distracting.
3. Know the location of the testing center and arrive early to avoid being rushed and anxious. Be prepared. Wear comfortable clothes, anticipate a hot or cold room, and have available your registration materials, number-two pencils, erasers, and snacks for energy.
4. Attitude is critical. Approach the examination with the conviction that you have diligently prepared, and are ready and confident! A positive internal dialogue often translates to positive results, so always maintain a sense of pride and accomplishment.
5. Sometimes a quick scan of the complete test is helpful. Avoid scanning questions at this point. If scanning escalates your anxiety, it is probably best to eliminate it.
6. Read, listen to, and follow all directions and be sure you understand them. Do not assume anything.
7. Wear a watch and know the time limits. Proportion your time but avoid being a compulsive clock watcher.
8. Ignore others and your surroundings so your concentration remains undisturbed.
9. Be careful about giving the impression that you are dishonest. Avoid keeping "one eye" on the proctor and the other on your material.
10. You don't have to finish first! Pace yourself. Stay the allotted time. Leave time for checking at the end. Think that the first students finished were probably not prepared.
11. Maintain your pace; standardized tests require that you progress quickly to the end. Skip questions that require time and return to them later. Guess when you are quite unsure and keep moving. Change answers only when you are sure you were wrong initially.
12. If you become frustrated and your concentration lapses, sit back, close your eyes, relax, and regroup.
13. If your frustration persists, scan material you have already completed. It may help you get back on track.
14. Expect "off the wall" questions. Note them, guess if you have to, and keep moving.
15. Avoid premature closure and rushing to judgment. Read the whole question and all answer choices before making a selection.
16. Accept questions at face value and avoid thinking too much or reading too much into questions. Most questions are straightforward and simple. They are not a trick.
17. Break complex questions into parts, then begin with the part you understand and work from there.
18. There is no penalty for guessing; be a gambler. If you can eliminate some choices, you will drastically improve your chances of guessing the correct answer.

A POSITIVE APPROACH TO ANSWERING QUESTIONS AND TO TEST TAKING

A positive, competitive approach and attitude are qualities of a successful individual. Hand in hand, however, goes a fund in knowledge. Nothing succeeds like knowledge of the subject matter for test taking. Indeed, the suggestions on test taking are all built on knowledge, which is strongly reinforced by your confidence, it, in turn, being supported by an understanding of the process involved in the successful answering of questions.

In this section, several specific questions will be selected from the Model Tests and will be examined not only for content but also for the process involved in the selection of the correct answer.

General Key Rules for Answering Questions

1. Are there specific disclaimers? *Best, all, none,* or some variety of negatives that separate the correct answer from the multiplicity of possible answers are the types of disclaimers to look for.
2. Are there specific qualifying words or topics that can be underlined? Sometimes these are the same as the disclaimers in item 1.
3. Are there similarities of choices in the answers? These similarities may allow elimination of choices.
4. Can some choices, such as the choice *all of the above,* be eliminated? Sometimes opposite choices help in the selection and in the narrowing down of the answers to one out of two possibilities.
5. If you can, sometimes a quick drawing or a formula will clarify the questions and initiate and aid in recall.
6. Remember, and keep in mind at all times, that all multiple-choice questions are really TRUE or FALSE decisions on a statement. Sometimes, in some cases, when in a quandary, they can best be answered by "I don't know" and "I'll proceed to the next question and not disturb my pace and concentration."
7. *Be positive!* If you have no good answers for several questions in a row, you positively *must forget them.* Do not dwell on failure, but have confidence in how much you know!

Application of Test-Taking Hints

We will use specific examples and apply our principles.

EXAMPLE: Model Examination B; Chemistry, Question 6

6. Glucose is NOT a(an):
   (A) aldose.
   (B) reducing sugar.
   (C) disaccharide.
   (D) sugar possessing optical activity.
   (E) monosaccharide.

ITEM 1:   Note the specific disclaimer *NOT.* This is an obvious and common one in test questions. You should *underline* this word.
ITEM 2:   Glucose is the topic of the question and should be *underlined.*
ITEM 3:   Similarity or dissimilarity of choices! There is a strong *dissimilarity* between choice (C): *dis*accharide and choice (E): *mono*saccharide. In fact, at this point, the answer is obvious to the knowledgeable individual. Since glucose is a *mono*saccharide, it cannot be a *dis*-accharide; for the purpose of analyzation and this review, let us continue.
ITEM 4:   Can choices be eliminated? Since both (C) and (E) cannot be true, *one* must be eliminated.

ITEM 5: A quick drawing to stimulate and help recall:

$$
\begin{array}{c}
\text{H} \qquad \text{O} \\
\diagdown \quad \diagup\diagup \\
\text{C} \\
| \\
\text{H---C---OH} \\
| \\
\text{etc.,} \\
| \\
\text{CH}_2\text{OH}
\end{array}
$$

ITEM 6: All multiple-choice questions are TRUE or FALSE statements!

For statement (A): "Glucose is NOT an aldose."

FACT: An aldose is an aldehyde carbohydrate. Look at the structure in item 5! This is indeed an aldehyde:

So, the choice is apparently true, but remember the disclaimer *NOT*. In this context, the answer for (A) is FALSE.

For statement (B): "Glucose is NOT a reducing sugar."

FACT: A reducing sugar is one that must be oxidized while reducing a metal ion $(\text{Cu}^{2+} \_\_ \text{Cu}^{+})$(a gain of electrons is reduction). Remember the disclaimer *NOT*. In this context, the answer for (B) is FALSE.

For statement (C): "Glucose is NOT a disaccharide."

FACT: A disaccharide is a carbohydrate that may be hydrolyzed to a simpler carbohydrate. Carefully examine the sketch. Can this compound be hydrolyzed (split by water) into a smaller carbohydrate? Remember the disclaimer *NOT*. In this context, the answer for (C) is TRUE. During an examination with stress on speed and limited time, you would not wish to continue working on this question. Here, however, to continue the analyzation of the process, please go on to the next statement.

For statement (D): "Glucose is NOT a sugar possessing optical activity."

FACT: An optically active compound requires an asymmetric carbon atom and no plane of symmetry. Examine the formula, and note carbon atom 2. Remember the disclaimer is *NOT*. In this context, the answer for (D) is FALSE.

For statement (E): "Glucose is NOT a monosaccharide." Note the formula, and the opposite of choice (C). Remember the disclaimer *NOT*. In this context, the answer for (E) is FALSE.

In summary, we arrive at:

(A)	FALSE	(D)	FALSE
(B)	FALSE	(E)	FALSE
(C)	TRUE		

So, the answer is (C). Wow! That's easy if you know all the facts, but what if you don't? Suppose your array of answers was:

(A)	FALSE	(D)	FALSE
(B)	I DON'T KNOW.	(E)	FALSE
(C)	TRUE		

or a variation such as:

(A)	I DON'T KNOW.	(D)	I DON'T KNOW.
(B)	I DON'T KNOW.	(E)	I DON'T KNOW.
(C)	TRUE		

or:

(A)	FALSE	(D)	FALSE
(B)	FALSE	(E)	FALSE
(C)	I DON'T KNOW.		

The answer (C) is obvious in all three sets of answers above. However, what about:

(A)	FALSE	(D)	FALSE
(B)	I DON'T KNOW.	(E)	FALSE
(C)	I DON'T KNOW.		

Without additional information or a hunch or a gut feeling (which is a subliminal input), our advice would be to *let it go!* Pick one of the two, (B) or (C), and move on. You have a 50–50% chance of being right. The more "I don't know" answers for possible choices, the lower the probability of being right. So, for a particular examination, without additional information, decide to *always select* the first "I don't know" answer. This will cut through the random answer position on examinations. Remember that the answers on the key are randomly distributed. By adopting the above system, you put a degree of constancy into your pattern, and you don't float likewise. Your chances are drastically enhanced.

We will look at one more question from the chemistry section of the first part of Model Examination B, using the same analytical techniques but in a less detailed way.

EXAMPLE: Model Examination B; Chemistry, Question 9

9. Alcohols have higher boiling points than do alkyl halides of the same chain lengths because:
   (A) alcohols are more polar.
   (B) alcohols have higher molecular weights.
   (C) alcohols form ethers.
   (D) alcohols form intermolecular hydrogen bonds.
   (E) All of the above.

KEY WORDS: Underline <u>Alcohols</u>, <u>higher boiling points</u>, <u>alkyl halides</u>, and <u>same chain lengths</u>.

(A) false. Alkyl halides are more polar.
(B) false. Halides have higher molecular weights than do alcohols.
(C) false. The statement is true, but this is a chemical property not dealing with the physical property of a boiling point.
(D) true. Compare CH_3OH to CH_3Cl
(E) "All of the above" can't be true if (A) is false.

In summary, we arrive at:

(A)	FALSE	(D)	TRUE
(B)	FALSE	(E)	FALSE
(C)	FALSE		

MCAT SCIENCE REVIEW

The purpose of this section is to help the student review some key material quickly, to place some of his or her information in perspective, and to help identify areas of weakness and strength. No attempt has been made to cover all of the material in the subject matter; but it is hoped that after the student has worked through the practice examinations and has studied the explanations to the questions, this section will amplify for him or her the highlights and essentials that are expected baseline knowledge for all educated people. A brief presentation such as this cannot cover all areas in sufficient depth. Some areas are omitted and others are presented only in a simplified manner. The individual who is well prepared will sometimes recognize compromises that must be made for the sake of brevity. This section should not be used as a substitute for a good general text in the areas but it should be used as a guide and in conjunction with a text so that the student may efficiently prepare for the MCAT. Again, we urge the student to begin preparation for the examination early and to be conscientious and thorough.

REVIEW OUTLINE

Biology

1. The Cell—Its Structure and Function
   * Size
   * Composition of Protoplasm
   * General Structure of Membranes in Cells
   * Mechanisms Moving Molecules Across Membranes of Cells
   * Prokaryotic Versus Eukaryotic Cell Structure

2. Structure and Function of Viruses
   * Viral Life Cycles

3. Nucleic Acids and Nucleotides
   * Nucleotide Structure
   * Nucleotide Functions
   * Nucleotide Functions in Cells
   * RNA (Ribonucleic Acid) Structure
   * RNA Functions
   * DNA (Deoxyribonucleic Acid) Structure
   * Genetic Information Flow in Cells
   * Protein Structure
   * Protein Function
   * Control of Use of Genetic Information
   * Overview of Genetic Regulation in Prokaryotes and Eukaryotes

4. DNA Replication
   * DNA Replication in Prokaryotes (*E. coli*)
   * DNA Replication in Eukaryotes
   * Chromosomal Replication Patterns in Eukaryotes
   * Tangle Prevention During DNA Replication in Prokaryotes and Eukaryotes
   * DNA Repair in Prokaryotes and Eukaryotes

5. Overall Genetic Organization of Prokaryotic Cells
   - Transcription in Prokaryotes
   - Post-Transcriptional Processing of RNA in Prokaryotes
   - Translation in Prokaryotes

6. Overall Genetic Organization of Eukaryotes Cells
   - Transcription in Eukaryotes
   - Post-Transcriptional Processing of RNA in Eukaryotes
   - Translation in Eukaryotes

7. Classification of Living Organisms

8. Organization of the Human Body
   - Organ Systems
   - Four Basic Tissues
   - Terms of Planes, Positions, Directions, and Relationships

9. Skeletal System
   - Axial Skeleton
   - Appendicular Skeleton
   - Characteristics of Bone
   - Joints

10. Muscular System
    - Classification
    - Skeletal Muscles
    - Muscle Attachment and Function
    - Terms to Describe Movement
    - Muscle Names
    - Structural Organization of a Muscle Fiber
    - Myofilaments
    - Sarcoplasm
    - Excitation
    - Contraction
    - Muscle Twitch
    - Tetanus
    - Energy Sources
    - Types of Muscle Fibers

11. Circulatory System
    - Functions
    - General Components and Structure
    - Course of Circulation
    - The Heart
    - Blood

12. Respiratory System
    - Removal of Inhaled Particles
    - Pulmonary Ventilation
    - Inspiration and Expiration
    - Positive and Negative Pressure Breathing
    - Neuronal Control and Integration of Breathing
    - Gas Exchange in the Alveoli
    - Oxygen Transport
    - Carbon Dioxide Transport
    - Chemical Regulation of Respiration

13. Urinary System
    - Structure of the Kidney
    - Tubular Passageways
    - Functions of the Kidney and Uriniferous Tubules
    - Hormonal Control of Secretion and Resorption

14. Integumentary (Skin) System
    - Skin
    - Glands
    - Hair
    - Nails

15. Digestive System and Nutrition
    - Nutrition
    - The Digestive System
    - The Major Digestive Glands
    - General Functional Schema of the Digestive Tube (ingestion, digestion, egestion)
    - Intestinal Motility
    - Innervation of the Intestinal Tract
    - Summary of Digestive Juices
    - Hormones of the Digestive Tract
    - General Digestion of the Major Food Groups

16. Nervous System
    - Nervous Tissue
    - The Neuron
    - Classification of Neurons
    - Groups of Neurons
    - Supportive Elements
    - Supportive Elements of the Peripheral Nervous System
    - The Central Nervous System
    - The Peripheral Nervous System
    - Reflex Arc

17. Organs of Special Sense
    - The Eye
    - The Ear
    - The Olfactory System
    - The Gustatory System

18. Endocrine System
    - The Pituitary Gland (Hypophysis)
    - The Thyroid Gland
    - The Parathyroid Glands
    - The Pancreas
    - The Adrenal Glands
    - The Testes
    - The Ovaries
    - Menstrual Cycle
    - Female Contraception
    - The Placenta
    - The Pineal
    - The Prostaglandins
    - The Small Intestine

19. Reproductive System
    - Reproductive Organs
    - Hormonal Control
    - Gametogenesis and Meiosis

- • Mature Gametes
- • Other Modes of Reproduction

20. Overview of Development
- • Stages in Development
- • Mechanisms Used to Form the Body Pattern During Development

21. Development in Humans
- • Fertilization
- • Cleavage
- • Blastocyst Formation
- • Implantation in the Uterus
- • Second Week
- • Second Month
- • Fetal Membranes and Placenta
- • Fetal and Neonatal Circulation
- • Multiple Pregnancy

22. Defense Against Foreign Organisms and Abnormal Cells
- • Barrier Layers
- • Clot Formation
- • Innate Defense Mechanisms
- • Specific Immune Mechanisms
- • Patterns of Specific Immune Responses
- • Cytoxic T Lymphocyte Responses
- • Antibody Structure
- • Helper T Lymphocytes
- • Antigen-Presenting Cells
- • Development of T Lymphocytes
- • Positive and Negative Selection of T Lymphocytes in the Thymus
- • Development of B Lymphocytes
- • Reactive Lymphoid Organs

23. Genetics
- • Mendelian Characteristics
- • Polygenic Traits
- • Paternity Exclusion and Reassignment of Misassigned Infants

24. The Animal Kingdom
- • Distribution of Living Organisms
- • Interrelationships of Animals
- • Population Dynamics
- • Major Environment—Habitats
- • Learning, Conditioning, Rhythms

25. Evolution
- • Key People and Concepts
- • Mechanisms of Evolution on a Small Scale (Microevolution)
- • Mechanisms of Evolution on a Large Scale (Macroevolution)
- • Speciation
- • Other Patterns of Macroevolution
- • The Concept of Species
- • Reproductive Isolation
- • The Rate of Evolution
- • Artificial Selection
- • The Hardy-Weinberg Law of Equilibrium
- • Mutations
- • Migration
- • Factors in Reproductive Isolation Between Species

Chemistry

1. General Chemistry
   - The Atom
   - Components of the Atom
   - Placement of Electrons—Energy Levels
   - Periodic Table
   - Gases
   - Liquids and Solids
   - Phase Changes
   - Chemical Compounds
   - Balanced Chemical Equations
   - Solutions
   - Acids and Bases, pH, and Buffers
   - Electrochemistry
   - Thermodynamics
   - Rate Processes in Chemical Reactions

2. General Principles
   - Characteristics of Mixtures and Compounds
   - Reactions
   - Role of Enzymes in a Reaction
   - Temperature of Conversion Factors
   - Formulas and Laws

3. Organic Chemistry
   - General Considerations
   - The Alkanes
   - The Cycloalkanes
   - The Alkenes
   - The Alkynes
   - Aromatic Compounds
   - The Grignard Reagent
   - Alcohols
   - Amines
   - Amides
   - Aldehydes and Ketones
   - Carboxylic Acids
   - Esters
   - Ethers
   - Final Remarks

4. Biochemistry
   - Areas of Biochemistry
   - pH and Buffers
   - Amino Acids, Peptides, and Proteins
   - Enzymes
   - Carbohydrates
   - Lipids
   - Nucleotides and Nucleic Acids; Biosynthesis of Nucleic Acids and Proteins

Physics

1. Frequently Encountered Physics Problems and Their Answers
   - Accelerated Motion
   - Forces and Motion
   - Projectile Motion
   - Friction
   - Work and Power
   - Energy
   - Momentum
   - Uniform Circular Motion
   - Fluids at Rest
   - Gravity
   - Temperature Calculations and Measurement
   - Heat
   - Thermodynamics
   - Electrostatics
   - Electricity
   - Electric Circuits
   - Electric Energy
   - Alternating Current
   - Machines and Mechanical Advantage
   - Simple Harmonic Motion
   - Waves
   - Sound Waves
   - Light Rays
   - Mirrors
   - Lenses
   - Composition of the Atom
   - Radioactivity
   - Nuclear Energy
   - Photons
   - Atomic Energy Levels

BIOLOGY

The Cell—Its Structure and Function

The cell is the basic unit of structure and function and basis of all life; all cells come from pre-existing cells.

Size

Most cells are between 10 and 100 μm (micrometers) in diameter. Measurements are made utilizing the following units:

$$
\begin{aligned}
1 \text{ cm} &= 10 \text{ mm} \\
1 \text{ mm} &= 1000 \text{ μm} \\
1 \text{ μm} &= 10{,}000 \text{ Å (angstrom units)}
\end{aligned}
$$

Average sizes of structures may be listed as follows:

cells about	10 μm	(100,000 Å)
mitochondria about	1 μm	(10,000 Å)
bacteria about	1 μm	(10,000 Å)
viruses about	0.1 μm	(1,000 Å)
macromolecules about	0.01 μm	(100 Å)
molecules about	0.001 μm	(10 Å)
hydrogen ion about	0.0001 μm	(1 Å)

Resolution is commonly defined as the ability to discriminate two points and visualize them as two points, even though they are extremely close together. With the unaided eye these points might appear as one point, but the microscope can aid in resolving them as two. The resolution is dependent on the wavelength of the light source and can be calculated to be about one-half the wavelength. Examples of resolving power are:

human eye about 0.1 mm (100 μm)
light microscope about 0.2 μm (2,000 Å)
electron microscope about 2–5 Å

Composition of Protoplasm

Protoplasm is made up mainly of proteins, carbohydrates, fats, salts, and water; its average elemental composition is

Oxygen 75+%	Potassium about 0.3%
Carbon 10+%	Chlorine about 0.1%
Hydrogen 10%	less than 0.1%—sodium,
Nitrogen 2+%	calcium,
Sulfur about 0.2%	magnesium,
Phosphorus about 0.3%	iron, etc.

General Structure of Membranes in Cells

Every living cell has a *plasma membrane,* which serves as the permeability barrier between the cell and its environment. A eukaryotic cell also contains membranes that separate different compartments within the cell. All of these membranes consist of *lipid* (primarily phospholipid) *bilayers* with associated *proteins*. Some proteins are associated with the surface of the membrane whereas other proteins extend across the lipid bilayer. Membrane surfaces which face away from the cytoplasm in eukaryotic cells may have numerous *oligosaccharide groups* (polymers of sugars) attached to proteins and lipids. The oligosaccharide-bearing components are especially numerous on the external surface of the plasma membrane.

When viewed at high magnification by routine transmission electron microscopy, most membranes in a cell appear as two dark lines separated by a light zone. The complex is approximately 10 nm (100 Å) in thickness.

Lipid Bilayers in Membranes

When mixed with water, phospholipids (both glycerophospholipids and sphingolipids) and glycolipids spontaneously form bilayer structures as a result of the strongly polar phosphate-containing or sugar-containing "head" of each molecule associating with the water and the non-polar alkyl "tails" of the fatty acyl groups aggregating by hydrophobic interactions.

Glycerophospholipids contain a glycerol linked to two fatty acyl groups and one phosphate group. The phosphate group may in turn be linked to further groups such as ethanolamine (in phosphatidyl ethanolamine), choline (in phosphatidyl choline), serine (in phosphatidyl serine), or inositol (in phosphatidyl inositol).

Sphingolipids contain a sphingosine linked to one fatty acyl group and are usually linked to a phosphate plus a choline (sphingomyelin), a sugar (ceramides), or to a complex oligosaccharide (gangliosides). Sphingolipids are absent from most prokaryotes and occur primarily in the outer face of the plasma membrane in eukaryotes.

Lysophospholipids have one fatty acyl group removed, cutting the ratio of nonpolar to polar structure in half. Conversion of phospholipids to lysophospholipids promotes conversion of phospholipid bilayers into micelles and may destabilize membranes.

Substitution of *cis-unsaturated fatty acids* for *saturated fatty acids* decreases the closeness of the packing in the nonpolar layer, increasing fluidity in the layer and increasing movement of small polar molecules across the layer.

The addition of *cholesterol* to a lipid bilayer reduces fluidity of the lipids and reduces penetration of small polar molecules across the bilayer.

Membrane Proteins

Peripheral membrane proteins are attached to integral membrane components (lipids or proteins) by noncovalent bonds. Peripheral proteins may be removed from a membrane by milder treatments than are required to remove integral membrane proteins.

Integral membrane proteins cannot be released from a membrane without breaking covalent bonds or disrupting the lipid bilayer.

Some integral membrane proteins are anchored to the lipid bilayer by covalent linkage to a lipid, usually a fatty acyl group (frequently a myristyl group), a prenyl group (frequently a farnesyl group), or a phospholipid (usually a glycosylphosphatidylinositol [GPI] anchor).

Transmembrane integral membrane proteins contain one or more protein domains which extend across the lipid bilayer. Most transmembrane domains appear to adopt alpha helical secondary structure and consist primarily of amino acids with hydrophobic side chains. Some transmembrane integral membrane proteins form ion channels across the membrane, others are active transport or facilitated diffusion carriers, and still others are receptors for growth factors or hormones. The functions of many membrane proteins are unknown.

Some membrane proteins appear to be free to diffuse in the plane of the membrane, whereas other membrane proteins (particularly receptors) have restricted mobility or can be clustered in response to stimuli, usually by interaction with cytoskeletal elements. The current model of membrane organization is called the fluid mosaic model because of the freedom of movement of lipids and some proteins in the membrane.

Membrane Function

The primary function of a membrane in a cell is to control movement of materials from one compartment to another. Several processes are involved in these movements. Simple diffusion occurs in any fluid, whereas carrier-mediated processes are peculiar to biological membranes.

Simple Diffusion (Passive Movements) in Fluids

Concentration gradients consisting of differences in concentration of a component in a fluid can drive a net movement of that component. Each component in any fluid will diffuse from regions of high concentrations of that component toward regions of low concentration of that component. This movement, called simple diffusion, is the result of random movements of each particle in the fluid, and occurs whether the component is charged or not.

Electrostatic gradients (potential fields) can drive net movements of charged particles such as ions in a fluid. Charged components in a fluid will be attracted to opposite charges and repelled by similar changes. Therefore, if a potential field is present, positively charged particles will move toward the negative pole and negatively charged particles will move toward the positive pole.

Because both concentration gradients and electrostatic forces act on charged components, the sum of the forces acting on a charged component can be described as an *electrochemical gradient*.

Simple Diffusion Across Lipid Bilayers

Because a biological membrane is composed of a lipid bilayer containing associated proteins, the movement of materials across the membrane is determined by the properties of the lipid bilayer unless movement occurs through a channel or by means of a carrier molecule.

Very small molecules which carry no net charge (water, oxygen, carbon dioxide) cross lipid bilayers relatively easily by simple diffusion, regardless of the polarity of the molecules. These molecules do not require carriers or channels to cross membranes.

Moderate-sized nonpolar molecules with no net charges (benzene, steroids) cross bilayers readily. These molecules have much more trouble moving through the water to get to the membrane than they have crossing the membrane. Small nonpolar molecules move relatively easily in water, but large nonpolar molecules such as fatty acids or triglycerides may primarily move through blood or tissue fluid complexed with a lipoprotein and may be taken up by cells through a receptor-mediated endocytosis mechanism which recognizes the protein component of the lipoprotein and takes up the lipid along with the protein.

Polar molecules up through three carbons in size and with no net charges cross bilayers moderately rapidly. These molecules usually cross membranes without requiring channels or carriers.

Polar molecules in the size range of biological monomers (five and six carbon sugars) and with no net charges cross lipid bilayers very slowly, usually too slowly to support metabolic processes. These molecules must therefore cross membranes by way of a channel or by way of a carrier-mediated mechanism.

Ions and polar macromolecules cross lipid bilayers very slowly, if at all. These ions or molecules must therefore cross membranes by way of a channel or by way of a carrier-mediated mechanism. Many types of macromolecules may initially be taken into cells through receptor-mediated endocytosis, then cross the membrane of the vesicle formed during endocytosis after alteration of the macromolecule.

Mechanisms Moving Molecules Across Membranes of Cells

1. Simple Diffusion

Materials that cross lipid bilayers rapidly enough to meet the needs of cells usually cross cellular membranes by simple diffusion. These materials always move down their electro-chemical gradient and the rate of movement increases as the electrochemical gradient increases over the full range of reasonable concentrations. Water, oxygen, and carbon dioxide usually cross membranes by simple diffusion.

Osmosis is a special case of simple diffusion. Because of the extensive interactions between solutes and water, the presence of solutes in water reduces the effective concentration of free water. Water will therefore diffuse from areas of lower solute concentration (*hypotonic* = lower solute concentration, therefore higher water concentration) to areas of higher solute concentration (*hypertonic* = higher solute concentration, therefore lower water concentration). When this occurs across a membrane that allows water to cross more easily than most solutes, substantial changes in volume occur. Multicellular animal cells normally operate in *isotonic* body fluids (same total solute concentration as inside the cells). Placing most animal cells in a hypertonic environment causes the cells to shrink. Placing the cells in a hypotonic environment causes the cells to swell and burst.

2. Facilitated Diffusion

Materials that cross lipid bilayers too slowly to meet cellular needs but which are being moved down their electrochemical gradient are usually moved by facilitated diffusion. This process may use either a channel or a uniporter carrier (both usually proteins). In either case, however, the movement is down the component's electrochemical gradient and shows saturation kinetics (increasing the gradient beyond a point causes no further increase in transport).

3. Active Transport

Materials that cross lipid bilayers too slowly to meet cellular needs but which are occasionally or frequently being moved up their electrochemical gradient are moved by active transport. This process uses a protein carrier which moves the component independently of its electrochemical gradient because the carrier consumes energy (usually adenosine triphosphate, or ATP) to make its conformational changes directional. Like facilitated diffusion, active transport shows saturation kinetics (increasing the component concentration beyond a point causes no further increase in transport). Unlike facilitated diffusion, active transport is (a) sensitive to the concentration of the component on only one side of the membrane (the "loading" side), (b) insensitive to the concentration of the component on the other side of the membrane, and (c) usually saturates at relatively low component concentrations.

Once a reliable concentration gradient of one component has been established by active transport, its concentration gradient may in turn be used to drive additional coupled active transport mechanisms (sometimes called secondary active transport). If the coupled component moves in the same direction as the gradient component, the process is a *symport* process. If they move in opposite directions, the process is an *antiport* process.

MECHANISMS MOVING MOLECULES ACROSS CELL MEMBRANES

I. *Passive transport* (does not require energy expenditure)	1. Concentration gradients drive a net force and each component in any fluid will diffuse from regions of higher concentrations toward regions of lower concentrations.
	2. Electrostatic gradients cause charged particles to be attracted to opposite charges and repelled by similar charges.
Simple diffusion	Water, oxygen, carbon dioxide (dissolved gases), and lipid soluble molecules cross easily through the phospholipid bilayer of a membrane.
Osmosis (a special case of simple diffusion)	Water diffuses from areas of lower solute concentration (hypotonic) to areas of higher solute concentration (hypertonic).
Facilitated diffusion	A channel or uniporter carrier is used; the movement is down the component's electrochemical gradient and shows saturation kinetics.
II. *Energy-requiring transport*	Materials are moved up their electrochemical gradient using cellular energy.
Active transport	A protein carrier moves the particle independently of its electrochemical gradient; the carrier consumes energy (usually ATP).
Endocytosis	Process whereby the cell membrane engulfs extracellular material, moves it into the cell, and forms membrane-bound vesicles.
Exocytosis	Manufactured and modified materials are secreted by this process and eliminated from the cell.

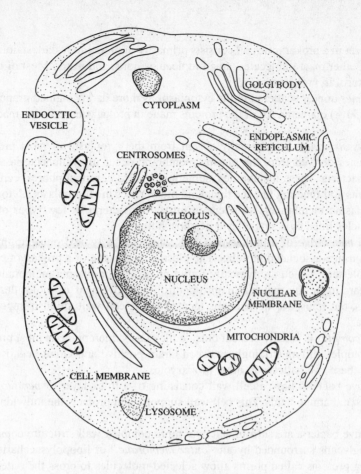

Diagram of eukaryotic cell.

Prokaryotic Versus Eukaryotic Cell Structure

All living cells can be categorized as prokaryotic or eukaryotic on the basis of their structural organization.

Prokaryotic cells have no nuclear envelope separating the nuclear material from the cytoplasm. Organisms with prokaryotic cellular structure are unicellular, so each cell is an organism. Prokaryotic organisms frequently occur in loosely organized colonies.

Eukaryotic cells contain a nuclear envelope which separates their nuclear compartment from their cytoplasmic compartment. Organisms with eukaryotic cellular structure may be unicellular (protistans) or multicellular (fungi, plants, and animals). Multicellular eukaryotes contain multiple cell types in organized patterns.

Prokaryotic Cell Structure

A typical prokaryotic cell consists of a *nuclear area* or *nucleoid* surrounded by *cytoplasm*. The cytoplasm is bounded by a *plasma membrane,* which is in turn typically surrounded by a *cell wall complex.*

Nuclear Area

The nuclear area contains a chromosome consisting of a circular DNA molecule anchored at one location to the plasma membrane, but which is otherwise free in the cytoplasm. The DNA is usually complexed with proteins and other molecules, but is not organized into the nucleosomal histone-DNA complexes typical of eukaryotic nuclear DNA. In routine transmission electron micrographs, the nuclear area is usually lighter staining than the adjacent cytoplasm. The DNA in the nuclear area contains most of the genetic information in a prokaryotic cell, although smaller episomes or plasmids may also be present in the cell. Plasmids frequently contain genes conferring resistance to antibiotics.

Cytoplasm

The cytoplasm in a prokaryotic cell consists primarily of moderately dark staining cytosol containing proteins, other macromolecules, small molecules, ions, and water. Most of the metabolism occurs in the cytosol in prokaryotes.

Free ribosomes appear scattered in the cytoplasm as more darkly stained granules of approximately 25 nm (250 Å) diameter. All of the proteins made in prokaryotic cells are made on free ribosomes.

Membranous structures are normally absent from the cytoplasm of most prokaryotic cells. Internal membranes derived from the plasma membrane occur in cyanobacteria and some other photosynthetic bacteria. These membranes, sometimes called chromatophores, contain the photosynthetic pigments and function like the thylakoid membranes in chloroplasts. Cytoplasmic infoldings from the plasma membrane also occur in nitrifying bacteria. A few types of bacteria have cytoplasmic vesicles lined by a single layer of phospholipids.

The *plasma membrane* of a prokaryotic cell consists of a typical phospholipid bilayer with embedded and surface-associated proteins. The plasma membrane of a prokaryotic cell lacks glycolipids and cholesterol which are typically found in eukaryotic plasma membranes. The plasma membrane appears to be the major structure controlling movement of molecules in and out of prokaryotic cells, but transport mechanisms located in the cell wall are also important in Gram-negative bacteria.

A *cell wall complex* is usually present outside the plasma membrane in most prokaryotic cells. The cell wall complex differs strikingly between Gram-positive and Gram-negative bacteria, and may differ from these two patterns in other prokaryotes.

Gram-positive bacteria have a cell wall consisting of a thick layer of *peptidoglycans,* which consist of sugars and amino acids. This cell wall supports and protects the individual cell which it surrounds.

Gram-negative bacteria are surrounded by a more complex wall structure consisting of a thin layer of peptidoglycans surrounded by an *"outer membrane"* of lipopolysaccharide and protein. Channel-forming proteins called porins allow selected molecules to cross the outer membrane. A fluid-filled *periplasmic space* containing enzymes lies between the peptidoglycan layer and the plasma membrane and between the peptidoglycan layer and the outer membrane. The lipopolysaccharides of the outer membrane cause it to resist passage of water-soluble molecules which are not transported through the porins. As a result, the outer membrane of the cell wall in Gram-negative plays a greater role in controlling passage of materials than the cell wall in Gram-positive bacteria.

Prokaryotic cells may have structures extending outward from the cell wall complex. *Flagella* consist of a protein rod (about ¹⁄₁₀ as thick as a eukaryotic flagellum and lacking microtubules in its core) attached to the cell by a hook (bent structure) and a swivel (basal rotational mechanism). Flagella are responsible for movement of the cell.

Pili are hollow protein tubes which attach bacteria to surfaces and transfer DNA between cells during conjugation (mating).

Many prokaryotic cells have a *capsule* or *slime layer* consisting of a loose polysaccharide gel located outside the cell wall complex. This layer protects parasitic bacteria against host defense mechanisms.

Eukaryotic Cell Structure

A typical eukaryotic cell consists of a nucleus surrounded by cytoplasm containing ribosomes, a cytoskeleton, and numerous membranous organelles. The cytoplasm is bounded by a plasma membrane which may, in turn, be surrounded by a cell wall complex in plants, fungi, and some protistans or by extracellular matrix materials in animals.

Eukaryotic Nuclear Structures

The nuclear compartment (nucleus) is separated from the cytoplasmic compartment by a *nuclear envelope* consisting of two layers of membrane and perforated by nuclear pores. The outer membrane of the nuclear envelope complex is chemically similar to endoplasmic reticulum, whereas the inner nuclear membrane has inserted proteins which connect with the nuclear lamina (containing intermediate filament-like lamin proteins) which in turn connects to the nuclear matrix.

The nuclear contents (nucleoplasm) can exchange materials with the cytoplasmic contents (cytosol) by diffusion and selective transport through *nuclear pores*. Small molecules (diameter <9 nm) move through nuclear pores by simple diffusion. Proteins move from the cytosol into the nucleus by active transport through nuclear pores. Targeting is by short amino acid sequences which are in different locations in different proteins. Transfer RNA molecules are directionally transported from the nucleus into the cytosol, probably through nuclear pores and probably by active transport. Messenger RNA molecules are directionally transported from the nucleus into the cytosol through nuclear pores, probably by active transport. Efficient export requires a 5' methylated guanine cap and release from the spliceosome complexes (normally when splicing out of introns is complete). Ribosomal subunits are directionally transported from the nucleus into the cytosol, probably through nuclear pores and probably by active transport.

The *nucleolus,* which is visible in most eukaryotic cell nuclei during interphase, contains small amounts of DNA (most of the rRNA genes) and larger amounts of RNA (mostly rRNA) and proteins (rRNA processing proteins and ribosomal proteins). The nucleolus is the location of rRNA synthesis and assembly of ribosomal subunits from rRNA and from proteins imported from the cytoplasm.

Eukaryotic Chromosome Structure

Nuclear DNA in eukaryotes is organized into *chromosomes*. Chromosome number, shape of the condensed chromosomes during mitosis and meiosis, and DNA content of each chromosome are consistent among the normal members of a species. Chromosome number, shape, and DNA content may vary widely between species and even between some closely related species. Each unreplicated chromosome appears to contain a single linear DNA molecule.

Functional eukaryotic chromosomes appear to contain three essential components. These three components have been assembled and shown to constitute a functional artificial chromosome in yeast cells.

1. A *centromere sequence* is necessary to integrate the chromosome into the spindle during either mitosis or meiosis. A normal chromosome would contain a single functional centromere.
2. At least one *replication initiation sequence* is needed to initiate DNA replication in the chromosome. Isolated replication initiation sequences are referred to as *autonomously replicating sequences.* Most natural eukaryotic chromosomes contain multiple replication initiation sequences.
3. A *telomere sequence* is needed at each end of the chromosome to allow replication without loss of genetically critical sequences. Telomeres consist of simple repeated sequences added by telomerase enzymes in actively dividing cells.

Chromatin Structure

Each unreplicated eukaryotic chromosome contains a single linear DNA molecule which is complexed with proteins to form *chromatin,* consisting of protein and DNA in an approximately 2:1 ratio by weight.

Histones are the most numerous category of proteins in chromatin, comprising approximately half of the chromatin protein and occurring in approximately a 1:1 ratio to DNA by weight. Histones contain numerous amino acids with side chains containing basic functional groups, resulting in a net positive surface charge which binds ionically to the negatively charged phosphate groups in DNA.

Histone classes H2A, H2B, H3, and H4 aggregate with DNA to form *nucleosomes*. Each nucleosome contains two molecules of each histone class comprising a protein core and has two "turns" of DNA (approximately 146 nucleotide pairs) wound around the outside.

Nucleosomes appear to form at close spacing on most chromosomal DNA regions unless nucleosome assembly is inhibited by regulatory proteins bound to the DNA. As a result, regions of DNA which are transcriptionally active usually contain extensive regions of DNA between nucleosomes and appear as lighter-staining *euchromatin* when viewed by light and electron microscopy. Histones of class H1 (or H5 in some cells) bind to the DNA between closely spaced nucleosomes to aggregate the DNA into 30 nm diameter chromatic fibers which predominate in darker-staining *heterochromatin*.

Condensed chromosomes, which form during mitosis and meiosis, contain a poorly characterized *scaffolding* which further compacts the 30 nm diameter condensed nucleosome aggregates. The composition of the scaffolding is unclear, but Topoisomerase II enzymes occur bound to DNA at intervals. The topoisomerase functions as an enzyme which reduces DNA coiling during replication, but labeled antibody staining shows that topoisomerase remains in the scaffolding when histones are removed, which suggests that topoisomerase may be part of the scaffolding structure.

Eukaryotic Cytoplasm

1.   *Cytosol.* The largest functional compartment in eukaryotic animal cells is the *cytosol* or fluid cytoplasm between recognizable cytoplasmic organelles. The cytosol consists primarily of moderately dark staining material containing proteins, other macromolecules, small molecules, ions, and water. Glycolysis and many other general metabolic processes occur in the cytosol.

2.   *Free ribosomes.* These organelles appear scattered in the cytosol as more darkly stained granules of approximately 25 nm (250 Å) diameter. All of the proteins that will function in the cytosol, nucleus, and peroxisomes are made on free ribosomes. Proteins that will be imported from the cytosol into mitochondria and chloroplasts are also made on free ribosomes. Free ribosomes which are engaged in protein synthesis are organized into *polyribosomes (polysomes)* which may appear as clusters, linear arrays, or rosettes in routine electron micrographs.

3.   *Smooth endoplasmic reticulum (sER).* This organelle consists of irregular tubes and flattened sacs or cisterni of cytoplasmic membrane and has no ribosomes on its cytoplasmic surfaces. Endoplasmic reticulum (both sER and rER) provides the surfaces on which synthesis of phospholipids and part of the synthesis of steroids occurs. Enzymes associated with sER are also involved in detoxifying many foreign molecules such as drugs.

4.   *Secretion and Endocytosis Apparatus.* Rough endoplasmic reticulum, Golgi bodies, lysosomes, secretory vesicles, and numerous types of transport vesicles may be viewed as an integrated functional system which manufactures, modifies, and moves proteins and other molecules which may be secreted by exocytosis or taken into the cell by endocytosis.

    a.   *Rough Endoplasmic Reticulum (rER).* This consists of flattened sacs of cytoplasmic membrane with ribosomes associated with the cytoplasmic surface. The ribosomes on rER are the site of synthesis of proteins which will be "packaged" by the Golgi bodies. These proteins include lysosomal enzymes and proteins which will be secreted by the cell. The ribosomes on the rER do not appear to be permanently attached, but a ribosome attaches to rER if the polypeptide currently being synthesized by the ribosome carries a signal sequence of amino acids near its amino terminal end that triggers uptake of the polypeptide into the rER. After the polypeptide is taken into the rER, the initial oligosaccharide groups are added to glycoproteins prior to their transfer to Golgi bodies.

    b.   *Golgi bodies.* They consist of stacks of flattened sacs of smooth cytoplasmic membranes. The stack of membrane sacs in a Golgi body is polarized. One surface receives vesicles from the rER and is called the cis face. The other surface buds off vesicles which carry materials to lysosomes, secretory vesicles, and the plasma membrane and is called the trans face. Golgi bodies are called dictyosomes in plant cells. In animal cells with a single large Golgi body, the Golgi body is usually located near the pair of centrioles which are found next to the nucleus.

    Proteins synthesized on ribosomes associated with rER enter the Golgi by transfer of membrane vesicles from the rER to the cis face of the Golgi apparatus. Endoplasmic reticulum-resident proteins are retrieved by receptors which recognize their signal sequence and are routed back to the rER.

    While in the Golgi body, oligosaccharides on glycoproteins are modified by removal and substitution of sugars and by addition of sialic acid. Lysosomal enzymes are selected by recognition of their signal peptide and tagged with mannose-6-phosphate residues added to their oligosaccharides. Glycosaminoglycans are assembled onto core proteins to form proteoglycans. In addition, ceramides in the lipid bilayers of membrane vesicles which fused with the Golgi body are modified into sphingomyelin or into gangliosides.

    Lysosomal enzymes are recognized by receptors for mannose-6-phosphate and are transferred in vesicles from the trans Golgi face to lysosomes. Secretory granule components are recognized through mechanisms which are unclear and are transferred in vesicles from the trans Golgi face to secretory granules. Once in secretory granules, the components are concentrated and proteins may be processed by proteolytic enzymes. Many other components are transferred in vesicles from the Golgi trans face to the plasma membrane and released in the process of constitutive secretion.

   c. *Secretory vesicles.* These are spherical sacs of membrane containing materials which will be secreted from the cell by exocytosis.

   d. *Lysosomes.* These are spherical sacs of membrane containing hydrolytic enzymes (digestive enzymes) which function in acidic environments (usually about pH 4.5 to 5.0). Lysosomal enzymes usually function in digestion of material brought into the cell by phagocytosis or in digestion of damaged organelles.

5. Mitochondria. These organelles are approximately 0.5 μm in diameter and contain two layers of membrane. The outer membrane is smooth while the inner membrane is folded into finger-like or shelf-like cristae. The fluid space inside the inner membrane is called the matrix. Most of the ATP synthesis during aerobic cellular respiration occurs in mitochondria. The Krebs cycle occurs in the matrix. Electrons collected by flavin adenine dinucleotide (FAD) or nicotinamide adenine dinucleotide (NAD) are passed along the electron transport system, many of whose enzymes are integral membrane proteins in the inner membrane, and generate a proton (hydrogen ion) gradient across the inner membrane which is used as an energy source to convert ADP into ATP. Mitochondria are also involved in several parts of steroid synthesis and interconversion.

   Mitochondria are partially genetically autonomous and appear to arise by division of existing mitochondria. Mitochondria contain circular DNA molecules and prokaryote-like ribosomes which are involved in synthesis of a subset of the proteins which are present in the mitochondria. Most of the mitochondrial proteins are encoded by nuclear DNA and are synthesized on free ribosomes in the cytoplasm. Mitochondrial proteins are imported from the cytosol into the intermembrane space and the matrix in mitochondria by transmembrane transport complexes. Proteins are targeted to mitochondria by recognition of signal peptide sequences within the polypeptide chain of the protein.

6. Cytoskeleton. The cytoskeleton consists of the components that alter cell shape and that anchor and move organelles in cells. The cytoskeleton includes microfilaments, microtubules, intermediate filaments, and related structures.

   a. *Microfilaments.* These contain actin protein subunits assembled into very thin filaments (5 nm diameter). Microfilaments are usually associated with myosin and other proteins. Microfilaments are bundled into much larger stress fibers in some cell types. Microfilaments are capable of contraction, usually by sliding past each other due to interaction with myosin or some other "motor" protein.

   b. *Microtubules.* These contain alpha and beta tubulin protein subunits assembled into very small tubules (25 nm diameter). Microtubules are rigid tubes which can support cell shape or serve as a surface along which to move organelles inside the cell. Microtubules are rearranged to form the mitotic spindle during mitotic cell division. Microtubules appear to be organized and oriented by microtubule organizing centers associated with centrioles and several other cellular structures.

   c. *Intermediate filaments.* These contain one of a family of intermediate filament proteins assembled into fibers with a diameter of approximately 10 nm. Five major classes of intermediate filaments have been identified based on protein composition. Intermediate filaments may contain desmin, cytokeratin, vimentin, neurofilament, or glial fibrillary acidic protein. Each type of intermediate filament protein occurs in a different set of cell types. Intermediate filament fibers can be bent but resist stretching. They mechanically link desmosomal (macula adherens) cell–cell junctions across cells and may have additional functions.

   d. *Centrioles.* Each centriole is a cylinder of 9 triplets of microtubules. Centrioles occur in the center of the *centrosome* region next to the nucleus in animal cells and from which most of the microtubules in the cytoskeleton originate. The centrioles are duplicated and are associated with the ends of the mitotic spindle during mitosis. Basal bodies of eukaryotic cilia and flagella have the same structure as centrioles and appear to be the organizing structures for the axoneme in the cilium or flagellum.

   However, centrioles may have no function of their own. Centrioles are always associated with pericentriolar *microtubule organizing centers* in the cytoskeleton. The microtubule organizing centers appear to be essential to formation and spatial organization of microtubules. Because fully functional microtubule organizing centers without associated centrioles have been well documented in plant cells and in early mouse embryos, the function of the centrioles themselves is in question.

7. *Cytoskeleton-Associated Cell Surface Appendages.* Cilia, flagella, and microvilli are cell surface appendages with core structures containing cytoskeletal components.

    a. *Cilia and flagella.* Both have a core axial structure (the axoneme), which contains a cylinder of nine doublets of microtubules with an additional pair of single microtubules in the center. This "nine doublets plus two" pattern of microtubules makes these organelles easy to recognize when viewed in cross section by transmission electron microscopy. Both cilia and flagella have an outer covering of plasma membrane. Many flagella have dense-staining axial structures between the axoneme and the plasma membrane. Both cilia and flagella are motile. The flagellum in a sperm cell moves the cell through its environment. The cilia on epithelial cells of the trachea move the mucus layer which forms the cell's environment past the cell.

    b. *Microvilli.* These are small finger-like projections of the cell surface. Typical microvilli are usually less than 2 μm long and less than 0.5 μm in diameter. Microvilli contain only microfilaments (no microtubules) and cytosol and have an outer covering of plasma membrane. Microvilli are frequently an adaptation to increase surface area for absorption of solutes.

8. *Peroxisomes.* The organelles are membrane-lined vesicles which typically contain catalase which generates hydrogen peroxide used to detoxify various organic molecules. Peroxisomes are also involved in beta oxidation of fatty acids, and are involved in photorespiration and the glyoxylate cycle in plant cells. Peroxisomes import all of their enzymes from the cytosol by recognition of a short recognition peptide sequence. The translocation complex, which moves the enzymes across the peroxisome membrane, has not been described.

9. *Inclusions.* Inclusions in eukaryotic animal cells may include lipid droplets, glycogen granules, and melanin granules.

    a. *Lipid droplets.* These are spherical aggregates of lipid. Although the outer layer of the lipid droplet may contain phospholipids, a typical membrane structure does not appear to separate the lipid droplet from the cytoplasm. Lipid droplets appear as dark spheres when viewed by transmission electron microscopy and appear as empty spheres in routine light microscopic (LM) preparations.

    b. *Glycogen granules.* They occur as clusters in cytoplasm. Glycogen granules are easily visible by transmission electron microscopy and are usually very darkly stained and larger than ribosomes in routine preparations. Glycogen granules are not visible by LM, but glycogen can be demonstrated by LM using periodic acid Schiff (PAS) staining.

    c. *Melanin granules.* They are membrane-bound vesicles containing melanin. Melanin granules occur in cells near the basal layer in epidermis of skin and the pigmented cells at the rear of the retina of the eye. Melanin granules in epidermal cells are made in melanocytes and transferred into the epidermal cells.

10. *Plasma Membrane.* The plasma or cell membrane in a eukaryotic cell is a typical cellular membrane consisting of a lipid bilayer with integral and peripheral proteins. Many animal cell plasma membranes have the following additional features.

    a. The *outer face* of the plasma membrane is enriched in *glycolipids,* some of which are gangliosides with extensive oligosaccharide groups.

    b. Many of the transmembrane proteins, lipid-anchored proteins, and peripheral proteins associated with the outer face of the plasma membrane are *glycoproteins* with attached oligosaccharide groups.

    c. The oligosaccharides of the glycoproteins and lipids from the "fuzzy coat" or *glycocalyx* associated with the outer face of the plasma membrane. Although all of the functions of the glycocalyx are not known, glycocalyx oligosaccharides are the ligands for the lectin-like P-selectin receptors involved in initial binding of neutrophils to endothelial cells as the neutrophils leave blood vessels during inflammatory reactions. Likewise, the sialic acid units (which do not occur on bacteria) on the oligosaccharides help prevent complement-mediated damage to body cells during destruction of bacteria by complement. The glycocalyx on absorptive cells in the small intestine contains digestive enzymes which hydrolyze small fragments of molecules.

11. *Cell–Cell Junctions.* These are structures which join adjacent cells in multicellular animals. Junctional structures can be categorized as occluding junctions, attachment junctions, or communicating junctions.

a. *Occluding junctions* or *zonula occludens*. These are regions in which the outer layers of the plasma membranes of associated cells appear fused (no extracellular space). A zonula occludens complex usually occurs as a band around the apical ends of epithelial cells in a sheet epithelium. Zonula occludens complexes prevent passage of materials through the extracellular space between cells and allow an epithelium to serve as a barrier.

b. *Attachment junctions*. These may include several types of junctions. *Zonula adherens* typically occur adjacent to zonula occludens junctions. Associated cells appear to be attached by a band of dense material in the intercellular space which is associated with dense material on the cytoplasmic surface of each membrane. The cytoplasmic dense material is in turn associated with microfilaments of the cytoskeleton. Zonula adherens junctions form a mechanical attachment between cells which protects the zonula occludens junctions in epithelial cells.

Macula adherens may occur as *desmosomes* joining two adjacent cells or as *hemidesmosomes* joining a cell to its basal lamina. In a macula adherens junction, a spot of dense material in the intercellular space between attached cells (desmosome) or between a cell and its basal lamina (hemidesmosome) is associated with a spot of dense material on the cytoplasmic surface of the plasma membrane of each cell involved. The cytoplasmic dense material is attached to intermediate filaments of the cytoskeleton of the attached cells. Macula adherens junctions form mechanical attachments between the connected structures (cell–cell or cell–basal lamina).

c. *Communicating junctions*. These allow ions to move from the cytoplasm of one cell to the cytoplasm of an adjacent cell. A *nexus* or *gap junction* is a region (usually spot-like) in which the plasma membranes of opposed cells maintain a precise apparent gap (about 2 nm) which actually contains protein channels that cross both membranes. Nexus junctions allow rapid ionic communication between the connected cells.

Eukaryotic Extracellular Materials

1. Cell Walls. These structures consist of layers of extracellular material (cellulose, pectins, etc. in higher plants and chitin in fungi) which surround individual cells. A cell wall supports the individual cell which it surrounds and helps support the body of the higher plants and fungi.

COMPARISON OF PROKARYOTIC AND EUKARYOTIC CELL STRUCTURE

Structure	Prokaryotic Cell	Eukaryotic Cell	
		Animal	Plant
Cell wall complex	+	−	+
Plasma membrane	+	+	+
Nuclear area (nucleoid)	+	−	−
Nucleus	−	+	+
Ribosomes	+	+	+
Endoplasmic reticula (sER and rER)	−	+	+
Golgi bodies	−	+	+
Secretory vesicles	−	+	+
Lysosomes	−	+	+
Mitochondria	−	+	+
Cytoskeleton	−	+	+
• microfilaments	−	+	+
• microtubules	−	+	+
• intermediate filaments	−	+	+
• centrioles	−	+	−
Cilia and flagella	−*	+	−
Microvilli	−	+	−
Peroxisomes	−	+	+
Chloroplasts	−	−	+

* Many bacteria have flagella, but they are protein rods unrelated to the membrane covered flagella containing microtubules that occur in eukaryotic cells.

2. *Extracellular Matrix.* The material located between cells in multicellular animals is referred to as extracellular matrix. Unlike a cell wall, extracellular matrix does not usually appear as a series of layers around individual cells. Animal extracellular matrix usually contains fibrous proteins or glycoproteins such as collagen and elastin plus complex polysaccharides such as glycosaminoglycans. Extracellular matrix in bone is hardened by adding calcium and phosphate ions. Extracellular matrix is the major structural component in the connective tissues which give shape to the bodies of most higher animals.

Cell Division—Mitosis

For purposes of convenience, mitosis is divided into prophase, metaphase, anaphase, and telophase; the process, however, is a continuous one. The major events during the phases are:

1. *Prophase.* Chromosomes become distinct and nucleolus (nucleoli) disappear(s); centriole(s) and asters and spindle appear; nuclear membrane disappears.
2. *Metaphase.* Chromosomes move to the equator of the cell and duplicate.
3. *Anaphase.* The two chromatids split apart and start migration toward the poles of the spindle; the spindle loses its definition.
4. *Telophase.* Chromosomes lengthen and become less distinct; nucleoli reappear. The next period of growth and rest is known as *interphase.*
5. *Interphase.* Cell growth; protein synthesis; DNA synthesis; chromosome duplication.

Mitosis in human cells. The four phases of mitosis are shown, with the major structures noted. The chromatids appear in prophase, then line up in the cell center in metaphase. One set of 46 chromosomes move to each daughter cell in anaphase, and the splitting of the cell in telophase completes the process.

Methods of Examining the Cell

1. Histological Methods

a. *Microscopy.* Microscopes are usually classified according to the type of energy source. Besides the straight line microscope and the electron microscope, the researcher utilizes polarization, phase contrast, interference, ultraviolet, and X-ray microscopes.

b. *Stains.* Dyes are used in solution to stain generally the nucleus and/or cytoplasm, or specifically, particular cell components. Dyes in general are neutral salts having both acidic and basic radicals. A basic dye exhibits its coloring property because of the basic radical it possesses. Structures stained by it are designated as basophilic—the nucleus, for example. An acidic dye exhibits its staining property because of the acidic radical. Structures delineated by it are acidophilic—the cytoplasm, for example.

Examples of stains routinely employed:

1. Hematoxylin, a common histologic stain, stains nuclei blue;
2. The common histological stain eosin (H&E) and other acidic dyes, such as picric acid, stain the general cytoplasm;
3. Iron hematoxylin, which stains chromosomes, mitochondria, Golgi complex, and contractile elements of muscle cells black or dark blue;
4. Carmine, which stains nuclei red-purple;
5. Basic aniline dyes, such as toluidine blue, azure A and methylene blue, which stain mucopolysaccharides metachromatically;
6. Mallory's connective tissue (CT) stain, which stains collagen fibers bright blue, nuclei red or orange, and various cell components blue, red, orange, or purple;
7. Reticular fibers, which are argyophilic, are stained brown by silver impregnation methods.

2. Histochemical Methods

Tissues are composed of various chemicals such as proteins, carbohydrates, lipids, inorganic salts and miscellaneous substances, and various tests are used to detect these chemicals. *Examples:*

1. Proteins (with tyrosine)—yellow color with picric acid;
2. Enzymes—various tests for phosphatases, lipases, oxidases, esterases, and dehydrogenases;
3. Carbohydrates—glycogen by periodic acid Schiff (PAS) test results in a magenta or purple color; glycoproteins give a positive PAS magenta color. Basal laminae and reticular fibers are strongly PAS positive;
4. Lipids—Sudan dyes or osmic acid;
5. Nucleic acids—Feulgen reaction is specific for DNA, but not for RNA, which can be detected by ribonuclease. Both DNA and RNA are basophilic (because they are both acids).

3. Fixation

The fixative must modify the cell to resist further treatments and also to make further treatments possible. Fixatives may be classified as either coagulant or noncoagulant. Examples of each are:

1. *coagulant:* methanol, ethanol, acetone, nitric acid, hydrochloric acid, picric acid, trichloroacetic acid and mercuric chloride;
2. *noncoagulant:* formaldehyde, glutaraldehyde, osmium tetroxide, potassium dichromate, acetic acid, and potassium permanganate.

Fixatives can also be subclassified into two categories. The following are examples:

1. *additive:* osmium tetroxide, formaldehyde, and glutaraldehyde;
2. *nonadditive:* methanol, ethanol, and acetone.

4. Method of Preparation

1. *Fixation:* a piece of tissue is placed in a fixative solution, which kills and preserves the cells in the tissue with as few structural changes as possible;
2. *Dehydration:* water is usually removed from the tissues by passing it through a series of increasing strengths of alcohol solutions;
3. *Embedding:* embedding places the tissues in a solid medium, usually paraffin or plastic;
4. *Sectioning:* tissue is cut into sections with a thickness of 5 microns or 5000 nm for light, and about 60 nm for electron microscopic evaluation;
5. *Staining:* sections are stained with colored dyes for light microscopy and heavy metals for electron microscopy to enhance visualization.

Quick Recall Test Questions and Answers

Choose the Best Answer

1. If a cell were put into a solution of greater osmotic pressure than its protoplasm:

   A. water would pass out through the plasma membrane faster than in.
   B. water would pass in through the plasma membrane faster than out.
   C. the cell would swell.
   D. no unequal rates would be experienced.
   E. the result could not be predicted.

2. Messenger RNA receives its instructions from:

   A. ribosomes.
   B. endoplasmic reticulum.
   C. DNA in the nucleus.
   D. cytoplasm.
   E. the Golgi zone.

3. During metaphase of mitosis:

   A. there is a dissolution of the chromosomal material.
   B. the centrioles with asters are at the opposite poles.
   C. the cell membrane starts to reappear.
   D. the nuclear membrane disappears.
   E. there is a slowdown in metabolic activity.

4. Resolution—the ability to discriminate between two points that are close together—depends on the wavelength and the numerical aperture of the objective lens used. In which of the following statements are the lens and resolution incorrectly paired?

   A. The human eye resolves 100 μ.
   B. The light microscope resolves 0.2 μ.
   C. The transmission electron microscope resolves 3–5 Å.
   D. The opthalmoscope resolves 1 μ.
   E. The scanning electron microscope resolves 70–100 Å.

5. The process by which a cell takes up material into membrane bound vesicles is known as:

   A. phagocytosis.
   B. active transport.
   C. exocytosis.
   D. endocytosis.
   E. transfer.

6. Microvilli would most likely be located on the surface of a cell that carries out which of the following processes?

   A. secretion
   B. protection
   C. motility
   D. absorption
   E. conduction

7. Unlike facilitated diffusion, active transport is:

   A. sensitive to the concentration of the component on only one side of the membrane (the "loading side").
   B. insensitive to the concentration of the component on the other side of the membrane.
   C. known to saturate at relatively low component concentrations.
   D. all of the above.
   E. none of the above.

8. These paired terms all relate to histological techniques. Which one is an incorrect match?

   A. hematoxylin—specific for enzymes
   B. eosin—general stain for cytoplasm
   C. periodic acid Schiff reaction—demonstrates carbohydrates
   D. Feulgen stain—DNA affinity
   E. osmic acid—stains lipids

9. The fluid-mosaic cell model of the cell membrane depicts it as:

   A. a bilayer of lipid between two layers of protein.
   B. a bilayer of lipid with integral and peripheral proteins.
   C. a bilayer of protein between two layers of lipid.
   D. alternating layers of protein and lipid (jelly roll).
   E. purely protein in composition.

10. Which of the following cell organelles or structures produces chemical energy via the electron transport chain?

    A. mitochondria
    B. rough endoplasmic reticulum (rER)
    C. smooth endoplasmic reticulum (sER)
    D. peroxisomes
    E. free ribosomes

11. The process by which a cell can move a substance from a point of lower concentration to a point of higher concentration (against the diffusion gradient) is called:

    A. osmosis.
    B. plasmolysis.
    C. turgor pressure.
    D. active transport.
    E. passive transport.

12. Which of the following structures is/are NOT considered a modification of the cell membrane?

    A. basement membrane
    B. terminal bars
    C. desmosomes
    D. intercalated discs
    E. microvilli

13. If a cell is viewed by microscope under low power and then under high power, and no fine adjustment is necessary to see it clearly, the microscope is considered:

    A. achromatic.
    B. bifocal.
    C. parfocal.
    D. unifocal.
    E. apochromatic.

14. The internal structure of a eukaryotic cilium or flagellum, no matter what the organism, has the same fibrillar arrangement, consisting of _____ pairs of tubules.

    A. 7 outer and 2 inner
    B. 9 outer and 2 inner
    C. 11 outer and 2 inner
    D. 9 outer and 1 inner
    E. 9 outer and 3 inner

15. Cellular "digestive" or "suicide" packages is a common description for:

    A. mitochondria.
    B. Golgi zones or Golgi bodies.
    C. lysosomes.
    D. centrosomes.
    E. multivesicular bodies.

16. Of the following, which is not considered a membranous organelle?

    A. ribosome
    B. endoplasmic reticulum
    C. Golgi body

    D. mitochondrion
    E. lysosome

17. The smallest unit possessing the capability to maintain life and to reproduce is:

    A. an organ.
    B. a cell.
    C. DNA.
    D. RNA.
    E. a nucleus.

18. All of the following are characteristic of prokaryotic cells EXCEPT:

    A. cell wall complex.
    B. plasma membrane.
    C. nuclear area.
    D. ribosomes.
    E. rough endoplasmic reticulum.

DIRECTIONS: For questions 19–22, refer to the responses labeled A–D below. For each question, choose the letter response that is most closely associated with the given item. You may use a letter choice more than once, or not at all.

    A. possesses hydrolytic enzymes
    B. functions in protein synthesis
    C. condenses (packages) secretory products
    D. functions in energy production

19. Mitochondrion

20. Lysosome

21. Golgi apparatus

22. Rough endoplasmic reticulum

23. Which of the following is highly developed in a cell that is metabolically very active and has a high energy (ATP) requirement?

    A. lysosomes
    B. rough endoplasmic reticulum
    C. Golgi apparatus
    D. mitochondria
    E. peroxisomes

24. In mitosis the chromosomes are located on the equator of the cell during:

    A. prophase.
    B. metaphase.
    C. anaphase.
    D. telophase.
    E. interphase.

Answers

1. **A.** If a cell is placed in a hypertonic solution, water from within it will cross the semipermeable membrane and leave the cell, and the cell will shrink. If a cell is placed in a hypotonic solution, water from without will enter the cell and it will swell. In an isotonic solution, as many molecules of water will enter as will leave the cell and the cell will remain the same.

2. **C.** The whole activity is controlled by its genetic components, which are located in the nucleus.

3. **B.** During metaphase of mitosis the centrioles with asters are at the opposite poles; the chromosomes move to the equator of the cell and duplicate.

4. **D.** The common resolving powers of the eye, light microscope, and electron microscope have been correctly stated. The opthalmoscope provides a good light source and a little magnification but certainly does not help much to improve the resolving power of the eye.

5. **D.** Rough endoplasmic reticulum, Golgi bodies, lysosomes, secretory vesicles, and numerous types of transport vesicles may be viewed as an integral functional system which manufactures, modifies, and moves proteins and other molecules that may be secreted by exocytosis or taken into the cell by endocytosis (pinocytosis).

6. **D.** Microvilli are small, finger-like projections of the cell surface. Typical microvilli are usually less that 2 μm long and less than 0.5 μm in diameter. Microvilli contain only microfilaments (no microtubules) and cytosol, and have an outer covering of plasma membrane. Microvilli are frequently an adaptation to increase the surface area for absorption of solutes.

7. **D.** The characteristics of active transport are delineated.

8. **A.** Hemotoxylin is a very common histologic stain; it stains nuclei blue. It is routinely used with eosin (H&E) to stain the general cytoplasm. All other techniques are correctly matched.

9. **B.** All membranes consist of lipid (primarily phospholipid) bilayers with associated proteins. Some proteins are associated with the surface of the membrane, whereas other proteins extend across the lipid bilayer. Membrane surfaces which face away from the cytoplasm in eukaryotic cells may have numerous oligosaccharide groups (polymers and sugars) attached to proteins and lipids.

10. **A.** Most of the ATP synthesis during aerobic cellular respiration occurs in mitochondria. The Krebs cycle occurs in the matrix. Electrons collected by flavinadenine dinucleotide (FAD) or nicotinamide adenine dinucleotide (NAD) are passed along the electron transport system, many of whose enzymes are integral membrane proteins in the inner membrane, and generate a proton (hydrogen ion) gradient across the inner membrane which is used as an energy source to convert ADP into ATP.

11. **D.** Active transport requires energy and allows a cell to move material from a point of lower concentration to a point of higher concentration.

12. **A.** Directly underlying epithelium is found a homogeneous, noncellular material, composed of reticular fibers and protein polysaccharides, which serves to bind down the tissue; this structure is the basement membrane.

13. **C.** In a parfocal optical microscope the objective lenses are so constructed or mounted that one may change from one to another and the image remains focused; the lenses have focal points in the same plane.

14. **B.** The internal structure of a cilium or flagellum is composed of 9 outer and 2 inner pairs of tubules.

15. **C.** Lysosomes contain hydrolytic enzymes and are also known as digestive bags, etc.

16. **A.** Ribosomes can be free floating or they may be attached to the endoplasmic reticulum which is then called rough endoplasmic reticulum (RER).

17. **B.** The cell is the basic unit of structure and function and the basis of all life; all cells come from preexisting cells.

18. **E.** Prokaryotic cells have no rough endoplasmic reticulum. (See table on p. 17.)

19. **D.** Mitochondria are the biochemical powerplants of the cell. They recover energy from foodstuffs

(via the Krebs cycle and respiratory chain) and convert it (via phosphorylation) into ATP (adenosine triphosphate). In this manner they produce the energy necessary for the metabolic processes.

20. **A.** Lysosomes contain acid phosphatase and other hydrolytic enzymes. These enzymes are enclosed by a membrane and are released when needed into phagocytic vesicles, etc.

21. **C.** The Golgi complex is prominent in glandular cells and is thought to function in the production, concentration, packaging, and transportation of secretory material.

22. **B.** Ribosomes are attached to the membranes of the endoplasmic reticulum which is designated as rough ER. Ribosomes are responsible for synthesis of proteins.

23. **D.** Most of the ATP synthesis during aerobic cellular respiration occurs in mitochondria. The Krebs cycle occurs in the matrix. Electrons collected by flavin adenine dinucleotide (FAD) or nicotinamide adenine dinucleotide (NAD) are passed along the electron transport system, many of whose enzymes are integral membrane proteins in the inner membrane, and generate a proton (hydrogen ion) gradient

across the inner membrane which is used as an energy source to convert ADP into ATP. Mitochondria are also involved in several parts of steroid synthesis and interconversion.

24. **B.** For purposes of convenience, mitosis is divided into prophase, metaphase, anaphase, and telophase; the process, however, is a continuous one. In metaphase, chromosomes move to the equator of the cell. The major events during the phases are:

1. *Prophase*. Chromosomes become distinct and nucleolus (nucleoli) disappear(s); centriole(s) and asters and spindle appear; nuclear membrane disappears.

2. *Metaphase*. Chromosomes move to the equator of the cell.

3. *Anaphase*. The two chromatids split apart and start migration toward the poles of the spindle; the spindle loses its definition.

4. *Telophase*. Chromosomes lengthen and become less distinct; nucleoli reappear. The next period of growth and rest is known as interphase.

5. *Interphase*. Cell growth; protein synthesis; DNA synthesis; chromosome duplication.

Structure and Function of Viruses

All typical viruses contain *nucleic acid* encoding the genetic information carried by the virus. The type of nucleic acid used by a particular category of virus will be consistent but varies widely among categories of viruses. The nucleic acid may be DNA or RNA and may be linear or circular. DNA and RNA may be either single- or double-stranded in viruses.

Viruses which require unusual replication enzymes such as RNA replicase or reverse transcriptase frequently carry copies of those enzymes bound to the nucleic acid in the virus particles.

Typical viruses contain a protein *capsid* or *capsule,* usually surrounding the nucleic acid. The protein subunits in the capsid are usually arranged to form either a polyhedron or a helix. The capsid may contain a single type of subunit or several types. Likewise, the capsid may contain a single layer of protein subunits or multiple layers.

Many viruses contain accessory structures attached to the capsid or additional layers outside the capsid. Bacteriophages may have a "stalk-like" apparatus at one end of the polyhedral capsid which is involved in passing the nucleic acid across the bacterial cell wall.

Eukaryotic animal cell viruses frequently contain a lipid bilayer structure outside of the capsid. This lipid bilayer is derived from the host cell plasma membrane and envelops the virus as the virus is budded off from the host cell surface. The lipid bilayer usually contains viral proteins which were encoded by viral nucleic acid, synthesized on host cell ribosomes, and inserted into the host cell plasma membrane prior to budding off the viruses.

Viral Life Cycles

A virus is only capable of reproduction while in a suitable host cell. Numerous reproductive patterns have been described in different viruses.

Bacteriophages (viruses infecting bacteria) typically follow one of two strategies or pathways, since release of viruses from the host bacterial cell is constrained by the bacterial cell wall. In a *lytic* replication strategy or pathway, the virus rapidly replicates after entering a host cell, then triggers lysis of the host cell to release the assembled viruses. In a *lysogenic* strategy or pathway, a DNA copy of the viral nucleic acid (the provirus) becomes incorporated into the host cell chromosome where it is replicated along with the adjacent host DNA. The integrated virus may cause little alteration in host cell phenotype or may cause detectable changes in host phenotype. A virus following a lysogenic strategy must shift to a lytic strategy in order to replicate new virus particles and release them from the host cell. In many of the bacteriophages studied so far, environmental insults which damage the bacterial host trigger the integrated *provirus* to exit the host DNA and follow a lytic reproductive strategy.

Animal cell viruses may follow similar patterns of rapid replication leading to death of the host cell or of incorporation into a host chromosome. Incorporated viral DNA may cause no detectable phenotypic changes or may cause changes as fundamental as loss of growth regulation resulting in cancer. In animal cell hosts, an intermediate strategy is also possible because the viruses can be budded from the host cell surface without killing the cell. As a result, viral replication can occur at moderate rates in infected cells for extended periods. As an example, macrophages infected with HIV-1 may survive for extended periods and serve as sources of viruses to infect nearby CD4+ T lymphocytes in lymphoid organs.

Retroviruses are single-stranded RNA viruses that infect animal cells. These viruses use reverse transcriptase to make DNA copies of the viral RNA, after which the DNA copies become incorporated into host chromosomes. Because the viral DNA is somewhat transcriptionally active, these viruses frequently alter the phenotype of infected cells. At one point, some retroviruses (including HIV-1) were thought to be capable of remaining incorporated for 10 years or more, but more recent observations indicate that HIV-1 is replicating actively in lymphoid organs during the period between infection and development of clinical AIDS. This raises the possibility that some incorporated retroviruses may not remain incorporated for as long as was previously assumed. Retroviruses are important as inducers of a number of cancers in experimental animals and a rare form of T-cell leukemia in humans. In addition, HIV-1 and HIV-2 are responsible for essentially all cases of acquired immunodeficiency syndrome (AIDS).

Quick Recall Test Questions and Answers

Choose the Best Answer

1. The genome of a typical virus may be either DNA or RNA, each of which may be single-stranded or double-stranded.

   A. TRUE
   B. FALSE

2. Typical viruses contain a protein capsid which surrounds the viral nucleic acid. The polypeptide subunits in the capsid may be arranged in a helical or polyhedral pattern.

   A. TRUE
   B. FALSE

3. Many eukaryotic animal cell viruses have a lipid bilayer surrounding the protein capsid. The lipids in the bilayer are synthesized by viral enzymes before the virus leaves the host cell.

   A. TRUE
   B. FALSE

4. Although typical viruses normally replicate inside a host cell, many viruses can replicate themselves outside of their normal host cell if they are provided with an external source of ATP.

   A. TRUE
   B. FALSE

5. A typical bacteriophage following a lytic type of reproductive strategy will insert its DNA into the host cell chromosome before turning on viral replication leading to lysis of the host cell.

   A. TRUE
   B. FALSE

6. The enzyme which catalyzes the initial replication of the viral genome during infection of a eukaryotic cell by a typical retrovirus is:

   A. RNA polymerase.
   B. reverse transcriptase.
   C. DNA polymerase I.
   D. DNA polymerase II.
   E. DNA polymerase III.

7. Bacteriophages are:

   A. quite dangerous to humans.
   B. grown by innoculation of sterile broth.
   C. reproduced only in living cells.
   D. used as a source of vaccine against many bacterial diseases.
   E. used in the production of vaccine against specific viral agents.

Answers

1. A. Although a single type of virus will have a single type of nucleic acid, examples of viruses with any possible type and configuration of nucleic acid exist.

2. A. Although a virus may contain additional coats derived from the plasma membrane of the host, the nucleic acid is typically surrounded by a polyhedral (or more rarely a helical) protein capsid.

3. B. The first sentence in this statement is true, but the second sentence is false. Although proteins in viral lipid layer typically include proteins coded by viral genes, the lipids are typically derived from the plasma membrane of the host cell and are therefore synthesized by host cell enzymes in the rough endoplasmic reticulum and Golgi apparatus.

4. B. This statement is false because viral replication requires numerous host cell enzymes, host cell ribosomes, and other host cell components. Therefore replication of viruses can occur only inside host cells.

5. B. This statement is false because in a lytic cycle the viral DNA is not typically inserted into the host cell chromosome. Insertion into the host cell chromosome is typical of a lysogenic strategy or process.

6. B. The correct answer is reverse transcriptase, which catalyzes assembly of DNA using an RNA template (RNA genome of the retrovirus in this case). RNA polymerase catalyzes assembly of RNA using a DNA template. DNA polymerase III catalyzes replication of DNA in prokaryotes. DNA polymerases I and II catalyze DNA synthesis during DNA repair in prokaryotes.

7. C. A bacteriophage is a virus that is a parasite of bacteria; sometimes lysis of the bacteria cell is a result.

Nucleic Acids and Nucleotides

DNA (deoxyribonucleic acid) and *RNA* (ribonucleic acid) are nucleic acids which are polymers of nucleotides, electron carriers such as *FAD, NAD,* and *NADP* are dinucleotides, and high energy phosphate carriers such as *ATP, CTP, GTP,* and *UTP* are single nucleotides.

Nucleotide Structure

Nucleotides are the monomers which are assembled to produce more complex nucleic acids. Each nucleotide consists of three components.

1. *Pentose Sugar.* Each nucleotide contains one five-carbon sugar which is either ribose (ATP, FAD, NAD, NADP, and RNA) or deoxyribose (DNA).
2. *Nitrogenous Base.* Each nucleotide contains one nitrogenous base which may be either a purine or a pyrimidine. Pyrimidines consist of a 6-membered ring containing carbon and nitrogen atoms. Pyrimidines include cytosine (C), uracil (U), and thymine (T). Purines consist of a similar 6-membered ring fused to a 5-membered ring. Purines include adenine (A) and guanine (G).
3. *Phosphate.* Each nucleotide contains one (MP), two (DP), or three (TP) phosphate groups. The letter code for the nitrogenous base plus the letter code for the number of phosphates can be used to designate a nucleotide. For example, a nucleotide with adenine and one phosphate is AMP.

Energy Transfer by Nucleotides

If more than one phosphate group is present on a nucleotide, the bonds attaching the extra (second or third) phosphates to the nucleotide are less stable and can be easily hydrolyzed to release the energy used to make those bonds and make that energy available to other processes in the cell. As a result, nucleotide triphosphates are the primary energy source used to supply energy-consuming reactions in cells. ATP is the most widely used nucleotide triphosphate and is used for a wide variety of reactions. UTP is used in biosynthetic reactions involving additions of sugars. GTP is used to provide energy for protein shape changes by G proteins involved in receptor-triggered reaction sequences and protein synthesis.

Positional Nomenclature

Locations of atoms on nucleotides are specified relative to the carbon atoms in the ribose or deoxyribose ring.

1. The purine or pyrimidine is attached to the *1' carbon* on the sugar.
2. The phosphate group is attached to the *5' carbon* on the sugar.
3. The hydroxyl group on the *3' carbon* on the sugar is reacted with the phosphate group on the adjacent nucleotide when a nucleotide is added to a DNA or RNA chain.

Nucleotide Functions

Nucleotides may be polymerized into *linear chains* of any length by covalently attaching (by a modified dehydration synthesis) the 3' carbon (using its attached hydroxyl) of the sugar of one nucleotide to the phosphate on the 5' carbon of the adjacent nucleotide. This arrangement creates polarity in chains of nucleotides.

The end of the chain with a free (unreacted) hydroxyl on the 3' carbon of the terminal nucleotide is called the *3' end* of the chain. Most reactions which add nucleotides to a DNA or RNA chain can react only with the 3' end of the existing chain. DNA synthesis catalyzed by DNA polymerase enzymes and RNA synthesis catalyzed by RNA polymerase enzymes follow this pattern.

The end of the chain with a free (unreacted) phosphate on the 5' carbon of the terminal nucleotide is called the *5' end* of the chain. The 5' end (or a structure near the 5' end) of a messenger RNA molecule must be recognized by a ribosome before the ribosome can assemble on the messenger RNA during initiation of protein synthesis (translation).

Base Pairing by Nucleotides

Nucleotides may base pair with complementary nucleotides by forming hydrogen bonds between their nitrogenous bases. Stable base pairs consist of a purine paired with a pyrimidine. Two patterns of base pairing occur normally.

1. Adenine base pairs with uracil or thymine by forming two hydrogen bonds.
2. Guanine base pairs with cytosine by forming three hydrogen bonds.

Nucleotide Functions in Cells

1. Nucleotide triphosphates transport energy from energy-generating chemical reactions to energy-consuming reactions within the same cell.
2. Nucleotide triphosphates serve as monomers for the synthesis of RNA and DNA.
3. Nucleotides may be modified into chemical signals for use within a cell. Cyclic AMP is an example.

RNA (Ribonucleic Acid) Structure

RNA is a polymer of *ribonucleotides* (*ribose* is the 5⁻ carbon sugar). The purine bases in RNA are adenine and guanine. The pyrimidine bases in RNA are cytosine and *uracil*. (Ribose is replaced by deoxyribose and uracil is replaced by thymine in DNA. Adenine, guanine, and cytosine occur in both RNA and DNA.)

RNA usually consists of a *single linear* chain of nucleotides. However, RNA chains may fold and form base pairs between regions of the same chain where complementary sequences occur, resulting in "hairpin" loops. Double-stranded RNA occurs as the genetic material in some viruses.

RNA Functions

Messenger RNA (mRNA) codes for the amino acid sequence (primary structure) of polypeptide chains in proteins.

Transfer RNA (tRNA) carries amino acids (as aminoacyl groups on the tRNA) into protein synthesis and uses the nucleotide sequence in a mRNA to determine where to insert the amino acid carried by the tRNA into the forming polypeptide chain. The amino acid–RNA linkage in the aminoacyl tRNA is formed using energy from nucleotide triphosphates and contains the energy needed to form the peptide bond joining the amino acid to the peptide.

Ribosomal RNAs (rRNA) form the structural framework of the ribosomal subunits, and a loop of one of the rRNA molecules appears to be capable of catalyzing the formation of peptide bonds.

Several *ribonucleoprotein (RNP) particles* containing small RNA molecules are involved in RNA and protein processing. Small nuclear ribonucleoproteins (snRNPs) which contain small RNA molecules remove introns from mRNA in eukaryotes. The signal recognition particle which recognizes membrane and secretory polypeptides forming on ribosomes is a cytoplasmic ribonucleoprotein containing a small RNA.

DNA (Deoxyribonucleic Acid) Structure

DNA is made of *deoxyribonucleotides* (*deoxyribose* is the 5-carbon sugar). The purine bases in DNA are adenine and guanine. The pyrimidine bases in DNA are cytosine and thymine.

The nucleotides within a single DNA chain or strand are joined by *covalent bonds* linking the 3' carbon on one nucleotide with the phosphate on the 5' carbon of the adjacent nucleotide.

A DNA molecule usually consists of *two linear chains* of nucleotides and is referred to as *double-stranded,* although single-stranded DNA occurs in some viruses. The two strands in a DNA molecule run in opposite directions (have opposite polarity), so the 3' end of one strand is next to the 5' end of the other strand. The two strands in a DNA molecule are most frequently twisted into a right-handed *helix.* Other possible twisting patterns such as Z form DNA appear to occur less frequently.

The two chains or strands in a DNA molecule are paired by *hydrogen bonds* between complementary base pairs (A-T, G-C). Because the hydrogen bonds between the base pairs are much weaker than the covalent bonds which join the nucleotides within a single strand, the two strands can be separated without breaking the strands. This feature is used during DNA replication and during RNA synthesis.

Genetic Information Flow in Cells

Genetic information *(genotype)* is stored in cells in the form of the sequence of deoxyribonucleotides in DNA. The double-stranded nature of DNA allows repair of damage as long as both strands are not damaged in the same location.

Genetic information is transmitted accurately from cell to cell during mitosis and from parent to offspring during reproduction because the deoxyribonucleotide sequence in the parental DNA molecules determines the deoxyribonucleotide sequence in newly formed DNA molecules during *DNA replication* (except when mutations occur).

Point mutations result from unrepaired mistakes in DNA replication or misrepaired damage in nonreplicating DNA. A point mutation is a change in the sequence of deoxyribonucleotides in DNA.

Conversion of genetic information into a cellular phenotype requires a sequence of events.

Transcription (RNA Synthesis). The deoxyribonucleotide sequence in regions of DNA (genes) codes for (serves as a template for) the ribonucleotide sequence in mRNAs. The bases in RNA can hydrogen bond to the bases in DNA, so one base in DNA specifies one base (complementary to it) in RNA.

Translation (Protein Synthesis). The ribonucleotide sequence in regions of DNA (genes) codes for (serves as a template for) the ribonucleotide sequence in mRNAs codes for the amino acid sequence in proteins (polypeptides). A three nucleotide codon in the mRNA base pairs with the complementary three nucleotide anticodon on an aminoacyl tRNA to allow the aminoacyl group (one amino acid) on the aminoacyl tRNA to be added to the polypeptide (protein) being synthesized. Therefore, a three nucleotide unit in mRNA functions as one codon to specify one amino acid in a polypeptide. A polypeptide in turn forms all or part of a protein.

The proteins form cellular structures and/or perform or catalyze cell functions. Proteins directly or indirectly produce the *phenotype* of a cell.

The phenotype of a cell consists of the structures and functions of the cell. Cell structures consist of proteins plus other molecules whose synthesis is catalyzed by proteins. Cell functions are either performed by proteins, by molecules whose synthesis was catalyzed by proteins, or are catalyzed by proteins (enzymes). Because most chemical reactions in cells do not occur unless they are catalyzed by enzymes, every function in a cell is either directly or indirectly dependent on the protein composition of the cell. The proteins in the cell therefore directly or indirectly interact with the environment of the cell to produce the phenotype of the cell.

Protein Structure

Proteins are made of 20 different types of amino acids which share a common "backbone" structure consisting of an *amino group* covalently bonded to a carbon atom (the alpha carbon) which is in turn covalently bonded to a *carboxylic acid (carboxyl) group*. Each of the 20 different types of amino acids differs in the "side chain" structure attached to the alpha carbon.

One amino acid in a polypeptide chain in a protein is specified by a sequence of three nucleotides in a *messenger RNA (mRNA)*. This three nucleotide *codon* is translated through the mediation of a *transfer RNA (tRNA)*.

The *amino acid sequence* of each polypeptide chain (its primary structure) interacts with the polypeptide's environment and with other functional components in the cell in which the polypeptide was made to determine further modifications and eventual assembly of a functional protein.

1. Many if not most polypeptides must be altered by removal of one or more amino acids from the amino-terminal end, because the functional polypeptide in a protein does not have a methionine in the amino-terminal position. Methionine is the first amino acid (N-terminal) in all newly synthesized polypeptides because the methionine codon is also the initiation codon for protein synthesis.

2. Many polypeptides require addition of prosthetic groups (such as the heme groups in hemoglobin) before the polypeptide becomes functional.

3. A polypeptide must fold into a functional shape during or after its synthesis. Chaperone proteins are required for correct folding of many polypeptides.

4. Altered forms of many polypeptides and proteins are selectively degraded by proteosomes, frequently in response to ubiquitin attachment to the polypeptide or protein.

5. A functional protein may consist of a single polypeptide chain or may contain two or more polypeptides.

6. Many proteins are activated or inactivated by phosphorylation catalyzed by protein kinases.

7. Many proteins can interconvert between two or more shapes in response to allosteric interactions. An allosteric interaction causes a shape change in a protein in response to the binding of a molecule to a location outside the normal active site of the protein.

Protein Function

Proteins serve many types of functions in cells. *Structural proteins* form all or parts of cell structures such as ribosomes, chromosomes, mitotic spindles, and cell membranes. *Enzymes* are almost all proteins and are required to catalyze most chemical reactions in cells, including DNA synthesis, RNA synthesis, protein synthesis, carbohydrate synthesis, and lipid synthesis. Most cellular reactions will not occur under normal intracellular conditions without access to the appropriate enzyme. *Transport proteins* serve as carriers or channels to allow molecules to move across cell membranes to enter cells, leave cells, or move from one part of a cell to another. *Signal* or *regulatory proteins* respond to changes in a cell by changing their interactions with critical components such as DNA, thereby altering cell functions.

Control of Use of Genetic Information

Prokaryotic cells do not use all of their genetic information all of the time, and most eukaryotic cells in complex organisms never use more than a small part of their genetic information. Therefore, use of genetic information in a cell is normally restricted and may change over time.

Cells in a complex organism all contain the same genetic information (because they were all produced from the fertilized egg by mitosis), but may have thousands of different phenotypes. Those phenotypes occur in a well-defined pattern that makes up the body of the organism. Therefore, cells can selectively use parts of their genetic information during development.

In many cases, use of regions of DNA is regulated by regulatory proteins which are produced or activated in response to signals from the cell's environment. Some regulatory proteins make DNA available for coding for RNA, others may make DNA inaccessible for coding for RNA, and some control use of mRNA after it has been produced.

Overview of Genetic Regulation in Prokaryotes and Eukaryotes

1. *Transcriptional regulation* is the primary regulatory mechanism in prokaryotes and developing eukaryotes and is a major mechanism in adult eukaryotic cells, but post-transcriptional mechanisms can alter or modify the resulting phenotype.

2. Regulation through *differential RNA processing* is not a major mechanism in prokaryotes but has been documented in several eukaryotic systems.

3. Regulation through *differential mRNA transport* is impossible in prokaryotes but may occur in some adult eukaryotic cells and is probably a major mechanism leading to cytoplasmic localization of mRNA in developing eukaryotes.

4. Regulation through *differential mRNA degradation* probably occurs in both prokaryotes and eukaryotes, but the effects of poly-A tail length and 3' untranslated sequences on this process in eukaryotes are well documented.

5. Regulation through *differential translation* of different mRNAs occurs in prokaryotes, but the most spectacular cases have been documented in developing eukaryotes.

6. Regulation through post-translational modification of proteins occurs in both prokaryotes and eukaryotes.

Quick Recall Test Questions and Answers

Choose the Best Answer

1. ATP is a:

   A. polysaccharide.
   B. fat.
   C. nucleotide.
   D. protein.
   E. phospholipid.

2. A molecule containing ribose, phosphate, purines, and pyrimidines is a:

   A. protein.
   B. fat.
   C. phospholipid.
   D. carbohydrate.
   E. nucleic acid.

3. Energy is routinely released from ATP (in cells) by:

   A. converting the entire molecule to CO_2 and water.
   B. hydrolyzing the adenine from the ribose.
   C. hydrolyzing one or two phosphates from the molecule.

4. If one strand of a DNA molecule contains the sequence 3'A-C-G-T-A5', the other strand of the DNA molecule could contain the sequence _____ at the same location.

   A. 3'A-C-G-T-A5'
   B. 3'A-C-G-U-A5'
   C. 5'T-G-C-A-T3'
   D. 5'U-G-C-A-U3'
   E. 3'C-A-T-G-C5'

5. Amino acids are joined to each other to form polypeptides by condensation (dehydration synthesis) of the _____ functional group on the amino acid at the growing end of the polypeptide with the _____ functional group on the next amino acid to be added to the chain.

   A. carboxyl, hydroxyl
   B. hydroxyl, carboxyl
   C. carboxyl, amino
   D. hydroxyl, hydroxyl
   E. hydroxyl, amino

6. In the primary structure of a protein, amino acids are joined together by:

   A. peptide bonds.
   B. phosphodiester bonds.
   C. glycosidic bonds.
   D. hydrophobic bonds.

7. The sequence of amino acids in a polypeptide chain is the _____ structure of the protein.

   A. primary
   B. secondary
   C. tertiary
   D. quaternary

8. Enzymes are composed mainly of:

   A. polysaccharides.
   B. lipids.
   C. proteins.
   D. nucleic acids.
   E. oligosaccharides.

9. During protein synthesis, transfer RNA:

   A. transfers genetic information from the nucleus to the cytoplasm.
   B. binds to codons on a mRNA to determine where the amino acid carried on the tRNA belongs in the protein.
   C. transfers completed proteins from the nucleus to the cytoplasm.
   D. binds to DNA to pick up genetic information which is then used by ribosomes in the cytoplasm to assemble proteins.

10. Transfer RNA carries _____ to the site of _____ synthesis.

    A. nucleotides, DNA
    B. nucleotides, RNA
    C. amino acids, protein
    D. amino acids, DNA
    E. amino acids, RNA

11. Most amino acids are specified by codons containing _____ in mRNA.

    A. a single nucleotide
    B. pairs of nucleotides
    C. triplets (sets of three) of nucleotides
    D. sets of 4 nucleotides
    E. sets of 5 nucleotides

12. The codons which specify the sequence of amino acids in a protein occur in:

    A. rRNA.
    B. mRNA.
    C. tRNA.
    D. ribosomes.

Answers

1. **C.** ATP has the typical structure of a nucleotide, consisting of a nitrogenous base (adenine), a 5-carbon sugar (ribose), and one or more phosphate groups (three in the case of ATP).

2. **E.** Ribose, phosphate, purines, and pyrimidines occur in RNA, which is a nucleic acid.

3. **C.** Converting the molecule to CO_2 and water releases energy but destroys the energy carrier, so this process is not used routinely. Hydrolyzing the adenine from the ribose does not release useful energy in most circumstances. Hydrolyzing the third or second phosphate releases useful energy and the remaining part of the molecule may be re-phosphorylated by many energy-releasing reactions.

4. **C.** A DNA strand contains T (thymine) instead of U (uracil), which occurs in RNA, so choices **B** and **D** can be eliminated. A correct DNA strand must have the opposite orientation (since the strands in DNA are antiparallel) and must contain the complementary sequence to the strand in the question (T to pair with A, G to pair with C, C to pair with G, and A to pair with T). Only choice **C** meets these criteria.

5. **C.** The carboxyl and amino groups are reacted to form a peptide bond through a series of steps which attach the amino acid to a transfer RNA and then eventually transfer the amino acid to the polypeptide.

6. **A.** Phosphodiester bonds join nucleotides in RNA or DNA, glycosidic bonds join sugars in oligosaccharides or polysaccharides, and hydrophobic "bonds" are involved in protein folding and lipid-lipid attraction.

7. **A.** Secondary structure involves the local shape of the polypeptide (alpha helix, etc.), tertiary structure involves the overall shape of the polypeptide (globular, etc.), and quaternary structure involves joining two or more polypeptides to form a functional protein.

8. **C.** Most catalytic macromolecules (enzymes) are proteins, although a few catalytic macromolecules are RNA (nucleic acid).

9. **B.** tRNA serves as the temporary link between mRNA and an amino acid so that the amino acid carried by the tRNA is inserted into the correct place in a growing polypeptide chain.

10. **C.** See the answer to question 9.

11. **C.** Each amino acid is specified by one or more codons. Each codon contains three nucleotides and base-pairs (by hydrogen bonds) with the anticodon on the tRNA carrying the amino acid.

12. **B.** The codons in mRNA base-pair with anticodons in tRNA.

DNA Replication

DNA Replication in Prokaryotes (E. coli)

Synthesis of new DNA strands during DNA replication is catalyzed by *DNA polymerase III*. The nucleotide sequence of the new strand is determined by base pairing with a *template strand of DNA*. The energy to form the bonds is derived from hydrolysis of two of the three phosphates attached to the *deoxyribonucleotide* which is being added to the DNA strand. DNA polymerase can only use a single-stranded DNA template, can only "read" the template strand in the 3' → 5' direction, can only assemble a new strand in the 5' → 3' direction, and can only add nucleotides to the 3' end of an existing strand of nucleotides.

In addition to catalyzing assembly of DNA strands, DNA polymerase also checks each deoxyribonucleotide after inserting it and removes it if the base pairing is incorrect.

Two additional types of DNA polymerase (I and II) in *E. coli* cells are used in DNA repair.

Initiation of DNA Replication in Prokaryotes

Initiation of DNA synthesis is not totally understood, but appears to occur at specific points on the DNA called replication initiation sites. A special set of proteins apparently separate the two DNA strands at the replication initiation site, allowing the components of the replication complex to assemble. An RNA primer generated by DNA Primase associated with the initiation complex is also necessary to allow initiation of synthesis of the "leading" strand.

Continuation of DNA Replication (Elongation) in Prokaryotes

Once begun, DNA replication is catalyzed by a large complex of associated enzymes called a *replisome* or *replication complex*. A replication complex consists of a minimum of six enzymes, most of which are not physically associated except during DNA replication. Much of this complexity is made necessary by the characteristics of DNA polymerase.

1. *DNA Helicase* separates the two strands of the DNA molecule that will be replicated so that each strand can serve as a template for the synthesis of a new strand. ATP is hydrolyzed as the helicase moves along the DNA.
2. One *DNA Polymerase III* moves along the separated DNA strand which has a 3' "free end" and uses that strand as a template. This DNA polymerase synthesizes a continuous new strand complementary to the template strand and follows closely behind the helicase. This new strand is called the *leading strand* and the DNA polymerase which catalyzes its formation is called the *Leading Strand DNA Polymerase*.

   The other original DNA strand runs in the wrong direction to be used continuously as a template by DNA polymerase since the "free end" of the strand is the 5' end. As a result, the DNA polymerase copies this strand in a series of short (about 200 nucleotides) strands, each formed while the DNA polymerase is moving in the opposite direction from the helicase. Each of the segments must be initiated by forming an RNA primer to create a new strand with a free 3' end to which DNA polymerase III may add nucleotides, after which the RNA primer must be removed and the ends of the adjacent new segments ligated (joined). From the time that the segments are synthesized until the ligase catalyzes their joining, experimental dissociation of the hydrogen bonds holding the new strand to the template strand releases the segments as *"Okazaki fragments,"* named for their discoverer.

   Due to the complex events, replication of the template strand with the 5' free end is delayed slightly relative to replication of the leading strand. The strand being formed in segments is called the *lagging strand* because its replication lags behind the other strand. The following enzymes are involved in lagging strand replication.
3. *Single-strand DNA Binding Protein* (ssb protein in *E. coli*) binds to and protects single-stranded regions of DNA exposed in the lagging strand.
4. *DNA Primase* synthesizes a short segment of RNA complementary to the template strand of DNA. The RNA primer is usually about 10 nucleotides in length, and a new primer is made approximately 200 nucleotides after the last primer segment.
5. The *Lagging Strand DNA Polymerase III* adds deoxyribonucleotides to the 3' end of the RNA primer, moving along the template strand until it contacts the 5' end of the next RNA

primer. The DNA polymerase then releases the DNA and somehow "leapfrogs" back up the DNA template to the next RNA primer.

6. A *DNA Repair Complex* (containing DNA Polymerase I) then treats the RNA primer segments in the same way that the repair complex treats any other structurally abnormal segment of DNA. The abnormal part (the ribonucleotides) are removed and replaced with normal components (deoxyribonucleotides).

7. *DNA Ligase* then joins the free ends of adjacent segments of the new DNA strand to form a continuous strand.

Termination of DNA Replication in Prokaryotes

Termination of DNA replication, like initiation of DNA replication, is not completely understood. In some prokaryotes, termination apparently occurs at precise points on the DNA, possibly due to a protein bound to the DNA. In other systems, termination appears to occur when two replication complexes moving in opposite directions along the DNA collide.

DNA Replication in Eukaryotes

Synthesis of new DNA strands during DNA replication in eukaryotic cells is similar to the process in prokaryotes, but several differences have been reported. Synthesis of the new DNA strands is catalyzed by *DNA polymerase alpha* (lagging strand) and *DNA polymerase delta* (leading strand). This represents a major difference from prokaryotes in which two molecules of the same type of polymerase are involved. DNA repair uses a separate enzyme (DNA polymerase beta) as is the case in prokaryotes. DNA replication in mitochondria uses a single type of polymerase (DNA polymerase gamma) which is distinct from the nuclear enzymes and apparently functions in a prokaryotic pattern.

The rest of the mechanism appears similar to the process in prokaryotes. The nucleotide sequence of the new strand is determined by base pairing with a template strand of DNA. The energy to form the bonds is derived from hydrolysis of two of the three phosphates attached to the deoxyribonucleotide which is being added to the DNA strand. Both DNA polymerases can only use a single-stranded DNA template, can only "read" the template strand in the $3' \rightarrow 5'$ direction, can only assemble a new strand in the $5' \rightarrow 3'$ direction, and can only add nucleotides to the 3' end of an existing strand of nucleotides. Error checking of inserted nucleotides appears to occur in eukaryotic DNA replication, but the isolated nuclear DNA polymerases lack the exonuclease activity responsible for error checking in prokaryotes.

When a nucleic acid sequence is written out, it is assumed that the 5' end is first and the 3' end last unless otherwise noted. Therefore, ATGTGCA is 5'-ATGTGCA-3' and the Watson-Crick complementary sequence is TGCACAT (5'-TGCACAT-3' or 3'-TACACGT-5')—not TACACGT, which would be the wrong polarity. This is true of all nucleic acid pairings, including DNA-DNA, DNA-RNA and codon-anticodon interactions.

Chromosomal Replication Patterns in Eukaryotes

Initiation of replication occurs at numerous points within each region of a eukaryotic chromosome. Different parts of the same chromosome are replicated at different points in the S (DNA synthesis) phase of the cell cycle. A cluster of simultaneously active replication origins is called a *replication unit*.

In mature body cells, initiation appears to occur at specific points on the DNA called *replication initiation sites* or *replication origins* (called *autonomous replicating sequences* in yeast). In oocytes and some early embryonic cells, initiation appears to occur at much larger than normal numbers of sites on each chromosome, and injected bacterial DNA is replicated at the same time as chromosomal DNA is replicated, thus indicating that initiation is apparently occurring irrespective of the nucleotide sequence in the DNA. The proteins involved in either case have not been clearly identified.

Termination of DNA replication, like initiation of DNA replication, is not well understood in eukaryotes. Some mechanism of precise termination is essential because of the multiple initiation points which do not operate simultaneously and which could easily lead to excess replication.

Nonsimultaneous replication of the DNA molecule extending from end to end in a chromosome requires a mechanism to prevent repeated replication of any parts of the DNA during any one S phase. Mammalian cells appear to achieve this through an unknown inhibitor of DNA replication which is associated with replicated regions of chromosomes from the time of their replication during S phase until the cell divides. The evidence for this is that fusing a cell in S phase with a cell in G2 fails to trigger DNA replication in the G2 nucleus. However, fusing a cell in S phase with a cell in G1 triggers DNA replication in the G1 nucleus.

Tangle Prevention During DNA Replication in Prokaryotes and Eukaryotes

Excessive twisting of DNA or interlocked loops of DNA are prevented by *topoisomerase* enzymes which fall into the same categories in prokaryotes and eukaryotes.

Type I topoisomerases occur in both prokaryotes and eukaryotes. Although the detailed mechanisms differ, these enzymes all temporarily clip one strand of a double-stranded DNA to allow untwisting.

Type II topoisomerases also occur in both prokaryotes and eukaryotes. These enzymes cut both strands of one DNA double-stranded helix to allow a second double-stranded helix to pass through. This is used to separate interlocked loops in prokaryotes and in mitochondria. Topoisomerase II is bound to nuclear DNA at intervals and may attach DNA to the chromosomal scaffolding as well as to reduce tangling during replication.

DNA Repair in Prokaryotes and Eukaryotes

Repair of damage to DNA can occur by at least three fundamentally different pathways in *E. coli* (and presumably other prokaryotes) and in some eukaryotes. Two of these three mechanisms occur in other eukaryotes.

1. *Photoreactivation. Pyrimidine dimers* produced by ultraviolet light can be repaired by *photoreactivation* without excision of components. The enzyme that catalyzes the repair is called DNA photolyase or *photoreactivating enzyme* and is the product of a single gene. The enzyme uses visible light energy to remove the covalent bonds generated by the UV light. This system is active in many prokaryotes and plants, but is absent in many animals including humans.

2. *Base Excision Repair.* Some single damaged nitrogenous bases (especially uracil) can be removed from their deoxyribose by a glycosylase enzyme, after which one or more nucleotides in the damaged area are removed and replaced. This process is called *base excision repair* and occurs in both prokaryotes and eukaryotes.

3. *Nucleotide Excision Repair.* This more generalized process can remove almost any type of damage as long as one of the two DNA strands is undamaged. In this case, a stretch of nucleotides is removed, then replaced by a new strand whose assembly is catalyzed by a DNA polymerase. Methylation of the older DNA strand in the molecule is apparently used to decide which is the preferable template strand when a mismatch occurs without obvious damage. This process occurs in both prokaryotes and eukaryotes, but the size of the region that is excised differs in different organisms.

Quick Recall Test Questions and Answers

Choose the Best Answer

1. In most prokaryotes, initiation of DNA replication appears to occur:

   A. at specific sites on the DNA which are used in each replication cycle.
   B. at random locations on the DNA which change from one replication cycle to the next.

2. Initiation of replication in prokaryotes and eukaryotes appears to use a similar mechanism in which protein factors (different in each case) bind to the initiation sequences on the DNA and separate the strands to allow replication.

   A. TRUE
   B. FALSE

3. The enzyme (catalyst) for DNA replication is:

   A. DNA.
   B. mRNA.
   C. DNA polymerase.
   D. RNA polymerase.
   E. part of the structure of the ribosome.

4. The template (information source) for DNA replication is:

   A. DNA.
   B. mRNA.
   C. DNA polymerase.
   D. RNA polymerase.
   E. part of the structure of the ribosome.

5. The raw material (reactant) for DNA replication is:

   A. DNA.
   B. deoxyribonucleotide monophosphate.
   C. deoxyribonucleotide triphosphate.
   D. ribonucleotide monophosphate.
   E. ribonucleotide triphosphate.

6. DNA replication in prokaryotes:

   A. produces both new strands continuously by adding nucleotides to the end of the strands.
   B. polymerizes nucleotides into short segments, then joins the segments using a ligase enzyme to form both new strands.
   C. produces one new strand continuously by adding nucleotides to the end of the strand and polymerizes nucleotides into short segments, then joins the segments using a ligase enzyme to form the other new strand.

7. The enzyme which catalyzes the replication of the leading strand during DNA replication in *E. coli* is:

   A. RNA polymerase.
   B. reverse transcriptase.
   C. DNA polymerase I.
   D. DNA polymerase II.
   E. DNA polymerase III.

8. The enzyme which catalyzes the replication of the lagging strand during DNA replication in *E. coli* is:

   A. RNA polymerase.
   B. reverse transcriptase.
   C. DNA polymerase I.
   D. DNA polymerase II.
   E. DNA polymerase III.

9. Initiation of synthesis of a new DNA segment complementary to the lagging strand template requires synthesis of ____ before the Okazaki fragment of DNA can be extended from its 3' end.

   A. an RNA primer
   B. a DNA primer
   C. a protein primer
   D. a cluster of single-stranded DNA binding proteins
   E. a new DNA polymerase

10. The function of DNA ligase in DNA replication in prokaryotes is to:

    A. join adjacent Okazaki fragments on the lagging strand.
    B. fill in the gaps created by primer removal on the lagging strand.
    C. synthesize RNA primers on the lagging strand.
    D. add deoxyribonucleotides to the new leading strand.

11. The function of topoisomerases I and II in DNA replication in prokaryotes is to:

    A. join adjacent Okazaki fragments on the lagging strand.
    B. fill in the gaps created by primer removal on the lagging strand.
    C. synthesize RNA primers on the lagging strand.
    D. add deoxyribonucleotides to the new leading strand.
    E. remove excess twisting of the DNA molecules.

12. A mutation which caused loss of the 3'→5' exonuclease proofreading activity from *E. coli* DNA polymerase III but had no effect on the catalysis of phosphodiester bond formation would ____ the rate of DNA replication and would ____ the mutation rate in the bacteria.

   A. have no effect on, have no effect on
   B. slightly increase, increase
   C. slightly reduce, decrease
   D. slightly increase, decrease
   E. slightly reduce, increase

13. Photoreactivation-type DNA repair involves:

   A. chemical reversal of the damage without removal of bases or nucleotides.
   B. removal of a single base followed by excision and replacement of a segment of nucleotides.
   C. removal and replacement of a segment of nucleotides.

14. Base excision-type DNA repair involves:

   A. chemical reversal of the damage without removal of bases or nucleotides.
   B. removal of a single base followed by excision and replacement of a segment of nucleotides.
   C. removal and replacement of a segment of nucleotides.

15. Nucleotide excision-type DNA repair involves:

   A. chemical reversal of the damage without removal of bases or nucleotides.
   B. removal of a single base followed by excision and replacement of a segment of nucleotides.
   C. removal and replacement of a segment of nucleotides.

Answers

1. **A.** Initiation occurs at specific sites, typically one per chromosome in prokaryotes.

2. **A.** Although the specific proteins involved probably differ, the processes involved in initiation appear to use similar mechanisms.

3. **C.** DNA polymerase enzymes of different types catalyze chromosomal replication and DNA replication during DNA repair processes.

4. **A.** Each existing DNA strand in a DNA molecule serves as a template for assembly of a new strand of DNA (catalyzed by DNA polymerase) during DNA replication.

5. **C.** DNA contains deoxyribonucleotides, not ribonucleotides (that is why its called DNA instead of RNA). The extra two phosphates on each deoxyribonucleotide are removed when the nucleotide is added to the new DNA strand and provide the energy to form the new phosphodiester bond.

6. **C.** The continuously formed strand is the leading strand, and the strand made in segments is the lagging strand. The discontinuous replication of the lagging strand is caused by the lack of a form of DNA polymerase which can add to the 5' end of a growing DNA strand, so only the existing strand with the correct orientation is replicated continuously.

7. **E.** Separate molecules of DNA polymerase III catalyze replication of the leading strand and the lagging strand in *E. coli*.

8. **E.** Separate molecules of DNA polymerase III catalyze replication of the leading strand and the lagging strand in *E. coli*.

9. **A.** Remember that DNA polymerase can only add nucleotides to existing strands, but RNA polymerase enzymes (like the primase) can initiate new strands.

10. **A.** DNA ligase is needed to join the DNA fragments (called Okazaki fragments, after their discoverer) resulting from the lagging strand replication.

11. **E.** Type I topoisomerases primarily reduce twisting. Type II topoisomerases may also allow separation of interlocked loops of DNA.

12. **B.** This mutation should slightly speed up replication, because the enzyme would not be degrading any mispaired bases in the newly synthesized DNA strand. As a result, however, the frequency of new mutations would be greatly increased.

13. **A.** Photoreactivation usually achieves repair without excision of entire nucleotides.

14. **B.** Base excision repair begins with removal of one or more damaged bases, usually followed by excision of the rest of the nucleotides associated with the damaged bases.

15. **C.** Nucleotide excision usually involves removal of a patch of nucleotides surrounding the damaged region in the DNA.

Overall Genetic Organization of Prokaryotic Cells

The DNA in prokaryotic cells is located in the cytoplasm, so DNA replication, RNA synthesis (transcription), and protein synthesis (translation) occur in the same cellular compartment.

In some cases a single structural gene (DNA coding a mRNA which codes for one polypeptide) is controlled as a single unit. In most cases, a single promoter (binding site for RNA polymerase to initiate RNA synthesis) controls a series of structural genes which are transcribed as a single mRNA with a series of translation initiation and termination points. The mRNA is translated to form all or some of the enzymes for a biochemical pathway. A cluster of structural genes controlled by a single promoter is called an *operon*.

Translation of a mRNA molecule typically begins before transcription of the mRNA is complete. This allows very rapid changes in cellular phenotype through transcriptional control mechanisms.

In most cases of both single gene units and operons, access to the promoter by RNA polymerase is controlled by one or more regulatory proteins which respond to conditions in the cell.

Cytoplasmic proteins have rapid access to DNA because the DNA is not separated from the cytoplasm by a nuclear membrane. Therefore, proteins which alter transcription can act very quickly after they are altered by cytoplasmic conditions.

Transcription in Prokaryotes

RNA synthesis (transcription) in prokaryotes follows the general pattern typical of all RNA synthesis in normal cells. The template or sequence information source is one of the two nucleotide strands in a DNA molecule, the enzyme which catalyzes the process is RNA polymerase, and the reactants which combine to form the new RNA strand are ribonucleotide triphosphates containing adenine, guanine, cytosine, or uracil. Release of two of the three phosphates from each nucleotide as it is bonded to the chain provides the energy for bond formation. The process of transcription may be subdivided into initiation, elongation, and termination phases. Locations on the DNA are described relative to the RNA polymerase movement during transcription. The polymerase moves toward downstream locations and away from upstream locations.

Initiation of Transcription in Prokaryotes

Prokaryotes typically use a single type of *RNA polymerase* (the core enzyme) in combination with multiple *sigma factors* for initiation of RNA synthesis. RNA polymerase complexed with one of the sigma factors binds to a *promoter sequence* on the DNA just upstream of the starting point for RNA synthesis. The position and orientation of the DNA sequence in the promoter regions determines the position and orientation of the RNA polymerase, which in turn determines the location of the starting point for RNA synthesis and determines which DNA strand serves as a template. Because each sigma factor recognizes a different promoter sequence, a prokaryote can use availability of different sigma factors to switch large-scale processes such as nitrogen metabolism, heat shock responses, or sporulation on or off.

Control of Initiation of Transcription in Prokaryotes

In an actively growing prokaryote, most of the operons which are used are transcribed by RNA polymerase which initiates RNA synthesis complexed to a single type of sigma factor (sigma 70 in *E. coli*). Two types of control systems control initiation of RNA synthesis in these operons.

1. *Activator Proteins*. Many promoters do not bind the RNA polymerase-sigma factor complex effectively unless an *activator protein* is bound upstream of the promoter. These operons are not fully active unless the activator protein is available in a form that can bind to the activator site on the DNA. Availability of functional activator protein is controlled by interactions between the protein and critical molecules in the cytoplasm.

   As an example, the lac operon (like several other metabolic operons) in *E. coli* requires binding of the catabolite activator protein (CAP) to a site just upstream of the promoter. Active metabolism due to abundant glucose results in low cyclic AMP levels in the cytoplasm. Because CAP requires cyclic AMP for activity, CAP is inactive under these conditions. As a result, turning on the other transcription control system in the lac operon results in very little transcription as long as glucose is readily available. Starvation increases cyclic AMP levels, resulting in active CAP. Under these conditions, the activator site is usually complexed with CAP, so turning on the other control system results in very rapid transcription.

2. *Repressor Proteins.* Many operons have a protein-binding sequence called an *operator sequence* located downstream of and overlapping the promoter. The operator sequence binds a *repressor protein* which prevents transcription of the operon. Availability of functional repressor protein is controlled by interactions between the protein and critical molecules in the cytoplasm.

In the case of the lac operon in *E. coli,* the unaltered repressor protein binds to the operator sequence. Therefore, the lac operon is normally totally turned off regardless of the status of CAP. However, when lactose is available in the cell's environment, binding of lactose or related molecules inactivates the repressor protein. In the absence of active CAP, this results in a low rate of transcription of the genes in the lac operon. In the presence of active CAP, the result is active transcription of the genes in the operon.

At the beginning of the initiation process, the complex of the RNA polymerase core enzyme plus the appropriate sigma factor initially binds to the double-stranded DNA to form a closed complex in which the two DNA strands are still held together by base-pair hydrogen bonding. The closed complex becomes an open complex when the polymerase binds more tightly to the DNA and forces the two DNA strands apart along a short region. Synthesis of the new RNA strand begins in the open complex. Only the DNA strand oriented in the correct direction ($3' \rightarrow 5'$) is used as a template.

The Elongation Phase of Transcription in Prokaryotes

As each ribonucleotide triphosphate base-pairs with the exposed bases on the DNA template, the 3' hydroxyl on the previously added nucleotide binds to the proximal (next to the sugar) phosphate on the newly base-paired ribonucleotide, forming the new phosphodiester bond and releasing the terminal two phosphates (which provides the energy to form the bond).

At about the point that the new RNA chain reaches ten nucleotides in length, the sigma factor is released from the RNA polymerase, the core enzyme becomes more compact, and one or more elongation factors may bind to the RNA polymerase. Elongation continues from the time the RNA polymerase leaves the initiation site just downstream of the promoter until the RNA polymerase encounters a termination sequence. As the RNA polymerase moves along the DNA, the newly formed RNA strand is separated from the DNA template strand and the two DNA strands reassociate.

Termination of Transcription in Prokaryotes

Sites at which transcription terminates in prokaryotes frequently contain nucleotide sequences in the RNA which allow base-pairing to form a hairpin loop. In many cases the loop is enriched in guanine and cytosine and the RNA just downstream of the loop is rich in uridine. Sites of this type appear to cause termination without intervention of protein termination factors and are called *rho-independent termination sites*. Termination sites which lack the guanine and cytosine-rich region in the hairpin loop and lack the adjacent uridine-rich region typically require a protein termination factor called *rho* for efficient termination. These sites are called *rho-dependent termination sites*. In either case, when termination occurs, the RNA polymerase detaches from the DNA and releases the RNA strand.

Post-Transcriptional Processing of RNA in Prokaryotes

mRNA Processing in Prokaryotes

Messenger RNA in prokaryotes is usually translated without modification, in most cases with translation beginning before transcription has been completed.

rRNA and tRNA Processing in Prokaryotes

Ribosomal RNAs and tRNAs are typically transcribed as large RNA molecules which are then cut apart by ribonucleases to release the functional RNAs. Ribosomal RNA genes in *E. coli* occur in at least six transcriptional units, each containing one 16S, one 23S, and one 5S rRNA gene separated by intervening spacer RNA regions. Most of these transcriptional units also contain one or two tRNA sequences. The remaining tRNAs are transcribed singly or in clustered units which must be cut apart.

Both rRNAs and tRNAs also require modification of numerous bases on the nucleotides prior to becoming functional. The functions of base modification in rRNAs are unclear, but modified bases in some tRNAs may be essential in causing the anticodon to pair with the correct set of codons.

Initial Assembly of Ribosomes in Prokaryotes

In prokaryotes, ribosomal RNA processing and assembly with ribosomal proteins to form the large and small subunits occurs in the cytoplasm. Ribosomal RNAs are cut out of the large initial transcripts produced from each of the seven or more ribosomal RNA transcription units by ribonuclease enzymes. Extensive modification of bases (by methylation) occurs in all three size classes of rRNA. In *E. coli,* 16S rRNA is assembled with 21 proteins to form the 30S small ribosomal subunit. The larger 23S rRNA plus the small 5S rRNA are assembled along with more than 30 proteins to form the 50S large ribosomal subunit.

Translation in Prokaryotes

Translation (protein synthesis) requires *mRNA* to serve as the template or amino acid sequence information source, *ribosomes* to serve as the assembly surface and catalyst for peptide bond formation, and *aminoacyl groups on tRNA* to serve as the reactants. Attachment of the amino acid to a tRNA to form an aminoacyl tRNA creates a high-energy bond which provides the energy to form the peptide bond. The three nucleotide anticodon on the tRNA "reads" the three nucleotide codon on the mRNA by base-pairing with it and thereby places the amino acid carried by the tRNA (the aminoacyl group) in the correct location in the growing polypeptide.

Aminoacylation of tRNAs

Aminoacyl groups are attached to tRNAs by *aminoacyl synthetase* enzymes. Each amino acid appears to be attached to its tRNAs by a single type of aminoacyl synthetase which distinguishes that amino acid from the other 19, some of which may be very similar chemically. The aminoacyl synthesase must also clearly distinguish the one or more tRNAs which carry that amino acid from all other tRNAs. All aminoacyl synthesase enzymes appear to use the same reaction mechanism to attach the aminoacyl group to the tRNA. The linkage between the aminoacyl group and the tRNA contains sufficient energy to drive the formation of a peptide bond when the aminoacyl group is transferred during translation.

Initiation of Translation

In *E. coli,* three protein *initiation factors* and a special *formylmethionyltRNA initiator tRNA* (fMet-tRNAi) are required for initiation of translation. The small ribosomal subunit recognizes the 5' end of the mRNA and the fMet-tRNAi binds to the AUG *initiation codon* on the mRNA positioned in the P site on the ribosome. The larger ribosomal subunit then binds to the small subunit-mRNA-fMet-tRNAi complex, completing initiation.

The Elongation Phase of Translation

Elongation requires the aminoacyl-tRNA whose anticodon will base-pair to the next codon in the mRNA and three elongation factors. An elongation factor carries the next aminoacyl-tRNA into the A site on the ribosome, and a rRNA loop on the ribosome catalyzes formation of the new peptide bond.

Termination of Translation

Termination in *E. coli* requires one of two closely related *protein termination factors* which recognize the termination codons. The result of termination is release of the polypeptide from the tRNA to which it is attached, release of the ribosome from the mRNA, and dissociation of the small and large ribosomal subunits.

Quick Recall Test Questions and Answers

Choose the Best Answer

1. Most of the genes in prokaryotes are organized into operons containing a regulatory complex which controls a series of DNA coding sequences for mRNAs or rRNAs and tRNAs.

   A. TRUE
   B. FALSE

2. The primary chromosome in a typical prokaryote:

   A. is a series of interlocked DNA circles.
   B. is a single circular DNA molecule.
   C. is a single linear DNA molecule with two free ends.
   D. is a series of linear DNA molecules, each with a pair of free ends.
   E. has a complex linear structure which is not well understood.

3. The enzyme (catalyst) for RNA synthesis in prokaryotes is:

   A. DNA.
   B. mRNA.
   C. DNA polymerase.
   D. RNA polymerase.
   E. part of the structure of the ribosome.

4. The template (information source) for RNA synthesis is:

   A. DNA.
   B. mRNA.
   C. DNA polymerase.
   D. RNA polymerase.
   E. part of the structure of the ribosome.

5. The raw material (reactant) for RNA synthesis is:

   A. DNA.
   B. deoxyribonucleotide monophosphate.
   C. deoxyribonucleotide triphosphate.
   D. ribonucleotide monophosphate.
   E. ribonucleotide triphosphate.

6. When mRNA is synthesized by an RNA polymerase:

   A. both DNA strands serve as templates to produce two types of RNA.

   B. one of the DNA strands serves as a template and the other strand is not used.
   C. both DNA strands are averaged to determine the RNA sequence.

7. RNA polymerase in *E. coli*:

   A. can initiate new RNA strands and add nucleotides to the 5' end of existing RNA strands.
   B. can initiate new RNA strands and add nucleotides to the 3' end of existing RNA strands.
   C. can initiate new RNA strands and add nucleotides to either the 3' end or the 5' end of existing RNA strands.
   D. cannot initiate new RNA strands but can add nucleotides to the 5' end of existing RNA strands.
   E. cannot initiate new RNA strands but can add nucleotides to the 3' end of existing RNA strands.

8. RNA polymerase attaches to the ___ region of a prokaryote operon to begin RNA synthesis.

   A. operator
   B. promoter
   C. repressor
   D. structural gene
   E. inducer

9. An appropriate sigma factor is required for ____ in prokaryotes.

   A. initiation of transcription
   B. initiation of translation
   C. elongation during transcription
   D. elongation during translation
   E. termination of both transcription and translation

10. The functions of the promotor region in a prokaryotic operon include:

   A. serving as a template for the synthesis of messenger RNA.
   B. serving as the source of information for the synthesis of repressor proteins.
   C. serving as an attachment site for RNA polymerase.
   D. serving as a binding site for repressor proteins.
   E. coding for the amino acid sequence of one or more enzymes.

11. In an inducible operon (i.e., the lac operon in *E. coli*), the repressor protein coded by the regulator gene binds to the ____ to inactivate the operon.

    A. promotor
    B. operator sequence
    C. regulator gene
    D. first structural gene in the operon
    E. last structural gene in the operon

12. The enzyme (catalyst) for protein synthesis in prokaryotes is:

    A. DNA.
    B. mRNA.
    C. DNA polymerase.
    D. RNA polymerase.
    E. part of the structure of the ribosome.

13. The template (information source) for protein synthesis in prokaryotes is:

    A. DNA.
    B. mRNA.
    C. DNA polymerase.
    D. RNA polymerase.
    E. part of the structure of the ribosome.

14. The raw material (reactant) for protein synthesis in prokaryotes is:

    A. mRNA.
    B. part of the structure of the ribosome.
    C. free amino acid.
    D. aminoacyl tRNA.
    E. part of the structure of the ribosome.

15. In prokaryotes, most amino acids are specified by ____ in mRNA.

    A. a single type of codon
    B. several different types of codons

16. Initiation of translation in *E. coli* (a prokaryote) involves all of the following EXCEPT:

    A. recognition of the mRNA by the small ribosomal subunit.
    B. three initiation factors.
    C. fMet-tRNA.
    D. attachment of the small ribosomal subunit to the large ribosomal subunit.
    E. two releasing factors.

17. Attachment of the aminoacyl groups to tRNA molecules in prokaryotes is catalyzed by:

    A. a single form of enzyme which can attach any amino acid to any tRNA.
    B. a single form of enzyme for each amino acid which can attach that amino acid to any tRNA which recognizes a codon for that amino acid.
    C. a single form of enzyme for each tRNA which can attach the amino acid for which the tRNA recognizes a codon.
    D. multiple forms of enzymes for each tRNA which can attach the amino acid for which the tRNA recognizes a codon.

18. Initiation of protein synthesis on a prokaryotic mRNA occurs:

    A. wherever a ribosome attaches to the mRNA (randomly along the molecule).
    B. at the first AUG codon in the mRNA molecule after each ribosome attachment point.
    C. at the poly-A tail on the mRNA.
    D. at the first nonsense (termination) codon on the mRNA.
    E. at the first AAA codon in the mRNA molecule after each ribosome attachment point.

Answers

1. **A.** Operon organization appears to be typical of most prokaryotic genes.

2. **B.** The primary or main chromosome and the episomes or plasmids in prokaryotes are typically circular.

3. **D.** RNA polymerase is the catalyst for all genome-encoded RNA synthesis. Most prokaryotes contain a single type of RNA polymerase, whereas eukaryotes typically contain three nuclear RNA polymerases.

4. **A.** The nucleotide sequence in most RNA (except poly-A "tails") is coded by DNA.

5. **E.** RNA contains ribonucleotides, not deoxyribonucleotides (that is why its called RNA instead of DNA). The extra two phosphates on each ribonucleotide are removed when the nucleotide is added to the new RNA strand and provide the energy to form the new phosphodiester bond.

6. **B.** A single strand of the DNA serves as a template for RNA synthesis. If promoters are located appropriately to initiate RNA synthesis using both strands of DNA in a given region (e.g., in the DNA of some viruses), only one strand can be used by one RNA polymerase at a time.

7. **B.** RNA polymerase can add to the 3' end of existing strands (as can DNA polymerase), but unlike DNA polymerase, RNA polymerase can initiate new strands.

8. **B.** The promoter is the region of DNA recognized by RNA polymerase (in prokaryotes) or by a cluster of transcription initiation factors (in eukaryotes), leading to initiation of RNA synthesis (transcription).

9. **A.** The sigma factor is required for initiation and is then released, so it is not needed for elongation or termination.

10. **C.** Repressor protein binding sites in some operons may overlap the promoter region, but the promoter region is defined by RNA polymerase binding.

11. **B.** The operator sequence is defined by repressor protein binding. The operator sequence may partially overlap the promoter and/or the first structural gene in some operons.

12. **E.** A loop of rRNA appears to catalyze peptide bond formation.

13. **B.** The sequence of nucleotides in mRNA (read in groups of three as codons) determines the sequence of amino acids in the polypeptide being synthesized.

14. **D.** The aminoacyl group on tRNA is ready to participate in protein synthesis. A free amino acid would have to be activated and attached to tRNA as an aminoacyl group before it could be used in protein synthesis.

15. **B.** Almost all amino acids are specified by two or more codons.

16. **E.** Releasing factors are involved in termination of translation instead of initiation. All of the other choices are involved in initiation.

17. **B.** In both prokaryotes and eukaryotes, a single enzyme appears to load a particular amino acid onto all tRNAs which can carry that amino acid.

18. **B.** The AUG codon is the anticodon for methionine. In prokaryotes, the first methionine codon after each ribosome attachment point on an mRNA serves as the initiation codon and binds initiator tRNA carrying N-formylmethionine.

Overall Genetic Organization of Eukaryotic Cells

Because the nuclear DNA in eukaryotic cells is separated from the cytoplasm by the nuclear envelope, DNA replication and RNA synthesis (transcription) occur in a different compartment (the nucleus) from protein synthesis (translation), which occurs in the cytoplasm. In addition, nuclear DNA exists in complex chromatin structures and extensive processing of most RNA types occurs between their transcription and their function. Additional complexity results from large amounts of nuclear DNA for which the functions are unknown and the presence of DNA-based genetic systems in mitochondria and chloroplasts which function in an integrated fashion with the nuclear genetic system.

Several functionally distinct categories of DNA can be described in eukaryotes.

1. *Protein-coding DNA.* Some DNA regions code for functional amino acid sequence-coding regions of mRNA molecules. In most eukaryotic cells, each structural gene coding for the mRNA which is translated into a single polypeptide typically has its own promoter and associated genetic control regions. This differs strikingly from the operon organization typical of most genes in prokaryotes.

About 50% of apparent protein-coding genes occur as single copies per haploid genome and have no closely related protein-coding genes in the genome.

About 50% of apparent protein-coding genes occur as families containing 2 to 1,000 closely related but nonidentical versions per haploid genome. In very closely related genes, the proteins have very similar properties; in less closely related gene families, however, the proteins may have evolved into very different functional roles while retaining recognizable sequence homology.

Histone genes are apparently unique among protein-coding genes in that histone genes occur as a cluster which is tandemly repeated 20 to 50 times.

2. *RNA-coding DNA.* Genes that code for structural RNAs typically occur in tandemly repeated units in eukaryotes. Large rRNA molecules are coded by 250 copies of a tandemly repeated cluster. 5S rRNA genes occur in about 2,000 copies and are located separately from other rRNA genes. Transfer RNA genes vary, with most types occurring in 10 to 100 copies.

3. *Noncoding DNA.* More than 70% of the DNA sequences in a multicellular eukaryote are not represented in functional mRNA, rRNA, or tRNA molecules in the cytoplasm.

Some of this DNA has known functions. *Regulatory protein-binding sequences* may or may not be transcribed, depending on their location relative to the structural gene sequence. This DNA has clear functions, however, independent of its transcription because it is involved in regulation of transcription of nearby structural genes. *Intron* and *spacer DNA* sequences are transcribed but they are removed during processing and do not appear in the cytoplasm as parts of functional RNAs. The functions of most of these sequences are not understood. Some spacer DNA regions may serve simple mechanical connection functions.

Other categories of DNA lack obvious functions. *Mobile (transposable) element DNA* has no known functions that benefit the cells which contain it. The Alu sequence in humans comprises 6% of the nuclear DNA, but appears to be defective copies of the 7SL gene which now function as *retroposons* (transposable elements which utilize RNA copies in the same way as retroviruses). The normal copies of this gene encode the RNA component of the signal recognition particle in protein synthesis. The L1 transposable element comprises about 4% of the nuclear DNA and codes for a reverse transcriptase. This transposable element also is a retroposon. Numerous other mobile elements occur in much lower numbers of copies per cell.

Simple sequence DNA has some identified functions (telomeres) but many regions have no known function. Satellite DNA located near centromeres is puzzling because it occurs in large numbers of copies (suggesting some important function), but shows rapid changes (indicating that mutations have no harmful effects).

Transcription in Eukaryotes

RNA synthesis in eukaryotes is mechanistically similar to the process in prokaryotes. The *template* or sequence information source is one of the two nucleotide strands in a *DNA molecule*; the enzyme, which catalyzes the process, is one of the three types of *RNA polymerase* in eukaryotes (each type catalyzes synthesis of a different class of RNA); and the *reactants*, which combine to form the new RNA strand, are *ribonucleotide triphosphates* containing adenine, guanine, cytosine, or uracil. The process of transcription may be subdivided into initiation, elongation, and termination phases.

Eukaryotic RNA Polymerase Enzymes

Eukaryotic cells typically contain three distinct RNA polymerase core enzymes (Pol I, Pol II, and Pol III). Each core enzyme transcribes a distinct class of genes and responds to a distinct set of transcription factors. The core structure of all three RNA polymerases is much more complex than in prokaryotic RNA polymerase.

Enzyme	RNA Pol I	RNA Pol II	RNA Pol III
Genes transcribed	Class I	Class II	Class III
Gene products (after processing)	rRNA	mRNA U1–U5 snRNP	tRNA, 5S rRNA, U6 snRNP

Initiation of Transcription in Eukaryotes

The promoter sequences in Class I and Class II genes are primarily upstream of the starting point for transcription. The promoter sequences in most Class III genes are downstream of the starting point for transcription.

TATA binding protein is involved in initiation of at least some genes in all three classes, but the other transcription initiation factors appear to be distinct for each class of genes.

Multiple proteins are required for initiation of transcription of genes in all three classes. These transcription initiation factors bind to the DNA in the promoter region, after which RNA polymerase of the appropriate type binds to the DNA-protein complex.

Regulation of Initiation of Transcription in Individual Class II Genes

Regulatory sequences for class II genes may be located near the upstream end of the promoter region, far upstream of the promoter, downstream of the promoter within introns in the structural gene, or downstream of the structural gene.

Regulatory DNA sequences which bind proteins that increase transcription of the associated genes are called *enhancers* and the proteins which bind to the enhancers are called *gene activator proteins*. Many gene activator proteins act by directly interacting with the complex of general transcription factors, apparently as a result of loop formation by the intervening DNA.

Regulatory DNA sequences which bind proteins that decrease transcription of the associated genes are called *repressor binding sites* and the proteins which bind to the enhancers are called *gene repressor proteins*. Repressor proteins may act by blocking enhancer functions or by inhibiting general transcription factor complex formation at the promoter.

A single structural gene may be associated with large numbers of regulatory sequences, each of which leads to activation or inhibition of transcription of the gene under a particular set of conditions.

The Elongation Phase of Transcription in Eukaryotes

The elongation phase of transcription appears identical in prokaryotes and eukaryotes. As each ribonucleotide triphosphate base-pairs with the exposed bases on the DNA template, the 3' hydroxyl on the previously added nucleotide binds to the proximal (next to the sugar) phosphate on the newly base-paired ribonucleotide, forming the new phosphodiester bond and releasing the terminal two phosphates (which provides the energy to form the bond). As the RNA polymerase moves along the DNA template, the DNA strands are separated just ahead of the active site for RNA synthesis. Just behind the active site, the RNA strand is separated from the DNA template and the DNA strands are allowed to re-form complementary base pairs. Elongation continues from the time the RNA polymerase leaves the initiation site until termination occurs.

Termination of Transcription in Eukaryotes

Termination of transcription of class I genes appears to depend on sequences located downstream from the termination site. The mode of action of these sequences is unclear, but at least one soluble protein is needed.

Termination patterns in class II genes are unclear due to the very rapid processing of the transcripts which removes the 3' end in preparation for poly-A addition. Some class II genes appear to contain adenine and thymine-rich regions just downstream of the termination point. These structures resemble the rho-dependent termination signals in *E. coli*.

Termination of transcription of the 5S rRNA gene (a class III gene) occurs within a series of uridines following a guanine- and cytosine-rich region. This resembles the rho-independent termination sequences in bacteria, but in the eukaryotic 5S gene, mutations which prevent hairpin loop formation in the G-C region, do not alter termination. The mechanism is unclear, but at least in vitro no additional protein factors appear to be essential and the interaction must therefore be between the transcribed RNA and the RNA polymerase III itself.

Post-Transcriptional Processing of RNA in Eukaryotes

Post-Transcriptional Alteration of rRNA (Class I Genes)

Large ribosomal RNAs (5.8S, 18S, 28S) are transcribed as a single large (45S) RNA molecule which is the cut apart by nucleases to release the functional RNAs. Ribosomal RNA genes occur as tandemly repeated transcription units, with clusters of tandem repeated units on 10 chromosomes in diploid human cells. Each transcription unit contains one 18S, one 5.8S, and one 28S rRNA gene separated by intervening spacer RNA regions. Introns are not present within the 18S, 5.8S, or 28S structural genes in most eukaryotes, but some unicellular eukaryotes have introns in their large rRNA sequences and these introns are capable of removal by self-splicing. rRNAs undergo methylation and other modifications to numerous bases on the nucleotides prior to entry into the cytoplasm as part of a ribosome. The functions of base modification in rRNAs are unclear.

Assembly of Ribosomal Subunits

In eukaryotes, ribosomal RNA processing and assembly with ribosomal proteins to form the large and small subunits occurs in the nucleolus. Ribosomal RNAs are cut out of the large initial transcripts produced from each of the ribosomal RNA transcription units by ribonuclease enzymes. Extensive modification of bases (by methylation) occurs in all three size classes of larger rRNAs.

More than 100 different polypeptides synthesized in the cytoplasm move into the nucleus and into the nucleolus and complex with the 45S rRNA transcript before it is processed. These protein components include most, if not all, of the proteins that will be present in mature ribosomes, proteins involved in rRNA processing, and generalized RNA-binding proteins.

Approximately 30 min after synthesis of a 45S rRNA precursor, the 18S rRNA processed from the transcript has been assembled with approximately 33 proteins to form the 40S small ribosomal subunit and has been transported through a nuclear pore and into the cytoplasm where it becomes active.

Approximately 60 min after synthesis of a 45S rRNA precursor, the 5.8S and 28S rRNA from the transcript plus 5S rRNA synthesized elsewhere in the nucleus have been assembled with approximately 49 proteins to form a 60S large ribosome subunit and have been transported through a nuclear pore and into the cytoplasm where it becomes active.

Post-Transcriptional Alteration of mRNA (Class II Genes)

Processing of the RNA transcribed from a class II gene into a functional mRNA occurs within the nucleus and requires a series of modifications to the RNA.

1. Capping

Almost immediately after initiation of transcription, one of the three phosphates on the 5' nucleotide on the RNA is removed and a GMP (derived from a GTP) is attached using a 5'–5' linkage. Methyl groups are then added to the guanine in the terminal position and to the base (usually A or G) on the original 5' terminal nucleotide.

2. Polyadenylation

Just after the RNA polymerase II passes the poly-A addition signal on the DNA, the RNA transcript is cleaved at the signal. Poly-A polymerase then adds 100 to 200 adenosine nucleotides to the 3' end of the transcript to form the poly-A "tail." Different patterns of 3' cleavage and poly-A addition may produce different carboxy-terminal ends on the protein and different life spans for the mRNAs in the cytoplasm.

3. Intron Removal

The snRNPs U1, U2, U5, and U4/U6 plus other components assemble on the recognition sequences on each intron to form a spliceosome. The intron is excised in a loop or lariat form and the adjacent exons are ligated together. In many genes, intron removal may destroy over half of the original transcript. Different patterns of intron removal in different cells types lead to different protein coding sequences in mRNAs produced from identical transcripts.

4. Editing

mRNA nucleotide sequence can be changed by editing enzymes which change or delete nucleotides. Conversion of single bases has been documented for several human mRNAs, and extensive editing using guide RNAs has been demonstrated in trypanosomes. The full effect and extent of this process is not fully understood.

Transport of mRNA to the Cytoplasm

Transport of mRNA to the cytoplasm is delayed until splicing has removed all introns. As the mRNA then moves through a nuclear pore, spliceosomes and other nuclear proteins are removed and cytoplasmic RNA-binding proteins bind to the mRNA. Different mRNAs may be transported into different regions of the cytoplasm. In at least some cases, correct transport of mRNA depends on sequences in the 3' UTR (untranslated region between polypeptide termination and the poly-A tail).

Post-Transcriptional Alteration of 5S rRNA and tRNA (Class III Genes)

5S rRNA transcripts are the same length as the functional RNA in ribosomes and therefore undergo no length processing.

Transfer RNAs are formed from transcripts with excess nucleotides on both the 5' and 3' ends, and some eukaryotic tRNA transcripts contain an intron. Some tRNAs appear to form their typical hairpin loop structures and fold at least partially into the L-shaped tertiary structure prior to excision from the original transcript by a ribonuclease. Extensive modification of bases on the nucleotides may occur before or after excision. The 3' end created by excision requires addition of a CCA unit catalyzed by tRNA nucleotidyl transferase to provide the attachment point for the aminoacyl group.

In addition, modification of numerous bases occurs in most tRNAs after transcription. The timing of modification relative to excision is not clear. After processing, tRNA is apparently transported into the cytoplasm through nuclear pores.

Translation in Eukaryotes

Aminoacylation of tRNAs

This process in eukaryotes closely resembles aminoacylation of tRNAs in prokaryotes. Aminoacyl groups are attached to tRNAs by *aminoacyl synthetase enzymes*. Each amino acid appears to be attached by a single type of amino acyl synthetase which distinguishes that amino acid from the other 19, some of which may be very similar chemically. The aminoacyl synthetase must also clearly distinguish the one or more tRNAs which carry that amino acid from all other tRNAs.

Initiation of Translation

Initiation of translation in eukaryotes is more complex than in prokaryotes. In eukaryotes, at least 9 *initiation factors* are required, and the methionine on the initiator tRNA is not formylated. The initiation factors are proteins present in the cytoplasm.

The *initiator Met-tRNA (met-tRNA$_i$)* in both prokaryotes and eukaryotes is a tRNA distinct from the met-tRNA which is used to translate AUG codons in the interior of the mRNA. Methionine is attached to eukaryotic Met-tRNA$_i$ in the same way as any other aminoacyl group is attached, but Met-tRNA$_i$ is the only tRNA which can enter a ribosome at the P site to initiate translation.

The Elongation Phase of Translation

Each elongation reaction in eukaryotes is similar to the same event in prokaryotes in that it requires the *aminoacyl-tRNA* to fit the next codon in the mRNA and *elongation factors*. Several elongation factors are GTP-binding proteins which hydrolyze GTP to GDP during elongation.

Termination of Translation

Termination in eukaryotes uses a single *release factor*. The result of termination is release of the polypeptide from the tRNA to which it is attached, release of the ribosome from the mRNA, and eventual dissociation of the small and large ribosomal subunits.

Techniques available for isolation and characterization of DNA, RNA, and protein include "blots" which involve electrophoretic separation followed by transfer to nitrocellulose sheets and testing for complementary sequences or immunological binding.

1. The Southern Blot consists of restriction enzyme digests of DNA separated by gel electrophoresis, transferred (blotted) on to nitrocellulose sheets or similar material, and tested against a specific, labeled DNA probe for complementary sequences.
2. The Northern Blot consists of electrophoretically separated RNA molecules transferred on to nitrocellulose sheets and tested against labeled DNA probes. It is widely used to estimate the amount of a specific mRNA in a cell at different points in development.
3. The Western Blot involves the separation of proteins by gel electrophoresis, transfer to nitrocellulose sheets, and probing with labeled antibodies directed against specific proteins. The present confirmatory test for HIV infection is a Western Blot analysis directed against specific viral proteins in blood.

Quick Recall Test Questions and Answers

Choose the Best Answer

1. During interphase in a typical eukaryotic cell, the DNA coding for ribosomal RNAs is:

   A. in a single location on a single chromosome in the center of the nucleolus.
   B. in multiple locations on multiple chromosomes around the perimeter of the nucleolus.
   C. in multiple locations on multiple chromosomes in the heterochromatin along the inner surface of the nuclear envelope.
   D. in multiple locations on multiple chromosomes scattered throughout the euchromatin in the nucleus.
   E. in multiple locations on a single chromosome in the nucleoid

2. Introns are found:

   A. primarily in prokaryotic genes.
   B. primarily in eukaryotic genes.
   C. commonly in both eukaryotic and prokaryotic genes.

3. The DNA of eukaryotic cells is wrapped around histones to form structures called:

   A. nucleoli.
   B. nuclear matrix.
   C. nucleosomes.
   D. centromeres.

4. Eukaryotic genes which code for mRNA and tRNA are similar in that:

   A. they are transcribed by the same RNA polymerase.
   B. the promoter sequences are upstream of the transcription initiation point.
   C. multiple proteins must bind to the DNA before the RNA polymerase binds.

5. Compared with DNA binding proteins which activate or inactivate eukaryotic class II genes, DNA binding proteins which activate or inactivate bacterial operons typically bind to DNA that is:

   A. closer to the promoter.
   B. farther from the promoter.
   C. at a similar distance from the promoter.

6. The enzyme (catalyst) for protein synthesis in eukaryotes is:

   A. DNA.
   B. mRNA.
   C. DNA polymerase.
   D. RNA polymerase.
   E. part of the structure of the ribosome.

7. The template (information source) for protein synthesis in eukaryotes is:

   A. DNA.
   B. mRNA.
   C. DNA polymerase.
   D. RNA polymerase.
   E. part of the structure of the ribosome.

8. The raw material (reactant) for protein synthesis in eukaryotes is:

   A. mRNA.
   B. DNA.
   C. free amino acid.
   D. aminoacyl tRNA.
   E. part of the structure of the ribosome.

9. Ribosomes in eukaryotes contain:

   A. a single subunit.
   B. two identical subunits.
   C. one large and one small subunit.

10. In comparison with ribosomes in prokaryotes, ribosomes in eukaryotes contain:

    A. larger rRNAs and more proteins.
    B. smaller rRNAs and more proteins.
    C. larger rRNAs and fewer proteins.
    D. smaller rRNAs and fewer proteins.

11. In eukaryotes, most amino acids are specified by ____ in mRNA.

    A. a single type of codon
    B. several different types of codons

12. The release of the completed polypeptide chain from the ribosome occurs:

    A. wherever a ribosome bumps into another ribosome along the mRNA (randomly along the molecule).
    B. at the first AUG codon in the mRNA molecule.
    C. at the poly-A tail on the mRNA.

    D. at the first nonsense (termination) codon on the mRNA.

    E. wherever the mRNA forms a hairpin loop.

Answers

1. **B.** The rRNA-coding regions of the chromosomes (usually on multiple chromosomes) are associated with the outer region of the nucleolus, while the center is occupied by partially assembled ribosomes.

2. **B.** Introns occur primarily in genes in eukaryotes.

3. **C.** The DNA-histone complexes called nucleosomes form "string of beads" structures which occupy most locations in dispersed euchromatin and which occur in packed "solenoid" arrays in heterochromatin and condensed chromatin.

4. **C.** mRNA is produced by RNA polymerase II and tRNA is produced by RNA polymerase III. The promoter sequences in Class II genes (coding for mRNA) are upstream of (located 5' relative to) the starting point of RNA synthesis, whereas the promoter sequences of Class III genes (coding for tRNA) are downstream of (located 3' relative to) the starting point for RNA synthesis.

5. **A.** Prokaryotic regulatory proteins typically bind just downstream or just upstream of the promoter, but eukaryotic regulatory proteins typically utilize much more distant sites, many of which are believed to interact with the promoter by looping out the intervening DNA.

6. **E.** A loop of rRNA appears to catalyze peptide bond formation.

7. **B.** The sequence of nucleotides in mRNA (read in groups of three as codons) determines the sequence of amino acids in the polypeptide being synthesized.

8. **D.** The aminoacyl group on a tRNA is ready to participate in protein synthesis. A free amino acid would have to be activated and attached to tRNA as an aminoacyl group before it could be used in protein synthesis.

9. **C.** The subunits in eukaryotic ribosomes are larger than the corresponding subunits in prokaryotic ribosomes, but prokaryotes and eukaryotes each contain ribosomes composed of large and small subunits.

10. **A.** The larger ribosomes in eukaryotes contain larger rRNAs and more different proteins than the ribosomes in prokaryotes.

11. **B.** Almost all amino acids are specified by two or more codons.

12. **D.** Nonsense codons trigger releasing factors to terminate translation.

Classification of Living Organisms

Taxonomy is the classification of living organisms based on characteristics and ancestry. Two *kingdoms*—animal and plant—are easily distinguished. In general, members of the former consume food and are mobile while those of the latter are stationary and produce their own nutrients.

Several systems have evolved to classify the great variety of living organisms. One such system divides living things into five kingdoms based on: (1) the presence (eukaryotic) or absence (prokaryotic) of membrane-bound nuclei in the cells; (2) the number of cells forming the organism; and (3) the mechanism for nutrition. This five-kingdom classification system is shown in the following table.

FIVE-KINGDOM CLASSIFICATION SYSTEM

Kingdom	Characteristics	Examples
Monera	unicellular without organized nuclei; absorb or produce their own nutrients	bacteria, blue-green algae
Protista	unicellular with membrane-bound nuclei; ingest, absorb, or produce nutrients via photosynthesis	protozoans, algae
Fungi	multicellular with membrane-bound nuclei; absorb nutrients	mushrooms, molds
Plants	multicellular with membrane-bound nuclei and a cell wall; possess chlorophyll and undergo photosynthesis	flowering plants and trees; evergreens
Animals	multicellular with membrane-bound nuclei; ingest nutrients	mammals, birds, amphibians, fish, reptiles, insects, crustaceans, etc.

These kingdoms can be divided into three main groups based on the mode of nutrition—photosynthetic organisms (plants and algae), organisms which absorb their nutrients (bacteria and fungi), and organisms which engulf or ingest their nutrients (protozoa and animals).

Each kingdom is further divided into phyla (sing. phylum), which are subdivided as follows: phyla → into classes → into families → into genera → into species. Each of these groups may be divided into six additional subgroups.

All living organisms are given a scientific name using the combination of genus and species. Under this binomial naming system, the scientific name for a human is *Homo sapiens*. To illustrate the classification system a demonstration of how one classifies a human is given below:

CLASSIFICATION OF THE HUMAN

Classification Group		Distinguishing Features
Kingdom	Animalia	Consume food and are mobile.
Phylum	Chordata	Notochord, hollow nervous system (neural tube) dorsally positioned, gill slits in pharyngeal wall, heart ventral to digestive system.
Subphylum	Vertebrata	Segmental vertebral column.
Class	Mammalia	Mammary glands for nourishment of young; hair or fur; warm-blooded; diaphragm.
Order	Primates	Large cerebral hemispheres; opposable digits; nails; highly developed sense of sight—eyes directed forward; teeth specialized for different functions.
Family	Hominidae	Walk with two limbs (bipedal locomotion); binocular color vision.
Genus	Homo	Ability to speak and most highly developed and largest brain.
Species	sapiens	Large skull, high forehead, reduced size of brow (supraorbital) ridges, prominent chin; decreased amount of body hair.

Quick Recall Test Questions and Answers

Choose the Best Answer

1. All are distinguishing features of the phylum chordate EXCEPT:

   A. notochord.
   B. neural tube dorsally positioned.
   C. gill slits.
   D. heart ventral to digestive system.
   E. nutrients produced via photosynthesis.

2. Phyla may be subdivided into:

   A. classes.
   B. families.
   C. genera.

   D. species.
   E. all of the above.

Answers

1. **E.** The characteristics of the phylum chordata are listed; it belongs to the animal kingdom and does not carry out the process of photosynthesis.

2. **E.** Each kingdom is further divided into phyla, which are subdivided into classes, families, genera, and species. Each of these groups may be divided into subgroups.

Organization of the Human Body

A multicellular organism is composed of millions of cells organized into functional units (organs and systems) which are formed by various groups of similar cells (tissues) working together. These cells are embedded in intercellular substances and tissue fluids. A *tissue* consists of a group of cells performing a similar function. Four basic tissues compose the human (mammalian) body: epithelium, connective tissue, muscle and nerve tissues. The four basic tissues may be organized to form functional units known as *organs*. Each organ has a definite function which results from the combined functions of the various tissue components. Several organs which function together as a unit for a specified purpose make up an organ *system*. The animal *organism* is composed of several interrelated organ systems.

Organ Systems

The human body is composed of the systems listed in the following table.

ORGAN SYSTEMS IN THE HUMAN

System	Functions
Muscular	Produces motion of body parts and viscera.
Skeletal	Supports the body, protects organs, and produces blood cells.
Circulatory	Transports nutrients, wastes, gases (oxygen and carbon dioxide), hormones, blood cells throughout body; also protects body against foreign organisms.
Nervous	Responds to internal and external stimuli; regulates and coordinates body activities and movements.
Integumentary	Limits and protects the body as a whole; prevents excess loss of water and functions in regulating body temperature.
Digestive	Enzymatically breaks down food materials into usable and absorbable nutrients.
Respiratory	Functions in the exchange of gases (oxygen and carbon dioxide).
Urinary	Removes body wastes from bloodstream and helps regulate homeostasis of internal environment.
Reproductive	Perpetuates the living organism by the production of sex cells (gametes) and future offspring.
Endocrine	Regulates body growth and function via hormones.

Four Basic Tissues

1. Muscle Tissue

Muscle tissue is contractile in nature and functions to move the skeletal system and body viscera.

TYPES OF MUSCLE

Type	Characteristics	Location
Skeletal	Striated, voluntary	Skeletal muscles of the body
Smooth	Nonstriated, involuntary	Walls of digestive tract and blood vessels, uterus, urinary bladder
Cardiac	Striated, involuntary	Heart

2. Nervous Tissue

Nervous tissue is composed of cells *(neurons)* that respond to external and internal stimuli and have the capability to transmit a message *(impulse)* from one area of the body to another. This tissue thus induces a response of distant muscles or glands, as well as regulating body processes such as respiration, circulation, and digestion. Nervous tissue composes the central (brain and spinal cord) and peripheral (peripheral nerves, ganglia, and receptors) nervous systems and the special sensory receptors (eye, ear, taste buds, and olfactory region).

3. Epithelial Tissue

Epithelial tissue covers the external surfaces of the body and lines the internal tubes and cavities. It also forms the glands of the body. Characteristics of epithelial tissue (epithelium) are that it

(1) has compactly aggregated cells;
(2) has limited intercellular spaces and substance;
(3) is avascular (no blood vessels);
(4) lies on a connective tissue layer—the basal lamina;
(5) has cells that form sheets and are polarized;
(6) is derived from all three germ layers.

TYPES OF EPITHELIUM

Classification	Location(s)	Function(s)
Simple squamous epithelium	Endothelium of blood and lymphatic vessels; Bowman's capsule and thin loop of Henle in kidney; mesothelium lining pericardial, peritoneal and pleural body cavities; lung alveoli; smallest excretory ducts of glands.	Lubrication of body cavities (permits free movement of organs); pinocytotic transport across cells.
Stratified squamous keratinized epithelium	Epidermis of skin.	Prevents loss of water; protection.
Stratified squamous nonkeratinized epithelium (moist)	Mucosa of oral cavity, esophagus, anal canal; vagina; cornea of eye and part of conjunctiva.	Secretion; protection; prevents loss of water.
Simple cuboidal epithelium	Kidney tubules; choroid plexus; thyroid gland; rete testis; surface of ovary.	Secretion; absorption; lines surface.
Stratified cuboidal epithelium	Ducts of sweat glands; developing follicles of ovary.	Secretion; protection.
Simple columnar epithelium	Cells lining lumen of digestive tract (stomach to rectum); gall bladder; many glands (secretory units and ducts); uterus; uterine tube (ciliated).	Secretion; absorption; protection; lubrication.
Pseudostratified columnar epithelium	Lines lumen of respiratory tract (nasal cavity, trachea, and bronchi) (ciliated); ducts of epididymis (stereocilia); ductus deferens; male urethra.	Secretion; protection; facilitates transport of substances on surface of cells.
Stratified columnar epithelium	Male urethra; conjunctiva	Protection.
Transitional epithelium	Urinary tract (renal calyces and pelvis, ureter and urinary bladder).	Protection.

Epithelial cells may also have specializations at the cell surface. For example,

microvilli—fingerlike projections of plasma membranes. Mainly located at luminal surfaces of absorptive cells (brush border of proximal convoluted tubules and striated border of intestinal epithelium).

cilia—motile organelles extending into the luman consisting of specifically arranged microtubules. Mainly located in respiratory epithelium and part of female reproductive tract.

flagella—similar to cilia. Primary examples are human spermatozoa.

stereocilia—are actually very elongated microvilli.

4. Connective Tissue

Connective tissue is the packing and supporting material of the body tissues and organs. It develops from mesoderm (mesenchyme). All connective tissues consist of three distinct components: ground substance, cells, and fibers.

a. *Ground substance*. Ground substance is located between the cells and fibers, both of which are embedded in it. It forms an amorphous intercellar material. In the fresh state, it appears as a transparent and homogenous gel. It acts as a route for the passage of nutrients and wastes to and from the cells within or adjacent to the connective tissue. The ground substance is composed of mucopolysaccharides *(glycosaminoglycans)*, proteins, lipids, and water. The primary glycosaminoglycans found in the ground substance are chondroitin sulfate and hyaluronic acid, the latter present in greater quantity.

b. *Fibers*. The fiber components of connective tissue add support and strength. Three types of fibers are present: *collagenous, elastic,* and *reticular*.

Collagen fibers (white fibers) are the most numerous fiber type and are present in all types of connective tissue in varying amount. Collagen bundles are strong and resist stretching. They are found in structures such as tendons, ligaments, aponeuroses, and fascia, which are subjected to pull or stretching activities.

Elastic fibers (yellow fibers) are refractile fibers which are thinner (0.2 to 1 μm diameter) than collagen fibers. They are extremely elastic and are located in structures with a degree of elasticity, such as the walls of blood vessels (elastic arteries), true vocal cords, and trachea.

Reticular fibers are thinner (0.2 to 1 μm diameter) than collagenous fibers. They are arranged in an intermeshing network (reticulum) which supports the organ. Reticular fibers are inelastic. They are found in the walls of blood vessels, lymphoid tissues (spleen and lymph nodes), red bone marrow, basal laminae, and glands (liver and kidney).

c. *Cells*. The *cells* of connective tissue are primarily attached and nonmotile *(fixed cells),* but some have the ability to move *(wandering or free cells)*. The typical cells found in connective tissue are:

Fibroblasts constitute the largest number of cells present in connective tissue. In an actively secreting state, they are flattened stellate-shaped cells with an oval nucleus and basophilic cytoplasm due to the numerous rough endoplasmic reticulum. In the inactive state, they appear as elongated spindles with a more basophilic oval or elongated nucleus. In this state, they are referred to as *fibrocytes*. The latter are the main cellular constituents of connective tissue structures such as tendons and ligaments. Only the nuclei of fibrocytes are observed between the fibers since the cytoplasm is indistinct. The terms fibrocyte and fibroblast are often used interchangeably.

Mesenchymal cells are undifferentiated connective tissue cells which have the potential to differentiate into other types of connective tissue cells. They are primarily found in embryonic and fetal tissues; some are thought to be present in the adult abutting the walls of capillaries. They are smaller than fibroblasts and are stellate in shape. They are capable of moving by extending their cell processes into the gel-like ground substance.

Macrophages (histiocytes) may be fixed or free. Free macrophages may wander through the connective tissue by extending their cell processes. Fixed macrophages are very numerous in loose connective tissue. They are polymorphic in shape and contain an oval nucleus. They have the ability to engulf extracellular material (foreign matter or necrotic cells). Macrophages are difficult to distinguish except when they are actively phagocytosing material and thus contain many vacuoles.

Adipocytes (fat cells) are found in most connective tissue, either singly or in groups. If the connective tissue layer is primarily composed of fat cells, it is referred to as adipose tissue. An adipocyte is a round, large cell with a distinct, dense nucleus usually located at the periphery of the cytoplasm. The majority of the cytoplasmic (cell) volume is taken up by a large lipid droplet. Due to the clear appearing cytoplasm and dark nucleus at one pole, the cell has a signet ring appearance. Fat cells do not undergo mitosis.

Mast cells are ovoid cells with small round nuclei. The cytoplasm contains numerous coarse basophilic granules which also stain metachromatically and are soluble in water. The mast cell granules are composed of *histamine* and an anticoagulant known as *heparin*. Histamine dilates blood vessels and increases the permeability of capillaries, thus increasing interstitial fluid. Mast cells take part in the allergic response of the body. Mast cells are found in most connective tissue and are numerous in the respiratory tract and near small blood vessels.

Plasma cells have a characteristic eccentric nucleus which contains chromatin arranged in a definite pattern near the nuclear envelope. This pattern gives a "cartwheel or spoke wheel" appearance. The juxtanuclear cytoplasm appears clear and less basophilic due to the Golgi complex located in this area. Plasma cells are found in the lamina propira of the gastrointestinal tract. They function in protecting the body against bacterial invasion by secreting antibodies [immunoglobulins (IgG)] into the circulating blood.

Reticular cells are star-shaped cells which join via their processes to form a cellular network. They are found abutting reticular fibers in certain glands and lymphoid tissues.

Pericytes are located in the adventitia of blood vessels. They are believed to be multi-potential cells which may differentiate into various connective tissue cells as well as into smooth muscle cells.

Certain white blood cells or leukocytes migrate out of the blood into the extracellular ground substance. The main leukocytes found in the connective tissue are lymphocytes, monocytes, eosinophils, basophils, and neutrophils. The leukocytes in connective tissue are similar in structure and function to those in the blood. The agranular leukocytes migrate in large numbers under normal conditions. Lymphocytes accumulate in areas in response to chronic inflammation. Neutrophils also migrate in large numbers into the interstitium during an inflammatory response. Eosinophils occur in areas involved in allergic reaction, such as the respiratory tract.

Quick Recall Test Questions and Answers

Choose the Best Answer

1. Simple squamous epithelium is found in all of the following EXCEPT:

   A. lung.
   B. kidney.
   C. skin.
   D. blood vessels.
   E. pericardium.

2. Which of the following is NOT considered a basic tissue that makes up the human body?

   A. epithelium
   B. connective tissue
   C. bone
   D. muscle
   E. nervous tissue

3. Which of the following cells are multipotent and can differentiate into other types of cells?

   A. fibroblasts
   B. chondroblasts
   C. adipocytes
   D. mesenchymal cells
   E. endothelial cells

4. Ground substance found in connective tissue is composed of all of the following EXCEPT:

   A. chondroitin sulfate.
   B. hyaluronic acid.
   C. actinomyosin.
   D. mucopolysaccharides.
   E. proteins and lipids.

5. Epithelial cells may have specializations at the cell surface such as:

   A. microvilli.
   B. cilia and stereocilia.
   C. flagella.
   D. all of the above.
   E. none of the above.

6. Epithelial tissue:

   A. is derived from all three germ layers.
   B. is avascular.
   C. lies on a connective tissue layer—the basal lamina.
   D. has limited intercellular spaces and substance.
   E. is characterized by all of the above.

7. A group of cells subserving the same general function and bound together or united by varying amounts of intercellular substance and tissue fluids is called a (an):

   A. organ.
   B. tissue.
   C. system.
   D. organ system.
   E. ground substance.

8. Epithelial tissues may be characterized by:

   A. protection.
   B. secretion.
   C. absorption.
   D. all of the above.
   E. none of the above.

9. The outstanding features of connective tissue include:

   A. an orderly arrangement of cells into sheets.
   B. possessing a fairly large amount of intercellular material.
   C. making up the majority of the ducts of secretory organs.
   D. all of the above.
   E. none of the above.

10. The function of mast cells is related to the:

   A. secretion of immunoglobulins (IgG).
   B. phagocytic activity.
   C. allergic response of the body.
   D. secretion and storage of coagulants.
   E. constrictive properties of blood vessels.

11. The adult tissue which lines the human digestive and respiratory passageways is:

   A. epithelium.
   B. nervous tissue.
   C. blood.
   D. connective tissue.
   E. muscle.

12. The adult tissue which covers the surface of the human body is:

   A. epithelium.
   B. nervous tissue.
   C. blood.
   D. connective tissue.
   E. muscle.

13. The adult tissue which is capable of rapid transmission of signals among parts of the human body is:

   A. epithelium.
   B. nervous tissue.
   C. blood.
   D. connective tissue.
   E. muscle.

14. The adult tissue which supports the shape of the human body is:

   A. epithelium.
   B. nervous tissue.
   C. blood.
   D. connective tissue.
   E. muscle.

15. The adult tissue whose mechanical properties are due to the extracellular material in the tissue is:

   A. epithelium.
   B. connective tissue.
   C. nervous tissue.
   D. muscle.

16. The adult tissue which forms most glands is:

   A. epithelium.
   B. connective tissue.
   C. nervous tissue.
   D. muscle.

17. The adult tissue responsible for contraction during the heartbeat is:

   A. epithelium.
   B. connective tissue.
   C. nervous tissue.
   D. muscle.

18. The adult tissue which can generate the most mechanical force by contraction is:

   A. epithelium.
   B. nervous tissue.
   C. blood.
   D. connective tissue.
   E. muscle

Answers

1. **C.** The epidermis of skin is composed of stratified squamous epithelium.

2. **C.** The four basic tissues that compose the human body are epithelium, connective tissue, muscle, and nervous tissue. Bone is a member of the connective tissues.

3. **D.** Mesenchymal cells are undifferentiated connective tissue cells which have the potential to differentiate into other types of connective tissue cells. They are primarily found in embryonic and fetal tissues; some are thought to be present in the adult, abutting the walls of capillaries. They are smaller than fibroblasts and are stellate in shape. They are capable of moving by extending their cell processes into the gel-like ground substance.

4. **C.** Ground substance is located between the cells and fibers, both of which are embedded in it. It forms an amorphous intercellular material. In the fresh state, it appears as a transparent and homogenous gel. It acts as a route for the passage of nutrients and wastes to and from the cells within or adjacent to the connective tissue. The ground substance is composed of mucopolysaccharides (glycosaminoglycans), proteins, lipids, and water. The primary glycosaminoglycans found in the ground substance are chondroitin sulfate and hyaluronic acid; the latter is present in greater quantity.

5. **D.** Epithelial cell specializations at the cell surface may include microvilli, cilia and stereocilia, and flagella.

6. **E.** Besides the four characteristics listed, epithelial tissue has compactly aggregated cells, and has cells that form sheets and are polarized.

7. **B.** A tissue consists of a group of cells performing a similar function. The cells are embedded in intercellular substances and tissue fluids. Four basic tissues compose the human body: epithelium, connective tissue, muscle, and nervous tissue. The four basic tissues may be organized to form functional units known as organs.

8. **D.** Epithelium is a group of cells forming a tissue. Epithelium lines the gut, the respiratory system, and the genitourinary system, and forms the epidermis. It therefore can protect, secrete, and absorb.

9. **B.** Connective tissue, cartilage, and bone are basically supporting tissues. An abundance of non-living-formed substance is the feature that is common to the group as a whole. Cells are interspersed in the intercellular substance, and fibers are a constituent of the formed substance. Fibers and ground substance are called matrix.

10. **C.** The mast cell granules are composed of *histamine* and an anticoagulant known as *heparin*. Histamine dilates blood vessels and increases the permeability of capillaries, thus increasing interstitial fluid. Mast cells take part in the allergic response of the body. Mast cells are found in most connective tissue and are numerous in the respiratory tract and near small blood vessels. Plasma cell are found in the lamina propria of the gastrointestinal tract. They function in protecting the body against bacterial invasion by secreting antibodies (immunoglobulins, or IgG) into the circulating blood.

11. **A.** Epithelial tissue lines most naturally occurring spaces in the human body, including the spaces in the digestive and respiratory systems.

12. **A.** Epithelial tissue (the stratified squamous epithelium of the epidermis) lines naturally occurring surfaces on the human body.

13. **B.** Nervous tissue is responsible for transmitting rapid signals among body parts. Muscle tissue (cardiac or smooth types) may transmit rapid signals over smaller distances, and epithelial tissue in endocrine glands can transmit somewhat slower signals over long distances within the body.

14. **D.** Connective tissue in the form of bone and cartilage forms most of the skeleton which supports the overall shape of the human body, and fibrous connective tissues in the walls of organs support the shapes of the organs within the body.

15. **B.** Mechanical properties of connective tissues are almost totally due to extracellular matrix. Mechanical properties of epithelia, muscle tissues, and nervous tissues are primarily due to cytoskeletal components inside the cells in the tissues.

16. **A.** All exocrine glands are composed of epithelial tissues, as are some endocrine tissues. Some endocrine structures are modified nervous tissue structures (posterior pituitary, pineal).

17. **D.** Cardiac muscle contracts to produce the heartbeat, and modified cardiac muscle cells in the pacemaker region (sino-atrial node) initiate the contraction. Nervous tissue in the sympathetic and parasympathetic branches of the nervous system may modify the rate of the heartbeat but cannot initiate it.

18. **E.** Muscle tissue is specialized for contraction. Cells in some epithelia and some connective tissues may also contract, but generate much less force at the tissue level.

Terms of Planes, Positions, Directions, and Relationships

For descriptive purposes a standard body position, "the anatomic position," has been adopted. The anatomic position is the position of a person standing erect, feet together and parallel, face forward, arms at the sides, and palms forward (supinated).

TERMS OF PLANES

Plane	Definition
Midsagittal or median	A vertical plane in the antero-posterior direction which divides the body into equal right and left halves.
Sagittal	A vertical plane parallel to the midsagittal plane; it allows longitudinal slices that are parallel to the median plane.
Frontal or coronal	A vertical plane which passes from side to side; it is at right angles to the midsagittal plane and cuts the specimen into anterior and posterior components.
Transverse, horizontal, or cross	A horizontal plane at right angles to both the sagittal and frontal plane; it cuts the specimen into superior (upper or cephalad) and inferior (lower or caudad) portions. Cross sections of the specimen are obtained.

TERMS OF POSITIONS

Position	Description
Anterior or ventral	Toward the front of the body or belly side; (volar or palmar side are used in referring to the hand).
Posterior or dorsal	Toward the back (the dorsum) of the body.
Superior, craniad, or cephalad	In the direction of the head; nearer the head.
Inferior or caudad	In the direction of the feet; away from the head.
Superficial or external	Nearer the surface; without or nearer the outside of the body.
Deep or internal	Away from the surface; within or toward the inside or interior.
Medial	Nearer the midline of the body; toward the midsagittal plane or center.
Lateral	Farther from the midline; toward the side of the body or away from the midsagittal plane; to the side.
Proximal	Nearest a point of origin in general or nearest the trunk as far as the extremities are concerned; nearer the attachment to the body. Nearer the midline axis.
Distal	Farther from the point of origin of a structure or farther from the reference point or the midline axis.
Central	Toward the center of the body; toward the inside.
Peripheral	Away from the center of the body; toward the outside.
Plantar	The sole of the foot.

TERMS OF DIRECTION

Direction	Description
Rostral	In the direction of the nose (head).
Cranial	In the direction of the cranium.
Cephalic	In the direction of the head end of the body.
Caudal	In the direction of the tail end of the body or away from the head end.
Mesad	In the direction of the midline of a structure.
Lateral	In the direction away from the midline of a structure.

OTHER TERMS

Term	Description
Invagination	An inward bulging, depression, or pocketing (vagina) of a cavity or from a surface.
Evagination	An outward bulging (hernia) of an organ, etc. in a cavity or from a surface.
Ipsilateral or Homolateral	Referring to the same side of the body.
Contralateral	Referring to the opposite side of the body.
Origin	A muscle's proximal attachment, or its fixed or less movable end. The origin is not constant and can be reversed.
Insertion	The distal end; the less fixed and more movable end of a muscle attachment.
Antum	A cavity.
Condyle	A smooth, rounded articular surface.
Facet	A flat, smooth area—in vertebrae the articulating facet.
Epicondyle	A prominence or ridge above an articular surface (condyle).
Fossa	A shallow depression.
Hamulus	A hook-shaped process or eminence.
Hiatus	A slit or gap.
Meatus	A canal.
Sinus	A cavity in a bone (maxillary sinus); a venous blood channel in the cranium (cavernous sinus); or a cavity in a viscus, such as the pharynx (piriform sinus).
Spine	A pointed process.
Sulcus	A groove.
Trochlea	A pulley mechanism.
Tuberosity	A rough eminence, projection, or bump.
Foramen	A hole in a bone; in the cranium, the spinal cord passes through the foramen magnum.
Fissure	A slit between bones; between the parietal bones of the skull, the slit is the superior sagittal fissure.
Crest	A prominent, distinct area—the iliac crest.

Skeletal System

The skeletal system of vertebrates is an *endoskeleton*—that is, it is within the body—as compared to an *exoskeleton* characteristic of arthropods. The human skeletal system provides:

(1) support;
(2) protection of vital organs;
(3) sites for muscle attachment;
(4) storage sites of body calcium and phosphates; and
(5) sites for blood cell formation.

The *human skeleton* consists of bone and cartilage. The bones form the main rigid structure of the skeleton. The human skeleton consists of about 206 bones, some of which are fused while others are joined together at sites which permit various degrees of movement. The sites of junction, or articulation, whether movable or immovable, are known as *joints*.

The human skeleton is divided into an *axial skeleton* and an *appendicular skeleton*.

Axial Skeleton

The axial skeleton consists of 80 bones forming the trunk (spine and thorax) and skull.

Vertebral Column: The main trunk of the body is supported by the spine, or vertebral column, which is composed of 26 bones, some of which are formed by the fusion of a few bones. The vertebral column from superior to inferior consists of 7 cervical (neck), 12 thoracic, and 5 lumbar vertebrae, as well as a sacrum, formed by fusion of 5 sacral vertebrae, and a coccyx, formed by fusion of 4 coccygeal vertebrae. Each vertebra consists of a body anteriorly and an arched posterior region circumscribing an inner central canal, the *vertebral canal,* which extends from the foramen magnum at the base of the skull through the sacrum. The vertebral column functions to support the trunk of the body and to protect the spinal cord located in the vertebral canal. The vertebrae of the cervical, thoracic, and lumbar regions are separated from each other by round fibrocartilaginous articular discs known as *intervertebral discs*. The entire vertebral column is held together by ligaments.

Ribs and Sternum: The axial skeleton also contains 12 pairs of *ribs* attached posteriorly to the thoracic vertebrae and anteriorly either directly or via cartilage to the *sternum* (breastbone). The ribs and sternum form the *thoracic cage,* which protects the heart and lungs. Seven pairs of ribs articulate with the sternum *(fixed ribs)* directly, and three do so via cartilage; the two most inferior pairs do not attach anteriorly and are referred to as *floating ribs*.

Skull: The *skull* consists of 22 bones fused together to form a rigid structure which houses and protects organs such as the brain, auditory apparatus, and eyes. The bones of the skull form the *face* and *cranium* (brain case) and consist of 6 single bones *(occipital, frontal, ethmoid, sphenoid, vomer,* and *mandible)* and 8 paired bones *(parietal, temporal, maxillary, palatine, zygomatic, lacrimal, inferior concha,* and *nasal)*. The *lower jaw* or *mandible* is the only movable bone of the skull (head); it articulates with the temporal bones.

Other Parts: Other bones considered part of the axial skeleton are the *middle ear bones (ossicles)* and the small U-shaped *hyoid bone* that is suspended in a portion of the neck by muscles and ligaments.

Appendicular Skeleton

The *appendicular skeleton* forms the major internal support of the appendages—the *upper* and *lower extremities* (limbs).

Pectoral Girdle and Upper Extremities: The arms are attached to and suspended from the axial skeleton via the *shoulder (pectoral)* girdle. The latter is composed of two *clavicles (collarbones)* and two *scapulae (shoulder blades)*. The clavicles articulate with the sternum; the two *sternoclavicular joints* are the only sites of articulation between the trunk and upper extremity.

Each upper limb from distal to proximal (closest to the body) consists of hand, wrist, forearm, and arm (upper arm). The *hand* consists of 5 *digits* (fingers) and 5 *metacarpal* bones. Each digit is comprised of three bones known as *phalanges,* except the thumb which has only two bones. The

The axial skeleton. Eighty bones make up this portion of the skeleton. Numbers in square brackets indicate number of bones for each item.

wrist consists of eight *carpal* bones which articulate with metacarpals. The *forearm* consists of two bones, the *ulna* on the side of the fifth digit (little finger), and the *radius* on the thumb side. The articulation between radius and ulna at the wrist permits rotation of the radius over the ulna during pronation (palm facing backward) and supination (palm turned forward). The ulna articulates at the elbow joint with the *humerus* creating a hinge joint. The humerus, in turn, is connected to the shoulder girdle at the *glenoid cavity* of the scapula.

Pelvic Girdle and Lower Extremities: The lower *extremities,* or legs, are attached to the axial skeleton via the *pelvic* or *hip girdle*. Each of the two coxal, or *hip*, bones comprising the pelvic girdle is formed by the fusion of three bones—*ilium, pubis,* and *ischium*. The coxal bones attach the lower limbs to the trunk by articulating with the sacrum.

From distal to proximal the lower limb consists of foot, ankle, shank, and thigh. The *foot* consists of 5 digits *(toes)* and 5 *metatarsals*. The digits contain 3 *phalanges* each, except for the big toe, which has two, the *tibia* and *fibula*. The tibia is larger, is located medially, forms the shin, and articulates at the knee joint with the *femur (thigh bone)*. The knee joint is protected anteriorly by the kneecap, or *patella*. The femur articulates with the *acetabular fossa* of the coxal bone.

THE HUMAN SKELETAL SYSTEM

Part of the Skeleton	Number of Bones
Axial Skeleton	**80**
Skull	22
Ossicles (malleus, incus, and stapes)	6
Vertebral column	26
Ribs	24
Sternum	1
Hyoid	1
Appendicular Skeleton	**126**
Upper extremities	64
Lower extremities	64

APPENDICULAR SKELETON

Upper Extremity	Bones
Shoulder girdle	Clavicle and scapula
Arm	Humerus
Forearm	Radius (lateral) and ulna (medial)
Wrist	Eight carpal bones (proximal row: scaphoid, lunate, triquetrium, pisiform) (distal row: trapezium, trapezoid, capitate, hamate)
Palm	Five metacarpal bones
Digits	Thumb—two phalanges; fingers—three phalanges
Lower Extremity	**Bones**
Pelvic girdle	Pubic, ileum, and ischium (innominate bone)
Thigh	Femur
Leg	Tibia (medial) and fibula (lateral)
Foot	Seven tarsal bones (talus, calcaneus, navicular, cuboid, and three cuneiform bones)
Digits	Big toe—two phalanges; other toes—three phalanges

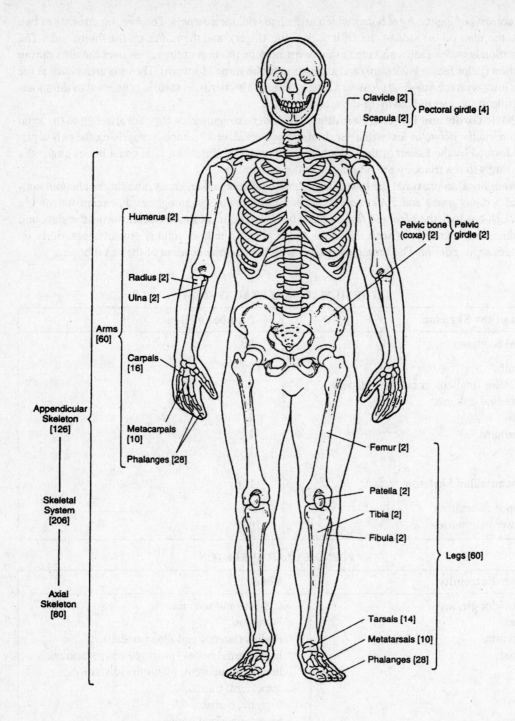

The appendicular skeleton. One hundred twenty-six bones make up this portion of the skeleton. Numbers in square brackets indicate number of bones for each item.

Characteristics of Bone

Bone is a specialized type of connective tissue consisting of cells *(osteocytes)* embedded in a calcified matrix which gives bone its characteristic hard and rigid nature. Bones are encased by a *periosteum,* a connective tissue sheath. All bone has a central marrow cavity. *Bone marrow* fills the marrow cavity or smaller marrow spaces, depending on the type of bone.

Types of Bone: There are two types of bone in the skeleton: *compact bone* and *spongy* (cancellous) *bone.*

Compact Bone. *Compact bone* lies within the periosteum, forms the outer region of bones, and appears dense due to its compact organization. The living osteocytes and calcified matrix are arranged in layers, or *lamellae.* Lamellae may be circularly arranged surrounding a central canal, the *Haversian canal,* which contains small blood vessels. This unit of a Haversian canal circumscribed by Haversian lamellae is known as an *Haversian system,* or *osteon.* Osteons are oriented along the longitudinal axis of the bone and communicate with each other, the periosteum, and the marrow cavity via oblique or transverse canals known as *Volkmann's canals.* Blood vessels enter and leave and are distributed throughout bone via the Haversian and Volkmann's canals. Irregular lamellae structures, the *interstitial lamellae,* are present between the Haversian systems. They are remnants of resorbed lamellar systems resulting from the remodeling of bone. The inner (next to marrow cavity) and outer (next to periosteum) limits of compact bone are formed by lamellar structures, the *inner (endosteal)* and *outer (periosteal) circumferential lamellae,* respectively. The Haversian systems are the major component of compact bone and lie between these two circumferential lamellae. The marrow cavity and Haversian canals are lined by *endosteum,* a thin layer of connective tissue. Both the endosteum and periosteum contain *osteogenic cells,* which can transform into bone-forming cells, or *osteoblasts.*

Spongy bone. Spongy bone consists of *bars, spicules,* or *trabeculae,* which form a lattice meshwork. Spongy bone is found at the ends of long bones and the inner layer of flat, irregular, and short bones. The trabeculae consist of osteocytes embedded in calcified matrix, which in definitive bone has a lamellar nature. The spaces between the trabeculae contain bone marrow.

Bone Cells: The cells of bone are osteocytes, osteoblasts, and osteoclasts. *Osteocytes* are found singly in *lacunae* (spaces) within the calcified matrix and communicate with each other via small canals in the bone known as *canaliculi.* The latter contain osteocyte cell processes. The osteocytes in compact and spongy bone are similar in structure and function.

Osteoblasts are cells which form bone matrix, surrounding themselves with it, and thus are transformed into osteocytes. They arise from undifferentiated cells, such as mesenchymal cells. They are cuboidal cells which line the trabeculae of immature or developing spongy bone.

Osteoclasts are found during bone development and remodeling. They are multinucleated cells lying in cavities, *Howship's lacunae,* on the surface of the bone tissue being resorbed. Osteoclasts remove the existing calcified matrix releasing the inorganic or organic components.

Bone Matrix: *Matrix* of compact and spongy bone consists of collagenous fibers and ground substance which constitute the organic component of bone. Matrix also consists of inorganic material which is about 65% of the dry weight of bone. Approximately 85% of the inorganic component consists of calcium phosphate in a crystalline form (hydroxyapatite crystals.) Glycoproteins are the main components of the ground substance.

MAJOR TYPES OF HUMAN BONES

Type of Bone	Characteristics	Examples
Long bones	Width less than length	Humerus, radius, ulna, femur, tibia
Short bones	Length and width close to equal in size	Carpal and tarsal bones
Flat bones	Thin flat shape	Scapulae, ribs, sternum, bones of cranium (occipital, frontal, parietal)
Irregular bones	Multifaceted shape	Vertebrae, sphenoid, ethmoid
Sesamoid	Small bones located in tendons of muscles	Patella (kneecap) in quadriceps femoris tendon

Joints

The bones of the skeleton articulate with each other at *joints,* which are variable in structure and function. Some joints are immovable, such as the *sutures* between the bones of the cranium. Others are *slightly movable joints;* examples are the *intervertebral joints* and the *pubic symphysis* (joint between the two pubic bones of the coxal bones). These contain fibrocartilage plates separating the articulating bones and have a slight gliding motion. The most common joints are *freely movable joints.* They are also referred to as *synovial joints* since their joint capsules are lined by a serous *synovial membrane* which produces a lubricating fluid—*synovial fluid*—between the articulating bones. The *capsule* is a fibrous connective tissue sheath which encases the joint. Another feature of synovial joints is that a thin layer of *hyaline cartilage* lines the articular surfaces of the abutting bones. The synovial joints can be classified according to the type of motion permitted by the structure of the joint.

TYPES OF JOINTS

Joint Type	Characteristics	Examples
Ball and socket	Permits all types of movement (abduction, adduction, flexion, extension, circumduction); it is considered a universal joint.	Hip and shoulder joints.
Hinge (ginglymus)	Permits motion in one plane only.	Elbow and knee, interphalangeal joints.
Rotating or pivot	Rotation is only motion permitted.	Radius and ulna, atlas and axis (first and second cervical vertebrae).
Plane or gliding	Permits sliding motion.	Between tarsal bones and carpal bones.
Condylar (condyloid)	Permits motion in two planes which are at right angles to each other (rotation is not possible).	Metacarpo-phalangeal joints, temporomandibular.

Adjacent bones at a joint are connected by fibrous connective tissue bands known as *ligaments.* They are strong bands which support the joint and may also act to limit the degree of motion occurring at a joint.

Quick Recall Test Questions and Answers

Choose the Best Answer

1. The skeletal system of vertebrates is an:

    A. axial skeleton.
    B. appendicular skeleton.
    C. endoskeleton.
    D. exoskeleton.
    E. ossicular skeleton.

2. Each statement concerning osteoclasts is correct EXCEPT that they:

    A. are multinucleated.
    B. lie in cavities known as Howship's lacunae.
    C. remove existing calcified matrix.
    D. are stimulated by parathyroid hormone.
    E. are stimulated by thyro-calcitonin.

3. The appendicular skeleton is composed of bones of the:

    A. cranium.
    B. vertebral column.
    C. pelvis.
    D. thoracic cage.
    E. upper and lower extremities.

4. The principal cells that form bone matrix are known as:

    A. osteoblasts.
    B. osteocytes.
    C. osteoclasts.
    D. interstitial lamella.
    E. Haversian systems.

5. Cells that are active in bone remodeling are:

    A. osteoblasts.
    B. osteocytes.
    C. osteoclasts.
    D. Haversian systems.
    E. interstitial lamella.

6. The main trunk of the body is supported by the spine or vertebral column. Concerning that structure, all of the following are true statements EXCEPT:

    A. The vertebrae are separated from each other by a fibro-cartilaginous disc.
    B. There are seven cervical vertebra but eight cervical nerves.

    C. The sacrum is made up of five fused vertebra.
    D. Each vertebra has a vertebral canal.
    E. The vertebral body is located posterior to the pedicles.

7. The true elbow joint (humero-ulna) is classified as a:

    A. ball and socket joint.
    B. hinge (ginglymus) joint.
    C. pivot joint.
    D. plane or gliding joint.
    E. condylar joint.

8. _____ give(s) origin to the skeletal system.

    A. Ectoderm
    B. Mesoderm
    C. Endoderm
    D. Ectoderm and endoderm
    E. Ectoderm and mesoderm

9. The human skeletal system provides:

    A. support and protection.
    B. sites for muscle attachment.
    C. storage sites for calcium and phosphates.
    D. sites for blood cell formation.
    E. all of the above.

10. All of the following are considered long bones EXCEPT the:

    A. humerus.
    B. femur.
    C. fibula.
    D. ulna.
    E. vertebral column.

11. One of the functions of human bone tissue is to:

    A. provide metabolic energy for movement.
    B. store calcium and phosphate.
    C. store potassium and chloride.
    D. form slippery surfaces at joints in the skeleton.

12. Compact bone tissue:

    A. is composed primarily of cells (little extracellular matrix).
    B. is composed primarily of extracellular matrix (with cells scattered throughout the matrix).
    C. contains only extracellular matrix (no living cells).

13. Cartilage:

    A. makes up most of the skeleton of adult mammals.

    B. forms the joint surfaces of many bones in the human skeleton.

    C. does not occur in the skeleton of adult humans.

Answers

1. **C.** The skeleton system of vertebrates is an endoskeleton—that is, it is within the body—in contrast to an exoskeleton characteristic of arthropods.

2. **E.** Osteoclasts are stimulated by parathyroid hormone and inhibited by thyro-calcitonin. Osteoclasts are found during bone development and remodeling. They are multinucleated cells lying in cavities, Howship's lacunae, on the surface of the bone tissue being resorbed. Osteoclasts remove the existing calcified matrix releasing the inorganic or organic components.

3. **E.** The appendicular skeleton forms the major internal support of the appendages—the upper and lower extremities (limbs).

4. **A.** The cells of bone are osteocytes, osteoblasts, and osteoclasts. Osteoblasts are cells which form bone matrix, surrounding themselves with it, and thus are transformed into osteocytes. Osteoclasts are cells found during bone development and remodeling.

5. **C.** Osteoclasts are cells involved in bone development and remodeling. Osteoclasts remove existing calcified matrix and release inorganic (calcium) or organic components to the system.

6. **E.** The main trunk of the body is supported by the spine, or vertebral column. Each vertebra consists of a body anteriorly and an arched posterior region circumscribing an inner central canal.

7. **B.** The humero-ulna permits motion in one plane only and is therefore a hinge joint.

8. **B.** Mesoderm is the germ layer of origin of the skeletal system.

9. **E.** The human skeletal system provides support, protection of vital organs, sites for muscle attachment, storage sites of body calcium and phosphates, and sites for blood cell formation.

10. **E.** The typically named long bones are the humerus, radius, ulna, femur, tibia, and fibula. The vertebral column is composed of vertebra which are small, irregular bones.

11. **B.** In addition to providing mechanical support for the body, the calcium and phosphate used to solidify the extracellular matrix in bone are used as metabolic reserves. Bone matrix is continually remodeled by resorption and deposition, allowing removal of calcium and phosphate from bone when they are needed and deposition of excess calcium and phosphate into bone matrix.

12. **B.** Compact bone consists of layers of extracellular matrix interspersed with scattered layers of spider-shaped osteocytes (bone cells).

13. **B.** Cartilage forms the articular surfaces of movable joints. Its slippery surface prevents excess wear in healthy joints. Cartilage also forms the supporting structures in the nose and ear and parts of the lower ribs.

Muscular System

Classification

A muscle cell not only has the ability to propagate an action potential along its cell membrane, as does a nerve cell, but also has the internal machinery to give it the unique ability to contract.

Most muscles in the body can be classified as striated muscles in reference to the fact that when observed under a light microscope the muscular tissue has light and dark bands or striations running across it. Although both skeletal and cardiac muscles are striated and therefore have similar structural organizations, they do possess some characteristic functional differences. Skeletal muscle contraction, for example, is made up of the contraction of many motor units. A motor unit consists of a single motor neuron coming from the spinal cord of the central nervous system and all the muscle fibers which it innervates (a few to 2,000).

In contrast to skeletal muscle, cardiac muscle is a functional syncytium. This means that, although anatomically it consists of individual cells, the entire mass normally responds as a unit and all of the cells contract together. In addition, cardiac muscle has the property of automaticity which means that the heart initiates its own contraction without the need for motor nerves. Motor nerves may alter this inherent rhythm but the resource for initiating the contraction lies within the special cardiac cells called pacemaker cells. Here an action potential is initiated and spreads to the other cardiac cells.

Nonstriated muscle consists of multiunit and unitary (visceral) smooth muscle. Visceral smooth muscle has many of the properties of cardiac muscle. To some extent it acts as a functional syncytium, e.g., areas of intestinal smooth muscle will contract as a unit. Smooth muscle is part of the urinary bladder, uterus, spleen, gallbladder, and numerous other internal organs. It is also the muscle of blood vessels, respiratory tracts, and the iris of the eye.

The basic contractile mechanism is probably the same in all muscle types although the structural organization of smooth muscle is very different from that of striated muscle. We will concentrate on skeletal muscle, knowing that what we discuss can be applied to cardiac muscle and to some extent to smooth muscle.

Skeletal Muscles

In order for the human being to carry out the many intricate movements that must be performed, approximately 650 skeletal muscles of various lengths, shapes, and strength play a part. Each muscle consists of many muscle cells or fibers held together and surrounded by connective tissue that gives functional integrity to the system. Three definite units are commonly referred to:

(1) endomysium—connective tissue layer enveloping a single fiber;
(2) perimysium—connective tissue layer enveloping a bundle of fibers; and
(3) epimysium—connective tissue layer enveloping the entire muscle.

Muscle Attachment and Function

For coordinated movement to occur, the muscle must attach to either bone or cartilage or, as in the case of the muscles of facial expression, to skin. The portion of a muscle attaching to bone is the tendon. A muscle has two extremities, its origin and its insertion; the origin is the relatively fixed attachment site, whereas the insertion is the end attached to a structure that will be moved when the muscle contracts. A pair of muscles usually control the movement of a joint; they are opposing or antagonistic muscles. For example, a flexor muscle is opposed by an extensor.

Terms to Describe Movement

Flexion is bending, most often ventrally to decrease the angle between two parts of the body; it is usually an action at an articulation or joint.

Extension is straightening, or increasing the angle between two parts of the body; a stretching out or making the flexed part straight.

Abduction is a movement away from the midsagittal plane (midline); to abduct is to move laterally.

Adduction is a movement toward the midsagittal plane (midline); to adduct is to move medially and bring a part back to the mid-axis.

Circumduction is a circular movement at a ball and socket (shoulder or hip) joint, utilizing the movements of flexion, extension, abduction, and adduction.

Rotation is a movement of a part of the body around its long axis.

Examples: a.   The atlas (1st cervical vertebra) rotates on the axis (2nd cervical vertebra).

             b.   The thigh may be rotated medially or internally; it may also be rotated laterally or externally.

Supination refers only to the movement of the radius around the ulna. In supination the palm of the hand is oriented anteriorly; turning the palm dorsally puts it into pronation. The body on its back is in the supine position.

Pronation refers to the palm of the hand being oriented posteriorly. The body on its belly is the prone position.

Inversion refers only to the lower extremity, specifically the ankle joint. When the foot (plantar surface) is turned inward, so that the sole is pointing and directed toward the midline of the body and is parallel with the median plane, we speak of inversion. Its opposite is eversion.

Eversion refers to the foot (plantar surface) being turned outward so that the sole is pointing laterally.

Opposition is one of the most critical movements in humans; it allows us to have pulp-to-pulp opposition, which gives us the great dexterity of our hands. In this movement the thumb pad is brought to a finger pad. A median nerve injury negates this action.

Muscle Names

The names of some muscles may appear strange; the naming, however, is based essentially on anatomical position, function, shape, or other feature. Here are some examples:

1. Position and Location:

a.	Pectoralis major and minor	pectoral region of thorax; the major is larger
b.	Temporalis	temporal region of head
c.	Infra- and supraspinatus	below and above spine of scapula
d.	External and internal intercostals	refers to their location in the intercostal spaces

2. Principal Action:

a.	Pronators (e.g., pronator quadratus) and supinators	pronation refers to palm down and supination to palm up; quadratus refers to the shape
b.	Flexors and extensors (e.g., flexor and extensor digitorum)	flexors and extensors of digits
c.	Levator scapulae	elevator of the scapula (shoulder)

3. Shape:

a.	Trapezius	trapezoid in shape
b.	Rhomboid major and minor	rhomboid in shape

4. Number of Divisions (Heads) and Position:

a.	Biceps brachii	two-headed muscle in anterior brachium (arm)
b.	Triceps brachii	three-headed muscle in posterior brachium (arm)

5. Size, Length, and Shape:

a.	Flexor pollicis longus and brevis	long and short flexors of the thumb
b.	Rhomboid major and minor	major is larger in size; rhomboid in shape.

6. Attachment Sites:

a.	Sternocleidomastoid	extends from sternum and clavicle (cleido) to mastoid process
b.	Sternohyoid	extends from sternum to hyoid bone

Structural Organization of a Muscle Fiber

A muscle fiber is a single muscle cell. If we look at a section of a fiber we see that it is complete with a cell membrane called the sarcolemma and has several nuclei located just under the sarcolemma—it is multinucleated. Each fiber is composed of numerous cylindrical fibrils running the entire length of the fiber.

The fibril exhibits light and dark bands—the "I" and "A" bands, respectively. The "I" band is bisected by the "Z" line and the "A" band by the "M" line. There is a somewhat lighter band within the "A" band that is called the "H" band. An even lighter area in the middle of the "H" zone on either side of the "M" line is called the "pseudo-H" band.

These striations are produced by the arrangement within the fibril of myofilaments which comprise the contractile machinery. A sarcomere, the area between two "Z" bands, is the functional unit of muscle; it is the region between two "Z" lines and consists of an "A" band and half of two abutting "I" bands. Refer to the illustration of the relaxed myofibril (page 73) for the positions of these lines and bands.

Myofilaments

1. The thick and thin myofilaments form the contractile machinery of muscle and are made up of proteins. Approximately 54% of all the contractile proteins (by weight) is myosin. The thick myofilament is composed of many myosin molecules oriented tail-end to tail-end. The head domains are oriented outward.

2. The second major contractile protein is actin, a globular protein. The thin myofilament contains two chains of F-actin arranged in a twisted fashion. This configuration gives the thin myofilament a certain periodicity. Associated with the thin myofilament along its entire length is the globular protein troponin. The presence of troponin along with tropomyosin-B inhibits myosin-actin interaction—it represses actomyosin formation. Calcium ions released following an action potential in the fiber membrane and T-tubules bind with troponin. Calcium-troponin binding removes the inhibition of actomyosin formation.

Sacroplasm

The sarcoplasm (cytoplasm of the muscle cell) contains Golgi complexes near the nuclei. Mitochondria are found between the myofibrils and just below the sarcolemma. The myofibrils are surrounded by smooth endoplasmic reticulum *(sarcoplasmic reticulum)* composed of a longitudinally arranged tubular network *(sarcotubules)*. The sarcotubules are continuous with dilated sacs called terminal cisternae. In skeletal muscle the terminal cisternae lie over the I–A junction of the sacromeres. The terminal cisternae of cardiac muscle are less well developed and are located adjacent to the Z discs. The terminal cisternae are in association with invaginations of the sarcolemma T-tubules.

The complex (terminal cistern-T-tubule-terminal cistern) formed at this position is known as a *triad*. The T-tubules function to bring a wave of depolarization of the sarcolemma into the fiber and thus into an intimate relationship with the terminal cisternae. The sarcoplasmic reticulum concentrates calcium ions (Ca^{2+}) within its lumen, but depolarization of the T-tubule membrane induces the nearby terminal cisternae of the sarcoplasmic reticulum to release this Ca^{2+} into the sarcoplasma among the myofilaments. The Ca^{2+} becomes associated with the troponin of the thin myofilament, bringing about contraction as on page 73.

Excitation

Contraction in a skeletal muscle is triggered by the generation of an action potential in the muscle membrane. Each motor neuron upon entering a skeletal muscle loses its myelin sheath and divides into branches with each branch innervating a single muscle fiber, forming a *neuromuscular junction*. Each fiber normally has one neuromuscular junction which is located near the center of the fiber. A *motor unit* consists of a single motor neuron and all the muscle fibers innervated by it. The *motor end plate* is the specialized part of the muscle fiber's membrane lying under the neuron.

The impulse arriving at the end of the motor neuron causes liberation of *acetylcholine* from vesicles in the neuron terminal. The acetylcholine acts at specific sites normally found only on the motor end plate section of the fiber membrane and increases the permeability of the motor end plate. The resulting Na^+ influx produces a depolarizing potential called the end-plate potential. This in turn depolarizes adjacent areas of the fiber membrane, triggering an action potential which is propagated in both directions from the central neuromuscular junction toward the fiber ends. Normally the magnitude of the end-plate potential is sufficient to discharge the muscle membrane, so that each impulse in the nerve ending produces a response in the muscle. The acetylcholine is rapidly destroyed by the enzyme *acetylcholinesterase* which is found in high concentrations at the neuromuscular junction.

Contraction

According to the sliding filament theory (Huxley) the sarcomere response to excitation involves the sliding of thin and thick myofilaments past one another making and breaking chemical bonds with each other as they go. Neither the thick nor thin myofilaments change in length. If we could imagine observing this contraction under a light microscope we would see the narrowing of the "H" and "I" bands during contraction while the width of the "A" band would remain constant.

The word *contraction* refers to those processes which are manifested externally by either a *shortening* of a muscle or by *tension development* in a muscle. If the muscle length is held constant, the contraction is referred to as an *isometric contraction*. In an isometric contraction the passive tension remains constant with the *active tension* being added to it to produce the *total tension* of the muscle.

If the muscle shortens during contraction, it is called an *isotonic contraction* and the total tension remains constant.

Events Leading to Muscle Contraction

1. Action potential of motoneuron.
2. Depolarization of motoneuron terminal.
3. Ca^{2+} enters motoneuron terminal.
4. Acetylcholine (ACh) released into synaptic cleft.
5. ACh diffuses across synapse.
6. ACh binds to receptors on muscle end plate; degradation of ACh by acetylcholinesterase.
7. Depolarization of muscle end plate (end plate potential).
8. Action potential in muscle.
9. Action potential invades transverse (T) tubule.
10. Ca^{2+} released from sarcoplasmic reticulum (SR).
11. Increased intracellular $[Ca^{2+}]$.
12. Ca^{2+} binds to troponin C on the thin filaments.
13. Action and myosin bind, forming cross bridges.
14. Cross bridges pivot.
15. Thick and thin filaments slide, producing muscle tension.
16. Ca^{2+} reuptake into sarcoplasmic reticulum by (Ca^{2+} ATPase).
17. Decreased intracellular $[Ca^{2+}]$.
18. Relaxation.

Muscle Twitch

A muscle's response to a single maximal stimulus is a *muscle twitch*. The beginning of muscular activity is signalled by the record of the *electrical activity* in the sarcolemma. The *latent period* is the delay between imposition of the stimulus and the development of tension.

Tetanus

When a volley of stimuli is applied to a muscle, each succeeding stimulus may arrive before the muscle can completely relax from the contraction caused by the preceding stimulus. The result is *summation,* an increased strength of contraction. If the frequency of stimulation is very fast, individual contractions fuse and the muscle smoothly and fully contracts. This is a *tetanus*.

Energy Sources

In any phenomenon including muscular contraction the energy input to the system and the energy output from the system are equal. Let us consider first the energy sources for muscular contraction. The immediate energy source for contraction is ATP which can be hydrolyzed by acto-myosin to give ADP, P_i, and the energy which is in some way associated with cross-bridge motion.

The ultimate source of this ATP is the ATP produced by the intermediary metabolism of car-bohydrates and lipids. Skeletal muscle has the biochemical machinery to utilize both. With mild exercise, oxygen availability after an initial period of adjustment is sufficient so that the aerobic pathways for ATP production can keep pace with the ATP utilization during the exercise—a new equilibrium is reached. During short-term, violent exertion, however, aerobic energy production cannot keep pace with energy utilization and even during the onset of mild exercise aerobic energy production initially lags behind energy utilization. Yet the ATP concentration remains constant. The reason is that there are stores of CP (creatine phosphate) in muscles and ATP levels can be main-tained at the expense of CP levels. In these cases of insufficient oxygen availability ("oxygen debt"), anaerobic pathways can produce enough additional ATP to permit those short-term bursts of exercise but lactic acid is generated. This incomplete oxidation produces substantially less energy than the complete aerobic oxidation to carbon dioxide and water.

SCHEMATIC OF SKELETAL (STRIATED) MUSCLE

Type of Muscle Fibers

Skeletal muscle fibers can be described, on the bases of structure and function, as follows:

1. *White (fast) fibers*—contract rapidly; fatigue quickly; energy production is mainly via anaer-obic glycolysis; contain relatively few mitochondria; examples are the muscles of the eye.
2. *Red (slow) fibers*—contract slowly; fatigue slowly; energy production mainly via oxida-tive phosphorylation (aerobic); contain relatively many mitochondria; examples are pos-tural muscles.
3. *Intermediate fibers*—have structural and functional qualities between those of white and of red fibers.

Quick Recall Test Questions and Answers

Choose the Best Answer

1. Of the elements listed, which is most essential for muscular contraction?

   A. sodium
   B. potassium
   C. magnesium
   D. calcium
   E. zinc

2. Sustained muscle activity leads to fatigue, which is accompanied by the accumulation of:

   A. ATP.
   B. ADP.
   C. Troponin.
   D. Acetylcholinesterase.
   E. Lactic acid.

3. Circumduction is a circular movement at a ball and socket joint and utilizes all the movements EXCEPT:

   A. flexion.
   B. extension.
   C. abduction.
   D. adduction.
   E. supination.

4. Moving the upper extremity away from the mid-sagittal plane and then back to the original position involves the movements of:

   A. supination and pronation.
   B. flexion and extension.
   C. inversion and eversion.
   D. abduction and adduction.
   E. dorsiflextion and plantarflextion.

5. Muscle contraction results when actin unites with:

   A. calcium ions.
   B. troponin.
   C. myosin.
   D. ATP.
   E. acetylcholine.

6. According to the sliding filament theory (Huxley), when a contraction is observed under the light microscope, the following occurs:

   A. there is a narrowing of the H band.
   B. there is a widening of the I band.
   C. there is a narrowing of the A band.

   D. there is a widening of the Z line.
   E. the pseudo-H band becomes very prominent.

7. Actin and myosin myofilaments are present in which muscle type?

   A. skeletal
   B. smooth
   C. cardiac
   D. all of the above
   E. none of the above

8. A Triad, in relation to skeletal muscles, refers to:

   A. the A and I bands and T-tubule collectively.
   B. one T-tubule and two adjacent terminal cisternae together.
   C. three Z bands in very close approximation.
   D. a sarcotubule, a T-tubule, and a terminal cisternae collectively.

9. A sustained contraction is called:

   A. tonus.
   B. a recovery period.
   C. tetanus.
   D. a contraction period.
   E. an "all or none" contraction.

10. Vigorous exercise will cause muscle fatigue which is primarily due to:

    A. the utilization and exhaustion of ATP.
    B. the accumulation of ADP.
    C. the accumulation of lactic acid.
    D. the accumulation of carbon dioxide.
    E. a sodium and potassium imbalance.

11. The state of a continuously mild or partial contraction of a muscle is denoted as:

    A. tetanus.
    B. tonus.
    C. an "all or none" contraction.
    D. a twitch.
    E. a reflex contraction.

12. Which of the following muscle types is not under the control of the autonomic (involuntary) nervous system?

    A. heart (cardiac)
    B. smooth

C. skeletal (striated)

D. arrector pili

13. If we examine the three types of muscles in respect to their characteristics, which of the series below is false?

	Characteristic	Cardiac	Skeletal	Smooth
A.	No. of nuclei	Several	Several	One
B.	Position of nuclei	Central	Central	Central
C.	Striations	Present	Present	Absent
D.	Control	Autonomic	Voluntary	Autonomic

14. The functional unit of a striated muscle is known as the sarcomere. A sarcomere on an electron micrograph is the region between:

A. two A bands.

B. two I bands.

C. two H bands.

D. two Z bands.

15. A fiber of striated (skeletal) muscle:

A. possesses only one nucleus.

B. possesses no clear Z bands.

C. possesses more than one nucleus.

D. has the same characteristics as smooth muscle.

E. possesses few mitochondria.

16. Which of the following is NOT true of normally functioning human skeletal muscle?

A. Contraction occurs only in response to a nerve impulse.

B. The plasma membrane of the muscle cells can conduct action potentials.

C. Cells maintain a state of partial contraction (due to spontaneous contractions) which is then adjusted to a state of greater or lesser contraction in response to nerve impulses from motor neurons.

17. A normal vertebrate skeletal muscle fiber (cell) is:

A. uninucleate and striated.

B. multinucleate and striated.

C. uninucleate and unstriated.

D. multinucleate and unstriated.

18. A normal vertebrate skeletal muscle fiber (cell):

A. produces rapid, brief contractions under direct somatic nervous system control (contracts only in direct response to a nerve impulse).

B. produces rapid, brief contractions under autonomic nervous system rate control (contracts

spontaneously at a rate which may be altered by autonomic nervous system activity).

C. produces slow, long-lasting contractions under direct somatic nervous system control (contracts only in direct response to a nerve impulse).

D. produces slow, long-lasting contractions under autonomic nervous system rate control (contracts spontaneously at a rate which may be altered by autonomic nervous system activity).

19. Prior to the contraction of a vertebrate fast-twitch skeletal muscle cell, the action potential passes along the motor axon and results in the release of ____ from the presynaptic ending when it reaches the synapse with the muscle cell.

A. adrenalin

B. sodium

C. acetyl choline

D. electricity

20. The sliding of the thick and thin myofilaments during the contraction of a vertebrate skeletal muscle cell is triggered by the ____ the sarcoplasmic reticulum.

A. release of calcium from

B. uptake of calcium by

C. release of sodium from

D. uptake of sodium by

21. The sliding of the thick and thin myofilaments during the contraction of a vertebrate fast-twitch skeletal muscle cell is powered by the ____ by the filaments.

A. synthesis of ATP

B. hydrolysis of ATP

C. synthesis of protein

D. hydrolysis of protein

ANSWERS

1. **D.** The sarcoplasmic reticulum concentrates calcium ions (Ca^{2+}). The Ca^{2+} becomes associated with the troponin of the thin myofilament, bringing about contraction.

2. **E.** In cases of insufficient oxygen availability ("oxygen debt") anaerobic pathways can produce enough additional ATP to permit short-term bursts of exercise but lactic acid is generated.

3. **E.** *Circumduction* is a circular movement at a ball and socket (shoulder or hip) joint, utilizing the movements of flexion, extension, abduction, and adduction.

4. **D.** *Abduction* is a movement away from the mid-sagittal plane (midline); to abduct is to move laterally.
Adduction is a movement toward the midsagittal plane (midline); to adduct is to move medially and bring a part back to the mid-axis.

5. **C.** In muscle contraction, first the actomyosin complex must be established; at that point ATP is hydrolyzed and the energy necessary is provided.

6. **A.** According to the sliding filament theory (Huxley) the sarcomere response to excitation involves the sliding of thin and thick myofilaments past one another. We see the narrowing of the "H" and "I" bands during contraction while the width of the "A" band would remain constant.

7. **D.** The basic contractile mechanism is the same in all muscle types.

8. **B.** The complex (terminal cistern-T-tubule-terminal cistern) formed is known as a *triad*. The T-tubules function to bring a wave of depolarization of the sarcolemma into the fiber and thus into intimate relationship with the terminal cisternae.

9. **C.** If more than two stimuli are given to a muscle in rapid succession, a partial fusion of all contractions results. The contractions occur before relaxation can take place or is completed. If a contraction is steadily maintained and no relaxation occurs between separate stimuli, the contraction is known as tetanus.

10. **C.** The cause of muscle fatigue is said to be the accumulated anaerobically produced lactic acid. Lactic acid may later be broken down into carbon dioxide and water for elimination, or it may be converted into glycogen and stored for future use.

11. **B.** Tonus refers to muscular activity in which a shortened condition is maintained for a prolonged period. Visceral muscle is the outstanding example of tonus. The word can be applied to any sustained process which is the result of probable regularly repeated excitation.

12. **C.** Skeletal (striated) muscle is under voluntary control. The autonomic nervous system innervates cardiac muscle, smooth muscle, and glands. Arrector pili musculature is associated with skin and is smooth musculature.

13. **B.** In skeletal muscle the nuclei are found peripherally. To complete the chart, the speed of contraction should also be mentioned. Skeletal muscle is the fastest working, smooth muscle is the slowest, and cardiac muscle occupies an intermediate position.

14. **D.** A sarcomere is the region between two Z bands. In simple terms, we are dealing with this unit: ZIAHAIZ. Contraction of the sarcomere is due to the fine filaments (actin) sliding between the thick filaments (myosin), pulling the Z bands to which they are attached with them. This pulls the Z bands closer together, and so the sarcomeres are shortened.

15. **C.** The striated muscle fiber is multinucleated.

16. **C.** Normally functioning skeletal muscle does not spontaneously contract. Contraction occurs only in response to somatic nervous system nerve impulses (action potentials).

17. **B.** Skeletal muscle cells are large and heavily multinucleated owing to their origin by fusion of myoblasts in the embryo. A typical skeletal muscle cell may contain hundreds of nuclei. These cells are also strongly striated as a result of the precise arrangement of the thick and thin myofilaments within each cell.

18. **A.** Skeletal muscle cells vary in the speed and force of their contractions, but produce faster and more forceful contractions than cardiac and smooth muscle. Skeletal muscle contractions occur in response to nerve impulses in the motor neuron controlling the particular muscle cell and are of brief duration.

19. **C.** In mammals, acetyl choline is the transmitter used in neuromuscular synapses.

20. **A.** Depolarization resulting from influx of sodium across the plasma membrane and transverse tubules of the muscle cell activates the sarcoplasmic reticulum (endoplasmic reticulum of the muscle cell) to release calcium ions. The calcium ions trigger the thin myofilaments to interact with the thick myofilaments.

21. **B.** Hydrolysis of ATP drives a conformational change in myosin that in turn drives sliding of the thick and thin myofilaments past each other.

Circulatory System

Functions

The circulatory system serves:

(1) to conduct nutrients and oxygen to the tissues;
(2) to remove waste materials by transporting nitrogenous compounds to the kidneys and carbon dioxide to the lungs;
(3) to transport chemical messengers (hormones) to target organs and modulate and integrate the internal milieu of the body;
(4) to transport agents which serve the body in allergic, immune, and infectious responses;
(5) to initiate clotting and thereby prevent blood loss;
(6) to maintain body temperature;
(7) to produce, carry, and contain blood;
(8) to transfer body reserves, specifically mineral salts, to areas of need.

General Components and Structure

The circulatory system consists of the heart, blood vessels, blood, and lymphatics. It is a network of tubular structures through which blood travels to and from all the parts of the body. In vertebrates this is a completely closed circuit system, as William Harvey (1628) demonstrated. The heart is a modified, specialized, powerful pumping blood vessel. Arteries, eventually becoming arterioles, conduct blood to capillaries (essentially endothelial tubes), and venules, eventually becoming veins, return blood from the capillary bed to the heart. (Malpighi [1661] demonstrated the capillary system.) The system is lined entirely by endothelium. Fluids (mostly water) which leave capillaries return as lymph to the bloodstream via lymphatic channels. The spleen, liver, and bone marrow function in the formation, destruction, and replacement of blood cells.

Systemic arteries originating from the left side of the heart (via the aorta) distribute oxygenated and nutrient-rich blood to the body. The systemic venous system returns deoxygenated blood to the heart. The pulmonary arterial circuit delivers this blood from the right side of the heart to the lungs and the pulmonary venous component returns oxygenated blood to the left side of the heart. Arteries travel away from the heart; veins come to it.

Course of Circulation

Systemic Route: The systemic route is made up of the arterial and venous systems.

a.   *Arterial system.* Blood is delivered by the pulmonary veins (two from each lung) to the left atrium, passes through the bicuspid (mitral) valve into the left ventricle and then is pumped into the ascending aorta; backflow here is prevented by the aortic semilunar valves. The aortic arch toward the right side gives rise to the brachiocephalic (innominate) artery which divides into the right subclavian and right common carotid arteries. Next, arising from the arch is the left common carotid artery, then the left subclavian artery; these two arise independently from the arch. In general the carotids split into external and internal carotids which supply the head, neck, and brain. The subclavians supply the upper limbs. As the subclavian arteries pass the first rib they are renamed axillary arteries. When the axillary arteries leave the axilla (armpit) and enter the arm (brachium) they are called brachial arteries. Below the elbow these main trunk lines divide into ulnar and radial arteries, which supply the forearm and eventually form a set of arterial arches in the hand which give rise to common and proper digital arteries. The descending (dorsal) aorta continues along the posterior aspect of the thorax giving rise to the segmental intercostal arteries. After passage "through" (behind) the diaphragm it is called the abdominal aorta. Branches are:

> inferior phrenic arteries to the diaphragm and adrenal gland;
> middle suprarenal (adrenal) artery to the adrenal;
> celiac artery to the stomach, part of duodenum, liver, and spleen;
> superior mesenteric artery to the small intestines, the cecum, ascending, and transverse colon;

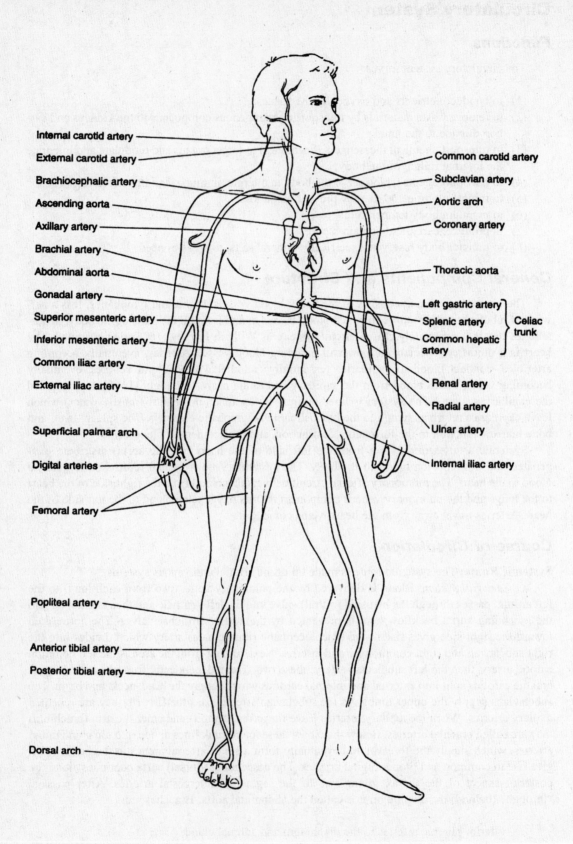

Internal carotid artery

External carotid artery

Brachiocephalic artery

Ascending aorta

Axillary artery

Brachial artery

Abdominal aorta

Gonadal artery

Superior mesenteric artery

Inferior mesenteric artery

Common iliac artery

External iliac artery

Superficial palmar arch

Digital arteries

Femoral artery

Popliteal artery

Anterior tibial artery

Posterior tibial artery

Dorsal arch

Common carotid artery

Subclavian artery

Aortic arch

Coronary artery

Thoracic aorta

Left gastric artery

Splenic artery

Common hepatic artery

Celiac trunk

Renal artery

Radial artery

Ulnar artery

Internal iliac artery

The major arteries of the human body, excluding the pulmonary arteries.

renal arteries to the kidneys and adrenals;

ovarian and testicular arteries to the respective gonads;

inferior mesenteric artery to the descending and sigmoid colon, and to the superior portion of the rectum;

lumbar segmental arteries to the abdominal wall.

At the pelvic rim the abdominal aorta divides into the right and left common iliac arteries. These divide into the internal iliacs, which supply the pelvic organs, and the external iliacs, which supply the lower limbs.

As the external iliac artery passes below the inguinal ligament into the thigh, its name changes to femoral artery. In the region posterior to the knee joint the artery is known as the popliteal artery; it divides into an anterior tibial artery to the anterior leg, a posterior tibial artery to the posterior leg, and a peroneal artery to the lateral aspects of the leg. The anterior and posterior tibial arteries eventually give rise to metatarsal and digital arteries for the supply of the dorsal and plantar aspects, respectively, of the foot.

b. *Venous system.* Veins are frequently multiple and variations are common. They return blood originating in the capillaries of peripheral and distal body parts to the heart. Tributaries converge and eventually all the blood of the body except that from the lungs and heart itself reaches the right atrium via the superior and inferior venae cavae.

The superior vena cava is formed in the following manner. The internal jugular veins, from the brain and deep face and neck, and the external jugular veins, from the superficial face and neck, join the subclavian veins, which receive the drainage of the upper limb and form right and left brachiocephalic (innominate) veins. The two brachiocephalic veins join to form the superior vena cava. Also joining the superior vena cava is the azygous system of veins, which drains the chest wall.

The inferior vena cava has the following origin. Femoral veins, from the lower limb, become in the abdominal cavity the external iliac veins, which receive the internal iliac veins from the pelvis and form the common iliac veins. The common iliac veins join to form the inferior vena cava. The inferior vena cava receives the renal veins, veins from the body wall, the right gonadal vein and the hepatic veins, from the liver, before passing through the diaphragm into the thorax to enter the right atrium of the heart.

Specific tributaries of the inferior vena cava (from below upward) include:

1. Lumbar veins
2. Right gonadal veins
3. Renal veins
4. Right suprarenal vein
5. Right phrenic vein
6. Hepatic veins

Hepatic Portal System: Blood draining the alimentary tract (intestines), pancreas, spleen, and gallbladder does not return directly to the systemic circulation, but is relayed by the hepatic portal system of veins to and through the liver. In the liver, absorbed foodstuffs and wastes are processed. After processing, the liver returns the blood via hepatic veins to the inferior vena cava and from there to the heart (right atrium).

Pulmonary Circuit: Blood is oxygenated and depleted of metabolic products such as carbon dioxide in the lungs. The pathway is as follows:

(1) Deoxygenated blood arrives in the right atrium and passes through the tricuspid valve into the right ventricle.

(2) It leaves the right ventricle via the pulmonary (trunk) artery and passes to the lungs; backflow is prevented by the pulmonary semilunar valves.

(3) In the capillary network of the lung, blood is oxygenated. It then leaves the lung via two pulmonary veins each from the right and left lung and passes to the left atrium.

(4) Blood passes through the bicuspid valve into the left ventricle and from there is expelled to the rest of the body via the ascending aorta; backflow is prevented by the aortic semilunar valves.

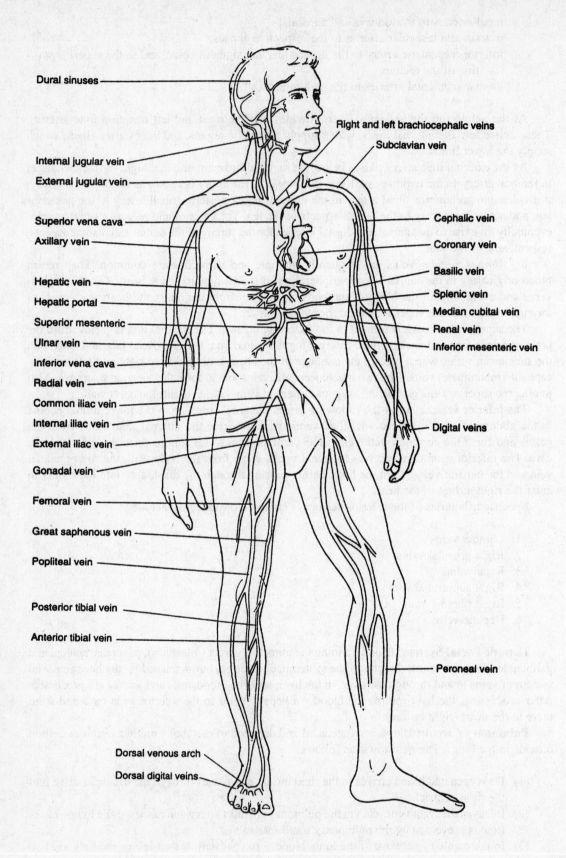

Dural sinuses

Right and left brachiocephalic veins

Subclavian vein

Internal jugular vein

External jugular vein

Superior vena cava

Cephalic vein

Axillary vein

Coronary vein

Hepatic vein

Basilic vein

Hepatic portal

Splenic vein

Superior mesenteric

Median cubital vein

Ulnar vein

Renal vein

Inferior vena cava

Inferior mesenteric vein

Radial vein

Common iliac vein

Internal iliac vein

External iliac vein

Digital veins

Gonadal vein

Femoral vein

Great saphenous vein

Popliteal vein

Posterior tibial vein

Anterior tibial vein

Peroneal vein

Dorsal venous arch

Dorsal digital veins

The major veins of the human body, excluding the pulmonary veins.

Lymphatic Drainage: A network of lymphatic capillaries permeates the body tissues. Lymph is a fluid similar in composition to blood plasma, and tissue fluids not reabsorbed into blood capillaries are transported via the lymphatic system eventually to join the venous system at the junction of the left internal jugular and subclavian veins. Like veins, lymphatics possess valves. Interposed along the course of some lymph vessels are lymph nodes. These nodes filter lymph and add lymphocytes to the circulation. Lymph nodes possess an outer cortex and an inner medulla. Lymphoid follicles are present in the cortex; irregular cords of lymphocytes make up the medulla.

The Heart

The heart is a highly specialized blood vessel which pumps 72 times per minute and propels about 4,000 gallons (about 15,000 liters) of blood daily to the tissues. It is composed of:

endocardium (lining coat; epithelium)
myocardium (middle coat; cardiac muscle)
epicardium (external coat or visceral layer of pericardium; epithelium and mostly connective tissue)
impulse conducting system

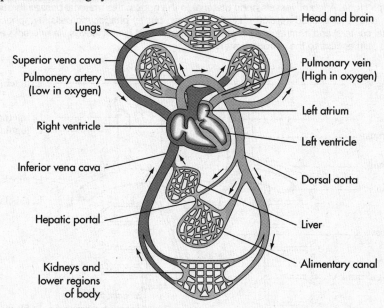

Distribution of blood in a complete double circulation. The relation of the capillaries to the arteries and veins cannot be shown in this diagram but is implied.

Mammals possess modified cardiac muscle fibers specialized for conduction (Purkinje system). The heart has an automatic rhythmic beat. Cardiac (autonomic) nerves exert an influence on heartbeat but serve only to change the force and frequency of the contractions in accordance with the physiologic needs of the organism.

Cardiac Nerves: Modification of the intrinsic rhythmicity of the heart muscle is produced by cardiac nerves of the sympathetic and parasympathetic nervous system. Stimulation of the sympathetic system increases the rate and force of the heartbeat and dilates the coronary arteries. Stimulation of the parasympathetic (vagus nerve) reduces the rate and force of the heartbeat and constricts the coronary circulation. Visceral afferent (sensory) fibers from the heart end almost wholly in the first four segments of the thoracic spinal cord.

Cardiac Cycle: Alternating contraction and relaxation is repeated about 75 times per minute; the duration of one cycle is about 0.8 sec. Three phases succeed one another during the cycle:

(a) atrial systole: 0.1 sec
(b) ventricular systole: 0.3 sec
(c) diastole: 0.4 sec

Afferent vessel

Cortex nodular
Germinal center
Trabecula
Medulla
Medullary sinus
Medullary cord
Reticulum
Capsule

Valve

Efferent vessel

Schematic of Lymph Node. Afferent vessels bring material to the nodes; this material passes through the reticulum of the nodes and is processed (foreign material is filtered out by phagocytic cells); lymphocytes (manufactured in germinal centers) and immunologic material are added and lymph leaves via efferent vessels (at the hilus) eventually to gain access to the venous system.

R. brachiocephalic v.

R. internal jugular v.
R. jugular trunk

R. subclavian trunk

R. subclavian v.

Superior vena cava

R. broncho-mediastinal trunk

Thoracic duct

L. brachiocephalic v.

L. internal jugular v.
L. jugular trunk

L. subclavian trunk
L. subclavian v.

L. broncho-mediastinal trunk

Diaphragm
Cisterna chyli
Lumbar trunk
Drainage of limbs, abdominal, pelvic viscera

Schema of Main Lymphatic Pathways. Note that the right jugular lymphatic trunk and the right subclavian lymphatic trunk form the right lymphatic duct. The left jugular lymphatic trunk and the left subclavian lymphatic trunk empty into the thoracic duct. The thoracic duct also receives the drainage from the lower limbs, abdomen, pelvis, perineum, and left thorax. The right head and neck specimen, the right upper extremity, and most of the right thorax drain via the right lymphatic duct. Both sides feed into the venous system at the junction (confluens) of the internal jugular and subclavian veins. Numerous variations exist.

The actual period of rest for each chamber is 0.7 sec for the atria and 0.5 sec for the ventricles, so, in spite of its activity, the heart is at rest longer than at work.

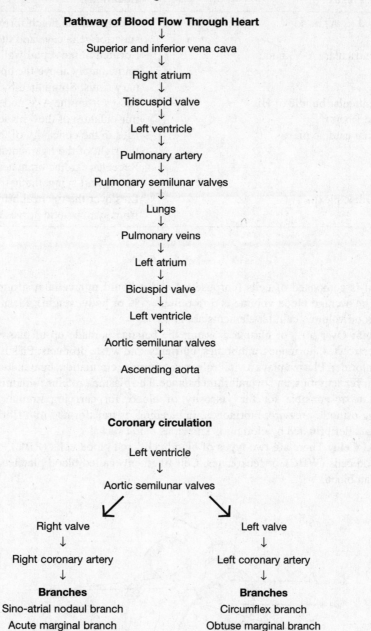

Pathway of Blood Flow Through Heart
↓
Superior and inferior vena cava
↓
Right atrium
↓
Triscuspid valve
↓
Left ventricle
↓
Pulmonary artery
↓
Pulmonary semilunar valves
↓
Lungs
↓
Pulmonary veins
↓
Left atrium
↓
Bicuspid valve
↓
Left ventricle
↓
Aortic semilunar valves
↓
Ascending aorta

Coronary circulation

Left ventricle
↓
Aortic semilunar valves

Right valve
↓
Right coronary artery
↓
Branches
Sino-atrial nodaul branch
Acute marginal branch
Posterior interventricular branch

Left valve
↓
Left coronary artery
↓
Branches
Circumflex branch
Obtuse marginal branch
Anterior interventricular branch

Coronary Veins:

1. Great cardiac vein accompanies anterior interventricular artery.
2. Small cardiac vein is in relation to marginal artery on the acute margin.
3. Middle cardiac vein accompanies posterior interventricular artery.
4. All veins are confluent in the coronary sinus, which empties into the right auricle.

CARDIAC NODES AND PLEXI

Node or Plexus	Location
Sino-atrial (S-A) node	Located in the notch formed by the superior vena cava and the right auricle.
Atrio-ventricular (A-V) node	Located in the septal wall of the right atrium immediately above the opening of the coronary sinus. Stimulated by the S-A node.
Atrio-venticular bundle of His (Purkinje fibers)	Passes from the A-V node into the musculature of the ventricular system.
Superficial cardiac plexus	Lies in the concavity of the aortic arch to the right of the ligamentum arteriosum. Receives cardiac branches from vagus nerves and sympathetic trunks.
Deep cardiac plexus	Lies over the tracheal bifurcation. Input from sympathetic nerves and vagus.

Blood

Blood is composed of cells (corpuscles) and a liquid intercellular ground substance called plasma. The average blood volume is 5 to 6 liters (7% of body weight). Plasma constitutes about 55% of blood volume; cellular elements about 45%.

Plasma: Over 90% of plasma is water; the balance is made up of plasma proteins and dissolved electrolytes, hormones, antibodies, nutrients, and waste products. Plasma is isotonic (0.85% sodium chloride). Plasma plays a vital role in respiration, circulation, coagulation, temperature regulation, buffer activities, and overall fluid balance. The plasma proteins (albumin, globulin, and fibrinogen) are responsible for the viscosity of blood, for carrying immune material, and for controlling osmotic pressure. Fibrinogen, in bleeding, is transformed into fibrin and helps form a clot. Plasma defibrinated by clotting is known as *blood serum.*

Blood Cells: There are two types of blood cells: red blood cells (RBC), or erythrocytes, and white blood cells (WBC), or leukocytes. Cell fragments called blood platelets are also present in mammalian blood.

Diagram of the heart.

a. *Erythrocytes—RBC.* These cells are biconcave discs about 7.7 micrometers in diameter. Mature cells lack a nucleus. The normal RBC hematocrit is about 36 to 45. The normal RBC counts are $5.2 \times 10^6/\text{mm}^3$ in males and $4.5 \times 10^6/\text{mm}^3$ in females. *Hemoglobin,* a complex molecule of iron and protein, is present in the cell. Red blood cells carry oxygen (in the form of oxyhemoglobin) from the lungs to the tissues and transport carbon dioxide from the tissues to the lungs. The membranes of the RBC carry Rh antigen and blood group antigens. Red blood cells have a life span of about 3 months. They are removed from the circulation by the spleen and replaced by new red blood cells formed in bone marrow. In the breakdown of hemoglobin, bilirubin is excreted and iron is retained.

b. *Leukocytes—WBC.* These cells differ from red blood cells by having nuclei and by exhibiting ameboid movement. A normal count of WBC in circulating blood is about 5 to 9 $\times$ $10^3/mm^3$. WBC contain phosphatases, liberate proteolytic enzymes, and function mainly in phagocytosis, proteolysis and antibody formation. An increase in the number of leukocytes is called *leukocytosis,* a decrease *leukopenia.*

There are two main types of leukocytes: nongranular and granular.

Non- or Agranular Leukocytes

1. *Lymphocytes* make up between 20 and 25% of total leukocytes and are seldom phagocytic. They originate from lymphoid tissue and bone marrow, function in immunologic responses and the detoxification of noxious substances, and are prevalent at sites of chronic inflammation. Some live several years.

2. *Monocytes* make up between 3 and 8% of total WBC. They are sometimes phagocytic and help in debridement.

Granular (possess abundant, specific granules) Leukocytes

1. *Neutrophils* make up about 65 to 75% of leukocytes. They are twice as large as a RBC and have a lobulated nucleus. They are the most active and phagocytic, providing the first line of defense against invading organisms. Dead neutrophils become *pus.*

2. *Eosinophils* make up about 2 to 5% WBC. They possess large red acidophilic granules and a bilobed nucleus. Large numbers are found at sites of parasitic infections and allergic reactions (specifically, in the respiratory and digestive tracts). Eosinophils function in the destruction of antigen-antibody complexes.

3. *Basophils* make up 0.5% or less of the total white blood cell count. They are rarely phagocytic. Basophils contain large quantities of basophilic granules. They are involved in immune phenomena, and produce heparin, which prevents the clotting of blood.

c. *Blood platelets.* These cytoplasmic structures are not true cells but are cell fragments characteristic of mammalian blood. (In lower vertebrates, cells called thrombocytes have a function similar to platelets.) Blood platelets average about 3 microns in diameter. About 250,000 to 350,000/mm³ are normally present. These structures arise by the fragmentation of cytoplasmic processes of giant bone marrow cells. Platelets agglutinate and adhere to regions of injured vessels; they plug wounds of blood vessels. They help physically in clotting and form thromboplastin (thrombokinase), an integral chemical component of clot formation.

FORMED ELEMENTS OF BLOOD
(8% OF BLOOD)

Cells	Number/Cubic Millimeter	Function
Erythrocytes (RBC)	5.2 million in males 4.5 million in females	carry oxygen to tissues carry carbon dioxide to lungs
Leukocytes (WBC)	5,000–9,000	phagocytosis, proteolysis, antibody formation
1. Lymphocytes	20–25% of WBC	detoxification, immunologic response
2. Monocytes	3–8% of WBC	phagocytosis, form macrophages
3. Neutrophils	65–77% of WBC	phagocytosis
4. Eosinophils	2–5% of WBC	allergic response, destroy antigen–antibody complexes
5. Basophils	0.5% of WBC	allergic response immune phenomena, produce heparin
6. Platelets (thrombocytes)	200,000–400,000	clotting

Composition of human blood in review

Whole blood					
Plasma 55%			Cellular elements 45%		
Water	Metabolites	Electrolytes	Red blood cells		
				Platelets	
					White blood cells
90%	- lipids - amino acids - carbohydrates - waste products	Na^+ K^+ Ca^{++} Mg^{++} CL HCO^-_3 HPO^{-2}_4 SO^{-2}_4			- lymphocytes - monocytes - neutrophils - eosinophils - basophils

Blood Clotting: Platelets contribute thromboplastin (thrombokinase), an enzymatically active substance. Thromboplastin interacts with calcium ions and prothrombin (a plasma protein). Prothrombin is an inactive precursor of the catalyst thrombin. In the presence of these components prothrombin is converted to thrombin. Subsequently thrombin reacts with the plasma protein fibrinogen, forming fibrin. Fibrin is an insoluble, coagulated protein which clots. A clot also contains blood cells. Diagrammatically we can represent clotting reactions as follows:

$$platelets \rightarrow thromboplastin$$
$$\downarrow$$
$$prothrombin + Ca^{2+} \rightarrow thrombin$$
$$\downarrow$$
$$fibrinogen \rightarrow fibrin.$$

Anticoagulants. An anticoagulant is a substance which prevents or retards coagulation of blood. Examples are: *heparin,* an acid mucopolysaccharide which occurs most abundantly in the liver; *aspirin* (acetylsalicylic acid), which also acts as an analgesic, antipyretic, antirheumatic compound; and the drug *Dicumarol,* a tradename for bihydroxycoumarin.

Blood Pressure: Blood pressure is usually measured by placing a sphygmomanometer cuff around the arm compressing the brachial artery and vein. Maximum blood pressure is obtained during ventricular contraction (systole) and minimum blood pressure indicates ventricular rest (diastole). The normal blood pressure listed for a young adult is 120 systolic and 80 diastolic (mm Hg).

Quick Recall Test Questions and Answers

Choose the Best Answer

1. Cardiac muscle makes up the greater portion of the:

   A. pericardium.
   B. epicaradium.
   C. myocardium.
   D. endocardium.

2. The most important function attributed to neutrophils and monocytes is to be active in:

   A. phagocytosis.
   B. the immunologic response.
   C. the allergic response.
   D. production of heparin.
   E. detoxification.

3. Blood is delivered to the right atrium by the superior and inferior vena cavas. From the right atrium blood passes to the right ventricle; in its passage it traverses the:

   A. tricuspid valve.
   B. pulmonary semilunar valve.
   C. bicuspid valve.
   D. aortic semilunar valve.
   E. valve of the inferior vena cava.

4. All of the following are branches of the ascending/aortic arch EXCEPT the:

   A. brachiocephalic artery (to the right).
   B. right common carotid artery.
   C. left common carotid artery.
   D. left subclavian artery.
   E. left coronary artery.

5. Heparin, an anticoagulant, is associated with cytoplasmic granules which are produced by the:

   A. lymphocytes.
   B. monocytes.
   C. neutrophils.
   D. eosinophils.
   E. basophils.

6. Blood is considered to be a specialized connective tissue. The ground substance, a constituent of the intercellular matrix of connective tissues, is specifically represented in the blood by:

   A. cells (corpuscles).
   B. fibrin.

C. thrombin.
D. blood plasma.

7. Eosinophils:

   A. make up between 20% and 25% of the total leukocytes.
   B. function in the destruction of antigen–antibody complexes.
   C. are classified as agranular leukocytes.
   D. possess basophilic granules and a bilobed nucleus.

8. Heartbeat is initiated by the:

   A. vagus nerve.
   B. sympathetic nervous system.
   C. A-V (atrio-ventricular) node.
   D. Purkinje system.
   E. S-A (sino-atrial) node.

9. The most numerous leukocytes are the:

   A. lymphocytes.
   B. monocytes.
   C. eosinophils.
   D. neutrophils.
   E. basophils.

10. The vital centers for control of heart rate, respiratory rate, and blood pressure are located in the

    A. pons.
    B. medulla.
    C. cerebellum.
    D. hypothalamus.
    E. midbrain.

11. Administration of which of the following compound(s) increases clotting time?

    A. heparin
    B. aspirin
    C. dicumarol
    D. all of the above
    E. none of the above

12. When a physician informs a patient that the blood pressure reading is 160/90, the physician refers to the:

    A. systolic blood pressure of the left ventricle.
    B. blood pressure in the veins of the arm.

C. systolic and diastolic pressures of the brachial artery.
D. systolic pressure of the aorta and diastolic pressure in the superior vena cava.
E. systolic pressure of the right ventricle.

13. A common experiment carried out in the physiology laboratory on the turtle heart involves first destroying the S-A node and observing the heart, and then destroying the A-V node and observing and recording the results. After these procedures it is found that the heart now:

A. beats faster.
B. exhibits no change in heart rate.
C. beats slower.
D. will stop beating.

14. Blood in the pulmonary vein is rich in:

A. oxyhemoglobin.
B. carbaminohemoglobin.
C. hemoglobin.
D. uric acid.
E. carbon dioxide.

15. Abnormal blood clots (thrombi) occur more frequently in people with:

A. prothrombin deficiency.
B. impeded venous blood flow.
C. vitamin K deficiency.
D. platelet deficiency.
E. none of the above.

16. Of the pairs below, which one is mismatched?

A. lymphatics—contain amino acids, salt, and water, but no blood corpuscles
B. hepatic portal vein—drains the intestinal tract and carries nutrients
C. inferior vena cava—carries oxygenated blood and has a low blood pressure
D. hypothalamus—secretes releasing factors that influence pituitary-target organ relationships
E. pulmonary veins—carry oxygenated blood

ANSWERS

1. **C.** The heart is a highly specialized blood vessel which pumps 72 times per minute and propels about 4000 gallons (about 15,000 liters) of blood daily to the tissues. It is composed of:
 endocardium (lining coat; epithelium)
 myocardium (middle coat; cardiac muscle)
 epicardium (external coat or visceral layer of pericardium; epithelium and mostly connective tissue)
 impulse conducting system

2. **A.** Both neutrophils and monocytes are phagocytic, helping to destroy foreign organisms.

3. **A. Pulmonary Circuit:** Blood is oxygenated and depleted of metabolic products such as carbon dioxide in the lungs. The pathway is as follows:

 (1) Deoxygenated blood arrives in the right atrium and passes through the tricuspid valve into the right ventricle.

 (2) Blood leaves the right ventricle via the pulmonary (trunk) artery and passes to the lungs; backflow is prevented by the pulmonary semilunar valves.

 (3) In the capillary network of the lung, blood is oxygenated. It then leaves the lung via two pulmonary veins each from the right and left lung and passes to the left atrium.

 (4) Blood passes through the bicuspid valve into the left ventricle and from there is expelled to the rest of the body via the ascending aorta; backflow is prevented by the aortic semilunar valves.

4. **B.** Blood is delivered by the pulmonary veins (two from each lung) to the left atrium, passes through the bicuspid (mitral) valve into the left ventricle, and then is pumped into the ascending aorta; backflow here is prevented by the aortic semilunar valves. The aortic arch toward the right side gives rise to the brachiocephalic (innominate) artery, which divides into the right subclavian and right common carotid arteries. Next, arising from the arch is the left common carotid artery, then the left subclavian artery; these two arise independently from the arch. In general the carotids split into external and internal carotids, which supply the head and neck and brain. The subclavians supply the upper limbs. As the subclavian arteries pass the first rib, they are renamed axillary arteries. When the axillary arteries leave the axilla (armpit) and enter the arm (brachium), they are called brachial arteries. Below the elbow these main trunk lines divide into ulnar and radial arteries, which supply the forearm and eventually form a set of arterial arches in the hand which give rise to common and proper digital arteries.

The descending (dorsal) aorta continues along the posterior aspect of the thorax giving rise to the segmental intercostal arteries. After passage "through" (behind) the diaphragm, it is called the abdominal aorta.

5. **E.** Basophils make up 0.5% or less of the total blood cell count. They are rarely phagocytic. Basophils contain basophilic granules, are involved in immune phenomena, and produce heparin, which prevents the clotting of blood. Heparin, an anticoagulant, occurs most abundantly in the liver. Other examples of anticoagulants are aspirin and the drug dicumarol.

6. **D.** Blood is composed of cells (corpuscles) and a liquid intercellular ground substance called plasma. The average blood volume is 5 to 6 liters (7% of body weight). Plasma constitutes about 55% of blood volume; cellular elements about 45%.
   Plasma: Over 90% of plasma is water; the balance is made up of plasma proteins and dissolved electrolytes, hormones, antibodies, nutrients, and waste products. Plasma is isotonic (0.85% sodium chloride). Plasma plays a vital role in respiration, circulation, coagulation, temperature regulation, buffer activities, and overall fluid balance. The plasma proteins (albumin, globulin, and fibrinogen) are responsible for the vicosity of blood, for carrying immune material, and for controlling osmotic pressure. Fibrinogen, in bleeding, is transformed into fibrin and helps form a clot. Plasma defibrinated by clotting is known as *blood serum*. There are two types of blood cells: red blood cells (RBC), or erythrocytes and white blood cells (WBC), or leukocytes. Cell fragments called blood platelets are also present in mammalian blood.

7. **B.** Leukocytes (WBC) differ from red blood cells by having nuclei and by exhibiting ameboid movement. A normal count of WBC in circulating blood is about 5 to 9 $\times$ 10³/mm³. WBC contain phosphatases, liberate proteolytic enzymes, and function mainly in phagocytosis, proteolysis, and antibody formation. An increase in the number of leukocytes is called *leukocytosis*, a decrease *leukopenia*. There are two main types of leukocytes: nongranular and granular.

Non- or Agranular Leukocytes:

(1) *Lymphocytes* make up between 20 and 25% of total leukocytes and are seldom phagocytic.

They originate from lymphoid tissue and bone marrow, function in immunologic responses and the detoxificiation of noxious substances, and are prevalent at sites of chronic inflammation. Some live several years.

(2) *Monocytes* make up between 3 and 8% of total WBC. They are sometimes phagocytic and help in debridement.

Granular (possess abundant, specific granules) Leukocytes:

(1) *Neutrophils* make up about 65 to 75% of leukocytes. They are twice as large as a RBC and have a lobulated nucleus. They are the most active and phagocytic, providing the first line of defense against invading organisms. Dead neutrophils become *pus*.

(2) *Eosinophils* make up about 2 to 5% WBC. They possess large red acidophilic granules and a bilobed nucleus. Large numbers are found at sites of parasitic infections and allergic reactions (specifically, in the respiratory and digestive tracts). Eosinophils function in the destruction of antigen–antibody complexes.

(3) *Basophils* make up 0.5% or less of the total white blood cell count. They are rarely phagocytic. Basophils contain large quantities of basophilic granules. They are involved in immune phenomena, and produce heparin, which prevents the clotting of blood.

8. **E.** Heartbeat is initiated by the S-A (sino-atrial) node.

9. **D.** The most numerous Leukocytes are the neutrophils (65–75%).

10. **B.** The medulla is a part of the brain stem and connects to the spinal cord at the foramen magnum. The following cranial nerves are associated with the medulla: (a) XII-hypoglossal nerve; (b) XI-spinal accessory nerve; (c) X-vagus nerve; (d) IX-glossopharyngeal nerve; (e) VIII-stato-acoustic nerve; and (f) portions of the facial nerve (VII). The vagus nerve (X) is the most important parasympathetic nerve. Stimulation of vagal fibers slows the heart rate; constricts the smooth muscles of the bronchial tree; stimulates secretion by the bronchial mucosa; and promotes peristalsis, gastric, and pancreatic secretions. Blood pressure control also involves aortic body,

carotid sinus, and carotid body receptor modulation by the glossopharyngeal (IX) and vagus (X) nerves.

11. **D.** An anticoagulant is a substance that prevents or retards coagulation of blood. Heparin is an acid mucopolysaccharide; it occurs most abundantly in the liver. Aspirin (acetylsalicylic acid) is an analgesic, antipyretic, antirheumatic compound that possesses anticoagulant properties. Dicumarol is a trademark for bishydroxycoumarin, an excellent anticoagulant.

12. **C.** Blood pressure is usually measured by placing the sphygmomanometer cuff around the arm to compress the brachial artery and vein. Maximum blood pressure is obtained during ventricular contraction (systole); in our case, 160. Minimum blood pressure indicates ventricular rest (diastole); in our case, 90.

13. **C.** The heart has its own rhythmicity. The rate of contraction and force of contraction, however, are modified by the sympathetic and parasympathetic influences. The S-A node is considered the pacemaker and initiates heartbeat; the A-V node will take over at a slower rate, and its own cardiac rhythmicity will keep the heart beating at a slower rate for some time in this experiment.

14. **A.** From the right ventricle blood is sent to the lungs via the pulmonary arteries; this blood is rich in carbaminohemoglobin and the CO_2 will be exchanged for O_2. Blood returns from the lungs to the left auricle via the pulmonary veins; this blood has been oxygenated and is rich in oxyhemoglobin. Blood then passes to the left ventricle and then out via the aorta to supply the tissues of the body.

15. **B.** Impeded or sluggish venous blood flow, especially of the veins of the lower extremity, can lead to the formation of blood clots. The disease, thrombophlebitis, is characterized by an inflammation of veins with thrombosis.

16. **C.** The inferior vena cava empties into the right atrium and carries deoxygenated blood; blood pressure is low at that point.

Respiratory System

The respiratory system is composed of a conduit for air and an air-blood interface for gaseous exchange in the alveoli of the lungs. The function of the lung is to facilitate movement of oxygen from the air into the pulmonary circulation and the movement of carbon dioxide from the body out. This is accomplished by simple diffusion from an area of high concentration to one of a low partial pressure.

The conducting passages of the respiratory system can be listed as:

(1) external (anterior) nares
(2) nasal cavity with conchae, meatuses, and sinuses
(3) internal (posterior) nares
(4) nasopharynx
(5) oropharynx (communicates with oral cavity and mouth anteriorly)
(6) laryngeal pharynx
(7) larynx (possesses false and true vocal cords)
(8) trachea
(9) primary (left and right) bronchi
(10) secondary (three named ones per lung—one per lobe) bronchi
(11) tertiary bronchi
(12) respiratory bronchioles
(13) alveolar ducts
(14) alveolar sacs
(15) alveoli

The human air passages.

The tracheobronchial tree (anatomic dead space) consists of about 16 generations of branches, while the respiratory unit is made up of an additional seven generations of respiratory bronchioles, alveolar ducts, and alveolar sacs for a total of 23 generations. The last seven are functional in gas exchange. (The upper parts of the respiratory system function in the removal of inhaled particles).

Removal of Inhaled Particles

Large particles are filtered by hairs and mucous material in the nose and respiratory tract. Air is also warmed and humidified. Mucus is continually moved by cilia toward the throat and expelled by swallowing, expectoration, or through the nose. No cilia are present in alyeoli; macrophages and leukocytes debride this area. Material so gathered is removed via the lymphatic system.

Pulmonary Ventilation

Respiratory refers to the gaseous exchanges which occur between the body as a whole and the environment. It entails:

(1) ventilation of the lungs
(2) gas exchange between lungs and blood
(3) transport of gases in the blood
(4) gas exchange between blood and interstitial fluids of the body

Ventilation must be adequate in environments ranging from sea level to high altitude and under degrees of physical activities ranging from sleep to exertion.

Respiratory minute ventilation is the amount of air that one inspires or expires each minute. It is equal to the amount of air inspired with each breath (the *tidal volume*) times the frequency (the number of breaths per minute). With each breath we normally inspire about 500 ml and breathe at a rate of 12 breaths per minute. The resting respiratory minute ventilation under these conditions is 6 1/min. During severe exercise, the respiratory minute ventilation may reach 80 to 100 1/min; this is an indication of the practical upper limit of our respiratory system. Thus a 15-fold increase in ventilation is possible, indicating that the respiratory system has considerable reserve.

Inspiration and Expiration

During inspiration the thoracic cavity expands, its volume increases, and air rushes into the respiratory tract due to the creation of negative pressure; the musculature involved is the diaphragm (innervated by the phrenic nerve) and the external intercostal muscles (innervated by intercostal nerves). During its contraction the diaphragm descends as much as 7 cm; the external intercostal muscles raise the rib cage. Relaxation of these muscles, the stabilization of the thoracic cage by the internal intercostal contraction of the abdominal musculature, plus the elasticity of the lung, return the organ to the pre-inspiratory resting phase. A normal breath involves a volume of about 500 ml. Normal expiration is passive and involves no great muscular contraction. When ventilation exceeds about 40 1/min, expiratory (abdominal) muscles come into play to speed up expiration. By contracting, they push on contents of the abdominal cavity which then push the diaphragm upward, forcing air out of the lungs.

Positive and Negative Pressure Breathing

Gases flow from regions of higher pressure to those of lower pressure. Thus, when the gas pressure in the alveoli is equal to that of the surrounding atmosphere, no movement of gas occurs. For inspiration to occur, the alveolar gas pressure must be less than the atmospheric pressure. There are two ways in which this pressure difference can be produced. The first is by positive pressure breathing as is the case when using a resuscitator. Here the pressure at the nose and mouth (the atmospheric pressure) is made greater than the alveolar gas pressure. The second method is by negative pressure breathing as is the case when using the iron lung. Here the alveolar gas pressure is lowered below atmospheric pressure.

Normal breathing is a form of negative pressure breathing. If we plot intra-alveolar pressure (intrapulmonary pressure) during inspiration and expiration, we see that enlarging the thorax and lungs enables the alveolar gas to expand until its pressure drops below that of the surrounding atmosphere and the inflow of gas then occurs. For expiration to occur, the alveolar gas pressure must be made greater than the atmospheric pressure. This is produced by the natural recoil of the lungs, during which time the alveolar gas is compressed until its pressure is above atmospheric pressure. Gas then flows out of the lungs. Resistance to respiration arises due to the elastic fibers of the lung itself and the surface tension phenomena (forces) present at any liquid-air interface.

Because the inner surface of the lung is lined with a fluid (surfactant, which has a low surface tension), surface tension forces play a role. As a result of this surface tension the alveolus will tend to collapse unless opposed by the inflating pressure. The amount of pressure needed to oppose surface tension and maintain inflation is determined by the Law of Laplace:

$$p = \frac{2T}{\text{radius}}$$

where p = the inflation pressure, T = surface tension forces, and radius means the radius of the alveoli.

With a plasmalike liquid lining the lungs (constant surface tension), as the radius decreases (deflation) the distending pressure increases. Also, smaller alveoli would require a greater distending force than the larger alveoli.

The density of the surfactant molecules at the liquid-air interface is such that at high lung volumes there are few surfactant molecules per unit of area and the surface tension is relatively high (like plasma). As deflation occurs, the surfactant molecules become more concentrated at the liquid air interface, and surface tension becomes relatively low (like surfactant). Thus, during deflation, the alveolar radius is decreasing, tending to increase the needed distending pressure, but the surface tension is becoming less, which tends to decrease the required distending pressure. The lung, therefore, has alveoli which will not collapse until very low pressures are reached (because the surface tension is low), and can have small and large alveoli existing side by side (because the surface tension is area dependent).

Absence of the ability to produce surfactant is a key element in hyaline membrane disease. Infants afflicted die of respiratory distress because their lungs collapse with each breath due to the high surface tension. Extreme muscular efforts are required for reinflation and respiration is very labored in these cases.

Neuronal Control and Integration of Breathing

Normal spontaneous breathing is under control of motor neurons (primarily the phrenic nerves to the diaphragm) which innervate the respiratory muscles. Brain impulses regulate and modulate the process. Voluntary activity originates in the cerebral cortex, automatic (autonomic) control rests in the pons and medulla of the brain.

The respiratory center, located in the medulla, has an inspiratory and an expiratory portion. The ventral portion produces forced and deep inspiration; the dorsal portion produces expiration.

Rhythmicity is spontaneous (12 to 15 times/minute) but is modulated by centers in the pons and medulla and by input from afferent vagal (stretch) receptors located in the lung. Stretching of the lung during inspiration reflexively limits the inspiratory drive.

Smooth muscle in the walls of the airways is innervated by parasympathetic and sympathetic nerves. Parasympathetic stimulation causes bronchoconstriction and an increase in airway resistance. Sympathetic stimulation produces relaxation. (Therefore, during an asthmatic attack it is helpful to inhale an aerosol containing a sympathomimetic drug, a drug that mimics the action of stimulating the sympathetic nervous system.)

Gas Exchange in the Alveoli

Abutting the alveoli (about 150 million/lung) is a large capillary bed providing an enormous diffusion area (about 90 m²) with an extremely thin barrier (about 5000 Å) for gaseous exchange. Gas exchange occurs only in the alveoli and not in the tracheobronchial tree; the nonfunctional space (anatomic dead space) volume comprises about 150 ml. The alveolar portion, known as the respiratory zone, has a volume of about 2,000 ml. The diffusion pathway for alveolar gas may be listed as:

(1) surfactant (lowers surface tension)
(2) alveolar epithelium
(3) interstitium (fused basement membranes)
(4) capillary endothelium (epithelium)
(5) plasma
(6) red blood cell

Oxygen Transport

Oxygen is transported mainly in the form of oxyhemoglobin. Normal hemoglobin (Hb) values are, respectively, 14 g/100 ml for women and 16 g/100 ml for men. Blood then contains an average of 15 g hemoglobin/100 ml blood; each gram of hemoglobin can combine with 1.39 ml of oxygen. Fully oxygenated blood can be calculated thus:

$$(15 \text{ g Hb}/100 \text{ ml blood}) \times (1.39 \text{ ml } O_2/\text{g Hb})$$

to contain 21 ml O_2/ml blood. This is known as the *oxygen capacity* of blood.

If the concentration of oxygen against the PO_2 is plotted, a sigmoid shaped curve, also called the *oxygen dissociation curve,* is obtained.

Four factors affect the affinity of hemoglobin for oxygen:

(1) pH
(2) temperature
(3) concentration of 2,3-diphosphoglycerate (DPG)
(4) carbon dioxide

A decrease in pH, an increase in temperature, or an increase in DPG will facilitate the release of oxygen in the tissue capillaries.

Actively metabolizing tissues have a higher temperature and produce metabolic acids (e.g., lactic acid) and carbonic acid via the reaction of released carbon dioxide and water. An increase in CO_2 and a decrease in affinity of hemoglobin for oxygen with a decrease in pH and an increase in carbamino Hb is called the *Bohr effect*. Most of the oxygen released is due to the decrease in PO_2 in the interstitial fluid but an extra amount is released due to these factors. Chronic hypoxia increases the amount of DPG and thus facilitates oxygen release by this mechanism.

Carbon Dioxide Transport

While some carbon dioxide remains in plasma, most diffuses into red blood cells. Here, it can be (1) transported in physical solution, (2) bound to the amino groups of hemoglobin as carbamino hemoglobin, or, most importantly, (3) converted to bicarbonate ions via its interaction with water to form carbonic acid, which almost completely dissociates into bicarbonate and hydrogen ions. This reaction occurs rapidly in red blood cells because the cells contain the enzyme carbonic anhydrase, which catalyzes the reaction.

The carbon dioxide in plasma can also be transported (1) in physical solution, (2) bound to the amino groups of plasma proteins (although the amount carried as carbamino compounds in plasma is small compared to the amount carried in red blood cells as carbamino hemoglobin), or (3) as bicarbonate ions. Few bicarbonate ions are produced in the plasma, however, because there is no carbonic anhydrase in plasma.

Bicarbonate ions produced in the red blood cells diffuse into the plasma because of the concentration gradient. However, the red blood cell membrane is not very permeable to cations so no positively charged ion can accompany the bicarbonate ions into the plasma. The result is that the inside of the red blood cell is slightly positive and so attracts negatively charged chloride ions from the plasma. This exchange of chloride for bicarbonate is referred to as the *chloride shift*. Thus, although bicarbonate is produced in red blood cells it is transported in plasma.

The hydrogen ions produced are buffered to a great extent by hemoglobin. The fact that reduced hemoglobin holds hydrogen ions more strongly than oxyhemoglobin means that, as oxygen is released to tissues, hydrogen ions generated by the addition of carbon dioxide can be taken up by the deoxygenated (reduced) hemoglobin. Slightly more hydrogen ions are produced than can be handled by the reduced hemoglobin produced. Thus, the pH of venous blood is slightly lower than that of arterial blood.

Because deoxygenated hemoglobin forms carbamino compounds much more readily than oxygenated hemoglobin does, venous blood can handle more CO_2 than can arterial blood.

The changes in the quantity of oxygen and carbon dioxide in the lungs are as indicated:

	Inspired Air, %	Expired Air, %	Change, %
Oxygen	20.96	16.02	4.94 loss
Carbon dioxide	0.04	4.48	4.44 gain

The carbon dioxide resulting from cellular metabolic activity diffuses into the blood because it is less concentrated there; here it then either combines with hemoglobin or is converted into carbonic acid:

$$CO_2 + H_2O \; H_2CO_3$$

The carbonic acid reacts with sodium in the plasma to form sodium bicarbonate:

$$H_2CO_3 + Na^+ \rightarrow NaHCO_3 + H^+$$

or it can react with potassium in the hemoglobin to form potassium bicarbonate:

$$H_2CO_3 + K^+ \rightarrow KHCO_3 + H^+$$

In the lungs the carbon dioxide is dissociated from the bicarbonate and hemoglobin and diffuses into alveolar space air for exchange.

Chemical Regulation of Respiration

Chemical stimulants of physiological importance that affect respiration are:

(1) increased arterial PCO_2 (hypercapnia),
(2) decreased arterial PO_2 (hypoxia),
(3) an increased arterial hydrogen-ion concentration (acidosis).

Arterial $[H^+]$ and PO_2 are monitored by carotid and aortic bodies which contain nerve endings that are sensitive to arterial pH and PO_2. The carotid bodies lie near the carotid sinus at the bifurcation of the common carotid arteries and send impulses through fibers of the glossopharyngeal nerves. The aortic bodies lie near the arch of the aorta; their neural fibers are part of the vagus nerves.

Increases in arterial PCO_2 are also sensed to some extent by these peripheral chemoreceptors (carotid and aortic bodies) but, more importantly, by a central chemosensitive area on the surface of the medulla overlying the medullary respiratory center. This central chemosensitive area, bathed in cerebrospinal fluid (CSF), is sensitive to changes in $[H^+]$ in the CSF. Although hydrogen ions poorly penetrate the blood-brain barrier which separates arterial blood and CSF, carbon dioxide can rapidly diffuse between the two fluids. Thus, arterial PCO_2 and CSF PCO_2 equilibrate. Once in the CSF, carbon dioxide reacts with water to form carbonic acid, which dissociates into bicarbonate and hydrogen ions. The central chemosensitive area is sensitive to the pH changes thus produced. In a similar manner (but of less importance) arterial PCO_2 alters arterial pH, which is best detected by the carotid and aortic bodies.

Oxygen lack stimulates ventilation solely by its effect on the peripheral chemoreceptors, but alveolar PO_2 must fall to low levels (50 to 60 membrane Hg) before ventilation begins to increase. However, some chemoreceptor discharge is present at normal oxygen tensions. Hypercapnia, which often accompanies hypoxia, will potentiate sensitivity of peripheral chemoreceptors to hypoxia. Hypoxia is the stimulus for increased ventilation observed at high altitudes.

Acidosis stimulates ventilation mainly via peripheral chemoreceptors. Arterial $[H^+]$ may also affect the central chemosensitive area but its influence there is slow in onset and much less pronounced. Hyperventilation driven by acidosis will "blow off" CO_2 and generate alkalosis in the CSF, which tends to depress ventilation. The results of these opposing forces is a lesser increase in ventilation than would occur with a constant arterial PCO_2. The effects of acidosis and either hypoxia or hypercapnia are additive with no complicated potentiation occurring.

Ventilation is much more sensitive to hypercapnia than to either hypoxia or acidosis. Changes in ventilation produced by hypercapnia are only slightly altered when the peripheral chemoreceptors are denervated, indicating the importance of the central chemosensitive area in monitoring CO_2. Hypoxia potentiates this CO_2 sensitivity.

Quick Recall Test Questions and Answers

Choose the Best Answer

1. Exchange in the lung of CO_2 and O_2 takes place in the:

   A. bronchi.
   B. bronchioles.
   C. alveoli.
   D. broncho-pulmonary segment.
   E. dust cells.

2. Blood pH is influenced by respiration; experimental hyperventilation in a physiology laboratory will result in the student's blood pH being:

   A. lowered.
   B. raised.
   C. unaffected.
   D. raised to pH6.

3. An area of the lung involved in gas exchange includes the:

   A. trachea.
   B. primary bronchi.
   C. alveolar ducts.
   D. pharynx.
   E. tertiary bronchi.

4. During exercise, an individual's tidal volume is 2L and her rate of breathing is 20 breaths/minute. Under these exercising conditions the respiratory minute ventilation is:

   A. 0.4 L/min.
   B. 1.0 L/min.
   C. 4.0 L/min.
   D. 10 L/min.
   E. 40 L/min.

5. Contraction of the diaphragm:

   A. decreases the volume of the thoracic cavity.
   B. makes the intra-alveolar pressure less than atmospheric pressure.
   C. is responsible for "positive pressure breathing."
   D. occurs during expiration.
   E. is accompanied by abdominal muscle contraction.

6. Respiratory distress in an infant (hyaline membrane disease) is associated with:

   A. high surface tension in the lungs.
   B. lungs that are more compliant than normal lungs (i.e., not as stiff).

   C. high concentrations of surfactant in the lungs.
   D. large alveoi collapsing before smaller ones.
   E. a decrease in the inflation pressure required to keep the lungs open.

7. Of the following, quantitatively the most important for transporting carbon dioxide is:

   A. carboxyhemoglobin.
   B. carbaminohemoglobin.
   C. carbonic anhydrase.
   D. dissolved carbon dioxide.
   E. bicarbonate ions.

8. Which of the following will facilitate the release of oxygen from the blood to the tissues?

   A. an increase in the partial pressure of carbon dioxide
   B. a decrease in temperature
   C. an increase in pH
   D. a decrease in diphosphoglycerate concentration

9. *Most* hydrogen ions produced when carbon dioxide is added to blood:

   A. are taken up by reduced hemoglobin molecules.
   B. are buffered by albumin and other plasma proteins.
   C. remain free and produce a large pH shift to the acid state.
   D. are buffered by bicarbonate ions in plasma.
   E. are removed by carbonic anhydrase.

10. The increase in ventilation that occurs at high altitude is stimulated by:

    A. hypercapnia.
    B. hypoxemia.
    C. decreased blood pH.
    D. cerebrospinal fluid acidosis.

Answers

1. **C.** CO_2 and O_2 exchange takes place in the alveoli of the lung.

2. **B.** Hyperventilation is abnormally rapid, deep breathing resulting in a loss of CO_2 and an increase in blood pH. A person would be in the state of respiratory alkalosis, since a decreased blood concentration of hydrogen ion is the result of pulmonary CO_2 elimination.

3. **C.** Gas exchange occurs only in the alveoli and not in the tracheobronchial tree. The alveolar portion, known as the respiratory zone, has a volume of about 2000 ml.

4. **E.** Respiratory minute ventilation, or the amount of air that we inspire or expire each minute, is equal to the amount of air inspired with each breath (the tidal volume) times the frequency (the number of breaths per minute). With each breath we normally inspire about 500 ml and breathe at a rate of 12 breaths per minute. The resting respiration minute ventilation under these conditions is 6 L/min.

5. **B.** During inspiration the thoracic cavity expands, its volume increases, and air rushes into the respiratory tract because of the creation of negative pressure; the musculature involved is the diaphragm (innervated by the phrenic nerve) and the external intercostal muscles (innervated by intercostal nerves).

6. **A.** Because the inner surface of the lung is lined with a fluid (surfactant, which has a low surface tension), surface tension forces play a role. As a result of this surface tension the alveolus will tend to collapse unless opposed by the inflating pressure.

7. **E.** While some carbon dioxide remains in plasma, most diffuses into red blood cells. Here, it can be (1) transported in physical solution, (2) bound to the amino groups of hemoglobin as carbaminohemoglobin, or, most importantly, (3) converted to bicarbonate ions via its interaction with water to form carbonic acid, which almost completely dissociates into bicarbonate and hydrogen ions. This reaction occurs rapidly in red blood cells because the cells contain the enzyme carbonic anhydrase, which catalyzes the reaction.

8. **A.** A decrease in pH, an increase in temperature, or an increase in DPG will facilitate the release of oxygen in the tissue capillaries. Actively metabolizing tissues have a higher temperature and produce metabolic acids (e.g., lactic acid) and carbonic acid via the reaction of released carbon dioxide and water.

9. **A.** Chemical stimulants of physiological importance that affect respiration are:
   (1) increased arterial PCO_2 (hypercapnia).
   (2) decreased arterial PO_2 (hypoxia).
   (3) increased arterial hydrogen-ion concentration (acidosis).

10. **C.** Oxygen lack stimulates ventilation solely by its effect on the peripheral chemoreceptors, but alveolar PO_2 must fall to low levels (50 to 60 mm Hg) before ventilation begins to increase. However, some chemoreceptor discharge is present at normal oxygen tensions. Hypercapnia, which often accompanies hypoxia, will potentiate sensitivity of peripheral chemoreceptors to hypoxia. Hypoxia is the stimulus for increased ventilation observed at high altitudes. Acidosis stimulates ventilation mainly via peripheral chemoreceptors. Arterial [H$^+$] may also affect the central chemosensitive area but its influence there is slow in onset and much less pronounced. Hyperventilation driven by acidosis will "blow off" CO_2 and generate alkalosis in the CSF, which tends to depress ventilation. The results of these opposing forces is a lesser increase in ventilation than would occur with a constant PCO_2. The effects of acidosis and either hypoxia or hypercapnia are additive with no complicated potentiation occurring. Ventilation is much more sensitive to hypercapnia than to either hypoxia or acidosis. Changes in ventilation produced by hypercapnia are only slightly altered when the peripheral chemoreceptors are denervated, indicating the importance of the central chemosensitive area in monitoring CO_2. Hypoxia potentiates this CO_2 sensitivity.

Urinary System

The urinary system has been charged by evolution with the protection of the *milieu interieur* of Claude Bernard, the great French physiologist. For organisms living in an aqueous environment, this protection requires a relatively simple mechanism, but for land dwellers such protection is critical for survival. Thus, we must think of excretion by way of the urinary tract as the end result of conservation of all useful circulating materials and simultaneous elimination of waste material. By contrast, excretion via the digestive tract is the end result of ingestion of either indigestible material or nutritional matter which remains unabsorbed. Overall then, the gut provides the nutrients to the blood, which is filtered by the kidney; the nutrients are then returned while waste is lost. Sugars, electrolytes, and amino acids are reclaimed from the filtrate at an efficiency of 95% or better. Given the large daily volume of digestive tract secretions, there is very efficient (almost 99%) water absorption in the gut but slightly lower efficiency of water absorption in the kidney, which must use a minimal volume of loss to solubilize the waste. Indeed, it is the ability to vary this efficiency of fluid absorption which accounts for the remarkable ability of the kidney to defend the osmolarity of the body fluids. The kidney also plays a critical role in adjustment of blood pH through its ability to vary urinary acid excretion and bicarbonate reabsorption. Finally, the kidney is a major factor in the maintenance of skeletal integrity through its ability to vary calcium and phosphate loss into the urine in response to vitamin D. It should not be forgotten that the kidney is the site of production of the 1,25-dihydroxy form of vitamin D, the most biologically active form of the vitamin.

Kidney

Ureter

Urinary bladder

The human urinary system in place in the human body. The dotted line represents the position of the diaphragm.

Structure of the Kidney

The kidney is a bean-shaped organ encased by a fibrous capsule and embedded within a fatty connective tissue and perirenal fascia. The kidney lies deep to the *peritoneum* (i.e., retroperitoneal) which lines the abdomino-pelvic cavity. It is approximately 10 cm long, 5 cm wide, and 3 cm thick. Its medial aspect, which is indented or concave, is known as the *renal hilus (hilum);* it is the location for the renal arteries and veins as well as for the renal pelvis. The hilus leads into a cavity, the *renal sinus,* within the kidney which contains fat, blood vessels, nerves, calyces, and renal pelvis.

The internal aspect of the kidney when bissected in a medial to lateral plane presents two zones; an outer *cortex* and an inner *medulla.* The medulla is adjacent to the renal sinus. The cortex is redder in appearance and has fine striations known as *medullary rays.* These striations are due to medullary structures (collecting tubules) extending into the cortex. The medulla consists of triangular (pyramidal) structures, *the renal pyramids,* separated by columns of cortical material known as *renal columns*. The bases of the renal pyramids face the cortex while the apices or *papillae* extend into the *minor calyces*.

The kidney is divided into functional *lobes,* each defined as one renal pyramid, its abutting cortex and part of the two adjacent renal columns. There are about 6 to 18 lobes. A *lobule* of a kidney is considered to be a medullary ray and the adjacent nephrons draining into the collecting ducts forming the ray.

The functional unit of the kidney is the *uriniferous tubule,* which consists of a *nephron* and a *collecting tubule* (duct) within the kidney. There are 1 to 3 million/kidney. The individual nephron is considered by many as the functional unit and the collecting tubule as a separate entity being part of the internal excretory pathway for urine.

Nephron: The nephron comprises the glomerulus and a tubular structure about 30–40 mm long and lined by epithelium. There is a remarkable similarity of the tubule to the gut, in that the epithelial lining of each segment of both structures is suited to its function. There is a much more important relationship between the two organs, however, in that the carrier proteins of the columnar epithelium are under the direction of the same genes, since inherited disorders of active transport in the nephron are often expressed in an identical fashion in the gut. The functionally sequential regions of the nephron are the glomerulus, the proximal convoluted and straight tubular segments, the loop of Henle (descending and ascending), and the distal convoluted tubule. The urine that exits the distal tubule enters the collecting duct and eventually finds its way to the renal pelvis and into the bladder.

Structure of the kidney and its fine structures. (a) A sagittal section of the kidney showing the entry and exit of the renal artery and renal vein, respectively. Note the minor calyx leading to the major calyx then to the renal calyx and the renal pelvis and ureter for the elimination of urine. (b) The renal cortex and renal medulla are enlarged and the nephron can be seen. The swollen portion is Bowman's capsule. Tubes lead down into the renal medulla then turn up back toward the cortex. Here they join with ducts leading down to the minor calyx. (c) A nephron expanded to show its details. Note the location of the capsule and how it leads to the proximal tubule, Henle's loop, the distal tubule, and the collecting duct. The peritubular capillary is not shown.

Bowman's capsule is embryonically formed by a capillary tuft (glomerulus) invaginating the blind end of a tubule, reflecting the outer layer back onto itself and forming the *visceral* and *parietal* epithelial layers. These layers are continuous with each other at the rim of the invagination, and the space between the layers is called *Bowman's space*. The original outer layer of epithelium, now in contact with the glomerulus, is the visceral layer and the two structures together form a unit called the *renal corpuscle (corpuscle of Malpighi)*. The entry and exit point of the corpuscular capillary arterioles is called the *vascular pole*, while the point at which Bowman's capsule is continuous with the proximal tubule is called the *urinary pole* of the renal corpuscle.

The visceral epithelial cell becomes a highly specialized *podocyte*, which has *pedicels (foot processes)* that are contiguous with the capillary endothelium. Thus, the structure called the *filtration barrier* is a complex of capillary endothelium which is fenestrated, a *basement membrane* interposed between the endothelium and the podocyte, and the membrane of each podocytic foot process; between each foot process is the *filtration slit*. It is imperative to a complete understanding of renal function to avoid the conclusion that the fluid which eventually enters the tubular opening is a simple filtrate—this despite the terminology. In fact, much of the selectivity of the so-called filtration barrier rests upon electrostatic charge determined by the chemical composition of the various membrane components. This concept of electrostatic regulation of membrane permeability is fundamental to other processes in the body, such as calcium channels which have become pharmacologically important in management of cardiovascular function, using calcium channel-blocking agents. The fluid which leaves the capillary arterioles to enter Bowman's capsule contains virtually all of the same soluble materials found in blood, including albumin. However, this fluid must get across the filtration barrier to reach the tubule, and in the process it gives up a great deal of the protein, which is returned into the blood.

Once crossing the barrier, the glomerular ultrafiltrate (as it is now called) enters the convoluted proximal tubule. Given the high concentrations (in relation to blood) of amino acids and glucose, as well as electrolytes and other soluble materials, it is clear that prior to excretion as urine, many changes will take place in this fluid. In very large measure, the columnar epithelial cells lining the proximal tubule are responsible for these changes, although the remainder of the nephron makes very important contributions as well.

Collecting Tubules: The route for the filtrate and exoretory product is from Bowman's space through the proximal convoluted tubule, descending thick and thin limbs of the loop of Henle, ascending thin and thick limbs, distal convoluted tubule and then into the collecting tubule. The latter unite and form 10 to 25 larger collecting ducts (papillary ducts of Bellini) which extend into the renal pyramids and terminate at the papillae.

The urine passes from the ends of these large collecting ducts into funnel-shaped collecting vessels, the *minor calyces,* into which the papillae extend. The 7 to 18 minor calyces empty into 2 to 3 *major calyces,* which are larger funnels that terminate in the *renal pelvis*. The renal pelvis is the terminal collecting site for urine in the kidney and is continuous with the ureter at the hilum of the kidney.

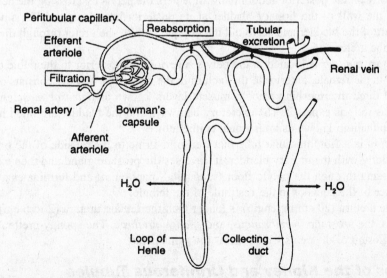

Activity at the nephron. Fluid passes from the bloodstream into the wall of Bowman's capsule during the process of filtration. The efferent arteriole becomes the peritubular capillary, and materials pass back into the capillary during reabsorption. The fluid passes through Henle's loop, then receives more materials from the peritubular capillary by tubular excretion. The blood then passes out a vein, while the fluid (urine) moves to the collecting duct.

THE NEPHRON AND ITS FUNCTION

STRUCTURE	FUNCTION	NATURE OF URINE
Renal corpuscle	Deliver blood; make ultrafiltrate.	Same as plasma, contains equivalent electrolytes, is isosmolar, very little albumin.
Proximal convoluted tubule	Active transport of sugars, amino acids, bicarbonate and electrolytes, passive water reabsorption, secretion of uric acid and other waste.	Diminished volume, isosmolar with plasma.
Descending loop of Henle	Passive diffusion of water, Na^+ and Cl^- out into medulla; water remains in medulla, while Na^+ and Cl^- diffuse back into loop.	Smaller volume, hypertonic with respect to plasma.
Ascending loop of Henle	Impermeable to water, Cl^- actively pumped to interstitium; Na^+ follows passively.	Little change in volume; becomes hypotonic.
Distal convoluted tubule	Reabsorption of Na^+, secretion of K^+, and H^+; regulated by aldosterone; excretion of fixed acids, net H excretion.	Decreased pH, lower Na^+, and very little bicarbonate, volume can change (see "Collecting ducts").
Collecting ducts	Variably permeable to water; regulated by antidiuretic hormone (ADH).	Both volume and osmolarity vary, depending upon ADH secretion by neurohypophysis.

Tubular Passageways

The *ureter* is a long muscular tube which connects the renal pelvis to the urinary bladder. It passes inferiorly on the posterior abdominal wall, enters the pelvis by crossing the pelvic inlet, and then pierces the wall of the urinary bladder at its posterior-lateral aspect. The smooth muscles which are part of the bladder and surround the oblique path of the ureter through the wall act as a sphincter of the ureter.

The *urinary bladder* is located in the pelvis superior and posterior to the pubic bone, anterior to the uterus in the female, anterior to the rectum in the male. The bladder consists of a thick wall composed of three intermeshing smooth muscle layers known as *detrusor muscles*. The bladder stores urine as well as expels it. The excretory pathways and the bladder are lined by the urinary type of the epithelium known as transitional epithelium.

The *urethra* is a fibromuscular tube that transmits urine to the outside of the body. It is continuous inferiorly with the urinary bladder. It traverses the prostate gland and then exits the pelvic cavity by passing through the pelvic floor (urogenital diaphragm) and terminates at the external urethral orifice of the penis or in the vestibule of the female.

The male urethra (20 cm in length) is longer than the female urethra (2 to 6 cm) and consists of three parts: the *prostatic, membranous,* and *spongy urethrae.* The spongy urethra is within the corpus spongiosum of the penis which forms the glans penis.

Functions of the Kidney and Uriniferous Tubules

The kidney, during the production of urine,

(a) excretes the waste products of metabolism;
(b) maintains the fluid volume of the extracellular regions of the body;

(c) excretes foreign materials from the body;

(d) regulates the type and concentration of salts retained in the body (maintain electrolyte balance);

(e) regulates the total body water;

(f) regulates the acid–base balance of the body.

The physiological processes occurring during the production of urine are

(a) *filtration*—the production of an ultrafiltrate of plasma within Bowman's space;

(b) *reabsorption*— the selective removal of material from the ultrafiltrate as it passes through the tubular nephron and the return of these substances into peritubular capillaries;

(c) *secretion*—the cells forming the nephron actively secrete material into the filtrate;

(d) *passive diffusion*—diffusion of fluids along the osmotic gradient.

Filtration: Once again, this process, as it occurs within the renal corpuscle, is not a simple event which merely depends upon pore size. It is certainly true that the filtration barrier prohibits intact red cells from following the fluid in which they are suspended. However, albumin, which is completely soluble in plasma, is also excluded from the capsular space to a very large extent—an exclusion which could only derive from the existence of an electrostatic barrier. Indeed, normal urine contains no albumin, although there are diseases of the filtration barrier which may result in excretion of up to 9 g of albumin per day. This gives a true sense of the tremendous efficiency of the kidney, which normally clears 25% of the total cardiac output of blood per minute, forming approximately 120–130 ml of filtrate per minute. Thus, in a day the kidneys will receive 5000 L for filtration, form about 170–180 L of ultrafiltrate, and put out approximately 1–2 L of urine—an ultimate efficiency of fluid retention of 99.8%, and clear proof that Claude Bernard was correct!

The factors in formation of the ultrafiltrate are:

(a) *filtration pressure* (about 25 mm Hg), which is the net pressure differential between the driving force within the glomerular arterioles and the total back pressure exerted by osmotic pressure of the blood + pressure within Bowman's space and the proximal tubule. Thus, fluid is driven outward from the capillary against the filtration barrier under pressure, where its contents either pass through the barrier or are selectively absorbed by the podocytes before they can enter the tubule.

(b) *pore size,* which prevents passage of protein with molecular weights > 70,000, as well as red and white blood cells.

The conseqence of these two factors is to produce an ultrafiltrate which is similar to plasma, is isotonic to blood, and contains most of the soluble elements of plasma, except for large quantities of albumin and cells.

Reabsorption: The ultrafiltrate, isotonic with plasma, enters the proximal tubule, which is lined with columnar epithelium; the cell surface (luminal) facing the tubular opening has many microvilli, called the brush border, precisely like the columnar epithelium of the proximal small intestine (jejunum). This surface is the site of the carrier, or transport proteins, which exhibit specificity for particular sugars and amino acids and which subserve active transport. This efficient system results in reabsorption of

(a) > 95% of filtered amino acids

(b) > 98% of filtered glucose

(c) 85% of the sodium, chloride, and bicarbonate

(d) calcium, magnesium, and phosphate

There is also a passive diffusion of 80–85% of the filtered water, which follows the concentration gradient established through the active transport of the solutes listed above. In addition, any trace amounts of albumin which escape the filtration barrier and enter the proximal tubule are taken up by pinocytosis, or are hydrolyzed by membrane-bound enzymes into smaller peptide units.

Secretion: The cells of the proximal tubule are also capable of secretion and routinely put out a number of substances into the urine forming in the lumen. These materials include creatinine, uric acid, antibiotics, drug metabolites, and radiopaque dyes. It should be recognized that the majority of these materials derive not from the renal parenchyma, but from the blood, so that secretion depends upon intracellular transport in a direction opposite to that for reabsorption. The secretion of urate becomes an important factor in evaluation of uric acid excretion in patients with gout.

Passive Diffusion: Although the passage of the ultrafiltrate through the proximal convoluted tubule results in dramatic decreases in solute within the lumen, there has also been fluid reabsorption in proportion. Thus, the urine which enters the descending loop of Henle remains isosmotic with plasma, although very much diminished in volume. The function of the loop, overall, is to produce urine which is hypertonic to plasma, a task that is accomplished by a countercurrent multiplier system. The basis for this process is the difference in water permeability between the descending (permeable) and ascending (impermeable) limbs of the loop. Thus, as the urine passes through the descending loop, Na^+, Cl^- and water pass through the wall by passive diffusion down a concentration gradient. Toward the end of the descending loop, the water which has left the tubular lumen continues to diffuse outward into the relatively hypertonic interstitium of the renal medulla, leaving the Na^+ and Cl^- to diffuse back into the loop, following a new concentration gradient. Effectively, the process succeeds in separating water from solute. In the ascending loop, the wall of the tubule is impermeable to water and is capable of actively pumping Cl^- out into the interstitium. Sodium ions follow chloride ions passively, thereby diminishing the tonicity of the urine and increasing the tonicity of the interstitium, since water cannot also passively diffuse. The creation of a hypertonic interstitium in the renal medulla is key to water reabsorption in the collecting duct system, a major regulatory system of the osmolarity of plasma which is under neuroendocrine regulatory control.

Elimination of Fixed Acids and Hydrogen Ions: Fixed acid is that quantity of acid which is produced by the cells but cannot be further degraded or eliminated through conversion to CO_2. The largest proportion of fixed acid is generally represented by phosphate, followed by lactate and beta-hydroxybutyrate. In contrast to the major body buffer system containing carbonic acid which can be converted to CO_2 and excreted easily by the lungs, these compounds are not volatile and will rapidly accumulate if not excreted by other means. In the distal tubule, the now-hypotonic urine containing these materials, whose pH is essentially the same as that of the ultrafiltrate, is made acid under normal circumstances. Reabsorption of Na^+ by exchange with K^+ and H^+ allows formation of mono- and dihydrogen potassium phosphates; simultaneously, the distal tubule generates NH_4^+ for production of ammonium phosphate salts and net excretion of hydrogen ions. The rate of exchange between sodium and potassium-hydrogen is regulated by *aldosterone*, a steroid hormone produced in the adrenal cortex.

Control of Water Reabsorption and Osmolarity: The pituitary gland, or neurohypohysis, regulates the plasma osmolarity by exerting control over water reabsorption at the level of the distal and collecting ducts. It does so by secretion of the *antidiuretic hormone* (ADH); since "diuresis" implies urinary fluid excretion, ADH diminishes urinary volume by increasing the permeability of the distal tubule and collecting ducts to water. Because of the hypertonicity of the medullary interstitium, water passes out of these structures into the interstitial space by passive diffusion and leaves concentrated urine behind. The increased water in the interstitium enters the circulation by way of the medullary vascular network (*vasa recta*) and reduces plasma osmolarity, thus inhibiting further ADH secretion. A frequent result of head trauma or severe cerebral hypoxia is the "syndrome of inappropriate ADH secretion," in which urine flow becomes very slow and plasma osmolarity decreases to dangerous levels.

As an important summary or overview, the kidney should be viewed as an organ which is a great deal more than a simple filter. Not only does it return biologically vital material to the body, but it regulates acid-base, electrolyte, and osmolar balances at the same time as it eliminates waste material into urine. It is also a highly metabolic organ which can help the liver in processes like gluconeogenesis and glycogenesis, as well as participating in partial detoxification of a number of harmful substances.

Hormonal Control of Secretion and Resorption

The simple cuboidal epithelium lining the distal convoluted tubule may also increase the Na$^+$ concentration in the interstitium by reabsorbing Na$^+$. At the same time, potassium ions (K$^+$) are excreted into the tubular lumen. The latter processes are regulated by *aldosterone,* a hormone produced by the adrenal cortex. The distal convoluted tubules also participate in maintaining the acid–base balance of the blood by adding hydrogen and ammonium ions into the filtrate.

The permeability of water through the walls of the distal convoluted tubules and collecting tubules is regulated by the *antidiuretic hormone* (ADH) secreted by the posterior lobe of the pituitary gland (neurohypophysis). The presence of this hormone makes these tubules more permeable to water. Because the interstitium of the renal pyramids is more highly concentrated (hypertonic) than the filtrate, water exits the collecting tubules and passes into the interstitium. This process continues along the length of the collecting ducts and results in concentrating the urine which therefore is *hypertonic*. The amount of water resorbed is regulated by ADH production. For example, an increase in ADH increases resorption of water resulting in a more hypertonic urine, whereas a decrease in ADH decreases resorption resulting in the excretion of more water and therefore, a diluted or hypotonic urine. Diuretic drugs counteract the action of ADH, causing less water resorption and increased urine volume. The osmotic gradient in the renal pyramids is also maintained by the *vasa recta* adjacent to the collecting tubules due to flow of water and Na$^+$ into and out of the vessel lumen. This establishes a countercurrent exchange system between the arterioles and venulae rectae.

Quick Recall Test Questions and Answers

Choose the Best Answer

1. Which of the following structure/function relationships is appropriately paired?

   A. glomerulus—produces ultrafiltrate isotonic to blood.
   B. proximal tubule—chloride ions are reabsorbed.
   C. loop of Henle (descending limb)—water diffuses out and urine becomes hypertonic.
   D. loop of Henle (ascending limb)—chlorine ions are actively reabsorbed and urine becomes hypotonic.
   E. All of the above are correctly paired.

2. Filtration in the kidneys results mainly from:

   A. blood flow (m/sec).
   B. reabsorption.
   C. blood pressure.
   D. secretion.
   E. osmotic phenomenon.

3. The functional unit of the kidney that is concerned with urine formation is the nephron; it consists of all of the following EXCEPT:

   A. Bowman's capsule
   B. proximal convoluted tubule.
   C. loop of Henle.
   D. distal convoluted tubule.
   E. minor calyx.

4. The kidney-filtered fluid leaving the distal convoluted tubule passes next through structures in which order?

   A. minor calyx → major calyx → urethra → urinary bladder
   B. collecting duct → minor calyx → major calyx → pelvis
   C. pelvis → ureter → urinary bladder → urethra
   D. descending limb of Henle → collecting duct → ureter → bladder
   E. proximal tubule → loop of Henle → collecting duct → minor calyx

5. A defining feature of active transport is:

   A. binding of solute to a carrier molecule.
   B. sterospecificity of substrate binding.
   C. existence of membrane pores.
   D. energy expenditure.

   E. the fact that it is more rapid than simple diffusion.

6. Which of the following structure—function relationships is NOT correct?

   A. glomerulus—produces ultrafiltrate isotonic to blood.
   B. proximal tubule—active reabsorption of glucose, sodium and potassium.
   C. descending limb—water diffuses out of lumen, urine becomes hypertonic.
   D. ascending limb—chloride ions are actively reabsorbed and urine becomes hypotonic.
   E. distal convoluted tubule—primary site of acidification and urine becomes hypertonic to blood plasma.

7. The kidney plays a role in:

   A. maintaining electrolyte balance.
   B. regulating acid-base balance.
   C. maintaining fluid volume of the extracellular regions.
   D. maintaining blood volume.
   E. all of the above.

8. Antidiuretic hormone (ADH) elicits its effect (conserving water) on the:

   A. glomerulus.
   B. proximal tubule.
   C. descending limb.
   D. ascending limb.
   E. distal convoluted and collecting tubules.

9. The _____ is a long muscular tube which connects the renal pelvis to the urinary bladder.

   A. urethra
   B. uriniferous tubule
   C. collecting tubule
   D. ureter
   E. nephron

10. The internal aspect of the kidney when bisected in a medial to lateral plane presents two zones:

   A. renal hilus and renal sinus.
   B. major and minor calyx.
   C. cortex and medulla.
   D. renal pyramids and columns.
   E. capsule and collecting tubules.

11. Major reabsorption of substances from the ultra-filtrate occurs in the proximal convoluted tubule and results in:

   A. the active reabsorption of all the glucose.
   B. the active reabsorption of 85% of the sodium chloride.
   C. the passive diffusion, due to the osmotic gradient, of 85% of the water from the filtrate.
   D. the active transport of all amino acids, ascorbic acid, and proteins.
   E. all of the above.

12. The ascending limb of the loop of Henle is:

   A. permeable to water.
   B. impermeable to water.
   C. permeable to Na^+ and Cl^-
   D. impermeable to Na^+ and Cl^-

13. Aldosterone is the most powerful mineralocorticoid. All of the following are true statements EXCEPT:

   A. It functions in the retention of water.
   B. It functions in the retention of sodium and chloride.
   C. It increases urinary loss of potassium and phosphorus.
   D. It is essential for life.
   E. It is under pituitary control.

14. The kidney in humans removes most waste products by:

   A. filtering fluid from blood, then resorbing the useful solutes.
   B. filtering fluid from the coelom, then resorbing the useful solutes.
   C. selectively transporting the waste products into the urine.
   D. selectively transporting the waste products into the feces.

15. The glomeruli of the human kidney are responsible for:

   A. selective resorption of water from the urine (controlled by antidiuretic hormone).
   B. resorption of glucose and amino acids from the urine.
   C. selective resorption of salt from the urine (controlled by aldosterone).
   D. establishment of a high salt concentration in the medulla of the kidney.
   E. ultrafiltration of water and solutes from blood plasma into the nephron.

16. The proximal convoluted tubules of the human kidney are responsible for:

   A. selective resorption of water from the urine (controlled by antidiuretic hormone).
   B. resorption of glucose and amino acids from the urine.
   C. selective resorption of salt from the urine (controlled by aldosterone).
   D. establishment of a high salt concentration in the medulla of the kidney.
   E. ultrafiltration of water and solutes from blood plasma into the nephron.

17. The loop of Henle of the human kidney is responsible for:

   A. selective resorption of water from the urine (controlled by antidiuretic hormone).
   B. resorption of glucose and amino acids from the urine.
   C. selective resorption of salt from the urine (controlled by aldosterone).
   D. establishment of a high salt concentration in the medulla of the kidney.
   E. ultrafiltration of water and solutes from blood plasma into the nephron.

18. The distal convoluted tubules of the human kidney are responsible for:

   A. selective resorption of water from the urine (controlled by antidiuretic hormone).
   B. resorption of glucose and amino acids from the urine.
   C. selective resorption of salt from the urine (controlled by aldosterone).
   D. establishment of a high salt concentration in the medulla of the kidney.
   E. ultrafiltration of water and solutes from blood plasma into the nephron.

19. The collecting ducts of the human kidney are responsible for:

   A. selective resorption of water from the urine (controlled by antidiuretic hormone).
   B. resorption of glucose and amino acids from the urine.
   C. selective resorption of salt from the urine (controlled by aldosterone).
   D. establishment of a high salt concentration in the medulla of the kidney.
   E. ultrafiltraction of water and solutes from blood plasma into the nephron.

Answers

1. **E.** All the pairings are appropriate. Review the material if you erred.

2. **C.** The peculiar features of renal circulation, such as the renal arteries originating directly from the aorta, the glomerulo-capillary arrangement, and differences in calibers of the afferent and efferent vessels indicate that blood pressure is of great functional significance for the production of urine. The vascular component probably plays an important role in the filtration process.

3. **E.** The nephron is a tubular structure about 30–40 mm long and lined by epithelium. It functions in producing an ultrafiltrate and then reabsorbing material from and excreting substances into the filtrate, resulting in an excretory product. It consists of several morphologically and physiologically different sections forming a continuous tubular unit. The regions of a nephron sequentially are: Bowman's capsule, proximal convoluted tubule, loop of Henle, and distal convoluted tubule. The latter is continuous with the collecting tubule (excretory duct) draining it. The loop of Henle extends into the medullary pyramid while the other three regions are found entirely in the cortex.

    Nephrons vary in their level or position in the cortex, with the cortical nephrons abutting the medulla. These vary in that the size of the renal corpuscle and the length of the loop of Henle are larger in the juxtamedullary nephrons.

4. **B.** The route for the filtrate and excretory product is from Bowman's space through the proximal convoluted tubule, descending thick and thin limbs of the loop of Henle, ascending thin and thick limbs and the distal convoluted tubule, and then moving into the collecting tubule. The latter unite and form 10 to 25 larger collecting ducts (papillary ducts of Bellini) which extend into the renal pyramids and terminate at the papillae.

    The urine passes from the ends of these large collecting ducts into funnel-shaped collecting vessels, the minor calyces, into which the papillae extend. The 7 to 18 minor calyces empty into 2 to 3 major calyces, which are larger funnels that terminate in the renal pelvis. The renal pelvis is the terminal collecting site for urine in the kidney and is continuous with the ureter at the hilum of the kidney.

5. **D.** Active transport makes it possible for a cell to maintain internal concentrations of small molecules that differ from concentrations in the immediate vicinity. The transport is "uphill" against the concentration gradient; the cell must expend energy to accomplish this phenomenon.

6. **E.** In the distal convuluted tubule, more sodium is lost. It is replaced by potassium, hydrogen, and ammonia. This area is also the primary site of acidification, and water is reabsorbed by osmosis.

7. **E.** The kidney, during production of urine,
    (a) excretes the waste products of metabolism;
    (b) maintains the fluid volume of the extracellular regions of the body;
    (c) excretes foreign materials from the body;
    (d) regulates the type and concentration of salts retained in the body (maintain electrolyte balance);
    (e) regulates the total body water;
    (f) regulates the acid-base balance of the body.

8. **E.** The permeability of water through the walls of the distal convoluted tubules and collecting tubules is regulated by the antidiuretic hormone (ADH) secreted by the posterior lobe of the pituitary gland (neurohypophysis). The presence of this hormone makes these tubules more permeable to water. Because the interstitium of the renal pyramids is more highly concentrated (hypertonic) than the filtrate, water exits the collecting tubules and passes into the interstitium. This process continues along the length of the collecting ducts and results in concentrating the urine, which therefore is hypertonic. The amount of water resorbed is regulated by ADH production. For example, an increase in ADH increases resorption of water, resulting in a more hypertonic urine; a decrease in ADH decreases resorption, resulting in the excretion of more water and therefore a diluted or hypotonic urine.

9. **D.** The ureter is a long muscular tube which connects the renal pelvis to the urinary bladder. It passes inferiorly on the posterior abdominal walls, enters the pelvis by crossing the pelvic inlet, and then pierces the wall of the urinary bladder at its posterior-lateral aspect. The smooth muscles which are part of the bladder and surround the oblique path of the ureter through the wall act as a sphincter of the ureter.

10. **C.** The internal aspect of the kidney when bissected in a medial to lateral plane presents two zones; and outer cortex and an inner medulla. The medulla is adjacent to the renal sinus. The cortex is redder in appearance and has fine striations known as medullary rays. These striations are due to medullary structures (collecting tubules) extending into the cortex. The medulla consists of triangular (pyramidal) structures, the renal pyramids, separated by columns of cortical material known as renal columns. The bases of the renal pyramids face the cortex while the apices or papillae extend into the minor calyces.

11. **E.** The functions of the proximal convoluted tubule are stated in responses **A** to **D**.

12. **B.** The loop of Henle functions by setting up the mechanism (countercurrent multiplier system) in the renal medulla for the production of hypertonic urine. The descending limb of the loop is permeable to water Na^+, and Cl^-. These materials pass through the walls according to osmotic gradients. Water diffuses out of the tubule lumen into the more concentrated (hypertonic) interstitial tissue of the renal pyramids; Na^+, and Cl^- diffuse passively into the tubule.

   The ascending limb of the loop differs in that its wall is impermeable to water. Therefore, water remains in the tubule. Also, chloride ions are actively reabsorbed and pumped into the interstitium surrounding the loop of Henle, as well as into the collecting ducts passing through the medullary pyramid. Sodium ions are thought to diffuse passively out of the tubules in conjunction with the Cl^-. This decrease in sodium chloride concentration of the filtrate results in a hypotonic filtrate at the distal end of the loop of Henle as it enters the distal convoluted tubule. The flow of the sodium chloride out of the tubule also increases its concentration in the surrounding interstitial tissue, which thus becomes hypertonic. This hypertonic interstitium is essential for production of hypertonic urine as the filtrate passes through the collecting ducts of the renal pyramid.

13. **E.** The zona glomerulosa of the adrenal gland is rich in lipids, especially cholesterol, from which the mineralocorticoids are formed. Aldosterone is the most powerful mineralocorticoid. Mineralocorticoids function in the retention of water, sodium, and chloride, and increase urinary loss of potassium and phosphorus by action on the renal tubules. This regulation of the electrolytes is essential to life. No pituitary control is present.

14. **A.** Urine is formed by filtering plasma components smaller than proteins from blood across the wall of the glomerulus into the nephron. As the fluid passes down the nephron, useful solutes are resorbed in the proximal and distal convoluted tubules and water is resorbed in the collecting duct.

15. **E.** The wall of the glomerulus is the filtering surface across which water and solutes smaller than proteins move from blood into the nephron.

16. **B.** The proximal convoluted tubules normally resorb essentially all of the sugars and amino acids from the urine. These useful solutes are actively transported across the epithelium from the urine to the surrounding connective tissue, where they are taken up into capillaries.

17. **D.** The loops of Henle establish a high salt environment in the medulla by exporting sodium and chloride ions from the ascending limb of each loop of Henle (which is carrying urine back up toward the cortex) and absorbing sodium and chloride ions into the descending limb of each loop of Henle (which is carrying urine down into the medulla). These processes have the net effect of moving sodium and chloride ions deeper into the medulla, creating a high salt environment through which the collecting ducts pass.

18. **C.** The distal convoluted tubules are the major site of hormonally controlled salt resorption.

19. **A.** The epithelium lining the collecting duct changes permeability in response to an antidiuretic hormone. When the permeability is high, as the urine moves down the collecting duct (which passes down through the medulla to the renal pelvis), water leaves the collecting ducts by osmosis (because of the high salt environment established in the medulla by the loops of Henle). As the permeability of the collecting ducts changes, urine may vary from approximately isotonic to blood plasma when the collecting duct epithelium allows little water resorption, to strongly hypertonic to blood plasma when the collecting duct epithelium allows maximum water resorption.

Integumentary (Skin) System

The skin and the specialized organs derived from the skin (hairs, nails, and glands) from the integumentary system.

Skin

The skin lines the external surface of the body. It is continuous with the mucous membranes of (1) the respiratory pathways via the nose; (2) the digestive tract via the mouth and anus; (3) the genitourinary system via urethra and/or vagina.

Functions: The skin functions by surfacing the body and thus protecting it from dehydration as well as from damage by the elements in the external environment. The skin also helps maintain normal body activities. The skin performs the following functions.

(1) Protects the body against dehydration. The skin is impermeable to water which, therefore, prevents loss of body fluids. This property permits humans, as well as other animals, to live in a nonfluid environment such as land.

(2) Protects the body against abrasive forces. The ability to withstand frictional forces also allows humans to walk and perform manipulatory skills with the hands.

(3) Protects the body against damage from toxic chemicals and extreme heat.

(4) Protects the body from the harmful effects of ultraviolet rays. This is primarily the function of the melanin pigment secreted by the melanocytes in the epidermis.

(5) Acts as a barrier to infectious organisms invading the body.

(6) Takes part in regulating the temperature of the body. The degree of heat loss or retention is regulated by neurovascular processes. The body is cooled by the evaporation of water (sweat) from its surface.

(7) Functions to excrete body wastes and fluids via the production of sweat by the sweat glands.

(8) Acts as a primary sense organ of the body for general somatic sensations, such as touch, pressure, heat, cold, and pain.

(9) Plays a role in the production of vitamin D through the action of ultraviolet light. The latter transforms vitamin D precursors (7-dehydrocholesterol) found in the skin into vitamin D.

Structure: Skin consists of the *epidermis* and *dermis (corium)*. Deep to the dermis and therefore, the skin, is the *hypodermis,* which is also known as the *subcutaneous* or *superficial* connective tissue of the body. The latter comprises loose connective tissue with various amounts of adipose cells (tissue).

Epidermis: The epidermis is derived from the ectoderm and is composed of a keratinized stratified squamous epithelium. The epidermis varies in thickness depending on the function of the specific region of the body. Its thickness is used to differentiate two types of skin: thick and thin.

Thick skin denotes skin with a thicker epidermis which contains more cell layers when compared to *thin skin*. The epidermis ranges in thickness from 0.07 mm to 1.4 mm. Skin itself (both epidermis and dermis) ranges from 0.5 mm to more than 4 mm. The epidermis, similar to other epithelial layers, is avascular and lies on a basal lamina (basement membrane). The latter separates it from the underlying dermis to which the basal layer of epidermis cells is anchored.

The epidermis consists of specific cell layers which differ in their morphology and function. The layers of the epidermis of thick skin (sole of foot and palm) from the basal lamina (dermis) to the free surface are:

(1) stratum basale or germinativum
(2) stratum spinosum
(3) stratum granulosum
(4) stratum lucidum
(5) stratum corneum

The combined layers of the strata basale and spinosum are also referred to as the *stratum malpighi* or *malpighian layer.*

In thin skin the stratum lucidum is absent and the stratum granulosum often appears as a discontinuous layer. The strata spinosum and corneum are always present as distinct layers but are thinner than in thick skin.

The layers of skin represent the different stages through which the epidermal cells (keratinocytes) pass as they undergo the process of keratinization from their origin in the stratum basale to their sloughing off as dead keratinized cells at the free surface.

The five layers of thick skin are characterized as follows:

1. Stratum basale
   a. Simple cuboidal to columnar epithelial cell layer resting on the basal lamina.
   b. Cells with the ability to divide (mitosis) and thus give rise to cells which migrate into the overlying stratum spinosum. This continuous process replenishes the keratinized epithelial cells which are shed from the surface.
   c. *Melanocytes,* which synthesize the brown pigment, *melanin,* in the form of pigment granules *(melanosomes).* Melanocytes have long cell processes which extend among the cells of the strata basale and spinosum. Via these processes they release and transfer melanosomes to the cells of the stratum malpighi. Increased exposure to UV light stimulates an increase in the secretion and release of melanosomes by the melanocytes, which results in the darkening of the skin (tanning). Dark color skin results from melanin, from carotene, a yellowish pigment, and from the degree of vascularity of the area, which adds a reddish-blue tint.
2. Stratum spinosum—consists of several layers of polygonal (polyhedral) cells which adhere to each other via desmosomes.
3. Stratum granulosum
   a. Consists of 3 to 5 layers of flat epithelial cells with pycnotic nuclei.
   b. Has a granular appearance due to the accumulation of irregular granules, the *keratohyalin granules,* within the cytoplasm. The granules are basophilic and are not encased by a membrane. The keratohyalin granules are associated with the numerous tonofilaments; both are involved in the production of keratin.
   c. The cells also contain *membrane-coating granules* (lamellated granules) composed of mucopolysaccharides and phospholipids. The latter are secreted into the intercellular regions surrounding the cells of the stratum granulosum. This intercellular matrix appears to block the passage of substances through the epidermis.
   d. The keratinocytes die in this stratum.
4. Stratum lucidum
   a. It is a homogeneous translucent layer separating the strata granulosum and corneum in thick skin.
   b. Consists of 3 to 5 layers of flat, elongated cells whose organelles and nuclei are indistinct or absent.
5. Stratum corneum
   a. Composed of layers of compressed, flat, cornified (keratinized) cells which lack nuclei and organelles. These scalelike cells are often referred to as *horny cells*.
   b. The most superficial horny cells slough off or desquamate constantly.

Dermis: The *corium,* or dermis, is the connective tissue layer between the epidermis and hypodermis. Depending on the region, its thickness may range from 0.5 mm to 4 mm. The border between these two strata is irregular in contour. This is caused by the irregular pattern of the surface of the dermis, to which the epidermis conforms. In a section perpendicular to the skin's surface, the dermis is seen to project into folds of the epidermis. These connective tissue projections are known as *dermal ridges* (or *papillae);* the epidermal regions between these ridges are the *epidermal* or *interpapillar pegs (ridges).* The dermal ridges are more numerous in thick skin (palm and soles), where greater abrasive forces occur. Because the epidermis follows the contours of the skin, the irregular contour of the dermis is projected onto the surface of the skin as ridges and grooves. The orientation and patterns of these surface grooves differ according to the skin region. They are very evident in the palm and fingers. The pattern is also extremely specific for each individual as is illustrated by the use of fingerprints to identify a person. These fingerprints, therefore, are actually the impressions of the grooves on the surface of the skin which represent the contour of the dermo-epidermal junction.

The dermis consists of two strata: the *papillary* and *reticular* layers.

Papillary layer. The *papillary layer* abuts the epidermis and forms the dermal ridges (papillae). It is thinner than the reticular layer and is composed of loose connective tissue. It consists of fine collagen, reticular, and elastic fibers associated with typical connective tissue cells (mainly fibroblasts and macrophages). The region abutting the basal cell layer is organized into a basement membrane. The processes of the basal cells anchor in the fibers of the membrane. The dermal ridges have extensive capillary networks. The epidermis is nourished by the diffusion of nutrients from this vascular bed. The papillary layer also contains encapsulated sensory receptors.

Reticular layer. The *reticular layer* is thicker and is composed of dense irregular connective tissue. The collagen and elastic fibers are thicker and coarser and form an interlacing network. Most fibers are primarily oriented parallel to the surface forming lines of skin tension called *Langer's lines,* which are important for surgical incisions. Capillaries are sparse. A rich nerve supply as well as encapsulated receptors are present in this layer. The reticular layer is the location of epidermal derivatives such as sweat and sebaceous glands and hair follicles. It also contains smooth muscles (arrector pili) associated with hair follicles and skeletal muscles in the head and neck (muscles of facial expression).

Glands

Glands are specialized organs derived from skin. There are two basic types: sebaceous and sweat.

Sebaceous Glands: Sebaceous glands are *simple branched alveolar (acinar) glands* with a *holocrine* mode of secretion. They are found in all areas of the body except the palms and soles. The excretory ducts of several glands open into the necks of a hair follicle.

The cells of the gland differentiate and become progressively larger as they accumulate lipid droplets in their cytoplasm. The cells eventually rupture releasing their lipid content and cell remnants into the lumen. The latter comprise the oily secretion of the sebaceous glands called *sebum,* which helps protect the skin from becoming extremely dry.

Sweat Glands: Sweat is a watery fluid containing ammonia, urea, uric acid, and sodium chloride. The production of sweat is important for the excretion of some body wastes and the regulation of body temperature and is under nervous system control.

There are two types of sweat glands: eccrine and apocrine.

Eccrine Sweat Glands: The *eccrine sweat glands* are simple, coiled tubular glands with a merocrine mode of secretion. These glands are the ones that are typically considered when discussing sweat glands. Up to 3 million are found distributed all over the body in humans, except at the margin of the lip, glans penis, and ear drums. The largest number occur in the thick skin of the palms and soles. The *secretory tubular* unit is very coiled and is located in the reticular layer of the dermis near the hypodermis.

Apocrine Sweat Glands: The *apocrine sweat glands* are very large glands which are thought to have a merocrine mode of secretion. They occur mainly in the hypodermis of the axilla, aerola of breast, labia majora, and scrotum. They are branched tubular glands whose secretory tubule is very dilated. Their secretory product is more viscous. The excretory ducts open into the hair follicles above the openings of this sweat gland.

The *ceruminous glands* of the external auditory canals, which secrete wax, and the *glands of Moll,* in the eyelid margin, are also considered to be apocrine sweat glands.

Hair

Hairs are long, filamentous keratinized structures derived from the epidermis of skin. The process of keratinization is similar to that in skin because cells divide, differentiate, and move toward the surface and become keratinized. Hairs are found covering the whole body except palms, soles, sides of fingers and toes, glans and prepuce of penis, clitoris, and labia minora.

Structure: A hair consists of a *shaft,* which extends above the skin surface, and a *root,* which lies within the skin. The root is encased by a tubular *hair follicle* composed of epidermal and dermal cell layers. At its deeper end, the follicle dilates and forms an invaginated *hair bulb* which is continuous with the root. The invaginated portion of the hair bulb contains a connective tissue papilla, the *dermal papilla,* which has a rich blood supply.

Hairs consist of three concentrically oriented epidermal layers: the *medulla, cortex,* and *cuticle.* The *medulla* forms the center of the hair and consists of two or three layers of cuboidal cells found only in coarse hair; these cornified cells contain soft keratin. The medulla is encased by the *cortex,* which constitutes the largest part of the hair. It consists of several layers of keratinized cells which contain numerous filaments embedded in an amorphous matrix. The latter form the *hard keratin* found in these compactly arranged spindle-shaped cells. Melanin granules are found in the cells of the cortex giving hair its coloration. Air in the intercellular region of these cells also affects the pigmentation of hairs. The *cuticle* surrounds the cortex and consists of a single layer of transparent, enucleated cells which form keratinized scales.

Hair Follicle: The *hair follicle* consists of two sheaths: the *epithelial root sheath* and the *connective tissue root sheath.* The epidermally derived epithelial root sheath abuts the cuticle and is subdivided into the *inner epithelial root sheath* and the *outer (external) epithelial root sheath.* The *inner epithelial root sheath* extends from hair bulb to the level of the excretory duct of the sebaceous glands. It comprises three layers: (1) the *cuticle root sheath,* abutting the cuticle; (2) *Huxley's layer;* and (3) *Henle's layer,* adjacent to the outer epithelial root sheath. These layers are composed of keratinized cells containing soft keratin. The cells of the inner epithelial root sheath arise from the *hair matrix* in the hair bulb and migrate upward from it.

The *outer epithelial root sheath* is continuous with the epidermis of the skin. Close to the hair bulb the outer epithelial root sheath consists of a simple cuboidal layer similar to the stratum germinativum.

The *connective tissue root sheath* (or *dermal root sheath*) is derived from the dermis and consists of three layers: (1) the *glassy membrane,* the innermost layer which is a noncellular translucent membrane that corresponds to the basal lamina deep to the epidermis; (2) the *middle layer,* similar to the papillary layer of the dermis, and consisting of fine connective tissue fibers arranged in a circular pattern; and (3) the *outer layer,* similar to the reticular layer and consisting of longitudinally arranged coarse collagen fibers.

Hair Growth: Growth of a hair depends on the viability of the epidermal cells of the hair matrix which lie adjacent to the dermal papilla in the hair bulb. The matrix cells abutting the dermal papilla proliferate and give rise to cells which move upward to become part of the specific layers of the hair root and the inner epithelial root sheath. The hair matrix, therefore, functions similarly to the malpighian layer of the epidermis in that it gives rise to cells which become cornified as they move toward the surface. Due to this upward movement of the cells arising from the hair matrix, the hair (root and shaft) grows outward. Hairs do not grow continuously but have specific growth and rest periods which vary according to the area of the body. Hair growth is influenced by growth hormone and the sex hormones.

Hair Musculature: Hairs are oriented at a slight angle to the skin surface and are associated with *arrector pili muscles.* These smooth muscle bundles extend from the dermal root sheath to a dermal papilla. Contraction results in the standing up of the hairs and raising of the skin surrounding the hair. This produces what is referred to as *gooseflesh* or *goose pimples.*

Nails

Nails are translucent plates of keratinized epithelial cells on the dorsal surface of distal phalanges of fingers and toes. The nail plate consists of a *body* and *root,* formed by compact layers of cornified epithelial cells similar to the stratum corneum. The *nail body* is the main portion of the plate lying on the *nail bed,* which is an epidermal layer consisting primarily of the malpighian cell layer. The proximal end of the body is continuous with the *nail root* at the *lunula.* The lunula is the crescentric whitish region at the proximal part of the nail.

Deep to the root and continuous with the proximal end of the nail bed is the *nail matrix.* The latter is a thickened stratum malpighi which gives rise to new cells that migrate upward and become keratinized. The matrix, therefore, functions in producing cornified cells composed of hard keratin which are added to the proximal end of the nail plate (root). This process increases the length of the nail. Nails increase in length at about 0.5 mm per week.

The *cuticle,* or *eponychium,* is a fold of the stratum corneum which extends over the surfce of the nail body in the area of the lunula.

A similar fold, the *hyponychium,* occurs deep to the distal free margin of the nail plate. The hyponychium is actually a thickening of the stratum corneum of the skin where the nail bed and epidermis of the skin are continuous.

THE INTEGUMENTARY SYSTEM

Organ	Major Function
Epidermis	Protection of the body; a barrier mechanism.
Dermis	Nourishes the epidermis by diffusion of nutrients; has sensory receptors.
Hair follicles	Produce hair.
Hair	Secondary sex characteristics; some protection.
Nails	Help in shaping the distal digits; some protection.
Sebaceous glands	Produce oily secretion which helps protect the skin from drying.
Sweat glands	Produce perspiration; control temperature of body.
Ceruminous glands	Secrete wax; protect auditory canals.
Superficial fascia	Stores fat.

Quick Recall Test Questions and Answers

Choose the Best Answer

1. Which is the correct sequence of epidermal maturation?

    A. stratum basale, stratum granulosum, stratum spinosum, stratum lucidum, stratum corneum
    B. stratum basale, stratum spinosum, stratum granulosum, stratum lucidum, stratum corneum
    C. stratum basale, stratum spinosum, stratum lucidum, stratum granulosum, stratum corneum
    D. stratum basale, stratum spinosum, stratum granulosum, stratum corneum, stratum lucidum

2. The reticular layer of the dermis contains all of the following EXCEPT:

    A. dense irregular connective tissue.
    B. collagen and elastic fibers.
    C. erector pili muscles.
    D. a rich capillary supply.
    E. hair follicles.

3. The stratum spinosum consists of several layers of polygonal cell which adhere to each other via:

    A. dermal ridges.
    B. gap junctions.
    C. terminal bars.
    D. desmosomes.
    E. basal lamina.

4. The stratum basale is also called the:

    A. epidermis.
    B. dermis.
    C. capillary layer.
    D. stratum corneum.
    E. stratum germinativum.

5. Certain cells of the skin produce a pigment that provides protection against ultraviolet irradiation. These cells are the:

    A. keratinocytes.
    B. fibroblasts.
    C. macrophages.
    D. melanocytes.
    E. eosinophils.

6. A common feature of sweat glands, salivary glands, and sebaceous glands is that they are:

    A. endocrine glands.
    B. exocrine glands.
    C. apocrine glands.
    D. merocrine glands.
    E. none of the above.

7. The eccrine sweat glands are classified as _____ glands.

    A. branched tubular
    B. simple coiled tubular
    C. simple branched acinar
    D. compound acinar

8. The dermis of the skin is derived from the embryonic germ layer known as the:

    A. neural crest.
    B. endoderm.
    C. mesoderm.
    D. ectoderm.

9. The cuticle, or eponychium, is a fold of the:

    A. stratum basale.
    B. stratum spinosum.
    C. stratum granulosum.
    D. stratum lucidum.
    E. stratum corneum.

10. The barrier which prevents bacteria from entering the human body by passing through the skin is the _____ tissue in the ____.

    A. epithelial, epidermis
    B. epithelial, dermis
    C. connective, epidermis
    D. connective, dermis
    E. adipose, hypodermis

11. Most of the mechanical strength of skin is due to the ____ tissue in the ____ .

    A. epithelial, epidermis
    B. epithelial, dermis
    C. connective, epidermis
    D. connective, dermis
    E. adipose, hypodermis

12. When sweat glands are actively secreting, heat loss from the body surface of a human is:

    A. increased.
    B. decreased.
    C. unchanged.

13. All of the cells in keratinocyte lineage (keritinized cells) in the epidermis are produced by mitotic division of cells in the:

    A. stratum germinativum.
    B. stratum granulosum.
    C. stratum lucidum.
    D. stratum corneum.
    E. dermis.

14. The papillary layer of the dermis in human skin contains:

    A. loose fibroelastic connective tissue.
    B. dense irregular fibroelastic connective tissue.
    C. dense regular collagenous connective tissue.
    D. dense regular elastic connective tissue.
    E. papillary glands.

15. The reticular layer of the dermis in human skin contains:

    A. loose fibroelastic connective tissue.
    B. dense irregular fibroelastic connective tissue.
    C. dense regular collagenous connective tissue.
    D. dense regular elastic connective tissue.
    E. reticular connective tissue.

16. The nail plate of a fingernail is produced from cells formed in the:

    A. eponchynium.
    B. hyponchynium.
    C. nail matrix.
    D. nail bed.

17. Eccrine sweat glands (typical sweat glands) usually occur attached:

    A. directly to the epidermis.
    B. to sebaceous glands.
    C. to hair follicles.

18. The hair shaft in a hair follicle contains cells produced by the:

    A. outer epidermal root sheath.
    B. inner epidermal root sheath.

    C. dermal root sheath.
    D. epidermal cells adjacent to the dermal papilla.

19. Sebaceous glands usually occur attached:

    A. directly to the epidermis.
    B. to eccrine sweat glands.
    C. to hair follicles.

20. Sebaceous glands use ____ secretory mechanisms.

    A. merocrine
    B. apocrine
    C. holocrine

ANSWERS

1. **B.** The epidermis consists of specific cell layers which differ in their morphology and function. The layers of the epidermis of thick skin (sole of foot and palm) from the basal lamina (dermis) to the free surface are:
    (1) stratum basale or germinativum
    (2) stratum spinosum
    (3) stratum granulosum
    (4) stratum lucidum
    (5) stratum corneum

2. **D.** The reticular layer is composed of dense irregular connective tissue. Capillaries are sparse. The reticular layer is the location of epidermal derivatives such as sweat and sebaceous glands and hair follicles. It also contains smooth muscle (arrector pili) associated with hair follicles and skeletal muscles in the head and neck (muscles of facial expression).

3. **D.** The stratum spinosum consists of several layers of polygonal (polyhedral) cells which adhere to each other via desmosomes.

4. **E.** The stratum basale is also called the stratum germinativum.

5. **D.** Melanocytes extend among the cells of the strata basale and spinosum. They produce pigment granules called melanosomes. Melanin is formed in the presence of tyrosinase in the melanosome; the starting product is carotene.

6. **B.** Sweat glands, salivary glands, and sebaceous glands are all exocrine glands.

7. **B.** There are two types of sweat glands: eccrine and apocrine. The eccrine sweat glands are simple, coiled tubular glands with a merocrine

mode of secretion; they are the typical sweat glands. The aporine sweat glands occur mainly in the hypodermis of the axilla, areola of the breast, labia majora, and scrotum and are branched tubular glands.

8. **C.** Whereas the epidermis is derived from ectoderm, the dermis and subcutaneous tissue under the skin is of mesodermal origin.

9. **E.** The cuticle is a fold of the stratum corneum which extends over the surface of the nail body in the area of the lunula. A similar fold, the hyponychium, occurs deep to the distal free margin of the nail plate. The hyponychium is actually a thickening of the stratum corneum of the skin where the nail bed and epidermis of the skin are continuous.

10. **A.** The epithelium provides the primary barrier to bacterial entry, since the cells are tightly joined to each other laterally.

11. **D.** The connective tissue in the dermis provides most of the mechanical strength of the skin. The strength is due to the extensive array of collagen fibers and other extracellular matrix components which make up most of the connective tissue. The dermis is the part of animal skin which is chemically preserved by tanning and used to make leather. The epithelium in the epidermis contributes some mechanical strength, but less than the dermis. The loose connective tissue and adipose tissue in the hypodermis contribute little mechanical strength, but allow the skin to move relative to the underlying structures.

12. **A.** Evaporation of the water transported to the body surface by the sweat glands removes heat from the body surface, leading to much more rapid heat loss. This process allows moving heat from the body surface into air which on a hot day may be warmer than the body surface.

13. **A.** Dividing cells in the stratum germinativum produce all of the keratinocyte lineage cells in the more superficial layers.

14. **A.** The connective tissue in the papillary layer is much less dense than in the deeper (and much thicker) reticular layer of the dermis. Like the reticular layer, it consists of collagen and elastic fibers plus other extracellular matrix components, so it qualifies as loose fibroelastic connective tissue (loose FECT).

15. **B.** The reticular layer makes up most of the dermis. It contains very large collagen fibers and large elastic fibers, most of which run roughly parallel to the skin surface but which are otherwise irregularly arranged. The cells are primarily fibroblasts. These characteristics are typical of dense irregular fibroelastic connective tissue.

16. **C.** Although the nail plate lies on top of the nail bed along the full length of the nail, production of the cells which differentiate into the nail plate appears to occur primarily in the root area where the epithelial part of the nail bed is referred to as the nail matrix.

17. **A.** Eccrine sweat glands usually are attached directly to the epidermis and are not usually associated with sebaceous glands or hair follicles.

18. **D.** The cells that form the hair shaft are produced by division of epidermal cells adjacent to the dermal papilla. The cells in the epidermal sheath around the hair do not contribute cells to the hair.

19. **C.** Although solitary sebaceous glands can occur, most sebaceous glands are attached to hair follicles.

20. **C.** Sebaceous gland cells fill with oily secretion and then are shed along with the secretion, so the mechanism is holocrine.

Digestive System and Nutrition

Nutrition

Every living organism is faced with a fundamental dilemma—how to simultaneously maintain its individual integrity while assimilating the essential fuels for life from the surrounding environment. Primitive single-celled organisms living in water literally bathe in their environment, while more complex beings such as we are must draw nutrients from our environment while guarding those which we already have assimilated. Thus, the heterotrophic, or animal cell has evolved a highly specialized structure known as the cell membrane which allows selection of those environmental nutrients necessary for metabolism, elimination of metabolic waste products, and physical delineation of the cell as a unit. In the human organism, composed of billions of cells which have differentiated into many distinct cell types, the function of the cell membrane has also become differentiated (e.g., nerve cells, muscle cells). Perhaps nowhere in the body is the relationship of cell function to structure more apparent than in the gastrointestinal tract and the kidney. Nonetheless, every cell must retain its individual integrity and find a nutrient supply, no matter how specialized its interior processes may become.

Nutrients, once assimilated, must be guarded against loss. Thus, it should not be surprising to find that the cell membranes of the early, or proximal portion of the intestine are very close in appearance and function to those of the early, or proximal part of the renal tubule. While the columnar epithelial cells of the jejunum are engaged in absorbing nutrients from within the intestinal passage and passing them into the blood, the columnar cells of the renal proximal tubule are responsible for protecting against loss of these same nutrients as they circulate through the kidney. In this section we will restrict ourselves to discussion of the function of the intestine, occasionally referring to significant similarities in the kidney.

Absorption of most nutrients within the intestine occurs only after *digestion* of the foods eaten. Thus, it is essential that the dinner we see and salivate over be broken down into its component elements on the scale of cell membranes before they can become useful to the body. Accordingly, nutrients are classified as *macro, micro,* or *trace* nutritional elements: macro elements include proteins, fats and complex carbohydrates, all of which require *digestion* prior to absorption; micro elements include materials like iron, calcium, and inorganic phosphate, which can be absorbed directly and for which there is a substantial daily need; trace elements include materials such as vitamins and elements like magnesium, selenium, and manganese. What follows is a more detailed examination of the broad issues raised above to provide a functional picture of the dual processes of digestion and absorption in achievement of a good nutritional state.

Unit for Measuring Value of Foods: A fundamental characteristic of all life is the need for energy production from nutrients; in humans this process occurs through oxidative combustion, the same basic process by which energy is released from wood or gasoline. As with wood and gasoline, a common end product is heat energy, which according to thermodynamic theory contributes to the *entropy*, or disorder, of the universe. Although we measure the energy value of wood and gasoline in British thermal units (BTUs), the unit commonly used to measure the energy value of foods is the *kilocalorie* (kcal). One kilocalorie is the amount of energy required to raise 1 kg (1,000 cc) of water one degree Celsius. In common parlance we speak of "calories," each one of which is $\frac{1}{100}$ of a kcal, or the energy necessary to raise 1 g (1 cc) of water one degree Celsius. Calories in the diet are derived exclusively from protein, fat, and carbohydrate, or the macronutrients. It is important to understand that, while these nutrient sources contain calories for energy production, the body can utilize their components for synthesis of many other molecules with minimal energy loss. Only when a molecule is completely utilized for energy production is its caloric value nutritionally relevant.

Proteins: These macromolecules are actually heteropolymers of L-amino acids, and their species-specific structures are rigidly controlled by the genome. Dietary protein in humans derives chiefly from animal and vegetable sources whose genomes differ significantly from that of the human. Accordingly, for humans to synthesize their own species-specific proteins, the dietary molecules must be reduced to their simplest component units (amino acids) and reutilized in human cells for synthesis of structural and enzyme proteins under direction of the human genetic code.

There are 21 naturally occurring amino acids, 8 of which humans cannot synthesize *de novo* or by using any molecule of similar structure; these are termed *essential amino acids*. The reason for our inability to construct these amino acids is that our genetic code does not include messages for the synthesis of the requisite enzyme proteins to establish the proper chemical bonds; thus, we must depend upon other organisms for production of these molecules, which are essential to our own lives. The remaining 13 amino acids can be made from other materials in human cells and, for this reason, are called *nonessential amino acids*. The relative amount of essential to nonessential amino acids, both in general and with respect to specific ones, varies widely with each dietary source; some proteins do not contain any of a given essential amino acid, so that without additional supply of the missing molecule from some other source, the protein cannot be reutilized by human cells and will, instead, be consumed for energy production.

Proteins are highly charged molecules and fall into two basic categories: *enzyme* and *structural*. All assume a three-dimensional conformation in aqueous solution, chiefly determined by the interactions of the charges with the water molecules but as well by internal bonds (e.g., disulfide bonds) between amino acids of the heteropolymer itself. Enzyme proteins act to reduce the energy required to cause a chemical reaction to occur by establishing transient bonds with a substrate molecule and creating a *transition state*, in the process altering its own conformation. It is this need to change conformation which renders enzymes susceptible to denaturation and "death"; hence the need for their constant resynthesis. Structural proteins are intrinsic parts of such components as cell membranes. Excellent examples of structural proteins are muscle actin and myosin; other structural proteins at the cell surface may function as receptor sites or antibody-binding sites.

A final point to touch on in this very brief summary is that protein is the sole source of dietary nitrogen. Even though we exist in an atmosphere comprising about 80% nitrogen, our bodies' only nitrogen source is the food we eat and the protein contained in it. Moreover, while we could not exist in human form without a nitrogen source, lacking the ability to "fix" atmospheric nitrogen, it is paradoxical that any nitrogen liberated from dietary protein is in the form of ammonia, a very potent neurotoxin. Since each amino acid comprising the protein we eat contains a minimum of one amino ($-NH_2$) group, the potential for ammonia toxicity with every meal is immense. We are, however, protected by two factors. The first is that most dietary protein is reutilized as intact amino acids, with the amino group acting as a sort of metabolic "lock" which prevents utilization for energy. The second is that the detoxification process in liver known as the "urea cycle" converts any liberated ammonia to the biologically inert compound called *urea*. Urea is excreted by the kidney into the urine, and a rough measure of kidney function can be obtained by assessing the *blood urea nitrogen*, or BUN. By contrast, if the liver has failed, the BUN will be low while the *blood ammonia* will be high. In each case, however, the abnormalities can be traced back to the breakdown or *catabolism* of amino acids for energy, since these compounds are the sole source of nitrogen.

Carbohydrates: These sugars, or saccharides, are generally present in the diet in single (mono-), dual (di-), or complex (poly-) saccharide form. The common dietary monosaccharides are fructose, glucose and galactose; disaccharides include sucrose (glucose + fructose) and lactose (glucose + galactose); ingested polysaccharides are usually starch and cellulose, both of which are large glucose polymers. The monosaccharides can be absorbed directly by the intestine, but the di- and polysaccharides must be enzymatically hydrolyzed into their monomer units. Nutritionally, the carbohydrates have important roles: The first is as a primary source of energy to offset the use of amino acids; the second is to supply the carbon skeletons for synthesis of nonessential amino acids; and the third is to serve as intrinsic components of many complex molecules called glycoproteins and glycolipids. Glycoproteins are important components of all cell membranes and glycolipids are especially important for normal function of the central nervous system. Regarding their use as a fuel, the caloric value of a gram of glucose is essentially identical to that of a gram of protein, from which one might correctly conclude that a diet which has more carbohydrate by weight than protein will ensure that all amino acids can be utilized for protein synthesis. Finally, the initial cellular steps in the breakdown of glucose result in two 3-carbon compounds which can be used for synthesis of fat (see below) as well as for amino acids. This is the reason that diets higher than normal in carbohydrate and total calories result in obesity.

Fats: The basic building block of dietary fat is the fatty acid, which is generally a straight- or simple-branched chain molecule comprising an even number of 12–18 carbon atoms and terminating in a carboxyl group. There are, of course, similar molecules which are either longer or shorter and are comprised of odd as well as even numbers of carbon atoms, but the bulk of dietary fatty acids are as described above, and are called *saturated fatty acids*. Further variation is seen in the C12–C18 compounds by virtue of insertion of one or more double bonds, a change which renders the compounds *unsaturated fatty acids*. Humans are able to synthesize saturated fatty acids starting from the common 2-carbon biochemical intermediate, acetyl-coenzyme A; unlike the situation with nitrogen, the human body has evolved enzymes capable of fixing carbon dioxide, thus permitting it to elongate a carbon chain as necessary. The system has limitations in the creation of double bonds, rendering certain unsaturated fatty acids essential in the diet.

Utilizing the 3-carbon triol fragment produced from glucose, called *glycerol*, the human body is able, by stepwise addition of fatty acids to each alcohol group, to create *triglycerides*. These mono-, di-, or triglycerides are simply one, two, or three fatty acids linked to the glycerol through ester bonding, created by an enzymatically-mediated reaction between the alcohol and carboxyl groups. It is also possible for humans to create, from the fundamental triglyceride structure, very complex macromolecules which are vital to the structure and function of various components of the central nervous system. It is worth noting that the bulk of the weight of the CNS, and specifically the brain, derives from the presence of simple and complex lipids.

In addition to the above, the human organism is capable of synthesis of cholesterol from acetyl-coenzyme A. Cholesterol is a molecule with a complicated ring structure from which many steroid hormones and compounds related to blood coagulation are derived. Cholesterol is also an important component of all cell membranes. This vital body molecule can be produced from almost any dietary macronutrient, so that dietary cholesterol restriction can go only so far in lowering an already elevated blood cholesterol level in prevention or treatment of coronary artery disease.

Nutritionally, fat is present in virtually all animal and plant constituents of the human diet, so that elimination of dietary fat is exceedingly difficult to accomplish. Moreover, the caloric, or energy value of fat is more than twice that of carbohydrate and protein; thus, reduction of fat may produce a diet too low in calories to meet daily energy requirements. In addition, because of the association between protein and fat, there is a risk of protein deficiency with draconian fat-reduction type diets.

Vitamins: Vitamins are a group of organic molecules which are derived from microorganisms and are essential for human nutrition. All vitamins undergo intracellular changes ("activation") which render them *cofactors*, in which form they interact with specific enzyme proteins to participate in the production of "transition states" of reactions. In their native form, as ingested, vitamins are not active and have no biological value *per se*. Once bound to an enzyme protein in the activated form, a vitamin molecule will remain in the body for as long as the integrity of the protein remains. Many vitamins are recycled by the body as well; both of these phenomena account for the very small daily quantities required by humans. Vitamins are essential to many key metabolic reactions, including 1-carbon transfer reactions involved in synthesis of DNA, so that deficiency, though rare in the Western world, can cause some striking diseases. Most authors tend to subgroup vitamins into those which are fat-soluble and those which are water-soluble, a classification that does little to describe their activities. It does have the advantage of explaining various aspects of secondary vitamin deficiencies, however, and we shall therefore follow the same classification.

Fat-soluble Vitamins

1. *Vitamin A(retinol, retinoic acid, retinal)*. The chief function of this compound is in the eye, where it supports dark vision and normal structure of the conjunctiva and cornea. Primary dietary sources of vitamin A are vegetables, fruits (beta-carotene, or two retinal molecules linked through their aldehydic groups) and animal liver (retinol, the storage form found chiefly in liver).

2. *Vitamin D (1,25-dihydroxycholecalciferol)*. Although originally described as a vitamin and identified as the antirachitic dietary factor, vitamin D is considered by many authorities to be a hormone. The human skin produces an activated cholesterol molecule utilizing the sun's ultraviolet radiation, from which 25-hydroxycholecalciferol is synthesized in liver. This material is essentially inactive in a biological sense, and must be carried in the blood to the kidney, where the enzyme necessary for 1-alpha-hydroxylation is expressed and the 1,25-dihydroxy compound produced. For this reason, severe kidney disease can result in rickets in children or osteomalacia in adults because

of the inability to produce the biologically active metabolite. Thus, it is important in such cases to distinguish between states of dietary deficiency, liver and/or kidney disease, and other disorders which may all resemble simple dietary D deficiency. The chief action of vitamin D is to enhance the synthesis of calcium-binding protein, which increases calcium and phosphate absorption by the intestine. The process enables the bone to produce *hydroxyapatite*, the crystalline material from which bone is constructed.

3. *Vitamin E (tocopherol)*. The chief function of vitamin E is as an antioxidant in cells throughout the body, suppressing the oxidation of polyunsaturated fatty acids by free radicals. Since the largest amount of these polyunsaturated fatty acids is found in membrane phospholipids, which in turn are present in large quantities in the central nervous system, vitamin E is now recognized as an important defense in maintenance of CNS integrity. It also acts in the same capacity in the red cell, protecting against excessive hemolysis. Vitamin E is known to increase sperm motility and to prevent second-trimester abortion in a number of animal species, although any such function in humans has yet to be demonstrated.

4. *Vitamin K (phylloquinone)*. A key element in the intrinsic coagulation pathway, vitamin K is essential for conversion of glutamate residues to gamma-carboxyglutamate in the prothrombin molecule, which then enables prothrombin to bind calcium, an essential step for its function in the coagulation cascade. Newborns are usually hypoprothrombinemic, resulting in a bleeding tendency; for this reason, it is standard neonatology practice to provide supplemental vitamin K by injection shortly after birth in order to maximize the ability of existing prothrombin to bind calcium.

Water-soluble Vitamins

1. *Thiamine (vitamin B_1)*. Thiamine, once activated, is a cofactor for many critical reactions, including those mediated by dehydrogenases; a pivotal step in energy production is the pyruvate dehydrogenase reaction, which converts a 3-carbon fragment of glucose (pyruvate) to acetyl coenzyme A. The acetyl CoA then either enters the tricarboxylic acid cycle or can be utilized for fatty acid synthesis. Another very important reaction in which thiamine participates is the transketolase step of the pentose phosphate shunt, which generates ribose-5-phosphate for nucleic acid synthesis. Thiamine is widely distributed in the normal human diet. Deficiency of thiamine results in the disease known as beri-beri.

2. *Riboflavin (vitamin B_2)*. Ingested riboflavin, derived predominantly from animal sources in the diet, is converted enzymatically to flavin mononucleotide (FMN) or to flavin adenine dinucleotide (FAD). Both of these cofactors are facile and reversible oxidation-reduction agents and are, therefore, predictably involved in many key mitochondrial reactions. Riboflavin is also a cofactor in production of niacin and pyridoxine to the limited degree possible in humans. The most remarkable fact is that riboflavin deficiency does not have a well-defined clinical state associated with it, as other water soluble vitamins do.

3. *Niacin (vitamin B_3)*. Niacin can be produced in limited quantities by humans from the dietary amino acid tryptophan. As already mentioned, riboflavin is a cofactor in this process. From the basic compound, nicotinic acid, activation produces nicotinamide adenine dinucleotide (NAD), and an additional phosphorylation reaction produces NADP. NAD is an important cofactor in oxidative metabolic pathways, such as the tricarboxylic acid cycle, while NADP is found in reductive pathways, such as the pentose phosphate shunt. Animal tissues are rich in both niacin and tryptophan. Deficiency of niacin causes the disease called pellagra.

4. *Pyridoxine (vitamin B_6)*. Pyridoxine comprises a pyridine nucleus which is substituted in one of three ways: It occurs in plant foods as pyridoxamine, and in animal foods as either pyridoxal (the aldehyde) or pyridoxol (the alcohol). While the alcohol-substituted form has no biological activity, it can be converted either to the aldehyde or the amine, both of which function as cofactors. Of all the water-soluble vitamins, pyridoxine is the one involved in the most diverse biochemical reactions, including amino acid transamination and decarboxylation, heme biosynthesis, and glycogenolysis. Another critical function is as a cofactor in conversion of L-glutamic acid to gamma-aminobutyric acid, or GABA, which is a key neurotransmitter substance in the brain.

Isolated B_6 deficiency is almost never seen in a clinical setting—it is usually part of a more global vitamin B complex deficiency.

5.   *Cobalamin (vitamin B_{12})*. Despite being involved as a cofactor in only two reactions in the human body, vitamin B_{12} is of critical importance. Cobalamin is synthesized exclusively by microorganisms and is, therefore, not present in plants, but can be found in relatively high concentration in animal liver. Unlike the other water-soluble vitamins, B_{12} is bound to a specific transfer protein produced in the stomach and called the *intrinsic factor*. When the bound B_{12} reaches the intestine, the complex is bound to specific cell surface receptors and taken up by pinocytosis. Once absorbed, cobalamin is hydroxylated to form hydroxycobalamin, the form in which it enters cells. Once intracellular in location, this compound enters one of two enzymatic conversion steps: within the cytosol it is converted to methylcobalamin, while in the mitochondrion it becomes adenosyl-cobalamin. As methylcobalamin, B_{12} is involved in reconversion of homocysteine to methionine, in the process generating tetrahydrofolate, which is a compound critical to methyl-group transfer and DNA synthesis. As adenosylcobalamin, B_{12} is involved in the transformation of methylmalonyl coenzyme A to succinyl CoA, a metabolic conversion required of a multitude of biologic subtrates for complete degradation. Failure to negotiate this enzymatic step results in severe clinical disease manifest as methylmalonic acidemia. Vitamin B_{12} deficiency can be due to many things and is manifested as the condition called pernicious anemia.

6.   *Folic Acid*. Folic acid is actually a group of compounds based upon a pteridine ring substituted with glutamic acid, linked through para-aminobenzoic acid. The number of glutamate residues, linked as a polypeptide chain, can be varied and the multiple compounds thus formed are called pteroylglutamates. The most active of the latter group is tetrahydrofolate, converted to 5-methylte-trahydrofolate in the liver and released as the chief circulating form of the vitamin. As mentioned earlier, folic acid is a key component of the 1-carbon transfer system so critical to nucleic acid synthesis. Indeed, it is this critical importance which lies at the bottom of the use of folic acid antagonists in the treatment of leukemias, where the synthetic rate of DNA is extraordinarily accelerated. Foods rich in folic acid include vegetables and fruits. Not only is folate deficiency a serious disorder in adults, causing a severe anemia; folate deficiency during pregnancy can adversely affect the neural growth plate of the fetus, resulting in neural tube malformations.

7.   *Biotin*. Biotin is the cofactor for CO_2 fixation, or carboxylation reactions. There are four such reactions, each at pivotal metabolic junctures. Fatty acid synthesis depends upon this process, which utilizes acetyl coenzyme A carboxylase to produce the 3-carbon malonyl CoA. A second biotin-dependent enzyme is propionyl coenzyme A carboxylase, which is the reaction producing methylmalonyl CoA (see above, vitamin B_{12}). A third is beta-methylcrotonyl CoA carboxylase, which is a step in leucine catabolism. The fourth is pyruvate carboxylase, a key enzyme in gluconeogenesis. The process by which biotin becomes a cofactor in these relationships is relatively unique and requires a separate enzyme (holocarboxylase synthase) to establish a bond between free biotin and a lysine residue in the carboxylase enzyme protein. Biotin is present in soy flour, yeast, egg yolk, and liver in high concentrations. Biotin deficiency results in loss of appetite, diminished activity, a skin rash and hair loss, and in its extreme form can mimic a genetic disease resulting in absence of the holocarboxylase synthase.

8.   *Pantothenic Acid*. A compound, pantothenic acid is an integral part of the coenzyme A molecule and functions as a cofactor in transfer of acyl groups. Acyl-group transfer is a key metabolic reaction in fatty acid synthesis and catabolism, amino acid catabolism and normal function of the tricarboxylic acid cycle. The presence of pantothenate in the coenzyme A molecule permits generation of a highly reactive thiol ester which serves as a thermodynamically favorable carrier for the acyl group. Pantothenic acid is widely distributed in foods. As with riboflavin, isolated pantothenate deficiency has not yet been described in humans.

9.   *Ascorbic Acid (vitamin C)*. Vitamin C qualifies as perhaps the best-known of the water-soluble vitamin group. However, it is unlike the other vitamins discussed above in that it does not bind chemically to a protein in order to function. Ascorbate has a valuable metabolic role as a mild reducing agent, since it donates hydrogen ions at precisely the proper energy level to maintain the reduced state of vital metal ions, especially copper and iron. In this capacity, vitamin C maintains the integrity of important metalloenzymes involved in collagen synthesis and steroidogenesis, as

well as maintenance of cytochromes and intestinal absorption of iron. Ascorbate is found in citrus fruits and green vegetables. Vitamin C deficiency causes scurvy, a disease in which many of the clinical findings—such as gingival hemorrhage and death, hemorrhage into old scars and refracture of old, healed fractures—point to a common effect on collagen metabolism.

Minerals: Upon leaving the ocean, land-dwelling organisms have had to evolve ways in which to carry with them adequate supplies of those minerals which are critical to the function of their enzyme systems. These include iron, calcium, and phosphorus as well as copper, magnesium, and many others. Generally speaking, a normal diet will supply adequate amounts of each essential mineral. Deficiencies result in clinical entities like anemia (iron), tetany (calcium), etc.

The Digestive System

Regionalization of the Embryonic Gut

1. Foregut (supplied mainly by celiac artery): pharynx, esophagus, stomach, and cranial portion of duodenum from which the primordia of the liver, gallbladder, and pancreas arise.

2. Midgut (supplied by superior mesenteric artery): caudal duodenum, jejunum, ileum, and ascending colon and two-thirds of transverse colon including the appendages cecum and vermiform appendix.

3. Hindgut (supplied by inferior mesenteric artery): distal third of transverse colon, descending colon, sigmoid colon, and rectum.

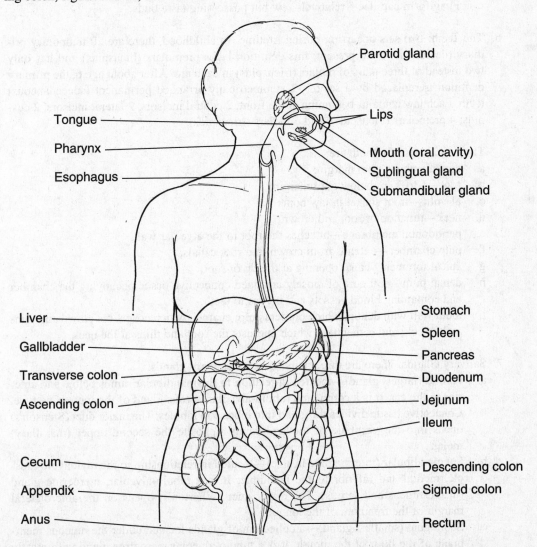

The human digestive tract relative to other structures of the body as seen from the ventral position.

Parts of the Adult Digestive Tract: The parts of the human intestinal tract may be listed in the following order: oral cavity (receives salivary gland secretions); oral and laryngeal pharynx; esophagus; cardiac sphincter; stomach; pyloric sphincter; duodenum (receives bile and pancreatic secretions); jejunum (absorption of nutrients); ileum (absorption of nutrients); cecum, ascending colon (water absorption); transverse colon; descending colon; sigmoid colon; rectum; and anal sphincter.

The Oral Cavity. The oral cavity is divided into:

1. Vestibule: the area between cheek and teeth.
2. The Lip: composed of a core of skeletal muscle and covered externally by skin.
3. The Cheek: structure similar to the lip.
4. Oral Cavity Proper: area from teeth to fauces.
5. The Tongue: composed primarily of a core of skeletal muscle and glands and covered by a mucous membrane. The anterior two-thirds of the upper (oral) portion is separated from the posterior one-third (pharyngeal) portion by the sulcus terminalis.

   Three types of lingual papillae appear as surface projections:
   a. Circumvallate papillae—located along the sulcus terminals and possessing taste buds;
   b. Filiform papillae—the most numerous;
   c. Fungiform papillae—relatively few but possessing taste buds.

6. The Teeth: two sets occurring during lifetime. In childhood, there are 20 temporary primary (deciduous) teeth present; this dentition lacks premolars (bicuspids) and has only two instead of three pairs of molars (tricuspids) in each jaw. After about age 6, the primary dentition is replaced by a set of 32 symmetrically arranged permanent (succedaneous) teeth. Each jaw contains beginning at the front: 2 central incisors, 2 lateral incisors, 2 cuspids, 4 premolars (bicuspids), and 6 molars (tricuspids).

   The basic parts of a tooth are:
   a. crown—above gum margin;
   b. root—1 to 3 cm below gum margin;
   c. alevolus—root socket in jaw bone;
   d. neck—junction of root and crown;
   e. periodontal membrane—attaches the root to the alveolar wall;
   f. pulp chamber—extends from crown into root canals;
   g. apical foramen—canal opening at the tip of root;
   h. dental pulp—soft core of loosely arranged connective tissue occupying the chamber and containing blood vessels and nerves to teeth;
   i. tooth wall with dentin, which borders pulp; enamel, which covers the crown and thins at the neck; and cementum, which encrusts the root and thins at the neck.

7. Salivary Glands: There are three pairs of major salivary glands.
   a. Parotid (largest gland)—located in relation to the mandibular ramus below and anterior to the ear. It is a compound tubulo-alveolar, serous gland of the merocrine type. Connective tissue divides the gland into lobes and lobules. The major duct (Stenson's) opens into the vestibule of the oral cavity opposite the second upper (maxillary) molar.
   b. Submandibular (intermediate in size)—located in relationship to the mylohyoid muscle, medial and inferior to the mandible. It is a tubulo-alveolar, merocrine gland (mixed-mucus and serous). The major duct (Wharton's) opens on the anterolateral margin of the frenulum of the tongue.
   c. Sublingual (smallest gland)—a collection of glands located under the mucous membrane of the floor of the mouth. It is a tubulo-alveolar merocrine gland with mostly mucous acini. The major duct (Bartholin's) empties on the side of the frenulum of the tongue, having joined the submandibular duct.

Tubular Digestive Tract. The adult tubular digestive tract has a general structural plan of mucosa, submucosa, muscular tunic, and adventitia.

1. Mucosa
   a. moist surface epithelium
   b. connective tissue (lamina propria)
   c. thin muscular layer (muscularis mucosae)
   d. villi (evaginations of the mucosa)
2. Submucosa
   a. connective tissue
   b. plexi of nerves and ganglion cells termed Meissner's plexus
   c. some areas may contain glands
   d. rich in blood vessels
3. Muscular tunic
   a. inner circular smooth muscle layer
   b. outer longitudinal smooth muscle layer
   c. Auerbach's myenteric plexus—between the two muscle layers is located a parasympathetic plexus of nerves associated with numerous ganglion cells
4. Adventitia
   a. connective tissue containing blood vessels, nerves, and lymphatics
   b. peritoneal covering (mesothelium) known as a serosa, located in some regions

Esophagus (about 10 to 12 in). The upper third of the esophagus features skeletal muscle (voluntary), the middle third both skeletal and smooth (involuntary) muscle, the lower third as the rest of the digestive tract only smooth muscle.

The Stomach. The stomach is highly vascular, contains gastric glands, and has smooth muscle fibers extending around the glands. There are two types of gastric glands: cardiac and fundic.

1. Cardiac glands secrete mucus
2. Fundic glands:
   a. mucous and epithelial cells—secrete mucus; this mucus protects against autodigestion and neutralizes acid to a small degree.
   b. parietal or oxyntic cells—secrete hydrochloric acid (HCI). Acid (pH below 5.5) is necessary to convert pepsinogen into pepsin; at pH 2, this reaction is almost instantaneous. Parietal cells secrete acid under the influence of the hormone gastrin (probably of greatest importance); parasympathetic mediation via acetylcholine; histamine; and the presence of foodstuffs, such as peptides and amino acids.
   c. chief (zymogenic) cells—secrete pepsinogen, the precursor of pepsin (proteolytic enzyme). These cells also secrete and release the hormone gastrin, as well as the protein called the *intrinsic factor* critical for vitamin B_{12} absorption.
   d. argentaffin cells—thought to secrete serotonin, a vasoconstrictor substance.

Small Intestine. The small intestine has three major regions:

1. Duodenum (10 in)
2. Jejunum (8.5 ft)
3. Ileum (12.5 ft)

The small intestine has mucosal surface modifications:

   a. Villi (projections of mucosa)—covered by simple columnar epithelium and having a core of connective tissue; they are broad in the duodenum, fingerlike in the ileum. In the core of the villus (in the connective tissue layer called the lamina propria) are found lymphocytes, eosinophils, plasma cells, macrophages, capillaries, and *lacteals* (lymphatic capillaries).
   b. Microvilli—present on columnar absorptive cells which cover the villi and line the crypts. This surface contains proteins (transport carriers) with high specificity for binding with sugars and amino acids. Some transport carriers are linked with the action of Na^+-K^+ ATPase at the opposite

surface (pole) of the epithelial cell, and the energy liberated by hydrolysis of ATP powers active transport (against a concentration gradient). A similar process occurs in the proximal renal tubule. The density of some of these intestinal carrier proteins is genetically-regulated.

Large Intestine (cecum, ascending, transverse, and descending colon)

Colon and Rectum

The Major Digestive Glands

Pancreas: The pancreas has both an exocrine and endocrine secretory function. Two excretory ducts are usually present and enter the second part of the duodenum. Exocrine glandular elements are arranged in acini. Acinar cells have a basal zone which is basophilic and an apical zone with zymogen granules which are the precursors of the enzymes in pancreatic juice—namely trypsin, chymotrypsin, amylase, and lipase. Acinar cells secrete

1. trypsinogen, which will be converted into trypsin.
2. chymotrypsinogen, which will be converted into chymotrypsin.
3. procarboxypeptidase, which will be converted into carboxypeptidase.

The above reactions are autocatalyzed (trypsinogen-trypsin). Trypsin, chymotrypsin, and carboxypeptidase attack proteins and polypeptides and eventually render amino acids which can be absorbed.

Pancreatic lipase, amylase, and proteases are controlled by the presence of foodstuffs and hormones. As acid chyme enters the duodenum from the stomach, secretin is released and fluid and bicarbonate are secreted.

Pancreatic juice

1. neutralizes the acid chyme in the duodenum and
2. provides enzymes for the digestion of proteins, carbohydrates, and fats.

Islets of Langerhans are the endocrine portion of the pancreas. The endocrine cell aggregations are interspersed irregularly among the acini. Three cell types can be identified:

1. A, or alpha, cells, which are presumed to form glucagon.
2. B, or beta, cells which are more numerous than A cells and produce insulin.
3. D, or delta, cells; their significance is uncertain but they might represent multipotent resting cells.

Liver: The liver, anatomically interposed between the intestine and the heart, has the following major functions:

1. Synthesis and storage of glycogen.
2. Maintenance of blood glucose homeostasis.
3. Production of glucose from amino acids, lactic acid, or glycerol (*gluconeogenesis*).
4. Synthesis of nonessential amino acids and catabolism of all, except the branched chain (which occurs chiefly in extrahepatic cells).
5. Detoxification of ammonia released from amino acids through synthesis of urea.
6. Fatty acid synthesis, storage, and metabolism of lipoproteins.
7. Fatty acid catabolism by the beta-oxidation cycle and production of ketone bodies (acetone, acetoacetate, beta-hydroxybutyrate).
8. Removal of bile pigment, derived from hemoglobin breakdown, from the blood and secretion into the bile.
9. Synthesis of albumin, the chief intravascular protein, and several proteins involved in coagulation.
10. Storage of many lipid-and water-soluble vitamins.
11. Detoxification of drugs and other harmful substances (cytochrome P450, glycine conjugation).
12. Embryonic hematopoietic (red blood cell producing) organ.

Gallbladder: *Bile,* which is a composite of *bile salts, bile acids* and *bile pigments,* as well as electrolytes secreted continuously by the hepatocytes, is collected and stored in the gallbladder. The bile salts and acids, synthesized from cholesterol, are critical for normal fat digestion in the intestine, since they enable micelle formation. Certain drugs and their hepatic metabolites are excreted in the bile. The ileum is extremely efficient in the reabsorption of bile salts, so that 95% of the amount excreted per day is returned to the liver via the cyclical path called the *enterohepatic circulation.* Since steroid hormone is made from the cholesterol nucleus, the 5% which is lost is a major excretory pathway for steroid hormone precursors.

General Functional Schema of the Digestive Tube (ingestion, digestion, egestion)

Oral Cavity: The oral cavity
a) Receives food and perceives taste, odor, texture, and temperature.
b) Grinds foodstuffs to facilitate the action of enzymes.
c) Adds enzymes, mucus, and moisture and shapes the bolus for the process of swallowing.

Pharynx and Esophagus: The oral and laryngeal pharynx, and the esophagus are essentially conduits for food to reach the stomach.

Stomach: Food is received, stored, and churned; digestive juices are added; and the digestive process started in the mouth is continued. Intrinsic factor (antipernicious anemia factor) is secreted.

Small Intestines: Digestion is completed and most absorption occurs in jejunum and ileum.

Large Intestines: The following occurs in the large intestines:

1. Water and electrolytes are reabsorbed to preserve that delicate balance in the body.
2. Food is propelled along for elimination (egestion).

Intestinal Motility

Intestinal motility facilitates

1. the mixing of food with secretions and enzymes,
2. the contact of foodstuffs with the intestinal mucosa, and
3. propulsion along the tube (peristalsis).

This process is controlled by the nervous system, hormonal secretions, and intestinal distension and similar phenomena.

Epinephrine (from the adrenal) inhibits contraction; serotonin (from the small intestines) stimulates contractions.

Innervation of the Intestinal Tract

The nerves supplying the intestinal tract affect smooth muscle, glands, endocrine tissue, and control motility and secretion. Motility or *peristalsis* is a wave of compression (contraction) that is followed by a regional relaxation. The gut musculature (smooth) is controlled by the autonomic nervous system.

Sympathetic Innervation: Effects of sympathetic innervation are:

1. some excitation of salivary secretion

2. decrease of motility and secretion in the stomach and small intestines due mainly to the vasoconstrictive action

3. inhibition of muscular contraction and intrinsic ganglion cell activity due to the release of the neurotransmitters epinephrine and norepinephrine

Parasympathetic Innervation: Effects of the parasympathetic innervation are:

1. stimulation of motility and secretion via its supply of the intrinsic plexi and the release of the neurotransmitter acetylcholine

2. release of gastrin

Summary of Digestive Juices

A key concept in understanding the secretions of the digestive tract is the necessity for reduction of most complex dietary molecules to their simplest units. Thus, proteins must be reduced to amino acids, complex carbohydrates to monosaccharides, and complicated lipids to fatty acids and triglycerides. This is necessary for rapid and efficient absorption when nutrients reach the intestine, and subsequently for easy transport via circulation to the liver.

Saliva: Saliva is protective and digestive. In this manner, it

1. dissolves food and passes it over the taste buds
2. lubricates food
3. starts starch digestion (contains amylase which breaks down 1,4-glycosidic bonds of glucose molecules as in starch)
4. contains antibacterial enzymes (lysozymes)

Saliva is composed of

a. water
b. electrolytes
c. enzymes (chiefly ptyalin, or salivary amylase)
d. mucin
e. glycoproteins
f. blood group proteins
g. gamma globulins

Ptyalin. Ptyalin (salivary amylase), produced mainly by the parotid, submandibular, and sublingual salivary glands, functions in the breakdown of starch into molecules of the disaccharide maltose.

Gastric Juice: The gastric juice is composed of

1. water
2. hydrochloric acid
3. inorganic salts
4. mucus
5. hydrolytic enzymes (pepsin, lipase)
6. intrinsic factor

The acidity of gastric juice facilitates the chemical hydrolysis of the peptide bonds in ingested protein, preparing it for further enzymatic breakdown. The total volume of gastric juice approximates 2–3 L per day, which serves to liquefy the ingested material and to assist solubilization.

Pepsin. Pepsin, a proteinase of gastric juice, is derived from its precursor pepsinogen, which is secreted by the chief cells of the gastric mucosa. Pepsin acts on protein substrates, breaking them down to amino acids, proteoses, and peptones.

Rennin. Rennin is secreted by the stomach. This enzyme splits some peptide bonds in casein to produce a calcium-precipitable paracasein.

Mucus. Mucus is composed of proteins, glycoproteins, polysaccharides, intrinsic factor, plasma proteins, and blood-group substances.

Intrinsic factor. Intrinsic factor, produced by the parietal cells of the stomach, is a muco-protein. It binds to vitamin B_{12} and "protects" it until it is absorbed in the ileum and then transported actively into the circulation.

Pancreatic Juice: Pancreatic juice contains proteolytic, lipolytic, and amylolytic enzymes.

Pancreatic amylase. Pancreatic amylase is an enzyme which hydrolyzes starch to maltose.

Steapsin. Steapsin, or pancreatic lipase, facilitates the digestion of fats.

Trypsinogen. Trypsinogen is secreted by the pancreas and converted by enterokinase to the active enzyme *trypsin*. Trypsin's substrates are proteins but specifically it further disintegrates proteoses and peptones.

Chymotrypsinogen. Chymotrypsinogen is the precursor in pancreatic juice of the enzyme *chymotrypsin*. Trypsin is active in this conversion. Chymotrypsin acts with trypsin to hydrolyze proteins and protein products to polypeptides and amino acids.

Bile: Bile is secreted by the liver, stored and concentrated in the gallbladder, and poured into the duodenum. It primarily contains bile salts (such as cholic acid, chenodeoxycholic acid, deoxycholic acid, and lithocholic acid), cholesterol phospholipids (lecithins), pigments (bilirubin), mucin and sodium, potassium, calcium, and other elements. It aids in the emulsification, digestion, and absorption of fat. It also contributes to the alkalinization of the intestinal contents.

Lacteals are found in the villi of the small intestines; they are part of the lymphatic system and function to take up chyle containing fat in lipoproteins.

Hormones of the Digestive Tract

Endocrine cells of the gut originate from the neural crest. Hormones of the gastrointestinal tract are produced by the mucosa of the stomach (gastrin) and by the small intestines (secretin and cholecystokinin). These gastrointestinal hormones are polypeptides which affect

1. water balance,
2. electrolyte balance,
3. enzyme secretions,
4. motility,
5. digestion,
6. absorption,
7. growth, and
8. hormonal release.

The general stimuli for their release are:

a. nervous activity;
b. physical extension;
c. chemical stimuli.

Specific stimuli for three key hormones are:

a. Gastrin—distension, vagal stimulation, and presence of proteins and amino acids.
b. Secretin—acid chyme (hydrogen ion) released when the pH falls below 4.5.
c. Cholecystokinin—presence of proteins and amino acids and of monoglycerides, and fatty acids.

Primary actions are as follows:

1. Gastrin
   a. stimulates gastric acid and pepsinogen secretion
   b. increases the distension of the stomach and gastric motility
2. Secretin
   a. stimulates the pancreas to secrete pancreatic fluid and bicarbonate
   b. stimulates biliary fluid secretion and bicarbonate
   c. potentiates the enzymatic response to cholecystokinin
   d. slows gastric motility and emptying
   e. stimulates pepsinogen secretion
   f. inhibits gastrin release
3. Cholecystokinin
   a. stimulates pancreatic enzyme secretion
   b. increases the pancreatic bicarbonate response to secretin
   c. increases the distensibility of the stomach and inhibits gastric emptying
   d. induces gallbladder contractions and emptying

General Digestion of the Major Food Groups

Carbohydrates: Starch digestion begins in the oral cavity under the influence of α-amylase and ends in the small intestines after exposure to pancreatic amylase. Products resulting from the above processes are further hydrolyzed by enzymes associated with the microvilli of the intestinal cells. For example: (1) maltase acts on maltose and maltotriose to yield glucose units; (2) sucrase acts on sucrose to produce glucose and fructose; and (3) lactase breaks down lactose to yield monosaccharide subunits.

SUMMARY OF CARBOHYDRATES DIGESTION

Organ	Food	Enzyme	End Product	Absorption In
Oral Cavity	Polysaccharides	Amylase	Glucose	All in small intestine
	Disaccharide (maltose)	Disaccharidase (maltase)	Glucose	↑
Stomach	NO DIGESTION			
Small Intestine	Polysaccharides	Intestinal and pancreatic amylase	Glucose	
	Disaccharides	Disaccharidases	Glucose	
	↕	↕		
	Maltose	Maltase	Glucose	
	Sucrose	Sucrase	Glucose and fructose	
	Lactose	Lactase	Glucose and galactose	↓
Large Intestine	CONTINUATION OF THE ABOVE PROCESSES (Essentially digestion is completed before large intestine)		Glucose, Fructose, and Galactose	Large Intestine

Proteins: Digestion begins in the stomach by the action of pepsin, which has a specificity for peptide bonds; it is inactivated by pancreatic juice. When products are transferred from the stomach to the duodenum, this stimulus results in the release of cholecystokinin (CCK) which is responsible for the release of pancreatic proteolytic enzymes such as (1) endo and exopeptidases, (2) trypsin, (3) chymotrypsin, and (4) elastase.

SUMMARY OF PROTEIN DIGESTION

Organ	Food	Enzyme	End Product	Absorption In
Stomach	Milk protein (Casein)	Rennin (In newborn)	Smaller peptides and a few amino acids	All in small intestine as amino acids
	Proteins (Casein)	Pepsin	↑	↑
Small Intestine	Proteins	Trypsin, chymotrypsin, carboxypeptidase —all secreted by the pancreas		
	Polypeptides, dipeptides			
		Intestinal aminopeptidase, dipeptidase, enterokinase	↓	↓

Fats: In the stomach, fat products are acted on by pepsin; when the products are released into the duodenum, cholecystokinin stimulates the pancreas to secrete lipases and the gallbladder to release its contents, which emulsify fat droplets resulting in the formation of micelles. The absorption is completed in the jejunum.

SUMMARY OF FAT DIGESTION

Organ	Food	Enzyme	End Product	Absorption In
Stomach	Fats	Absolute minimal digestion		All in small intestine
Small Intestine	Fats emulsified by bile	Intestinal and pancreatic lipase	Fatty acids and glycerol	

Quick Recall Test Questions and Answers

Choose the Best Answer

1. The enzyme ptyalin (salivary amylase) is produced mainly by the:

   A. chief cells of the stomach.
   B. cardiac glands of the stomach.
   C. argentaffin cells of the stomach.
   D. serous cells of salivary glands.
   E. acinar cells of the pancreas.

2. All of the following are liver functions EXCEPT:

   A. gluconeogenesis.
   B. lipid metabolism.
   C. glucogan synthesis.
   D. plasma protein synthesis.
   E. vitamin storage.

3. A surgeon can find the appendix by locating the:

   A. jejunum.
   B. cecum.
   C. colon (transverse).
   D. duodenum.
   E. right iliac fossa.

4. Bile, which is important in the digestion of fats, is produced by the:

   A. stomach.
   B. liver.
   C. duodenum.
   D. gallbladder.
   E. lacteals.

5. The gastric juice in the stomach:

   A. has a neutral pH.
   B. is alkaline.
   C. is acidic.
   D. contains trypsin.
   E. contains insulin.

6. The large intestine functions mainly in:

   A. absorption of water.
   B. excretion of water.
   C. absorption of sodium and potassium.
   D. finishing the digestive process.
   E. excretion of digestive enzymes.

7. One enzyme that is important in protein digestion is:

   A. ptyalin.
   B. trypsin.
   C. maltose.
   D. pancreatic lipase.
   E. rennin.

8. _____ is a zymogen or enzyme precursor.

   A. Pepsin
   B. Trypsin
   C. Pancreatic amylase
   D. Chymotrypsinogen

9. _____ is a proteinase with a pH optimum around 2.

   A. Pepsin
   B. Trypsin
   C. Pancreatic amylase
   D. Chymotrypsinogen

10. _____ has chloride ion as an activator.

    A. Pepsin
    B. Trypsin
    C. Pancreatic amylase
    D. Chymotrypsinogen

11. _____ can be activated by trypsin because of splitting of a single peptide bond.

    A. Pepsin
    B. Trypsin
    C. Pancreatic amylase
    D. Chymotrypsinogen

Match the letter of the nutrient deficiency disease in Column II with the deficient nutrient in Column I. Each letter may be used only once.

	Column I		Column II
12.	_____ vitamin A	A.	Kwashiorkor
13.	_____ vitamin B_{12}	B.	night blindness
14.	_____ vitamin C	C.	pernicious anemia
15.	_____ vitamin D	D.	pellagra
16.	_____ iodine	E.	beri-beri
17.	_____ niacin	F.	rickets
18.	_____ protein	G.	scurvy
19.	_____ thiamine	H.	goiter

Match the letter of the nutrient in Column II with the function in Column I. Each letter may be used only once.

	Column I		Column II
20.	_____ enhances the absorption of iron	A.	vitamin C
21.	_____ necessary for calcium's role in blood clotting	B.	vitamin D
		C.	vitamin K
22.	_____ needed for the synthesis of the protein that transports vitamin A from the liver	D.	copper
		E.	zinc
23.	_____ part of active cytochromeoxidase		
24.	_____ needed for the absorption of calcium in the intestine		

25. A pediatric patient fails to thrive, has most of his dietary nitrogen appearing in the feces, and has (by various tests) a normal small intestine mucosal surface. When a test protein is added directly to the small intestine, it is found that no significant amount of amino acids appears in the intestine or in the blood. However, addition of a trace amount of trypsin directly to the small intestine results in the complete hydrolysis of the protein with the rapid increase of amino acids in the portal blood supply. The problems of this infant are consistent with a deficiency in:

    A. lactase.
    B. enterokinase.
    C. chymotrypsinogen.
    D. trypsin.
    E. pancreatic flow of enzymes.

26. Which hormone causes contraction and emptying of the gall bladder?

    A. steapsin
    B. gastrin
    C. secretin
    D. cholecystokinin
    E. glucogan

27. The hormone which plays a key role in the secretion of pancreatic fluid and bicarbonate is:

    A. steapsin.
    B. gastrin.
    C. secretin.
    D. cholecystokinin.
    E. glucogan.

28. The nutritional value of the carotenoid provitamins lies in their conversion to:

    A. Vitamin A.
    B. Vitamin B_1.
    C. Vitamin C.
    D. Vitamin D.
    E. Vitamin K.

Answers

1. **D.** Ptyalin (salivary amylase), produced mainly by the parotid, submandibular, and sublingual salivary glands, functions in the breakdown of starch into molecules of the disaccharide maltose. Chief cells secrete pepsinogen, the precursor of pepsin. Cardiac glands secrete mucus. Argentaffin cells secrete seretonin. Acinar cells secrete zymogen granules, which are the precursors of the enzymes of pancreatic juice.

2. **C.** Please see summary of liver function in text (page 126).

3. **B.** The appendix is a blind sac originating from the cecum of the ascending colon (large intestines).

4. **B.** Bile is secreted by the liver, stored and concentrated in the gall bladder, and poured into the duodenum. It contains bile salts, cholesterol, lecithin, fat, pigments, and mucin. It aids in the emulsification, digestion, and absorption of fat, and contributes to the alkalinization of the intestines.

5. **C.** The gastric mucosa secretes hydrochloric acid, mucin, and the enzymes rennin, pepsin, and lipase. An average of 2 to 3 liters is secreted within a 24-hour time period. The pH of gastric juice usually varies from 0.9 to 1.5. This acidity allows pepsin to act while it inhibits ptyalin (salivary amylase). Food usually remains in the stomach for 3 to 4 hours.

6. **A.** One of the main functions of the large intestine is the reabsorption of water.

7. **B.** Trypsin is the enzyme that is functional in protein digestion. Ptyalin (salivary amylase) acts on starches while pancreatic lipase (steapsin) acts on fats. Maltose is not an enzyme but a sugar.

8. **D.** Chymotrypsinogen is the precursor in pancreatic juice of the enzyme chymotrypsin. Trypsin is active in this conversion. Chymotrypsin acts with trypsin to hydrolyze proteins and protein products to polypeptides and amino acids.

9. **A.** Pepsin is a proteinase of gastric juice (derived from its precursor pepsinogen), which is secreted by the chief cells of the gastric mucosa. The pH of the stomach varies around 1.5.

10. **C.** Pancreatic juice contains proteolytic, lipolytic, and amylolytic enzymes. Pancreatic amylase is the enzyme which hydrolyzes starch to maltose.

11. **D.** Chymotrypsinogen is the precursor in pancreatic juice of the enzyme chymotrypsin. Trypsin is active in this conversion. Chymotrypsin acts with trypsin to hydrolyze proteins and protein products to polypeptides and amino acids.

12. **B.** Vitamin A is formed from the carotenoid provitamins (yellow pigments of most vegetables and fruits). Deficiency causes poor dark vision adaptation, conjunctivitis, and keratinization of the cornea.

13. **C.** Despite being involved as a cofactor in only two reactions in the human body, vitamin B_{12} is of critical importance. Vitamin B_{12} deficiency can be due to many things and is manifested as the condition called pernicious anemia.

14. **G.** Vitamin C maintains the integrity of important metalloenzymes involved in collagen synthesis and steroidogenesis, as well as maintenance of cytochromes and intestinal absorption of iron. Vitamin C deficiency causes scurvy, a disease in which many of the clinical findings such as gingival hemorrhage and death, hemorrhage into old scars and refractures of old, healed fractures point to a common effect on collagen metabolism.

15. **F.** Vitamin D does not occur naturally and is manufactured in the animal body by the utilization of ultraviolet light. Deficiency mainly affects calcification of bones and teeth; rickets in the child and osteomalacia in the adult are consequences. The vitamin enhances the absorption of calcium and phosphorus from the intestinal tract.

16. **H.** A goiter is an enlargement of the thyroid gland not due to neoplasm or inflammatory disease. Endemic goiters are due to lack of intake of iodine (less than 10 µg/day) caused by deficiency in the soil and water. This interferes with hormone production and results in increased TSH production, thyroid compensatory hypertrophy, and eventual exhaustion of the gland.

17. **D.** Niacin is the functional group of the coenzymes NAD and NADP. Deficiency results in black tongue in canines and pellagra in humans. Dermatitis and neurological lesions are manifestations of pellagra.

18. **A.** Kwashiorker is a result of severe protein deficiency. It is characterized by anemia, edema, pot belly, depigmentation of the skin, loss or change in hair color, hypoalbuminemia, and bulky stools containing undigested food.

19. **E.** Vitamin B_1 is essential for the proper functioning of the nervous system; it is an antagonist to acetylcholine. Deficiency will result in beriberi in humans and polyneuritis in birds.

20. **A.** Vitamin C maintains the integrity of important metalloenzymes involved in collagen synthesis and steroidogenesis, as well as maintenance of cytochromes and intestinal absorption of iron.

21. **C.** Vitamin K is necessary for the production of prothrombin and thus for normal clotting to occur. Deficiency causes abnormally long

clotting times and hemorrhage.

22. **E.** Zinc is an essential component of nearly 100 different enzymes. It is a cofactor in dehydrogenenase, DNA polymerase, and carbonic anhydrase.

23. **D.** Copper is a prosthetic group of cytochrome oxidase. Animals that are copper deficient have defective collagen molecules lacking cross links. The collagen and elastin of major arteries weaken and rupture occurs. Copper is also essential for the proper utilization of iron.

24. **B.** The chief action of vitamin D is to enhance the synthesis of calcium-binding protein which increases calcium and phosphate absorption by the intestine, from which the bone produces hydroxyapatite, the crystalline material from which bone is constructed.

25. **B.** Trypsinogen is secreted by the pancreas and converted by enterokinase to the active enzyme trypsin. Trypsin's substrates are proteins, but specifically it further disintegrates proteoses and peptones. Chymotrypsin acts with trypsin to hydrolyze proteins and protein products to polypeptides and amino acids.

26. **D.** Cholecystokinin stimulates pancreatic enzyme secretion, increases the pancreatic bicarbonate response to secretin, increases the distensibility of the stomach and inhibits gastric emptying, and induces gallbladder contractions and emptying.

27. **C.** Secretin stimulates pepsinogen secretion, pancreatic fluid secretion, and bicarabonate, and biliary fluid secretion and bicarbonate; potentiates the enzymatic response to cholecystokinin; slows gastric motility and emptying; and inhibits gastrin release.

28. **A.** Vitamin A is formed from carotenoid provitamins (yellow pigments of most vegetables and fruits). Deficiency causes poor dark vision adaptation, conjunctivitis, and keratinization of the cornea.

Nervous System

The nervous system is usually divided into: (a) central nervous system (brain and spinal cord) and (b) peripheral nervous system (peripheral nerves and ganglia). The peripheral nervous system is divided into a somatic system and visceral (autonomic) system.

Nervous Tissue

Nervous tissue consists of neurons (nerve cells and their processes) and supportive elements. Neuroglia in the central nervous system and Schwann cells in the peripheral nervous system are the supportive elements.

The Neuron

The neuron is a cellular element and, as a highly specialized cell, it carries out the function of nervous transmission. The neuron is like many other cells within the body in that it consists of a nucleus with an associated nucleolus and a cytoplasm which is rich in organelles, the most prominent of which are the rough-surfaced endoplasmic reticulum (Nissl substance), mitochondria, and the Golgi apparatus. In addition to the above characteristics, it should be noted that neurons possess numerous cytoplasmic processes or appendages. In almost all of the many varieties of neurons, there are two kinds of processes: the *dendrites* and the *axon*.

The Dendrites:

1. are direct extensions of the cytoplasm.

2. are generally multiple.

3. provide an increased surface area, the dendritic zone, to allow for synaptic interaction.

The Axon:

1. There is only one per neuron.

2. This process arises from a conical elevation of cytoplasm which is devoid of rough-surfaced endoplasmic reticulum (Nissl) and this area is called the *axon hillock*.

3. It is usually thinner and longer than the dendrites of the same neuron.

4. It may be surrounded by a *myelin sheath* which is produced by the *oligodendrocytes* in the CNS and by the *Schwann cells* in the PNS. Discontinuities in this myelin sheath occur at intervals

A typical single multipolar neuron. (1) Proximal portion (in a lesion (cut) the process distal from the cell body could completely degenerate; retrograde degeneration would be detected in the proximal portion; however, with time the proximal portion has the capacity to regenerate in the PNS); (2) nucleus with nucleolus, containing the genetic material of the cell and directing the synthetic activity of the cell; (3) Golgi apparatus (zone), the packaging and contrating area of the cell's secretory activity; (4) dendrites—pick up an impulse and carry it toward the cell body; (5) endoplasmic reticulum (rough in this case—ribosomes are attached), the synthetic machinery of the cell (proteins, etc.); (6) cell membrane, semipermeable and the protector of the cell from its environment; (7) cytoplasm (specifically the area here is called axon hillock); (8) myelin sheath (formed by Schwann cells in the PNS and oligodentrocytes in the CNS), the insulator material of the axon; (9) direction of impulse conduction; (10 a, b) axon conducts impulses away from the cell body to contact other neurons, muscle cells, glands, or receptors of many types; (11) terminal branches of the axon.

known as the *nodes of Ranvier*. Though many axons are myelinated and are referred to as myelinated nerve fibers, numerous others possess no myelin ensheathment and thus are referred to as unmyelinated nerve fibers.

5.   At its ending, the axon transmits impulses: (a) to other neurons—the site of this impulse transmission being called a *synapse;* and (b) to effector cells such as muscle fibers or gland cells. The junction with skeletal muscle fibers constitutes a *motor end plate*.

The Action Potential: An impulse traveling along a neuron is an electrical phenomenon initiated by a temporary change in the permeability of the neuron's cell membrane. To understand this change, one must first examine the condition of a resting, or unstimulated, neuron. The membrane possesses specific sites for the active transport of sodium ions (Na^+) and potassium ions (K^+). At these sites, sodium is transported out of the cell, and potassium is transported inward. Both ions tend to return to their original positions through pores, but Na^+ ions are less successful than are K^+ ions. Thus, the unstimulated neuron accumulates a larger concentration of positive ions (both Na^+ and K^+) outside its membrane than in its cytoplasm. A voltmeter would measure this difference as about 70 mV, with the inside of the neuron being negative; this is called the *resting potential* or *membrane potential*.

A sufficient stimulus—whether it be mechanical, chemical, or electrical—causes a radical but temporary change in the permeability of the affected membrane region. The membrane possesses specific channels that can allow sodium to pass, and others for potassium; in a resting membrane both are closed. A stimulus causes the sodium channel to open, and accumulated sodium ions outside the membrane rush into the interior by diffusion. Their number is sufficient to reverse the interior charge, making it about 40 mV positive. This change, in turn, causes the potassium channels to open, allowing a loss of potassium ions from the cytoplasm. Thus, the initial gain of interior positive ions (Na^+) is countered by a loss of positive ions (K^+), and the cytoplasm once again is negatively charged. The charge reversal, from negative to positive to negative, occurs within only a few milliseconds. The phenomenon is termed an *action potential*.

Immediately after an action potential, the sodium and potassium channels close again, and the two types of ions are pumped back to their original sites. During this refractory period of several milliseconds, an additional stimulus will not lead to another action potential.

Initiation of the action potential at any point of a neuron's membrane acts as a stimulus to the adjacent membrane material; therefore, the effect is an action potential flowing along the membrane. The result is that the "message" moves quickly over the length of a motor neuron's axon. It is also the message that flows along and into a muscle fiber that has been stimulated by events at a motor end plate, because the membrane of a muscle fiber can act like that of a neuron.

The Synapse: The synapse is the site of contact between two neurons; it may be, and most commonly is, between an axon and a dendrite; however, contacts between an axon and the cell body and between axons and axons have also been observed. A typical synapse seen between an axon and dendrite (axodendritic synapse) has the following properties:

1.   As the axon terminal reaches the synaptic site, it forms a bulbous head called a *bouton*. This bouton, which constitutes the presynaptic element of the synapse, contains numerous mitochondria and specialized vesicles, the synaptic vesicles, which contain the various neurotransmitters (acetylcholine is the primary one).

2.   The dendrite, which constitutes the postsynaptic element of the synapse, is separated from the bouton by a cleft which varies in width from 150 to 200 Å.

3.   This axo-dendritic synapse is *not* a site where cytoplasmic continuity is established between the axon and the dendrite, as both the pre- and postsynaptic elements are separated by a cleft. However, via the process of synaptic vesicle release, this axodendritic synapse establishes a functional (chemical) continuity across the expanse of the cleft.

Classification of Neurons

Multipolar Neurons: Most abundant; somatic and visceral motor, and associational.

Pseudounipolar Neurons (occasionally referred to as **Unipolar Neurons**): Somatic and visceral *sensory* neurons; cell bodies are located in cranial sensory and dorsal root ganglia; peripheral process goes out to receptor and central process travels into the central nervous system.

Bipolar Neurons: Special *sensory* neurons; cell bodies are located in special sense organs; i.e., eye (retina), ear (spiral and vestibular ganglia), and nose (olfactory epithelium).

Groups of Neurons

Nucleus: cluster of nerve cell bodies *within* the central nervous system.
Ganglion: cluster of nerve cells bodies *outside* the central nervous system.
Cortex: layered arrangement of nerve cells bodies on the surface of the cerebrum and cerebellum (gray matter).

Supportive Elements

Neuroglia—Supportive Elements of the Central Nervous System: Neuroglia, the supportive elements of the central nervous system, are of several types:

1. Astrocytes. Astrocytes are fibrous and protoplasmic; their perivascular feet end on capillaries. They are located between capillary (or pia matter) and neurons and are implicated in the blood-brain barrier. Eighty percent of brain capillary surfaces are covered by perivascular end feet of astrocytes.

2. Oligodendrocytes. Oligodendrocytes function in the myelinization of central nervous system axons.

3. Microglia. Microglia are the phagocytic macrophage-like cells of the central nervous system.

Supportive Elements of the Peripheral Nervous System

1. Schwann (neurilemmal) Cells. These are involved in the myelinization of peripheral nervous system axons.

2. Satellite Cells. These cells surround nerve cell bodies in the ganglia (e.g., dorsal root ganglia) of the peripheral nervous system.

The Central Nervous System

The central nervous system is made up of the brain and the spinal cord.

Spinal Cord: Before one can appreciate the organization of the cerebral mass and brain stem, it is necessary to understand the basic structural organization found throughout the extent of the spinal cord.

Cross Section View. If one were to examine a cross section through any level of the spinal cord, the following would be seen:

1. A centrally located H-shaped mass which contains the cell bodies of multipolar neurons. This H-shaped mass is divided into dorsal and ventral columns, or *horns*. Cell bodies responsible for sensory phenomena are located in the dorsal horns, cell bodies for motor phenomena in the ventral horns. This H-shaped mass is collectively referred to as the *gray matter*.

2. Peripheral to this H-shaped mass, *white matter,* made up primarily of myelinated nerve fibers.

3. Entering the spinal cord at the apex of the dorsal horn, or column, is the dorsal root of the spinal nerve. The cell bodies of these fibers are pseudounipolar and are located in the dorsal root ganglion. The ventral root exits from the ventral horn of the gray matter. The cell bodies of these fibers are multipolar and located in the ventral horn.

4. White matter is divided into three masses of fibers known as *funiculi*. These three funiculi are:
    (a) the dorsal funiculus, located between the dorsal midline and the dorsal root,
    (b) the lateral funiculus, located between the dorsal and ventral roots, and
    (c) the ventral funiculus, located between the ventral root and the ventral midline.

Within each funiculus are found bundles of fibers (axons) called *tracts*. The fibers within a specific tract have a common origin, termination, and function and either descend or ascend in the cord.

5.   An orderly arrangement of gray and white matter that remains constant throughout the spinal cord, varying only in relative mass.

Intermediolateral Cell Column
Lateral Funiculus
Dorsal Horn (Gray Column)
Dorsal Funiculus
Dorsal Gray Commissure
Dorsal Medial Sulcus
Dorsal White Commissure
Dorsal Root (Afferent or Sensory)
Central Process
Dorsal Root Ganglion (Cell Body)
Peripheral Process
Spinal Nerve
Ventral Horn Cell
Ventral Root (Efferent or Motor)
Ventral Horn (Gray Column)
Synapse
Association Neuron
Ventral White Commissure
Ventral Canal
Ventral Median Fissure
Ventral Gray Commissure

Transverse section of spinal cord

Gross Anatomy and Relationships. The spinal cord viewed as a whole also has the following characteristics:

1.   It is cylindrical, about ½ inch in diameter and 18 inches in length, and has *cervical* and *lumbar enlargements* due to the involvement of these cord levels with the innervation of the upper and lower limbs, respectively.

2.   It runs within the bony *vertebral canal* but is shorter than the canal since vertebral column growth exceeds cord growth. The spinal cord ends at vertebral level L_1–L_2 (Lumbar 1–2).

3.   It is protected not only by the bony vertebral column but also by three connective tissue sheaths known collectively as the *meninges* (dura mater, arachnoid membrane, and pia mater). *Cerebrospinal fluid* is in the subarachnoid space (between arachnoid and pia) and bathes the cord and cushions it from shock.

4.   There are 31 pairs of *spinal nerves* that are connected to the cord by *dorsal* and *ventral roots*: 8 *cervical,* 12 *thoracic,* 5 *lumbar,* 5 *sacral,* and 1 *coccygeal.*

5.   The spinal nerves exit from the vertebral canal through *intervertebral foramina.*

6.   It is because the cord ends at vertebral level L_2 that *lumbar punctures* (spinal taps) can be done safely below that level. (Nerve roots arise from the cord and extend below this level to exit at the specific vertebral level. These roots are collectively called *cauda equina* and are deflected away from the needle and therefore are not damaged.)

The Brain: The brain is divided into three parts: the cerebrum (two cerebral hemispheres), the brain stem, and the cerebellum. The brain stem is, in turn, divided into the medulla, pons, midbrain, and diencephalon. Important facts about the structure and functions of each of the parts follows.

Cerebrum. The cerebrum consists of two hemispheres that are joined by a broad band of commissural fibers, the *corpus callosum*. Eminences on the surface are known as *gyri* and the furrows as *sulci* or *fissures*.

Each cerebral hemisphere is divided into five lobes:

1.   *frontal*—contains the major motor areas (motor speech area).
2.   *parietal*—is concerned with sensory impressions such as touch, pressure, and pain.
3.   *occipital*—is concerned with vision.
4.   *temporal*—is concerned with hearing.
5.   *insula*—is found deep within the Sylvian fissure.

The human brain as seen from the medial aspect. The spinal cord and vertebra are shown in relation to the brain.

The cerebrum is the seat of intelligence, consciousness and rational behavior and possesses areas for speech and writing.

A right lateral view of the cerebrum. Major areas and lobes, and the function they regulate are shown.

Medulla Oblongata. The medulla oblongata is structurally derived from the myelencephalon and is continuous with the spinal cord at the *foramen magnum* and extends to the caudal portion of the pons. The medulla controls movement of eyelids (in blinking), sneezing, coughing, chewing, swallowing, and vomiting, and contains centers for the autonomic control of respiration (breathing), heartbeat (rate and force), contracility of blood vessels, visceral movement (gastric juice production and peristalsis), and glandular secretion (salivation).

Pons. The pons is essentially a crossing and relay station for nerve tracts. It is a conduit through which the cerebral cortex communicates with the cerebellum. It contains the motor nuclei that exert control over facial expression and mastication, and it possesses cell bodies that control lacrimation and salivation, and it serves as a relay station of tactile sensation for the facial system.

Midbrain. The midbrain serves as a relay center for auditory and optic phenomena. It houses the oculomotor nucleus, which controls extraocular movements, and exerts autonomic control over pupillary constriction and the process of accommodation.

Diencephalon. The diencephalon is itself divided into the thalamus and the hypothalamus.

Thalamus.

1. Maintains the internal environment of the organism.
2. Processes all sensory input except olfactation.
3. Maintains a subconscious sense of comfort.
4. Serves as the main relay station between the cerebrum and the rest of the nervous system.
5. Serves in the integration of motor activities via its relay activity between the basal ganglia, the cerebellum and the cerebral cortex.

Hypothalamus. The hypothalamus regulates body temperature, osmotic balance, blood pressure, and sleep.

Cerebellum. The cerebellum is derived from the metencephalon. It integrates unconscious proprioceptive impulses, integrates and modulates vestibular functions and body equilibrium. The cerebellum is also responsible for muscular synergy of the body; it coordinates the smooth, accurate, and orderly sequences of muscular contraction and movement. Without cerebellar influence, muscle activity is disorganized and crude. There is, however, no conscious perception.

The Peripheral Nervous System

The peripheral nervous system is made up of a somatic portion and an autonomic portion.

Somatic Peripheral Nervous System: The somatic portion of the peripheral nervous system is made up of cranial nerves and spinal nerves.

Cranial Nerves. The cranial nerves are those peripheral nerves which leave the brain. It is customary to subdivide the cranial nerves into twelve pairs and to number and name these pairs as follows:

I.	Olfactory nerve	VII.	Facial nerve
II.	Optic nerve	VIII.	Vestibulocochlear (auditory) nerve
III.	Oculomotor nerve	IX.	Glossopharyngeal nerve
IV.	Trochlear nerve	X.	Vagus nerve
V.	Trigeminal nerve	XI.	Spinal accessory nerve
VI.	Abducens nerve	XII.	Hypoglossal nerve

The twelve pairs of cranial nerves as they emerge from the brain.

No.	Nerve	General Components	Peripheral Termination and Modality Supplied	Damage to Nerve Results in
I	Olfactory	Sensory	Nasal mucosa—olfaction	Anosmia; Parosmia
II	Optic	Sensory	Rods and cones of retina—vision	Visual field defects
III	Oculomotor	Motor	Superior, inferior, and medial rectus muscles and inferior oblique muscle—rotate eyeball	Strabismus or squint—deviation of the eyeball; Diplopia—double vision
		Motor	To a muscle which constricts pupil To ciliary muscle whose contraction thickens lens	Dilated pupil; Loss of light reflexes Loss of accommodation
IV	Trochlear	Motor	Superior oblique muscle—rotates eyeball	Strabismus and diplopia
V	Trigeminal	Motor	Muscles of mastication—mastication	Paralysis of the muscles of mastication
		Sensory	Skin of face and mucosa of mouth and nose—supplies sensation	Loss of sensation over the distribution of V; Loss of reflex; Tic douloureux—pain over the distribution of V
VI	Abducens	Motor	Lateral rectus muscle—moves eyeball laterally	Loss of the ability to abduct eyeball
VII	Facial	Motor	Muscles of facial expression	Facial paralysis (Bell's palsy); Expressionless face with a drooping mouth
		Sensory	Taste buds on the anterior two-thirds of the tongue	Loss of taste on the anterior two-thirds of the tongue
VIII	Vestibulocochlear	Sensory (Vestibular portion)	Cristae of semicircular canals—provide for equilibrium	Vertigo, nystagmus, and nausea
		Sensory (Cochlear portion)	Hair cells in the organ of Corti—provide for hearing	Deafness
IX	Glossopharyngeal	Motor	Parotid gland—provides for glandular secretion	Loss of secretion
		Sensory	Taste buds on the posterior one-third of the tongue	Loss of taste on the posterior one-third of the tongue
		Sensory	Epiglottis, root of tongue, soft palate	Loss of gag reflex
X	Vagus	Motor	Palate and pharyngeal constrictors and intrinsic muscles of larynx	Aphonia and dysphonia
		Motor	Via the cardiac and pulmonary ganglia to the cardiac muscle and to the smooth muscle and the glands of the pulmonary and gastrointestinal systems—provides for autonomic regulation of the above named organs	Automatic disturbances
XI	Spinal Accessory	Motor	Trapezius and sternomastoid muscles	Difficulty rotating head or raising shoulder
XII	Hypoglossal	Motor	Muscles of the tongue	Paralysis of tongue

Spinal Nerves. Thirty-one pairs of spinal nerves are connected to the spinal cord. Like any nerve, a spinal nerve is composed of nerve fibers (axons and their Schwann cell sheaths) coursing together outside the central nervous system. Spinal nerves are surrounded by well-organized protective sheaths, i.e., endoneurium, perineurium, and epineurium.

Spinal nerves contain both sensory and motor fibers.

a) Sensory:
   1) from receptors in skin and skeletal muscle (GSA—general somatic afferent),
   2) from receptors in smooth muscle in walls of organs and blood vessels (GVA—general visceral afferent).
b) Motor:
   1) to skeletal muscle (GSE—general somatic efferent),
   2) autonomic fibers to smooth muscle, cardiac muscle, and glands (GVE—general visceral efferent).

Sensory Pathway. A typical sensory pathway contains three neurons in a chain from the receptor on the surface of the body to consciousness in the cerebral cortex (Primary: 1°, Secondary: 2°, and Tertiary: 3° neurons).

1° neuron: has its pseudounipolar cell body in the dorsal root ganglion; its peripheral process goes out to the receptor through the spinal nerve; its central process follows the dorsal root and synapses in the CNS with a second-order (2°) neuron.

2° neuron: has its multipolar cell body in the central nervous system; those cell bodies concerned with pain and temperature are found within the spinal cord; those concerned with touch and pressure are localized in the medulla of the brain. The axon of this 2° neuron then crosses the midline and ascends to the thalamus, where it synapses with a third order (3°) neuron.

3° neuron: has its multipolar cell body in the thalamus; its axon ascends to the cerebral cortex.

Voluntary Motor Pathway. A typical voluntary motor pathway contains two neurons from the cerebral cortex to the effector organ in skeletal muscle.

Neuron 1: (upper motor neuron) has its multipolar cell body in the cerebral cortex; its axon descends, crosses in the medulla, and terminates in relation to lower motor neurons found in the ventral horn.

Neuron 2: (lower motor neuron) has its multipolar cell body in the ventral horn of the spinal cord; its axon (efferent fiber) leaves the spinal cord through the ventral root and follows the spinal nerve to the skeletal muscle, where it terminates as a motor end plate.

Autonomic Nervous System: The autonomic nervous system innervates all smooth muscle, cardiac muscle, and glands. The autonomic nervous system is divided into a sympathetic (flight and fight) component and parasympathetic (maintains homeostasis) component. The autonomic nervous system exerts important influences on the intrinsic eye musculature, skin glands, the cardiovascular, gastrointestinal, respiratory, endocrine, and reproductive systems.

Fear, rage, pain, and the like evoke sympathetic activity that mobilizes the resources of the body. Gastrointestinal activity is curtailed; heart rate and blood pressure increase and coronary arteries and bronchioles dilate.

1. dorsal root ganglion; 2. sympathetic chain ganglion; 3. terminal ganglion

Differences

Sympathetic	Parasympathetic
a. Thoracolumbar outflow (T1–L2)	a. Craniosacral outflow (cranial nerves III, VII, IX, X, and S2–S4)
b. Short preganglionic	b. Long preganlionic
c. Long postganglionic	c. Short postganglionic
d. Ganglia close to spinal cord	d. Ganglia close to organ
e. Emergency stress system	e. Steady-state system (homeostatic)
f. Epinephrine (neurotransmitter)	f. Acetylcholine (neurotransmitter)
g. Innervates skin	g. No skin innervation
h. Chain ganglion	h. No chain ganglion
i. Innervates adrenal gland	i. No adrenal innervation

Similarities of the two divisions: sympathetic (thoracolumbar), parasympathetic (craniosacral)

a.   Involuntary system: innervates smooth muscle, cardiac muscle, glands, and organs.

b.   Two neuron system: First neuron—inside CNS (preganglionic).
Second neuron—outside CNS in ganglion (postganglionic).

c.   Fibers run with cranial nerves, spinal nerves, and alone as splanchnic nerves.

SUMMARY ACTION OF THE AUTOMATIC NERVOUS SYSTEM

Organ	Sympathetic	Parasympathetic
Heart	Increases rate	Decreases rate
Vasculature	Constricts vessels	Dilates vessels
Blood	Increases pressure	Decreases pressure
Digestive (peristalsis)	Decreases rate	Increases rate
Bladder	Relaxes muscle	Contracts muscle
Bronchial Tree	Dilates	Constricts
Glands	Increases activity	Decreases activity

Reflex Arc

The typical pathway of a reflex may be outlined as follows: sensory receptor on dendrite of dorsal root ganglion cell → ganglion cell → axon of cell → dorsal root → dorsal horn of spinal cord → either directly to motor cell in ventral horn or via internuncial (association) neuron to ventral horn motor cell → axon via ventral root → spinal nerve → effector organ (e.g., muscle).

GENERAL TERMINOLOGY FOR DESCRIBING THE CRANIOSPINAL NERVES

General sensory or general somatic afferent (GSA)	Pain, temperature, and touch; proprioception, vibration, pressure, and discrimination	All spinal nerves; cranial nerves CN V, VII, IX, X
General visceral afferent (GVA)	Pain due to distension	All spinal nerves and CN X
Special sensory or special afferent (SSA)	Vision, equilibrium and hearing	CN II CN VIII
Special sensory or special visceral afferent (SVA)	Smell, taste	CN I CN VII, IX, X
Visceral motor or visceral efferent (GVE)	Smooth muscle, cardiac muscle, and glands	All spinal nerves; sympathetic component
	Levator palpebrae superioris, sphincter pupillae, and ciliary muscle of accommodation	CN III
	Lacrimal, submandibular, and sublingual glands	CN VII
	Parotid gland	CN IX
	Cardiac and smooth muscle	CN X
Somatic motor or general somatic efferent (GSE)	All skeletal muscle	All spinal nerves and CN III, IV, V, VI, VII, IX, XI, XII

Quick Recall Test Questions and Answers

Choose the Best Answer

1. The trochlear nerve (CN IV) supplies motor innervation to the _____, an extraocular muscle of the eye.

   A. superior rectus
   B. inferior rectus
   C. medical rectus
   D. inferior oblique
   E. superior oblique

2. Among the components of a reflex arc may be cited:

   A. sensory receptor on dentride.
   B. dorsal root ganglion cell.
   C. axon of dorsal root ganglion cell.
   D. dorsal horn of spinal cord.
   E. associational neuron.
   F. ventral horn motor cell.
   G. none of the above.
   H. all of the above.

3. The roots of the spinal nerves below the vertebral level of Lumbar 2 are known as the:

   A. cauda equina.
   B. conus medullaris.
   C. filum terminale internum.
   D. gray rami communicans.
   E. lumbosacral plexus.

4. Which is not a correct statement?

   A. The end of the spinal cord may be found opposite the disk between the L_1 and L_2 vertebrae.
   B. The spinal cord has a cervical enlargement which facilitates the innervation of the upper limb.
   C. Cerebrospinal fluid is produced by the choroid plexus and is found in the subarachnoid space.
   D. The three membranes known as meninges are the dura, arachnoid, and pia.
   E. Lumbar punctures are usually performed below the L_2 vertebral level.

5. Of the three types of neurons (classified according to the number of their processes) the cell bodies of _____ are found within the central nervous system (CNS).

   A. only unipolar (pseudounipolar)
   B. only bipolar
   C. only multipolar
   D. both unipolar and bipolar
   E. both bipolar and multipolar

6. Supportive elements of the nervous system include:

   A. astrocytes.
   B. oligodendrocytes.
   C. microglia.
   D. Schwann cells.
   E. all of the above.

7. An aggregation of nerve cell bodies inside the CNS is typically called a:

   A. clone.
   B. colony.
   C. Nissl zone.
   D. tract.
   E. nucleus.

8. The reflex arc is of utmost importance to human beings. Which of the following is NOT a component of the reflex arc?

   A. medulla
   B. dendrite (receptor)
   C. synapse
   D. ventral horn cell (effector)
   E. axon

9. In an auto accident the driver suffers complete sectioning of several anterior (ventral) roots of spinal nerves. What is the result of such a lesion to the regions supplied by those spinal nerves?

   A. no neural deficit
   B. loss of motor activity
   C. loss of sensation
   D. loss of sensation and motor activity
   E. loss of temperature and pain sensations

10. A patient awaiting selective surgery presents the following symptoms. Which of the following indi-

cate(s) a heightened activity of the sympathetic portion of the autonomic nervous system?

A. a yearning for water due to a dry mouth
B. sweaty palms
C. pale skin
D. all of the above
E. none of the above

11. Body temperature is regulated by the:

A. thalamus.
B. medulla.
C. pons.
D. cerebellum.
E. hypothalamus.

12. The cell bodies of the motor neurons are located in the spinal cord in the:

A. intermediolateral cell column.
B. dorsal root ganglia.
C. dorsal horn (gray matter).
D. ventral horn (gray matter).
E. ventral root ganglia.

13. After running to catch the bus for work, an individual experiences a rapid heart rate, an increase in respiratory rate, and an increase in blood pressure. We can attribute these changes to:

A. the peripheral nervous system.
B. the central nervous system.
C. the parasympathetic component of the autonomic nervous system.
D. increased metabolic rate.
E. the sympathetic component of the autonomic nervous system.

14. The part of the neuron that conducts impulses away from its cell body is called the:

A. axon.
B. dendrite.
C. node of Ranvier.
D. Schwann sheath.
E. nucleus.

15. The neurotransmitter acetylcholine is released by:

A. axon terminals.
B. dendrite terminals.
C. Golgi apparatus of neuron cell bodies.
D. Schwann cells.
E. the node of Ranvier.

16. A patient has suffered a cerebral hemorrhage that has caused injury and nonfunctioning of the primary motor area of his left cerebral cortex. As a result:

A. he cannot voluntarily move his right arm or hand or his right leg or foot.
B. he feels no sensation on the left side of his body.
C. reflexes cannot be elicited on the left side of his body.
D. he cannot voluntarily move his right arm or his left leg.
E. he feels no sensation on the right side of his body.

17. _____ give(s) origin to the nervous system.

A. Ectoderm
B. Mesoderm
C. Endoderm
D. Ectoderm and endoderm
E. Endoderm and mesoderm

18. The two cerebral hemispheres of the mammalian brain are connected via the:

A. corpus callosum.
B. posterior commissure.
C. anterior commissure.
D. anterior peduncle.
E. third ventricle.

19. The neurolemma of an axon is part of the:

A. nerve cell body.
B. Schwann cell.
C. node of Ranvier.
D. axoplasm.
E. axon hillock.

20. We speak of an aggregation of nerve cell bodies in the central nervous system as the site of a (an):

A. ganglion.
B. nucleus.
C. cranial nerve.
D. association area.
E. decussation.

21. Bell's palsy is associated with which cranial nerve?

A. CN III, oculomotor
B. CN V, trigeminal
C. CN VII, facial
D. CN IX, glossopharyngeal
E. CN X, vagus

ANSWERS

1. **E.** The trochlear nerve supplies the superior oblique muscle. All other muscles listed receive their innervation from the oculomotor nerve. Remember that the lateral rectus receives abducens nerve supply.

2. **H.** The typical pathway of a reflex may be outlined as follows: sensory receptor on dendrite of dorsal root ganglion cell → ganglion cell → axon of cell → dorsal root → dorsal horn of spinal cord → either directly to motor cell in ventral horn or via internuncial (association) neuron to ventral horn motor cell → axon via ventral root → spinal nerve → effector organ (e.g., muscle).

3. **A.** The roots below L_2 are collectively called the cauda equina and are deflected away from a needle during a lumbar puncture. The conus medullaris is the ending of the spinal cord. The filum terminale (pia mater) starts at the conus and anchors the cord to the dura at sacral level S_2. Gray rami connect the sympathetic chain with a typical spinal nerve.

4. **B.** The spinal cord viewed as a whole is cylindrical, about ½ inch in diameter and 18 in length, and has cervical and lumbar enlargements due to the involvement of these cord levels with the innervation of the upper and lower limbs, respectively.

5. **C.** Multipolar neurons are the most abundant; they are somatic and visceral motor, and associational in nature. They are found in the spinal cord and brain (central nervous system). Unipolar (pseudounipolar) neurons are somatic and visceral sensory neurons; their cell bodies are located in cranial sensory and dorsal root ganglia. Peripheral processes go out to receptors and central processes travel into the central nervous system. Bipolar neurons are special sensory neurons; their cell bodies are found in special sense organs, i.e., eye, ear, and nose.

6. **E.** Neuroglia, the supportive elements of the central nervous system, are of several types: astroytes, oligodendrocytes, and microglia. Supportive elements of the peripheral nervous system include Schwann cells and satellite cells.

7. **E.** This is a definition and should be memorized.

8. **A.** Reception via afferent (sensory) receptors, conduction via sensory fibers to the central nervous system (spinal cord), and propagation of the impulses to the efferent (motor) system will then result in appropriate action. Usually most reflex arcs include one association neuron in the spinal cord between their afferent and efferent fibers. The medulla is not a part of the spinal cord; it is a part of the brain, and usually reflex arcs do not utilize higher centers.

9. **B.** The cell bodies of the motor (efferent) system are located in the ventral horns (gray matter) of the spinal cord and their fibers leave the cord via ventral (anterior) roots which join with the dorsal (sensory) roots to form a spinal nerve. If a spinal nerve were sectioned, loss of both sensation and motor activity would be experienced. In this case only motor functions were interrupted.

10. **D.** The autonomic nervous system innervates all smooth muscle and glands. The autonomic nervous system is divided into a sympathetic (flight and fight) component and parasympathetic (maintains homeostasis) component. It exerts important influences on the intrinsic eye musculature; skin glands; and the cardiovascular, respiratory, endocrine, and reproductive systems. Fear, rage, pain, etc., evoke sympathetic activity which mobilizes the resources of the body. Gastrointestinal activity is curtailed; heart rate and blood pressure increase; and coronary arteries and bronchioles dilate.

11. **E.** Many activities are attributed to the hypothalamus. Lesions of this area may produce diabetes insipidus, obesity, sexual dystrophy, and loss of temperature control.

12 **D.** The gray matter of the spinal cord is divided into two components: motor and receptor. The motor part is comprised of the ventral and intermediolateral columns and gives rise to the ventral roots. Ventral horn cells supply voluntary muscles; intermediolateral cells give rise to preganglionic sympathetic fibers of the thoraco-lumbar system. The receptor portion is located in the dorsal horn. The white matter of the spinal cord is composed of nerve fibers in a network of connective tissue.

13. **E.** The sympathetic component of the autonomic nervous system mobilizes the body's reserve in case of emergencies.

14. **A.** Dendrites function in receiving information and conducting it toward the cell body. Axons carry that information away from the cell body and will synapse on dendrites of another neuron.

15. **A.** The chemical mediator of cholinergic nerve impulses is acetylcholine and is released by the axon terminals.

16. **A.** Control of these functions is due to crossing of the fibers, and control of the right side is by the left cerebral hemispheres.

17. **A.** Ectoderm is the germ layer of origin of the nervous system.

18. **A.** The corpus callosum connects the two cerebral hemispheres in the mammal; association fibers cross in this bundle.

19. **B.** The neurolemma of an axon is a part of the Schwann cell (outer membrane).

20. **B.** A group of nerve cell bodies is commonly considered to be the site of a nucleus.

21. **C.** The facial nerve innervates the muscles of facial expression. Facial paralysis (Bell's palsy) results in an expressionless face with a drooping mouth.

Organs of Special Sense

The Eye

The visual system is made up of the eye and complex nerve pathways for interpretation by the cerebral cortex and subcortical centers for the purpose of:

1. Refraction of light rays and the focusing thereof on the retina for the production of an image;
2. Conversion of light rays into a nervous impulse;
3. Transmission to visual centers of the brain for interpretation.

The visual system is composed of the following structures: eyelids, tearing apparatus (lacrimal gland), extrinsic muscles, eyeball, and optic nerve. We will concentrate on the eyeball and optic nerve.

Eyeball and Optic Nerve: The eye is nearly spherical and about 2.5 cm in diameter. The eyeball is composed of three coats—namely, an outer fibrous layer, a middle vascular and pigmented layer, and an inner or retinal layer—and the refractive elements—the cornea, the aqueous humor, the lens, and the vitreous humor.

Two clinical problems concerned with the size of the eyeball must be identified:

1. *myopia* (near-sightedness)—In this condition the eyeball is longer than normal and light rays come to focus in front of the retina.
2. *hyperopia* (far-sightedness)—In this condition the eyeball is shorter than normal and light rays come to focus in back of the retina.

Outer Layer. The outer fibrous tunic is the opaque *sclera* (white of the eye), which anteriorly becomes the transparent, nonvascular *cornea*. The sclera maintains the shape of the eye and gives attachment to the external ("extrinsic") ocular muscles. The cornea is composed of five layers and is one of the refractive elements.

Middle Layer. The middle vascular and pigmented tunic is the *choroid,* which anteriorly becomes the *ciliary body* and the *contractile iris*. The ciliary body, attached to the *lens* via the suspensory ligaments, aids in focusing light rays on the retina. Contraction of the ciliary muscles mediated by the parasympathetic portion (Edinger-Westphal nucleus) of the oculomotor nerve decreases the tension on the suspensory ligaments, allowing the lens to increase in thickness. The *pupil* is the central opening of the iris; its size is regulated by the amount of light present. Two smooth muscles regulate the opening; the constrictor, or sphincter pupillae, is innervated by the parasympathetic system (oculomotor nerve) and reduces the size of the pupil, while the dilator, or dilator pupillae, receives its innervation from the sympathetic system and enlarges the diameter of the pupil.

Inner Layer. The innermost tunic, the retinal layer, consists of ten layers of cells and fibers. Three layers are of neruonal importance:

a. rod and cone layer; here light energy is transformed into chemical and electrical energy;
b. bipolar cells, which allow for internal nerve impulse transmission;
c. ganglion cells which give rise to the *optic nerve*.

There are about 120 million rods and 6 million cones present per eye. The rods contain rhodopsin, or visual purple, which converts photons (basic unit of light) into chemical and then into electrical energy. Rhodopsin is formed from vitamin A; a deficiency of vitamin A may result in night blindness. Rods are very sensitive and function in dim light but yield no color discrimination. Cones contain iodopsin: they are concerned with bright light vision, visual acuity (scotopic vision), and color perception.

Bipolar cells make contact with many rods and cones to receive their impulses which they in turn transmit to the ganglion cells whose axons give rise to the optic nerve. It is estimated that the one million ganglion cells receive information from approximately 130 million rod and cone receptors.

The area at which optic nerve fibers exit is called the *optic disc* or *blind spot*. No photoreception takes place there but the central artery and vein of the retina may be observed there.

Directly in line (visual axis) with the center of the cornea is the *macula lutea*. This area exhibits a high concentration of cones, the center, known as the *fovea centralis,* is the area of most acute vision. The image formed on the retina is inverted, this is inverted again—corrected—by the brain.

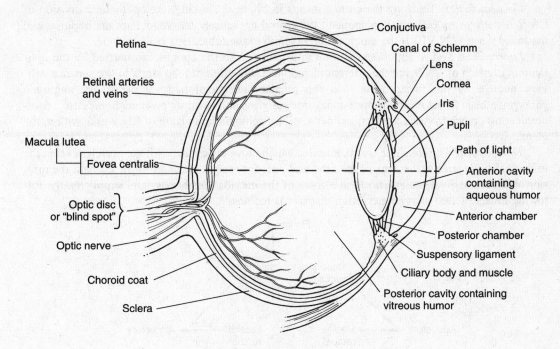

Longitudinal section of the eye.

Pathway for Seeing

Ganglion cells of the retina → optic nerve → optic chiasm (nasal retinal field fibers cross) → optic tract → lateral geniculate body → optic radiations → visual cortex (area 17 of occipital lobe of cerebrum).

Visual Reflex Pathways

Pupillary constriction due to exposure to bright light (involuntary reflex–parasympathetic response):

Retina → optic nerve → optic chiasm → superior colliculus → pretectum interneurons → Edinger–Westphal nucleus of oculomotor nerve (CN III), parasympathetic division → ciliary ganglion → constrictor pupillae muscle of iris.

Pupillary dilatation due to exposure to dim light (involuntary reflex–sympathetic response):

Optic pathways as above to midbrain → reticular formation to sympathetic nervous system → preganglionic fibers → superior cervical ganglion → postganglionic fibers → dilator pupillae muscle of iris.

Corneal (conjunctival or blink) reflex due to irritation of conjunctiva:

Afferent loop is ophthalmic of CN V; efferent path to orbicularis oculi utilizes the facial nerve (CN VII) and results in lid closure.

Pupillary light reflexes. When bright light is perceived by the retina, the optic nerve (afferent loop) brings the impulse to the brain. The efferent response, via the Edinger–Westphal complex of CN III, results in constriction of the pupils of both eyes.

Accommodation. Accommodation is accomplished by ciliary muscles, in conjunction with convergence of the eyes, which is accomplished mainly by the action of the medial rectus muscles. As the ciliary muscles contract, the tension on the suspensory ligaments holding the lens is lessened, permitting the lens to bulge for close vision. The afferent pathway ends in the Edinger–Westphal nucleus, and the efferent pathway is as described for the action of the sphincter pupillae muscle.

Corneal Reflex. Touching the cornea results in bilateral blinking; the ophthalmic division of CN V is the sensory (afferent) component; the central nervous system modulates the impulse, and the facial nerve (CN VII) is the motor (efferent) limb to the orbicularis oculi muscle.

Lacrimation Reflex. Emotional stimuli and irritation to the conjunctiva carried by the ophthalmic division of CN V are the afferent phenomena; the efferent loop starts in the superior salivary nucleus of the facial nerve. Via the greater superficial petrosal nerve, preganglionic parasympathetic fibers reach the pterygopalatine ganglion and synapse; postganglionics use a communicating branch to reach the lacrimal nerve of the ophthalmic division of CN V and, with it, the gland.

The Extrinsic Muscles. The are six muscles which move the eyeball. All the muscles except the inferior oblique arise at the apex of the orbit and pass forward at the sides of the eyeball; the inferior oblique muscle arises anteriorly in a fossa of the maxilla. For brevity and simplicity, the following muscle action–nerve innervation diagram is included.

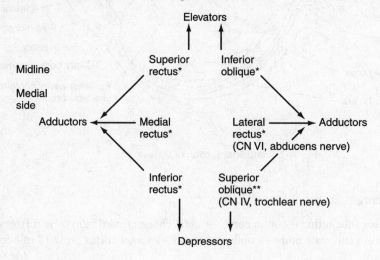

* Supplied by the oculomotor nerve.
** The first action of the superior oblique is to adduct, then depress; if it could function independently of all the others, the muscle could theoretically, at the end of its action, also abduct.

The Ear

The ear, which is located in the temporal bone, essentially serves in a dual capacity. It is an auditory organ for the sense of hearing (40–20,000 cycles/sec) and a vestibular organ monitoring the effects of gravity and position of the head. Hearing utilizes the cochlear mechanism; vestibular functions are modulated by the utricle, saccule, and the three semicircular canals.

Irritative lesions to the vestibular system may result in nystagmus, vertigo, nausea, incoordination, or any other disorders of equilibrium or posture.

The auditory functions of the ear are as follows:

1. reception and conduction of sound waves,
2. amplification of the waves,
3. transduction of the waves into nerve impulses,
4. transmission of the impulse to conscious centers.

The vestibular functions of the ear are as follows:

1. reception of stimuli and response to movements of the head and gravitational influences on the head.

2. nerve transmission to higher centers for reflex and postural adjustments to maintain equilibrium.

The ear is commonly divided into the external ear, the middle ear, and the inner ear.

The External Ear: The auricle, or pinna, is composed of skin molded on a complex elastic cartilage; it serves to gather and funnel sound waves into the external auditory meatus (canal), which terminates at the tympanic membrane, or eardrum. In the skin of the meatus are located fine hairs and large sebaceous glands. Coiled, tubular ceruminous glands are also present; they discharge a brownish secretion which in conjunction with the sebaceous products and desquamated cells produce a waxy product known as cerumen.

The Middle Ear: The middle ear is a cavity continuous superiorly with the mastoid air cells and inferiorly, via the auditory (Eustachian) tube, with the nasopharynx. The auditory tube is ordinarily closed and serves to equalize the internal and external pressures on the eardrum. Within the cavity are located three ossicles. From external (eardrum) to internal (oval window), they are respectively the malleus (hammer), the incus (anvil), and the stapes (stirrup). These small bones function in transduction: they translate the displacement of the tympanic membrane, produced by sound waves, into mechanical energy.

On the medial wall of the middle ear are the vestibular window (oval) and the cochlear window (round). The vestibular window houses the base of the stapes; the cochlear window is closed by a membrane. Movement of the eardrum sets up vibrations of the stapes in the oval window; these are transmitted to perilymph in the scala vestibuli (bony labyrinth). The movement is transferred to the endolymph in the cochlear duct (membranous labyrinth) and from there to perilymph in the scala tympani and then is dissipated through the movement of the membrane in the round window. Sound vibrations may be transmitted by surrounding bone in case of middle ear disease (deafness); therefore, the outer and middle ear are not absolutely essential for hearing.

The Inner Ear: The internal ear, located in the petrous portion of the temporal bone, consists of a complex series of fluid (endolymph)-filled sacs, the membranous labyrinth, housed within bony cavities (bony labyrinth), which are filled by perilymph. The interconnecting membranous channels serve static and kinetic senses (vestibular) as well as hearing (auditory).

The vestibular apparatus comprises three semicircular canals, utricle, and saccule.

The auditory mechanism is housed in the cochlear duct. Both senses are transmitted by the stato-acoustic nerve (cranial nerve VIII) to the brain. This nerve is also named "vestibulo-cochlear nerve"; in the past it had been called the "auditory nerve."

The Cochlea. The cochlear duct is a helical tube of about 2½ turns housed in its bony labyrinth. The duct separates the bony tube into two channels: the scala tympani and scala vestibuli. At the apex the scala tympani and scala vestibuli communicate at a point termed the helicotrema. The scala vestibuli begins at the oval window and the scala tympani terminates at the round window.

Pulsations are set up in the perilymph of the scala vestibuli by movements of the stapes at the oval window. They are propagated either via the helicotrema directly to the scala tympani or may pass through the vestibular membrane, activate movement in the endolymph of the cochlear duct, and then pass via the basilar membrane into the perilymph of the scala tympani. The pulsations stimulate the receptor (hair) cells located on the basilar membrane and elicit the phenomenon of hearing. Movements of the endolymph, varing with the volume and pitch of the sound waves are registered in specific regions of the organ of Corti. The cochlear division of the stato-acoustic nerve transmits the information to the medulla, then to the midbrain, the thalamus, and, finally, interpretation occurs in the cerebrum.

The Vestibular Apparatus. Head movements are perceived by the three semicircular canals, attached at right angles to the utricle. Displacement of the head causes endolymph to elicit a response in the sensory hair cells of the crista. Position with respect to gravity is monitored by movement of otoliths (calcium carbonate crystals) on the sensory hair cells, in the macula of the utricle and sacculus. The vestibular division of the stato-acoustic nerve (CN VIII) relays the informatin to the medulla, then to the cerebellum, where muscle coordination is elicited.

Semicircular Canals. There are three canals. Each possesses an ampulla with a modified, sensory epithelium (crista ampullaris) which is associated with neuronal reception. Each crista is stimulated by movements occurring in the plane of its specific canal. Rotational movement leads to a compensatory response of the eyes, head and limbs.

Utricle. The sensory epithelium is located in a region known as the macula. Gelatinous material in which are embedded crystals (otoliths) cover the hair cells. Any change in position of the head in space and any linear acceleration will result in pressure from the crystals on the hair cells and a compensatory reaction such as righting of the body and eye coordination.

Saccule. The morphology of the saccule is similar to that of the utricle. The saccule responds to vibrational stimuli.

The Olfactory System

The olfactory system may be visualized as a highly specialized mucous membrane located in the roof of each nasal cavity. Four primary odors—fragrant, acid, burnt, and rancid—are perceived. Olfactory stimulation is caused by gaseous and odiferous substances in solution. Olfactory seromucous glands secrete a watery fluid continuously. This allows for reception of dissolved substances and also lessens retention and lingering of stimulation. The receptive cells, bipolar ganglion cells, end in bulbous knobs that possess about ten olfactory hairs; these serve as the sensory receptors. The sense of smell is subject to fatigue; no structural differences are correlated with discrimination of different kinds of odors. Reception follows this route:

Bipolar cells of olfactory epithelium → olfactory bulb → olfactory tract (cranial nerve I) → olfactory stria → olfactory cortex.

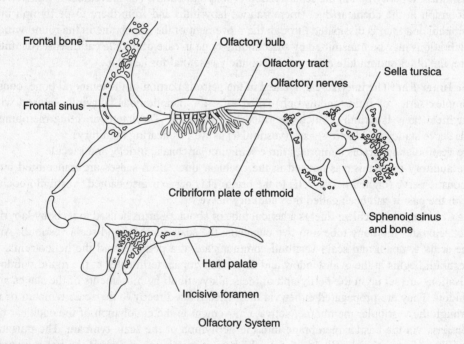

Olfactory System

The Gustatory System

In higher vertebrates the sense of taste is generally restricted to the oral cavity (tongue and epiglottic region). Taste buds are located in vallate, foliate, and fungiform papillae. The receptors in the taste bud are neuroepithelial cells. Substances must be in solution and the four modalities of taste—sweet, sour, salt, and bitter—are specific and regionalized. Sweetness is localized mainly on the tip of the tongue, sour and salt mainly on the central areas, and bitter on the back of the tongue.

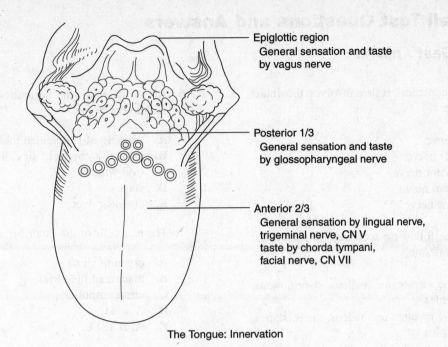

- Epiglottic region
  General sensation and taste
  by vagus nerve

- Posterior 1/3
  General sensation and taste
  by glossopharyngeal nerve

- Anterior 2/3
  General sensation by lingual nerve,
  trigeminal nerve, CN V
  taste by chorda tympani,
  facial nerve, CN VII

The Tongue: Innervation

NERVES OF THE TONGUE

	General Sensation	Taste	Motor
Anterior 2/3 Posterior 1/3 Epiglottic region of tongue	Lingual, trigeminal, CN V Glosspharyngeal, CN IX Superior laryngeal(internal brance), vagus, CN X	Chorda tympani, CN VII Glosspharyngeal, CN IX Superior laryngeal, CN X	Hypoglossal, CN XII Hypoglossal, CN XII

ORGANS OF SPECIAL SENSE IN BRIEF

Organ	Receptor	Stimulus	Location
Olfactory mucus membrane	Bipolar cells, olfactory epithelium	Gaseous or odiferous substances in solution	Nasal cavity, cribriform plate
Taste buds	Gustatory cells (neuroepithelial cells), vallate, foliate, fungiform papillae	Sweet, sour, salt, and bitter substances in solution	Tongue and epiglottic region
Eye	Rods and cones	Light waves	Eye
Ear: External	Pinna, tympanic membrane	Sound waves	Ear
Middle	Ossicular chain to oval window	Sound waves	Ear
Internal cochlea scala vestibula scala tympani basilar membrane	Organ of Corty	Pulsations (vibrations) converted to electrical stimulus	Ear
Vestibular apparatus semicircular canals (crista ampularis) utricle (macula) saccule	Hair cells	Movement (position of head), vibration	Ear

Quick Recall Test Questions and Answers

Choose the Best Answer

1. Eliciting the corneal reflex involves the intact fibers of the:

   A. optic nerve.
   B. trochlear nerve.
   C. oculomotor nerve.
   D. trigeminal nerve.
   E. abducens nerve.

2. Which of the following sequences is correct for sound transmission?

   A. tympanic membrane, malleus, stapes, incus, and cochlea
   B. tympanic membrane, malleus, incus, stapes, and cochlea
   C. tympanic membrane, auditory tube, middle ear, and inner ear
   D. tympanic membrane, incus, malleus, stapes, and cochlea
   E. tympanic membrane, malleus, incus, stapes, and semicircular canal

3. Turning the right eye upward and laterally involves which of the following muscles?

   A. superior rectus, superior oblique, and lateral rectus
   B. inferior rectus, inferior oblique, and superior oblique
   C. superior rectus, inferior oblique, and lateral rectus
   D. superior rectus, superior oblique, and medial rectus

4. Accommodation for near vision results from impulses originating in the brain and running in the:

   A. abducens nerve (cranial nerve VI).
   B. ophthalmic division of the trigeminal nerve (cranial nerve V).
   C. trochlear nerve (cranial nerve IV).
   D. optic nerve (cranial nerve II).
   E. oculomotor nerve (cranial nerve III).

5. Hearing utilizes the _____ mechanism.

   A. cochlear
   B. utricle
   C. saccule
   D. semicircular canal

6. All of the following structures are located in the middle ear except:

   A. opening of Eustachian tube.
   B. passage to mastoid air cells.
   C. oval window.
   D. stapes.
   E. cochlear duct.

7. The hair cells of the inner ear are located in the:

   A. organ of Corti.
   B. macula of the utricle.
   C. crista ampullaris.
   D. A and C.
   E. A, B and C.

8. The receptors (specialized neuroepithelium) for the perception of sound are the:

   A. spiral ganglion cells.
   B. hair cells of the macula.
   C. hair cells of the organ of Corti.
   D. cells of the crista ampularis.
   E. otoliths of the utricle.

9. The Eustachian tube provides a communication between the:

   A. inner ear and the cranial cavity.
   B. outer ear and middle ear.
   C. middle ear and mastoid air cells.
   D. middle ear and nasopharynx.
   E. middle ear and oropharynx.

10. Which of the following is the structure of the eye that is responsible for holding the lens in its normal position?

    A. iris
    B. cornea
    C. anterior chamber
    D. ciliary body
    E. fovea centralis

11. Three layers of neuronal elements are intimately involved in the transmission of light. The first component of that chain are the:

    A. ganglion cells.
    B. bipolar cells.
    C. rods and cones.
    D. connective tissue cells.
    E. neuroglia.

12. The vision of a near-sighted individual may be corrected by:

   A. a convex lens.
   B. a biconvex lens.
   C. a biconcave lens.
   D. none of the above.
   E. all of the above.

13. The region of the retina where vision is most acute is known as the:

   A. ciliary body.
   B. vitreous humor.
   C. conjunctiva.
   D. fovea centralis.
   E. aqueous humor.

14. Which of the following components of the eye is/are considered to refract light?

   A. cornea
   B. aqueous humor
   C. lens
   D. vitreous humor
   E. all of the above

15. Taste is mediated by all of the following cranial nerves except:

   A. trigeminal nerve (CN V).
   B. facial nerve (CN VII).
   C. glossopharyngeal nerve (CN IX).
   D. vagus nerve (CN X).

16. Sound vibrations received by the tectorial membrane are transmitted to the ossicular chain. The foot plate of the stapes is located in the:

   A. oval window (vestibular).
   B. round window (cochlear).
   C. helicotrema.
   D. organ of Corti.
   E. utricle.

17. There are about 120 million rods and 6 million cones present per eye. The rods are very sensitive and function:

   A. in colorful situations.
   B. in bright light.
   C. in dim light.
   D. where the intensity of light is no consideration.
   E. because they concentrate in the macula lutea.

18. The eyeball is composed of three coats—namely an outer fibrous layer, a middle vascular and pigmented layer, and an inner or retinal layer. The outer layer is comprised of the:

   A. extraocular muscles and sclera.
   B. sclera and cornea.
   C. iris and ciliary body.
   D. conjunctiva and choroid.
   E. conjunctiva and lens.

Answers

1. **D.** In order to elicit the corneal reflex the afferent (sensory) fibers of the ophthalmic division of the trigeminal nerve must bring the information to the central nervous system; the efferent (motor) reaction (blinking) is carried out via the facial nerve (contraction of the orbicularis oculi).

2. **B.** The auditory ossicles, malleus, incus and stapes, form a lever system which converts the vibrations of the air impinging on the tympanic membrane into mechanical energy to oscillate the foot plate of the stapes in the vestibular (oval) window.

3. **C.** The two elevators of the eye are the superior rectus and inferior oblique; the chief lateral deviator is the lateral rectus.

4. **E.** Accommodation involves narrowing of the pupil, bulging of the lens and adduction of the eyeball. The sequence starts in the Edinger–Westphal nucleus of CN III.

5. **A.** The ear, which is located in the temporal bone, essentially serves in a dual capacity. It is an auditory organ for the sense of hearing (40–20,000 cycles/sec) and a vestibular organ monitoring the effects of gravity and position of the head. Hearing utilizes the cochlear mechanism; vestibular functions are modulated by the utricle, saccule, and the three semicircular canals.

6. **E.** The middle ear is a cavity continuous superiorly with the mastoid air cells and inferiorly, via the auditory (Eustachian) tube, with the nasopharynx. Within the cavity are located the three ossicles. On the medial wall of the middle ear are the vestibular window (oval) and the cochlear window (round). The vestibular window houses the base of the stapes; the cochlear window is closed by a membrane.

7   **E.** Movements of the endolymph, varying with the volume and pitch of the sound waves are registered in specific regions of the organ of Corti. Head movements are perceived by the three semicircular canals, attached at right angles to the utricle. Displacement of the head causes endolymph to elicit a response in the sensory hair cells of the crista.

8. **C.** Pulsations are set up in the perilymph of the scala vestibuli by movements of the stapes at the oval window. Movements of the endolymph, varying with the volume and pitch of the sound waves, are registered in specific regions of the organ of Corti.

9. **D.** The middle ear is a cavity continuous superiorly with the mastoid air cells and inferiorly, via the auditory (Eustachian) tube, with the nasopharynx. The auditory tube is ordinarily closed and serves to equalize the internal and external pressures on the eardrum.

10. **D.** The middle vascular pigmented tunic is the choroid, which anteriorly becomes the ciliary body and the contractile iris. The ciliary body, attached to the lens via the suspensory ligaments, aids in focusing light rays on the retina. Contraction of the ciliary muscles mediated by the parasympathetic portion (Edinger–Westphal nucleus) of the oculomotor nerve decreases the tension on the suspensory ligaments, allowing the lens to increase in thickness.

11. **C.** The innermost tunic, the retinal layer, consists of ten layers of cells and fibers. Three layers are of neuronal importance:
    (a) rod and cone layer; here light energy is transformed into chemical and electrical energy;
    (b) bipolar cells, which allow for internal nerve impulse transmission;
    (c) ganglion cells which give rise to the optic nerve.

12. **C.** Anterior-posterior diameters of eyeballs vary. A long eye is considered near-sighted or myopic; light rays come to focus before they reach the retina; therefore, a concave lens is needed for correction. A short eye results in far-sightedness or hypermetropia; light rays would come to focus in back of the retina and, therefore, a convex lens is needed for correction.

13. **D.** Light must penetrate the retina to reach the rods and cones. The fovea centralis is the central portion of the macula lutea; it is the region of sharpest vision. It is thinner than the rest of the retina and only cones are present. Rods are absent from this area. Cones are regarded as color receptors, while rods are achromatic receptors of low intensity light.

14. **E.** The path of light starts at the cornea; it then enters the anterior chamber which contains the aqueous humor. Next it encounters the lens and then enters the posterior chamber filled with vitreous humor.

15. **A.** The nerve supply monitoring taste of the tongue is regionalized:
    (1) Anterior ⅔ of the tongue is supplied by the chorda tympani branch of the facial nerve (CN VII).
    (2) Posterior ⅓ of the tongue is supplied by the glossopharyngeal nerve (CN IX).
    (3) Epiglottic region is supplied by the vague nerve (CN X).
    The trigeminal nerve is responsible for monitoring general sensation from the anterior ⅔ of the tongue.

16. **A.** Pulsations are set up in the perilymph of the scala vestibuli by movements of the stapes at the oval window. The pulsations stimulate the receptor (hair) cells located on the basilar membrane and elicit the phenomenon of hearing.

17. **C.** Rods are very sensitive and function in dim light but yield no color discrimination. Cones contain iodopsin: They are concerned with bright light vision, visual acuity (scotopic vision), and color perception. Directly in line (visual axis) with the center of the cornea is the macula lutea. This area exhibits a high concentration of cones, the center, known as the fovea centralis, is the area of most acute vision.

18. **B.** The outer fibrous tunic is the opaque sclera (white of the eye), which anteriorly becomes the transparent, nonvascular cornea. The sclera maintains the shape of the eye and gives attachment of the external ("extrinsic") ocular muscles. The cornea is composed of five layers and is one of the refractive elements.

Endocrine System

Two systems modulate, integrate, and control the activities of the body: the nervous and endocrine systems. The response in nervous control is rapid whereas control via the endocrine system is fairly slow and longer lasting. The endocrine glands are ductless and secrete their products, called hormones, into the capillaries (bloodstream). Hormones are substances that are secreted into the bloodstream and travel to their target organs to elicit their effects. The product of the target organ may also feed back on the organ that stimulated its activity and production and thus manipulate its cycle of function. It may shut off the supply of stimulating hormone; this activity is called a negative feedback. The controlling mechanism can be thought of as a neuro-endocrine-somatic tissue relationship, or the brain affecting the pituitary gland, which in turn affects the target organs, which then elicit their effect upon the body tissues and cells. Hormones cannot be classified into one chemical class; they are, however, all organic substances and may be proteins, peptides, amino acids (or amino acid derivatives), and steroids, or prostaglandins (derivatives of essential fatty acids). Generally, the glands which produce protein hormones embryologically originate from the alimentary tract; they are the anterior pituitary, thyroid, parathyroids, and pancreas. Glands which produce steroid products are derived from the celomic mesothelium and are the testes, ovaries, and adrenal cortex. Glands whose products are small molecular weight amines arise from cells of nervous tissue derivation and are the neuro-hypophysis and the adrenal medulla.

This chapter gives the student a brief description of each endocrine organ, its products, and the results of hypo- and hypersecretion.

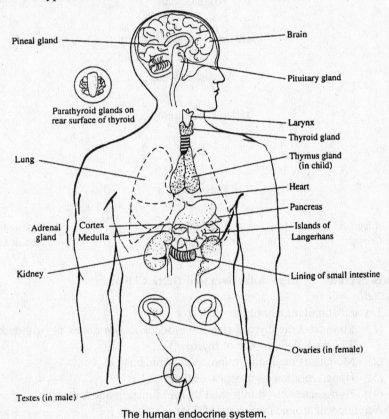

The human endocrine system.

The Pituitary Gland (Hypophysis)

The pituitary gland is commonly divided into an anterior and a posterior lobe according to origin. The anterior lobe (adenohypophysis) originates from the oral epithelium of the roof of the mouth in the embryo (Rathke's pouch), while the posterior lobe (neurohypophysis) is a downgrowth of the floor of the brain (in relation to the third ventricle and the hypothalamic areas).

Three cell types are found in the anterior lobe: chromophobes 50%; acidophils 40%; basophils 10%. Chromophobes are considered to be resting cells.

Hormones Secreted by Acidophils (Alpha Cells):

1. *Somatotropic hormone (STH)*
   a. Stimulates general body growth; acts on liver to produce somatomedins that act on epiphyseal cartilages
   b. Hypersecretion—before ossification is complete, giantism
      —after ossification is complete, acromegaly
   c. Hyposecretion—dwarfism
   d. Somatostatin—inhibits growth hormone production
2. *Lactogenic hormone* or luteotrophic hormone (LTH) or prolactin
   a. Promotes growth of breast which was already stimulated by estrogen and progesterone, especially during the last trimester of pregnancy
   b. Promotes and maintains lactation
   c. Helps in the maintenance of the corpus luteum
   d. Promotes maternal instinct
   e. Excessive levels in males result in hypogonadism

PATHWAY OF GROWTH HORMONE AND THE SOMATOMEDINS

(+) Stimulation   **(−) Inhibition**

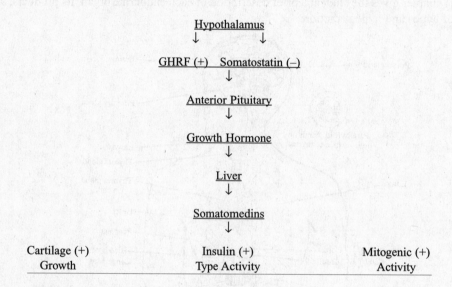

Hormones Secreted by Basophils (Beta and Delta Cells):

1. *Beta cells*
   a. Thyroid stimulating hormone (TSH)
      (1) Stimulates the thyroid gland to produce its hormones T_3 (triiodothyronine) and T_4 (tetraiodothyronine or thyroxin)
      (2) Modulates the iodide trapping mechanisms
      (3) Hypersecretion—goiter, exophthalmos
      (4) Hyposecretion—diminished thyroid function and lethargy
   b. Adrenocorticotropic hormone (ACTH)
      (1) Stimulates the adrenal cortex to produce glucocorticoids (cortisol, etc.)
      (2) Does *not* stimulate mineralocorticoid activity (aldosterone production)
      (3) Affects production of adrenal androgens
   c. Melanocyte stimulating hormone (MSH) or intermedin
      (1) Function poorly understood in humans
      (2) This hormone causes the dispersion of pigment in the chromatophores of the skin of cold-blooded vertebrates and a darkening of the skin results; the action of MSH allows for quick changes in the skin color in response to changes in the external environment.

2. *Delta cells*
   a. Luteinizing hormone (LH) in female Interstitial cell stimulating hormone (ICSH) in male
      (1) In the female this hormone is necessary for preovulatory development of the ovarian follicle, ovulation, and formation of the corpus luteum.
      (2) In the female it modulates the production of estrogen and progesterone.
      (3) In the male this hormone stimulates the interstitial cells of the testes, which results in a secretion of testicular androgens.
   b. Follicle stimulating hormone (FSH)
      (1) In the female this hormone stimulates the growth of the ovarian follicle.
      (2) In the male FSH stimulates the testes to produce sperm (spermatogenesis).

SCHEMA FOR PITUITARY FUNCTION

(Hypothalamus—Neurosecretory Cells)

Hormones of the Neurohypophysis:

The posterior lobe or neurohypophysis develops from the floor of the third ventricle of the brain. The function of this portion of the pituitary gland is to store and release the hormones oxytocin (produced by the paraventricular nucleus of the hypothalamus) and vasopressin or antidiuretic hormone (ADH, produced by the supraoptic nucleus of the hypothalamus). There is a binding protein neurophysis specific for each hormone.

1. *Oxytocin*
   a. Stimulates the contraction of the smooth muscle of the uterus and may play some role in the initiation of labor.
   b. Stimulates the ejection of milk by affecting the myoepithelial cells of the breast tissue (mammary gland).
2. *Vasopressin; antidiuretic hormone (ADH)*
   a. Acts upon the renal tubules to aid water resorption and thereby restricts diuresis; a lack of hormone results in the condition known as diabetes insipidus (the production of large volumes of dilute urine, polyuria).

GENERAL SCHEMA OF ENDOCRINE SECRETION

Hypothalamus
(Neurosecretory Cells)
↓
Axons from Hypothalamo-hypophyseal Tract
↓
Releasing Hormones Secreted
↓
Neurohypophysis Affected

The Pituitary Portal System: In humans the pituitary gland receives its blood supply via the right and left superior and the right and left inferior pituitary arteries from the internal carotid artery system. These vessels supply the hypothalamic areas, the pituitary stalk, and the posterior lobe. The anterior lobe, however, receives no arterial blood supply. The entire blood supply to the anterior lobe is derived from the pituitary portal veins. These veins arise from the capillary network of the median eminence and the infundibular stem. The vascular tufts of the primary capillary system are in close relationship with the nerve endings of the hypothalamo-hypophyseal tract. It is hypothesized that upon excitation these nerve fibers liberate their secretory products into this system, which then, via the portal veins, transports these neurosecretory products to the sinusoids of the anterior lobe. It is in this manner that the activity of the anterior lobe is governed by the hypothalamic areas.

Negative Feedback: The control of secretion of TRH, GnRH, and CRH is exerted by the concentration of the products of the target glands in the bloodstream. Therefore, hypothalamic and pituitary secretion is modulated (controlled) via a "Negative Feedback."

NEGATIVE FEEDBACK SCHEMAS

Schema 1

$(-)$ | → Neuron
　　　　↓　　Neurotransmitter
　　Endocrine Organ
　　　　↓　　Hormone
　　← Target Cell
　　　　↓
　　← Effect

Schema 2

$(-)$ | → Hypothalamus
　　　　↓　　Releasing Factor
$(-)$ | → Anterior Pituitary
　　　　↓　　Stimulating Hormone
　　← Endocrine Organ
　　　　↓　　Hormone
　　← Target Cell
　　　　↓
　　← Effect

Schema 3

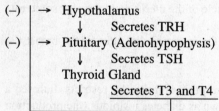

$(-)$ | → Hypothalamus
　　　　↓　　Secretes TRH
$(-)$ | → Pituitary (Adenohypophysis)
　　　　↓　　Secretes TSH
　　Thyroid Gland
　　　　↓　　Secretes T3 and T4

The Thyroid Gland

The thyroid gland is derived from the pharynx (the foramen cecum of the tongue). Its structural unit is the follicle; the follicle is composed of a unit of epithelial cells that surround a colloid space. Colloid is located extracellularly and contains thyroglobulin. The function of the thyroid gland is to produce colloidal material which contains the thyroid hormones (T_3 [triiodothyronine] and T_4 [thyroxin]) which affect the rate of metabolism of all the tissues of the body.

The iodides consumed in our food and water are absorbed and carried to the iodide pool in the extracellular fluid via the circulatory system. Five basic events can be identified in thyroid hormone production: (a) trapping iodide; (b) oxidation of iodide to organic iodine; (c) synthesis of hormone; (d) storage of hormone as the thyroglobulin moiety in the follicle; and (e) release of the hormone into the circulation. TSH from the anterior pituitary influences greatly the trapping mechanism; thiocyanates block this mechanism while thiouracil blocks the oxidation and synthetic steps. These compounds are classified as antithyroid agents.

The production of the hormone thyrocalcitonin has been implicated with the parafollicular cells or C cells of the thyroid gland. This hormone is an antagonist of parathyroid hormone and it functions to lower the serum calcium level and to enhance the deposition of calcium in bone. It lowers blood calcium levels by inhibiting bone resorption.

Action of Thyroid Hormone:
1. *Controls the rate of metabolism.*
2. *Controls the growth, maturation, and differentiation of the organism.*
3. *Influences nervous system activity.*

Problems Associated with Thyroid Function:
1. *Cretinism.* Congenital failure of proper development of the thyroid gland. The cretin is a dwarf—physically and mentally.
2. *Myxedema.* Acquired thyroid deficiency in the adult. This deficiency can be of two types:
    a. Thyroid deficiency due to thyroidectomy, neoplasms, thyroiditis, and so forth.
    b. A pituitary deficiency in the secretion of TSH.

The thyroid in these cases appears atrophic, hard, and fibrous. The clinical picture is the presentation of a patient who is fairly heavy, phlegmatic, and devoid of expression; his skin is rough and dry and sensitive to cold. The patient is sluggish mentally and physically. Laboratory tests would show a low basal metabolic rate, low protein bound iodine, and a high serum cholesterol level.

3. *Goiter.* Any enlargement of the gland not due to neoplasm or inflammatory disease. Endemic goiters are due to lack of intake of iodine (less than 10 μg/day) caused by deficiency in the soil and water. This interferes with hormone production, results in increased TSH production, thyroid compensatory hypertrophy, and eventual exhaustion of the gland.

4. *Hyperthyroidism.* Graves' disease. Increased activity by the organ. The patient exhibits loss of weight, nervousness, irritability, increased metabolic rate, rapid heart rate, sweating, and so forth. Exophthalmos, a protrusion of the eyeballs, is exhibited and thought to be due to an increased production of TSH. Hyperthyroidism may be an adjunct to the development of a goiter or may arise de novo.

The Parathyroid Glands

There are usually four parathyroid glands which are embedded in the thyroid gland. The parathyroid glands produce parathyroid hormone, which governs the metabolism of calcium and phosphorus. Calcium levels regulate parathyroid production of hormone. The parathyroids are essential to life; their removal results in cramps, convulsions, tremors, and eventually death due to tetany. The condition is due to the increased irritability of the muscular and nervous system caused by the decrease of calcium levels in the blood and body fluids. The activity of the parathyroids depends on the level of ionized calcium and phosphate ions in the serum.

Problems Associated with Parathyroid Function:
1. *Hypoparathyroidism.* This condition results in a decrease or urinary excretion of phosphorus and its concomitant rise in the serum; this results in a shift in the calcium-phosphorus serum levels and a decline in calcium resorption from bone. The fall in serum calcium will produce tetany. Low serum levels of calcium may also be influenced by deficient intake of calcium, deficiency of vitamin D in the diet, problems with intestinal absorption, or increased demand for calcium during pregnancy.

2. *Hyperparathyroidism.* Tumor is the most frequent cause of this condition. In this condition urinary phosphorus excretion is elevated and serum levels are decreased. Calcium resorption from bone is increased and serum levels rise. The glomerular filtrate is saturated and stones may form. Secondary renal disease may occur. Bones become decalcified and fractures result. Calcitonin lowers the blood calcium level.

The Pancreas

The pancreas is both an endocrine and exocrine gland. The endocrine portion to be discussed is located in the islets of Langerhans. The function of the islets of Langerhans is to produce insulin by the beta cells and glucagon by the alpha cells. A deficiency of insulin production results in the disease known as diabetes mellitus (elevated blood sugar level). The beta cells do not seem to depend on any outside trophic influences and the primary physiologic stimulus for insulin production seems to be the level of the blood sugar.

Insulin promotes the removal of glucose from the blood and also the conversion of glucose to glycogen in muscle and liver. It increases the rate of oxidation of glucose in the tissues, the conversion of carbohydrates into fats, the mobilization of fatty acids from adipose tissue, and the rate of protein synthesis.

Glucagon is the glycogenolytic hormone produced by the alpha cells of the pancreas; its principal action is to stimulate the conversion of glycogen to glucose by the liver. Glucagon also increases the peripheral utilization of glucose; therefore, it should not be referred to as simply the antagonist of insulin. Its secretion is controlled by the concentration of blood glucose and blood insulin levels. If insulin levels rise and blood glucose levels drop, glucagon secretion increases.

Two other cell types commonly associated with the islets are D cells, which produce somatostatin which inhibits glucagon release and decreases pancreatic exocrine functions, and F cells, which produce a polypeptide which inhibits pancreatic exocrine secretion and also decreases bile secretion.

The Adrenal Glands

The adrenal is composed of a cortex and a medulla. The cortex is derived from mesoderm of the Wolffian ridge in conjunction with the sex glands, whereas the medulla is of ectodermal, neural crest origin in conjunction with the anlage of the sympathetic nerve cells. In fetal life the adrenal is composed almost completely of cortex, but after birth the entire fetal cortex rapidly degenerates and is replaced by the adult cortex and medulla. The cortex, which produces the mineralocorticoids and glucocorticoids, is divided into three zones: (a) the most peripheral zona glomerulosa; (b) the intermediate zona fasciculata; and (c) the zona reticularis bordering the medulla. The function of the adrenal cortex is to produce the sex hormones: androgens, estrogens, and progesterone, and the corticosteroids: glucocorticoids and mineralocorticoids.

The zona glomerulosa is rich in lipids, especially cholesterol, from which the mineralocorticoids are formed. Aldosterone is the most powerful mineralocorticoid. Mineralocorticoids function in the retention of water, sodium, and chloride, and increase urinary loss of potassium and phosphorus by action on the renal tubules. This regulation of the electrolytes is essential to life. No pituitary control is present.

The zona fasciculata and reticularis are the sources of the glucocorticoids; i.e., 17-hydroxycorticosteroids. Corticosterone (hydroxycorticosterone), cortisone (compound E), and hydrocortisone; (cortisol or compound F) are the most widely known compounds. The levels of these hormones are increased by ACTH; they are gluconeogenic in nature. They convert amino acids into sugar instead of protein and in this way increase blood sugar and liver glycogen levels. Cortisone—in addition to influencing protein, carbohydrate, and fat metabolism—(a) affects the permeability of cell membranes; (b) interferes with the antigen-antibody response by inhibiting antibody formation; and (c) suppresses the inflammatory response. Cortisone, however, only relieves the symptoms of disease without influencing the cause.

The zona reticularis is responsible for the production of the sex hormones or 17-ketosteroids. The action of these hormones is no different from the action of the estrogens, androgens, and progesterone (the regular sex hormones produced by the testes and ovaries); i.e., they masculinize the body and increase the synthesis of amino acids and protein from nitrogen; they favor the retention of nitrogen, phosphorus, potassium, sodium, and chloride. ACTH has some control of these hormones.

Problems Associated with Adrenal Cortex Function:

1. Hypofunction or *chronic adrenal insufficiency.* Addison's disease. This condition is due to inadequate amounts of steroid hormones. Deficiency of glucocorticoids makes the patient easily susceptible to stress; deficiency of mineralocorticoids leads to a fall in serum sodium and rise in serum potassium. These patients lack proper resistance to infection and are easily dehydrated. Patients exhibit general languor and debility, a very weak heart, irritability of the stomach, and a peculiar change in skin color due to the deposition of melanin; this feature is highly characteristic.

2. Hyperadrenalism
   a. Overfunction of zona glomerulosa—aldosteronism (Conn's syndrome).
   b. Overfunction of zona fasciculata—(Cushing's syndrome).
   c. Overfunction of zona reticularis—adrenal virilism (Adrenogenital syndrome).

Schema 1

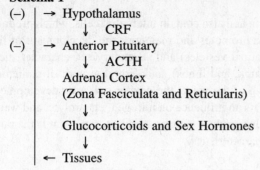

(–) → Hypothalamus
↓ CRF
(–) → Anterior Pituitary
↓ ACTH
Adrenal Cortex
(Zona Fasciculata and Reticularis)
↓
Glucocorticoids and Sex Hormones
↓
← Tissues

Schema 2

Adrenal Cortex
Zona Glomerulosa
_____
↓
Mineralocorticoids
_____
↓
Electrolytes (Sodium and Potassium) and
water balance is maintained by acting on
renal tubules and gastric mucosa
_____

Primary Aldosteronism—Conn's Syndrome:

Characterized by:

1. Periodic severe muscular weakness or paralysis.
2. Intermittent tetany and paresthesia.
3. Hypertension.
4. Renal disfunction.

Cushing's Syndrome:

Characterized by:

1. Painful adiposity of face, neck, and trunk (full moon face)
2. Excess hair growth in the female and preadolescent males.
3. Peculiar body striations.
4. Sexual dystrophy.
5. Muscular weakness and atrophy.
6. Hypertension.

Adrenal Virilism—Adrenogenital Syndrome:

Characterized by:

1. Excess hair growth.
2. Virilism.
3. Excessive muscularity.

The adrenal medulla is intimately connected with the nervous system and develops from the neural crest. The cells of the adrenal medulla are modified ganglion cells and receive stimulation from the preganglionic fibers whose cell bodies are located in the intermediolateral cell columns of the spinal cord in the thoracolumbar segments dealing with the sympathetic outflow of the autonomic nervous system. Sectioning of the splanchnic nerves to the adrenal medulla will result in cessation of secretion, while stimulation of these nerves enhances secretion markedly. The function of the adrenal medulla is to secrete the catecholamines adrenalin (epinephrine) and noradrenalin (norepinephrine).

In general these hormones help the body in frightful and stressful situations. They affect the vascular system (vasoconstriction), the heart (increased rate), respiration, carbohydrate metabolism (increased blood glucose levels), the pupillary dilators, the intestines, and uterine musculature.

A clinical picture of noradrenalism during which these pressor amines are produced in excess will show: (a) hypertension; (b) headache; (c) palpitation; (d) dyspnea; (e) weakness; and (f) chest and/or abdominal pain, etc.

The Testes

The testes function in the production of sperm and also contain interstitial cells, which produce the male sex hormone testosterone. Testosterone promotes and maintains the development of the male accessory genital organs (prostate and seminal vesicles) and secondary sex characteristics, i.e., beard growth, hair growth (pubic, axilla, trunk, and limbs), and scrotal growth. It maintains spermatogenesis, is responsible for the deepening of the voice, the greater muscular development of men, sex urge, and acne at puberty. It also exerts an influence on nitrogen, electrolyte, and water balance within the system. Both males and females produce estrogens and androgens; it is the ratio of the two which determines male and female characteristics.

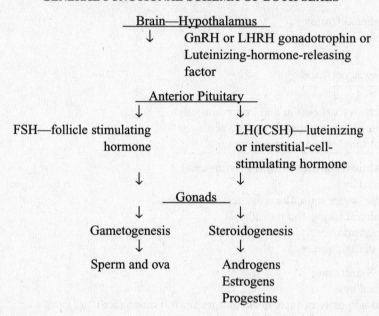

GENERAL FUNCTIONAL SCHEMA OF BOTH SEXES

Brain—Hypothalamus
↓   GnRH or LHRH gonadotrophin or Luteinizing-hormone-releasing factor

Anterior Pituitary
↓   ↓
FSH—follicle stimulating hormone   LH(ICSH)—luteinizing or interstitial-cell-stimulating hormone
↓   ↓

Gonads
↓   ↓
Gametogenesis   Steroidogenesis
↓   ↓
Sperm and ova   Androgens
             Estrogens
             Progestins

Steroidogenesis is similar in the ovary and the testis; the difference is in the predominance and quantity of the secretions. The androgen testosterone is the predominant secretion of the testis, while in the ovary the estrogen estradiol and the progestin progesterone predominate.

Actions of LH and FSH in the Male: These hormones act on the testis to promote:
1. adrogen secretion.
2. spermatogenesis.

Hormonal Control of Spermatogenesis:
1. Pituitary secretions regulate spermatogenic activities.
2. Interstitial-cell-stimulating hormone (ICSH) affects seminiferous tubules via androgen secretion.
3. FSH affects maturation of spermatids.
4. FSH and GH maintain spermatogenesis.

Androgenic and Anabolic Actions of Testosterone:
1. Maintenance of spermatogenesis.
2. Maintenance of structure and function of the accessory sex organs.
3. Promotion of secondary sex characteristics (size of genitalia, voice, glandular secretions, muscle development, and hair distribution).
4. Normal development and body growth.
5. Psychological balance.
6. Suppression of LH via feedback mechanism.

The Ovaries

Like the testes, the ovaries are endocrine glands. They have three functions: (a) they produce the female gamete (ovum); (b) they produce estrogens, which function in the preparation for fertilization of the egg and in the production of secondary female sex characteristics; and (c) they produce progesterone, which prepares the uterus for implantation. FSH from the pituitary initiates the development of the follicle and the production of estrogen; when the level of estrogen rises above a certain point, it shuts off FSH production, ovulation occurs, and LH and prolactin production take over in the development of the corpus luteum, which secretes progesterone. This hormone prepares the uterus for implantation of the fertilized egg; it promotes mammary gland development and prohibits additional ovulation. If fertilization does not occur, the corpus luteum regresses, progesterone production falls, and because maintenance of the lining of the uterus depends on progesterone, menstruation is the next phase of the cycle. If fertilization has occurred, the corpus luteum is maintained and secretes progesterone almost to the termination of the pregnancy.

Ovarian Cycle: It occurs from menarche to menopause, is typically 28 days long, and can be divided into two phases:

1. follicular or estrogenic
2. luteal or progestational

Menstrual Cycle

The ovarian cycle and the menstrual cycle of the uterus are integrated. The menstrual cycle can be divided into four phases:

1. menstrual phase (days 1–5);
2. proliferative or follicular phase (days 6–13), followed by ovulation (day 14);
3. secretory or luteal phase (days 15–25);
4. ischemic phase (days 26–28).

Uterine Changes during the Menstrual Cycle: Menses (days 1–5) involves the sloughing off of necrotic endometrium, blood, and uterine fluid, which is discharged as menstrual flow. During the proliferative phase (days 6–13), the primary hormonal stimulus is estrogen from the follicle, which promotes proliferation of uterine epithelium and glandular tissue. Ovulation generally occurs on day 14 of the cycle. During the postovulatory phase (days 15–25), the uterus is under the combined effects of estrogen and progesterone from the corpus luteum. This hormonal milieu promotes increased vascularity, further development of glands, their increased secretory activity (including glycogen accumulation), hypertrophy, and fluid accumulation. These changes prepare the uterus for implantation of a fertilized ovum, should fertilization occur. If fertilization does not occur, the corpus luteum begins to regress after day 25, leading ultimately to the onset of menses.

Hormonal Control of the Menstrual Cycle: The suppressed (and even declining) plasma gonadotropin (FSH and LH) levels during the follicular phase are due to the negative feedback inhibitory effects of estrogen being secreted from developing follicles. The small, abrupt rise in plasma estrogen is believed to trigger the ovulatory LH surge (by suspension of negative feedback or by positive feedback). During the luteal phase negative-feedback suppression is reestablished, but in this period feedback is due to the combined effects of estrogen and progesterone. Luteal failure occurs at about 26 days. It results in an abrupt withdrawal of estrogen and progesterone and hence in a release of feedback inhibition, which accounts for the rise in FSH and LH at the beginning of a new cycle.

Female Contraception

Female oral contraceptives represent combinations of synthetic progestational compounds (19-nortestosterone derivatives such as norgestrol and neorethindrone) with synthetic estrogen. The original rationale behind the pill was that the synthetic progestin in the presence of estrogen would block the ovulatory LH surge. The progestins are effective because they also cause the cervical mucus to produce an environment (like that in the luteal phase) hostile to sperm.

The Placenta

While the placenta is mainly concerned with support and nourishment of the developing embryo, it secretes estrogens, progesterone, and chorionic gonadotropin. Excess chorionic gonadotropin (similar to luteinizing hormone) is excreted in the urine and is the basis of most pregnancy tests. The estrogen production by the placenta inhibits FSH production and in this manner inhibits follicle development during pregnancy.

The Pineal

The pineal organ is a diencephalic outgrowth. Its products are melatonin, serotonin, and methylindoles. It has been linked to photoperiodism and seasonal breeding; experimental evidence now suggests that it produces an antigonadotropic substance. How the pineal influences the reproductive organs remains to be established. The pineal is considered a neuroendocrine transducer that modulates the functions of many different organs.

The Prostaglandins

Prostaglandins (PGs) are hormonelike substances that play a role in cellular metabolism. Their function, unlike that of hormones, is limited to immediate areas; in this respect they may be labeled as tissue hormones. These substances, which are derivatives of prostanoic acid, are C_{20} fatty acids containing a five-membered ring; they are found in almost every type of human and animal tissue and elicit a multitude of effects. Prostaglandins exert control over processes such as reproduction, inflammation, nerve impulse transmission, blood pressure and blood clotting, smooth muscle activity, and hormone secretion.

Major Actions of the Prostaglandins:

1. Lower blood pressure.
2. Modulate smooth muscle activity.
3. Inhibit the release of glycerol and fatty acid from adipose tissue.
4. Decrease nervous system excitability.
5. Modulate uterine smooth muscle.
6. Induce labor.
7. Modulate the bronchial tree.
8. Suppress gastric secretions.
9. Amplify pain response.
10. Stimulate renin secretion.
11. Modulate platelet aggregation.
12. Shrink swollen nasal passages.
13. Increase intraocular pressure.
14. Mediate inflammation.
15. Stimulate steroid production.
16. Promote sodium excretion.
17. Potentiate the pain-producing action of bradykinin.
18. Modulate norepinephrine release.

The Small Intestine

Food materials stimulate the secretion of certain hormones by the gastrointestinal mucosa and they may be summarized as follows:

1. Secretin: from duodenal mucosa—stimulates pancreatic juice secretion which is low in enzymatic content.

2. Pancreozymin: from duodenal mucosa—stimulates pancreatic juice secretion rich in enzymes.

3. Cholecystokinin: from duodenal mucosa—stimulates the contraction and emptying of the gallbladder.

4. Enterogastrone: from duodenal mucosa—inhibits motility and depresses the acid secretion by the stomach.

5. Gastrin: from pyloric region of stomach—enhances acid secretion by the stomach.

Quick Recall Test Questions and Answers

Choose the Best Answer

1. The most sensitive tests developed for the accurate detection of very small amounts of hormones to date are:

   A. bio-assays.
   B. immuno-assays.
   C. ascorbic acid depletion tests.
   D. flurometric assays.
   E. chromatographic assays.

2. Social stress will affect most severely the:

   A. pancreas.
   B. pineal.
   C. adrenal.
   D. parathyroid.
   E. thyroid.

3. Housed in the sella tursica is the:

   A. pineal organ.
   B. pituitary gland.
   C. olfactory bulb.
   D. optic chiasm.
   E. hypothalamus.

4. Follicle-stimulating hormone is to estrogen as luteinizing hormone is to:

   A. progesterone.
   B. testosterone.
   C. vasopressin.
   D. luteotrophic hormone.
   E. androgen.

5. Which of the following patterns would you expect to find in the blood one hour after a rich meal?

	Blood Sugar	Insulin
A.	high	low
B.	low	low
C.	high	high
D.	low	high
E.	no change	no change

6. During the follicular phase of a normal menstrual cycle, ovarian changes occur which are due to pituitary secretions of:

   A. FSH only.
   B. LH only.
   C. oxytocin.
   D. vasopressin.
   E. FSH and LH.

7. Growth hormone releasing factor is:

   A. a precursor of growth hormone.
   B. the same as growth hormone (somatotropin).
   C. a hypothalamic releasing factor.
   D. a dietary stimulant regulating positive nitrogen balance.
   E. an enzyme.

8. Glucagon, which is produced by the pancreas, and epinephrine, which is produced by the adrenal glands, are hormones which:

   A. raise blood sugar level.
   B. lower blood sugar level.
   C. do not affect blood sugar markedly.
   D. markedly increase liver glycogen.

9. Testosterone is produced by:

   A. spermatogonia of the testes.
   B. interstitial cells of the testes (Leydig cells).
   C. the glans penis.
   D. the prostate gland.
   E. Sertoli cells.

10. Hypersecretion of the hormone _____ will result in acromegaly (giantism).

    A. TSH—thyroid stimulating hormone
    B. STH—somatotropin (growth hormone)
    C. ACTH—adrenocorticotropic hormone
    D. thyroxin
    E. adrenalin

11. A lack of iodine in the diet usually is associated with which disorder?

    A. acromegaly
    B. goiter
    C. rickets
    D. skin rash
    E. tetanus

12. Each of the following is under control of the adenohypophysis EXCEPT the:

    A. thyroid.
    B. adrenal medulla.

C. testis.

D. adrenal cortex.

E. ovary.

13. The structure(s) responsible for the production of progesterone is/are:

A. ovarian follicle.

B. corpus albicans.

C. corpus luteum.

D. corpus spongiosum.

E. corpus cavernosum.

14. The pituitary (master) gland releases a gonadotrophic hormone which stimulates the production of testosterone by:

A. spermatogonia.

B. interstitial cells of Leydig.

C. Sertoli cells.

D. epididymis.

E. ductus deferens.

DIRECTIONS: For questions 15–20, choose the letter word or phrase that is most closely associated with the given item. You may use a letter choice more than once, or not at all.

A. Placenta

B. Hypothalamus

C. Adrenal cortex

D. Saliva

E. Pancreas

15. Chorionic gonadotropin

16. Relaxin

17. Cortisol

18. Ptyalin

19. Vasopressin

20. Maltase

DIRECTIONS: For questions 21–26, choose the letter word or phrase that most closely matches the description. You may use a letter choice more than once, or not at all.

A. Thyroid

B. Parathyroid

C. Thymus

D. Adrenal

21. Regulates the resorption of calcium from bone

22. Produces mineralocorticoids and glucocorticoids

23. Removal results in muscle spasms, tetany, and death

24. Oversecretion can cause an individual to have bulging eyeballs

25. Insufficiency can lead to mental and physical sluggishness

26. Plays a dominant role in the development of a competent immune system

27. Chromatin cells of the adrenal medulla are derived from:

A. the thyroglossal duct.

B. mesothelium of the Wolffian ridge.

C. endoderm.

D. neural crest ectoderm.

28. Which of the following hormones is the product of a pituitary acidophil (alpha cell)?

A. lutinizing hormone (LH)

B. follicle stimulating hormone (FSH)

C. thyroid stimulating hormone (TSH)

D. lactogenic hormone (LTH) or prolactin

E. melanocyte stimulating hormone (MSH)

29. All of the following may be considered as secondary sex characteristics of the male EXCEPT:

A. increase in sex drive.

B. external genitalia.

C. pattern of hair and beard growth.

D. development of a deeper voice.

E. skin pigmentation patterns.

Answers

1. **B.** Immuno-assays are the most sensitive of methods available for the detection of many substances.

2. **C.** Stress and strain will have a pronounced influence on the output of epinephrine and norepinephrine by the adrenal medulla. Activation of the sympathetic portion of the autonomic nervous system will result in increased activity by the adrenal medulla, which can be considered the site of the postganglionic cell bodies of that segment of the sympathetics.

3. **B.** The pituitary gland is located within the sella tursica.

4. **A.** FSH stimulates the production of estrogen by the developing follicle. LH stimulates the production of progesterone by the corpus luteum.

5. **C.** Langerhans described the beta cells (within the islets of Langerhans) of the pancreas, which produce insulin that affects the metabolism of glucose directly. Fat and protein are indirectly affected. After a meal the level of blood sugar rises, eliciting the production of insulin, which stimulates the absorption of glucose by the cells and helps in its conversion to glycogen. Insulin deficiency leads to high blood sugar levels and the disease called diabetes mellitus.

6. **E.** The pituitary and ovaries have a reciprocal effect upon each other. FSH (follicle stimulating hormone) from the pituitary elicits estrogen production from the developing follicle. When estrogen concentrations reach a certain blood level, it inhibits FSH production. At that time, the egg is discharged and the cells lining the follicle come under the influence of another gonadotrophin LH (luteinizing hormone) which influences the development of the corpus luteum.

7. **C.** The releasing factors that have been isolated and identified to date are produced in hypothalamic areas.

8. **A.** Glucagon is released into the bloodstream in response to diminishing blood sugar levels. The main action of glucagon is to promote liver glycogenolysis; as a consequence glycogen stores of the liver diminish. Epinephrine secreted by the adrenal medulla has the same general effect. Epinephrine is an important factor in the normal organism for counteracting the hypoglycemic action of insulin.

9. **B.** Most researchers feel that the interstitial cells of Leydig of the seminiferous tubules are the source of androgen and possibly testicular estrogen. The most potent androgen is testosterone.

10. **B.** Acromegaly and (or) giantism is due to overactivity of the alpha cells of the pituitary which secrete growth hormone. If a person is affected before puberty, he or she will develop into a fairly well proportioned giant. After maturity, an increase in the size of the hands and feet and massive development of the bones comprising the face are consequences. In the adult, strictly speaking, the term *acromegaly* must be applied to this condition.

11. **B.** Acromegaly is a result of pituitary oversecretion of growth hormone. Lack of iodine will result in goiter development of the thyroid gland. Rickets is due to a vitamin D deficiency. A skin rash is not a specific lesion that can be associated with only one specified cause, as can the others listed.

12. **B.** The adrenal medulla can be considered to house the post ganglionic neurons for part of the sympathetic portion of the autonomic nervous system and is responsible for epinephrine and norepinephrine production.

13. **C.** Progesterone is produced by the corpus luteum.

14. **B.** The interstitial cells are stimulated by ICSH (interstitial cell stimulating hormone), a gondadotrophin of the pituitary, to produce androgens. Testosterone is an androgen.

15. **A.** Chorionic gonadotropin is produced by the placenta and acts with other reproductive hormones to maintain pregnancy.

16. **A.** Relaxin is a product of the ovaries and placenta and functions in relaxing the pelvic ligaments during parturition.

17. **C.** Cortisol is produced by the adrenal and is active in the conversion of proteins to carbohydrates.

18. **D.** Ptyalin (salivary amylase) is found in saliva and initiates starch digestion.

19. **B.** Vasopressin (ADH) elaborated by the hypothalamus has an antidiuretic action on the kidney tubules.

20. **D.** Maltase, a component of saliva, participates in starch digestion.

21. **B.** It is believed by some that parathyroid hormone acts upon bone, eliciting changes in calcium and phosphrous. Osteoclasts are the cells stimulated by parathyroid hormone to facilitate

the resorption of calcium and phosphorus from bone. Administration of parathyroid hormone to animals without parathyroids results in an increase of phosphorus excretion in the urine, a fall in serum inorganic phosphorus levels, an increase in serum calcium, and an increase of calcium excretion in the urine.

22. **D.** The function of the adrenal cortex is to secrete sex hormone—androgens, estrogens, and progesterone; and corticosteriods—glucocorticoids and mineralocorticoids. These are all steriod hormones. The functional aspects of mineral and carbohydrate control by the adrenal are far more important than the influence it has on the reproductive organs (reproduction).

23. **B.** Tetany is a state of increased neuromuscular excitability caused by a decrease in serum calcium. This can exhibit itself by numbness, cramps, spasms, loss of consciousness, convulsions, and possible death.

24. **A.** Symptoms of hyperthyroidism can be listed as loss of weight, nervousness, irritability, rapid pulse, sweating, protrusion of the eyeballs (exophthalamus), and goiter.

25. **A.** Hypothyroidism results in sluggish mental and physical behavior. Pulse rate is down and skin appears dry.

26. **C.** Lymphocytes, which participate in such immunologic activities as delayed hypersensitivity reactions and graft rejection, are able to do so because of the influence of the thymus. Stem cells for this population are thought to pass through the thymus, and having come under its influence seed more peripheral lymphoid organs with their progeny. Removal of the thymus from newborn animals seriously impairs their immunologic system because of the lack of thymic influences.

27. **D.** The thyroglossal duct is the path that the thyroid gland takes in its descent from the base of the tongue to its final position in the neck. As far as the adrenal gland is concerned, the cortex has its origin from mesodeum while the medulla is derived from ectoderm, neural crest origin in conjunction with the anlage of the sympathetic nerve cells.

28. **D.** Luteinizing hormone and follicle stimulating hormone are products of delta cells. Thyroid stimulating hormone and melanocyte stimulating hormone are produced by beta cells. Lactogenic hormone is secreted by alpha cells.

29. **B.** At the time of puberty usually an increase in sex drive, beard growth, and development of a deeper voice are experienced. The external genitalia are part of the organism and will develop and grow as the organism does. They are genetically determined and are a primary characteristic of the male.

Reproductive System

Reproductive Organs

Male: Seminiferous tubules of the testis, epididymis, vas deferens, seminal vesicles, prostate, prostatic urethra, membranous uretha, penile urethra, glans penis.

Female: Ovaries, oviduct, uterus, vagina, the breasts (accessory organs containing mammary glands).

Hormonal Control

For a detailed discussion of the hormonal interactions concerning the reproductive system, the reader is referred to the section dealing with the endocrine system. However, the cyclic activity of the female organism is briefly summarized because it is of the utmost importance and quite difficult.

The reproductive cycle is under hormonal regulation; gonadotropic hormones of the pituitary (anterior lobe) stimulate the ovaries to produce a mature egg. The pituitary and ovaries have a reciprocal effect on each other. FSH (follicle stimulating hormone) from the pituitary elicits estrogen production from the developing follicle. When estrogen concentration reaches a certain blood level, it inhibits FSH production. At that time the egg is discharged and the cells lining the follicle come under the influence of another gonadotropin, LH (luteinizing hormone), which influences the development of the corpus luteum. The corpus luteum produces the hormone progesterone, which influences the wall of the uterus in preparation for implantation. As the concentration of progesterone rises, LH production is checked. If fertilization has occurred, the production of FSH is curtailed throughout the period of gestation through the production of estrogen by the placenta and ovary. If fertilization does not occur, the cycle begins anew.

Gametogenesis and Meiosis

The production of gametes, or sex cells—egg and sperm, is known as gametogenesis. Because an individual possesses an equal amount of genetic material from both parents and the same number of chromosomes as either parent, a reduction to one half that number must be accomplished in the development of the egg and sperm. Eggs and sperms are haploid; and a fertilized egg (zygote) possesses the diploid number of the parent again. The reduction occurs during meiosis.

The process of meiosis is best demonstrated in the following manner:

$$\underline{1,2} + \underline{1a, 2a}$$

The above unite in fertilization (form zygote) and the diploid adult somatic and primary germ cells are formed.

$$\downarrow$$
$$\underline{1, 1a, 2, 2a}$$

Primary germ cell in the adult undergoes spermatogenesis (male) or oogenesis (female); the result eventually will be haploid cells.
Tetrad formation

$$\downarrow$$
$$\underline{1, 1, 1a, 1a, 2, 2, 2a, 2a}$$

The first meiotic or reduction division occurs next, and results in the following:

$$\downarrow$$
$$\underline{1, 1a, 2, 2a} + \underline{1, 1a, 2, 2a}$$

Meiosis II occurs now and four haploid cells are produced.

$$\downarrow$$
$$\underline{1, 2 \quad 1a, 2a \quad 1, 2 \quad 1a, 2a}$$

Even though we have not indicated it, random assortment does occur during the process and chromosome combinations other than those illustrated are possible. In the human male four functional cells (sperms) are produced, while in the human female one functional cell (egg) and three polar bodies are produced. This is the general gamut of the process of meiosis.

Mature Gametes

Types of Eggs: Alecithal eggs have no yolk; examples are human and most other mammalian eggs. Microlecithal eggs have a small amount of yolk that is distributed equally; examples are sea urchin eggs. Telolecithal eggs have a large amount of yolk concentrated at one pole (lower or vegetal pole); examples are fish, reptile, and bird eggs. Centrolecithal eggs show a concentration of yolk in their center; insect eggs are the prime example.

Semen: In mammals semen is a fluid secreted by the male accessory sex glands, namely the prostate, seminal vesicles, and bulbourethral glands. Fructose is added by the prostate, as are acid phosphatase, citric acid, calcium, and fibrinolysin. The seminal vesicles add phosphorylcholine. The vas deferens is just a tube through which sperm are transported from the testes to the urethra. Between 3 and 4 ml of semen comprise one ejaculation, which contains between 300 and 400 million sperm cells.

Chromosomes: Forty-four autosomal chromosomes are present in every diploid cell of the human body. Mature gametes, however, are haploid. The total chromosome number of the human being is 46 (male 44 plus X and Y; female 44 plus X and X).

Other Modes of Reproduction

Budding, as in hydra, involves the multiplication of cells in one region of the organism and the organization of these cells into a new individual.

Binary fission or mitosis is a division of a cell into two equal parts and in this respect two new organisms (cells).

Parthenogenesis involves a mechanism in which a single cell is set apart for the purpose of reproduction. This cell has the capability to develop into a new organism.

A hermaphrodite possesses both male and female reproductive tissue.

Overview of Development

Stages in Development

Conversion of an animal egg into a functional multicellular organism normally involves a predictable series of stages.

Fertilization serves two functions. The egg must be activated (made capable of mitotic division) and the diploid condition in the nucleus in the egg must be restored. The embryo may be called a *zygote* from the time it is fertilized until it begins to cleave.

Cleavage is the process which converts the single-celled *zygote* (fertilized egg) into a solid multicellular embryo called a *morula*. Cleavage consists of mitotic cell divisions which are usually quite rapid owing to the reduction in the G1 phase of the cell cycle. These divisions therefore cause little increase in the total size of the embryo. At the end of cleavage a single large cell has been converted into many small cells. Any developmental information stored in regions of the egg cytoplasm is in separate cells at the end of cleavage. The cleavage pattern is frequently asymmetric when cytoplasmic information is being partitioned into specific cells.

Blastulation creates one or more spaces in the embryo into which cells can move during gastrulation. The *blastula* stage embryo differs from the morula in that the blastula contains a fluid-filled cavity called the *blastocoel*. The blastocoel is the space into which cells will move during *gastrulation* to convert the embryo into a multilayered structure. The blastocoel appears to form through loss of attachments among the cells in the center of the embryo, creating a space between the cells. At the end of the blastula stage, the embryo usually consists of what appears to be a single uniform layer of cells, although the layer may be many cells thick in some species.

The *blastocyst* stage in mammals is frequently equated with the blastula stage, but precedes the actual blastula stage. Blastocyst formation converts the solid morula stage into a hollow ball, but the space (blastocyst cavity) is not used for gastrulation. After the blastocyst stage, the cells in the inner cell mass form a disc which functions like the blastula stage in a bird embryo. Migration of cells converts the disc into a three-layered structure and involves an avian primitive streak-like structure, so the cell migration is clearly gastrulation and the preceding disc represents the blastula stage.

Gastrulation involves movements of cells, resulting in the conversion of the single-layered embryo into a three-layered embryo. At the end of gastrulation the embryo will typically have an external layer of *ectoderm*, a gut lining of *endoderm*, and a layer of *mesoderm* between the ectoderm and the endoderm. The primitive gut tube formed during gastrulation is called the *archenteron* ("old gut"). Gastrulation appears to involve major changes in the properties of the affected cells, since they have to alter their attachments to neighboring cells and become actively motile. The gastrulation pattern in complex animals is strongly correlated with the ancestry of the organisms in that organisms with a common ancestor usually have similar gastrulation patterns.

Organogenesis is the set of processes that convert the three-layered gastrula into a structure containing all of the organs which are necessary for survival as an independent organism (either larva or adult). Organogenesis varies in complexity with the complexity of the organism being formed. The known mechanisms involved in forming the body pattern which is expressed during gastrulation and organogenesis are described below.

Metamorphosis occurs only in organisms with larval stages and with abrupt transitions between stages. Organisms that have one or more larval stages in their life cycle form a larva during the organogenesis stage that follows cleavage. Conversion of the larva into the next larval stage or into an adult may be a gradual process or it may involve massive organogenesis from embryonic cell populations retained in the larva along with destruction of larval structures. Major conversions from one functional organism to another are called metamorphoses.

Mechanisms Used to Form the Body Pattern During Development

Three types of mechanisms used in generating the body pattern in developing organisms have been experimentally documented. Most organisms use at least two of these mechanisms at some point in their development, and many organisms probably use all three mechanisms.

Cytoplasmic information (probably in the form of mRNA or protein) is stored in specific areas of the egg cytoplasm during oogenesis (egg formation) in the ovary of many simple animals and perhaps in other organisms. Cytoplasmic information may be rearranged in response to fertilization. During cleavage, each area of cytoplasm ends up in a different cell. The informational molecules interact with the nucleus (probably turning specific genes on or off) to alter the cell's phenotype into the phenotype needed to form the appropriate part of the organism.

Use of cytoplasmic information as a pattern-generating mechanism can be easily demonstrated by removing individual cells from early embryos and noting which structures are missing later in development. If cytoplasmic information is the major mechanism involved, the parts normally formed by the missing cells will not form in the embryos from which the cells have been removed, but all other structures in the embryos will form normally.

This mechanism appears to be used most often in animals with relatively simple body patterns. Cytoplasmic information does not appear to be a major mechanism in birds or mammals. Most organisms that use cytoplasmic information also use cell-cell interactions to "fine-tune" formation of most complex organs.

Cell-cell interactions occur in all animal embryos that have been investigated so far. Cells in the developing embryo interact (through surface-surface interactions or by transferring chemical signals) to alter each other's phenotypes. This process is also called *induction*. Cell-cell interaction is frequently used to cause the parts of an organ to form in the correct relationship to each other but is not capable of generating an initial asymmetry in an embryo.

Cell-cell interaction can be experimentally detected by separating the cells between which interactions are suspected. If all cells involved still form their normal phenotypes after separation, cell-cell interaction (at least during the period following the separation) is clearly not essential in generating those phenotypes. Cell-cell interaction is also indicated if removal of one or more cells during cleavage results in failure to form structures normally created by neighbors of the cells that were removed. Cell-cell interaction appears to be the predominant identifiable developmental mechanism in vertebrates, especially in birds and mammals. The details of the mechanisms involved are unknown in most cases.

Cell-environment interactions have not been as thoroughly studied as cytoplasmic localization and cell-cell interactions, but have been demonstrated experimentally in several species.

Cell-environment interactions may be detected either by altering the environmental factors involved or by altering the orientation of the embryo relative to the factors and then observing the resulting developmental pattern. If cell-environmental interactions are involved, the orientation of the structure in the embryo will consistently follow the orientation of the environmental factor.

Embryos of birds and frogs appear to use gravity to produce initial differences between cells at the top (animal pole) and the bottom (vegetal pole) of the embryo.

Development in Humans

Fertilization

The development of a new organism starts with fertilization, the process during which the male and female gametes unite in the *ampulla* of the oviduct (Fallopian tube). The *diploid (2N)* number of chromosomes is achieved in this fusion. The egg (oocyte) is transported from the ovary down the oviduct by the *ciliary* movement and *peristaltic* action of the tube. Sperm pass quite rapidly from the vagina into the uterus, and then into the oviduct; they are propelled by the contractions of the musculature of the uterus and the oviduct.

Before fertilization can occur the spermatozoa must undergo *capacitation,* a process during which some of the protective coating of the head is removed. An *acrosome reaction* also occurs; during this process enzymes which are necessary to penetrate the protective barrier of the oocyte are released.

Of the approximately 350 million sperm deposited in a single ejaculation only about 350 reach the egg. Only one is necessary for fertilization but the others, it is thought, help in the dispersal of *corona radiata* cells (a circle, or "crown," of ovarian follicle cells that accompany the egg to this point) by release of enzymes such as hyaluronidase.

After passing through the corona radiata, the fertilizing sperm touches the *zona pellucida* surrounding the oocyte. The sperm next touches the oocyte cell membrane and fusion of both membranes occurs. The zona reaction then takes place; this prevents multiple sperm penetration. Upon entrance of the sperm, the secondary oocyte completes its second maturation division. The nucleus of the now mature ovum is known as the *female pronucleus*. When the male and female pronuclei come in contact, their nuclear membranes vanish, and the chromosomes intermingle. Fertilization is now complete, and the fertilized egg is known as a *zygote.*

Fertilization therefore consists of:

1. penetration of the corona radiata barrier,
2. penetration of the zona pellucida, and
3. fusion of sperm and oocyte plasma membranes.

Fertilization results in:

a. restoration of diploid number of chromosomes and variation of species,
b. determination of sex, and
c. activation of egg to begin development.

Cleavage

About 30 hours after fertilization, the zygote reaches the two-cell stage. Mitotic divisions rapidly increase the number of cells at this time; these small cells are termed *blastomeres* and the developing organism (now a solid ball) is called the *morula.* At approximately the 16-cell stage the zygote consists of centrally located cells, the *inner cell mass,* and a covering layer, the *outer cell mass.* The inner cell mass gives rise to the embryo proper, while the outer cell mass forms the *trophoblast,* which becomes the fetal component of the *placenta.* (In some species, cleavage of an ovum may occur without fertilization; the process is referred to as *parthenogenesis.*)

Blastocyst Formation

As the morula reaches the uterine cavity, fluid starts to accumulate internally between the inner cell mass and the outer cell mass and eventually forms a single cavity, the *blastocyst cavity*. The embryo is then referred to as the *blastocyst*. The inner cell mass (at this point located at one pole) now assumes the name *embryoblast,* and the outer cell layer, or *trophoblast,* at this time forms the epithelial wall of the *blastocyst*. By two weeks of gestation, the developing zygote has passed through the morula and blastocyst stages and has begun the implantation process by which it invades the uterine tissue to establish contact with the maternal circulation.

Implantation in the Uterus

Endometrium (uterine mucosa, an epithelium and underlying connective tissue) lines the uterus; *myometrium* forms the thick, middle muscular layer; and *perimetrium* covers the outside of the organ. When the blastocyst arrives the *uterine mucosa* is in the *secretory* or *progestational* phase. Uterine arteries are dilated, glands are enlarged, mucin and glycogen are being produced, and the tissue resembles a sponge. Implantation usually occurs either along the anterior or posterior wall of the uterus.

Second Week (Bilaminar Germ Disc Formation)

As the blastocyst embeds, the trophoblast differentiates into an inner *cytotrophoblast* and an outer *syncytiotrophoblast* layer. Syncytiotrophoblastic processes invade the endometrial epithelium and stroma. *Lacunae* (spaces) soon appear in the syncytiotrophoblast and fill with maternal blood and secretions; this nutritive material, called *embryotroph,* reaches the embryoblast by diffusion (a primitive uteroplacental circulation). The embryoblast differentiates into *endoderm* and *ectoderm* (two of the three primary germ layers) which form a flat disc known as the *bilaminar germ disc*. Between the cytotrophoblast and ectoderm layer the *amniotic cavity* develops, while beneath the ectoderm, the single layer of endoderm proliferates to form the definitive *yolk* sac. As development proceeds, the extraembryonic coelom, the cavity between the embryoblast and the trophoblast, expands and the large *chorionic cavity* is formed. Within the chorionic sac, the embryo and its amnion and yolk sac are suspended. Extraembryonic mesoderm lines this cavity and covers the embryoblast, thus connecting it to the trophoblast. As soon as blood vessels develop this connecting stalk will become the *umbilical cord*.

Highlighting this period is the development of the *primitive streak* on the surface of the ectoderm facing the amniotic cavity. The primitive streak functions as the *blastopore* during gastrulation. The cephalic end of this streak is known as the *primitive node*. During gastrulation, mesoderm cells segregate from the ectoderm layer and migrate between the ectoderm and endoderm by way of the primitive streak. In this manner the third primary germ layer, the *mesoderm* is formed between the ectoderm and endoderm except at the prochordal plate (buccopharyngeal membrane) and cloacal membrane.

The *allantois* appears as an outpocketing in the caudal end of the primitive gut around day 16. It stores excretory products in lower forms; it remains rudimentary in humans but plays a vital role as a source of vascular stem cells. During this period, formation of the *somites* from *mesoderm* and the initiation of the formation of the *central nervous system* from *ectoderm* begins. Mesoderm also gives rise to the blood vessels which eventually connect the placenta and the embryo.

Second Month (Germ Layer Differentiation)

During this period the main organ systems become established and external body features such as limb buds, face, ear, nose, and eyes become apparent.

Ectodermal Derivatives:

1. The *central and peripheral nervous system,* which develops in conjunction with the notochord. The notochord develops from the notochordal process and establishes a primitive axis for the embryo. (The nucleus pulposus of the intervertebral disc in the adult is the remnant of the notochord.) The established *neural plate* (composed of neuroectoderm above the notochord) forms a neural groove and neural folds and eventually becomes a *neural tube* giving rise to *brain vesicles* and the central canal

of the *spinal cord. Neural crest cells,* intermediate in position between the neural tube and surface ectoderm, develop into *dorsal root* and *cranial sensory* ganglia and their associated neurons.

2. *Placodes.* Many complex sensory structures begin their development as placodes, which are simple, localized ectodermal thickenings which invaginate into the underlying tissues and there differentiate into their definitive structures.

    a. An *otic placode* forms the *otic pit* and the *otic vesicle* giving rise eventually to organs of hearing and equilibrium.

    b. A *lens placode* under induction of the *optic vesicle* gives rise to the lens of the eye.

    c. A *nasal placode* gives rise to the *olfactory epithelium* of the nose.

3. The *epidermis,* including hair and nails, and subcutaneous connective tissue.

4. *Mammary glands,* the anterior *pituitary gland,* and the *enamel of the teeth.*

Mesodermal Derivatives: The sheet of mesoderm first gives rise to *paraxial mesoderm* (it will become the future paired *somites*), second to the *intermediate mesoderm* (it will become the future excretory units) and third to the *lateral plate* mesoderm (it will split into *somatic* and *splanchnic* [visceral] layers) which will line the intraembryonic *coelomic cavity.*

    a. *Somite Differentiation.* Somites are individual blocks of paraxial mesoderm arranged as paired chains along the length of the notochord and neural tube. Each somite will form bone, muscle, and dermis for a specific body segment. At the beginning 4 occipital, 8 cervical, 12 thoracic, 5 lumbar, 5 sacral, and 8–10 coccygeal pairs of somites are present; the first occipital and the last 5–7 coccygeal disappear at a later stage. As development proceeds each somite will be reorganized into a sclerotome, a myotome, and a dermatome.

    (1) *Sclerotome.* Initial cells become mesenchymal and migrate; later cells differentiate into:

        (a) *fibroblasts,* which give rise to reticular, collagenous, and elastic fibers of connective tissue;

        (b) *chondroblasts,* which give rise to cartilage;

        (c) *osteoblasts,* which give rise to bone of the vertebral column.

    (2) *Myotome.* Each myotome gives rise to the dorsal skeletal musculature of its segment.

    (3) *Dermatome.* Cells of this nature give rise to the dermis (skin) and subcutaneous tissue under the skin.

    b. *Intermediate Mesoderm Differentiation.* Cells in the cervical and thoracic region will give rise to *nephrotomes;* more caudally located cells form the *nephrogenic cord.* These will become the excretory units of the urinary system.

    c. *Lateral Plate Mesoderm*

    (1) *Somatic.* These cells form the lining of the intraembryonic coelomic cavity and give rise to the nonsegmental skeletal muscle of both wall and serous membranes which will eventually line the pericardial, pleural, and peritoneal cavities of the adult.

    (2) *Splanchnic.* These cells differentiate into *angioblasts,* which will give rise to blood cells and the cardiovascular and lymphatic systems. True blood formation starts in the second month and occurs in the liver, spleen, bone marrow, and lymph nodes.

Other Mesoderm Derivatives. Besides the structures described, mesoderm also gives rise to the gonads and their ducts, the cortex of the adrenal glands, and the spleen. It is also the source of the smooth muscle of the viscera.

Endodermal Derivatives: This germ layer provides

1. the epithelial lining of the gastrointestinal system,
2. the epithelial lining of the respiratory system,
3. the parenchyma of the tonsil, thymus, thyroid, parathyroid, liver, and pancreas,
4. the epithelial lining of the urinary bladder and urinary tract, and
5. the epithelial lining of the auditory (Eustachian) tube and the tympanic cavity (middle ear).

At 8 weeks the fetus stage has been reached and the dramatic changes leading to organ formation have occurred. The embryonic period now enters a phase of remarkable growth until the *conceptus* is ready for delivery.

DERIVATIVES OF THE GERM LAYERS

Ectoderm	Mesoderm	Endoderm
1. Epidermis of the skin • Hair and nails 2. Epithelium of the organs • Eye: retina, lens, cornea, and conjunctiva; lacrimal gland • Ear: external auditory meatus and membranous labyrinth • Nose: olfactory epithelium and glands of the nasal cavity and paranasal sinuses 3. Nervous system (central and peripheral) • Pia and arachnoid • Pineal gland and posterior lobe of pituitary • Adrenal medulla 4. Epithelium and glands of the lips, cheeks, gums, hard palate, and the parotid, submandibular, sublingual, and all minor salivary glands 5. Anterior lobe of pituitary gland 6. Enamel of the teeth 7. Muscles of the iris and the sweat glands 8. Epithelium of anal canal and vestibule of vagina	1. Connective tissue • Bone and cartilage 2. Synovial membranes 3. Lymphoid tissue • Tonsils and lymph nodes 4. Contents of the eye not developed from ectoderm 5. Middle and internal ear • Not membranous labyrinth or tympanic aspects 6. Dura and microglia 7. Teeth (except for enamel) 8. Cortex of adrenal gland 9. Serous membranes • Pleura, pericardium, peritoneum, and tunica vaginalis testis 10. Muscle • Striated, smooth, and cardiac 11. Endothelium of the cardiovascular and lymphatic system 12. Bone marrow, blood, and spleen 13. Urogenital organs	1. Epithelium of the digestive tract, tongue and taste buds, liver, biliary system, and pancreas 2. Epithelium of the thyroid, parathyroid, and thymus 3. Epithelium of the respiratory tract, larynx, trachea, bronchi, and alveoli 4. Epithelium of the genitourinary system

Fetal Membranes and Placenta

The fetal membranes are the: amnion, yolk sac, allantois, and chorion. While these membranes originate from the zygote, only the *yolk sac* and *allantois* contribute to embryonic structures.

The Amnion: The amniotic cavity is filled with fluid derived from the maternal circulation and from excretory products of the fetus. Amniotic fluid is swallowed by the fetus and taken up by the gastrointestinal system. The embryo, suspended by the umbilical cord, floats in the amniotic fluid. Amniotic fluid:

1. serves as a cushion and absorbs jolts,
2. allows the fetus to move,
3. helps in temperature regulation,
4. separates the amnion from the embryo,
5. provides a hydrostatic wedge during birth.

The Yolk Sac: The yolk sac is formed in the chorionic cavity and is connected to the umbilical cord. No yolk storage takes place in the human. However, the yolk sac plays a role in:

1. nutrient transfer before placental circulation is established,
2. blood cell development,
3. formation of the primordial germ cells.

The Allantois: This structure serves in the following manner:

1. it contributes to blood cell formation,
2. the allantoic blood vessels become the umbilical arteries and vein,
3. via the urachus the bladder is connected to the umbilicus.

The Placenta:
Structure. The placenta is composed of two parts:

1. the maternal part, derived from the endometrial decidua basalis,
2. the fetal part, derived from the chorionic villi.

Decidua. The decidua is the functional layer of the endometrium during pregnancy. Three zones are differentiated:

1. decidua basalis—this is the part deep to the conceptus, which forms the maternal placenta,
2. decidua capsularis—this is the part superficial to the conceptus and closest to the uterine cavity,
3. decidua parietalis—this is the term applied to the remaining portion of the uterine mucosa.

Chorionic Component. Originally the entire chorionic sac is covered by villi; however, around week eight, the villi not associated with the decidua basalis start to degenerate. The villi in relation to the decidua basalis increase in number and size and become the functional fetal portion of the placenta. The maternal and fetal components form an intimate anatomical and functional unit.

Function. Deoxygenated blood is carried from the fetus via the umbilical arteries to the placenta (villi). No mixing of maternal and fetal blood occurs. Exchange takes place over the endothelial barrier of the fetal vessels. Oxygenated blood passes into fetal placental veins, which form the umbilical vein, which supplies the fetus.

The main functions of the placenta are:

1. exchange of metabolic and gaseous products,
2. synthesis of glycogen, cholesterol and fatty acids,
3. synthesis of hormones,
4. transmission of antibodies.

Fetal and Neonatal Circulation

The cardiovascular system is designed to meet the needs of the fetus and at birth to adapt quickly to the demands of a new circuit and environment.

Fetal Circulation: Placenta → umbilical vein → ductus venosus of liver (half of the blood bypasses in this manner the hepatic circulation) → inferior vena cava → right atrium → foramen ovale, between right and left atria (blood bypasses the pulmonary circuit) → left atrium → left ventricle → ascending aorta → descending aorta → two umbilical arteries → placenta.

Blood that enters the right ventricle from the right atrium leaves via the pulmonary artery but bypasses the pulmonary circuit by passing through the ductus arteriosus, which connects the pulmonary artery to the aortic arch. In this manner blood reaches the aorta.

Changes at Birth: Due to a cessation of placental blood flow and the activation of the respiratory system because of pressure on the thoracic cavity and the replacement of amniotic fluid by air in the bronchial tree, certain changes are necessary:

1. ductus arteriosus closes due to muscular constriction of its wall,
2. blood flow through the lungs increases and results in a rise of pressure in the left atrium,
3. right atrial pressure drops due to cessation of placental circulation,
4. the above pressure differentials result in the closing of the foramen ovale and complete pulmonary circulation is established,
5. the umbilical arteries close,
6. the umbilical vein and ductus venosus close.

Adult Derivatives

Fetal structure		Adult structure
(1) umbilical vein	→	ligamentum teres
(2) ductus venosus	→	ligamentum venosuum
(3) umbilical arteries	→	(a) superior vesicle arteries
		(b) medial umbilical ligaments
(4) foramen ovale	→	fossa ovalis
(5) ductus arteriosus	→	ligamentum arteriosum

Multiple Pregnancy

Twinning: Twinning occurs in about 1% of normal births; about two-thirds are of the *dizygotic* (fraternal) twin type. The frequency of dizygotic twins increases with the age of the mother and is influenced by heredity. (No age correlation exists as far as *monozygotic* [identical] twins are concerned.) If a first pregnancy results in twins, subsequent twinning is about three to five times greater than in the normal population. The *genotype* of the mother seems to be the key determining factor in the frequency of twin births.

Monozygotic Twins (Identical Twins). A single oocyte and sperm are involved. Two inner cell masses form within a single trophoblast at the blastocyst stage. Each inner cell mass subsequently develops into an embryo. These embryos have a common placenta and chorionic cavity but possess separate amniotic cavities. These individuals have the same sex and blood groups, and a strong resemblance in external features. (Their phenotypes and genotypes are identical.)

Dizygotic Twins (Fraternal Twins). Two separate oocytes and two separate sperm are involved. Both zygotes are totally different genetically. They may or may not be of the same sex. These zygotes implant independently and develop their own placenta and membranes. (Fraternal twins are not identical in phenotype and genotype. They are no more similar than any other non-twin siblings.)

Triplets: Triplets occur once in about 8,000 pregnancies. They may result from:

1. one zygote and therefore be identical,
2. two zygotes, and therefore give rise to one set of identical twins and one independent infant,
3. three zygotes and result in three independent individuals.

Types of multiple births higher than triplets are rare but similar combinations do occur.

Quick Recall Test Questions and Answers

Choose the Best Answer

1. Which of the following does not contribute to the formation of semen?

   A. prostate
   B. seminal vesicles
   C. bulbo-urethral glands
   D. vas deferens
   E. sexual excitement

2. The human female has a karyotype of:

   A. 23 pairs of autosomes and an X and a Y.
   B. 23 pairs of autosomes and two X's.
   C. 22 pairs of autosomes and an X and a Y.
   D. 22 pairs of autosomes and two X's.
   E. 22 pairs of autosomes and two Y's.

3. During gametogenesis (spermatogenesis) in the male, the second meiotic division takes place between:

   A. the zygote and spermatid.
   B. the primary germ cells and haploid gametes.
   C. the secondary spermatocyte and spermatid.
   D. the spermatid and spermatozoan.
   E. the processes of capacitation and the acrosome reaction.

4. A hermaphrodite is characterized by being:

   A. both male and female.
   B. neither male nor female.
   C. can change his/her sex depending on conditions.
   D. sterile and asexual.
   E. very virile.

5. Human sperm and ova are similar in the respect that they:

   A. are haploid.
   B. both possess flagella, which give them good mobility.
   C. are approximately the same size.
   D. both carry the identical genetic information.
   E. are diploid.

6. Vasectomy is becoming a fashionable form of birth control in our society. In a vasectomy the _____ is/are cut, a portion is removed, and the stumps are sutured.

   A. epididymis
   B. vas deferens
   C. oviducts
   D. urethra
   E. seminal vesicles

7. The basic scientific finding that finally led to the development of the oral contraceptive (pill) used by many females in our society was that the pre-ovulatory surge of LH can be prevented by the administration of:

   A. FSH.
   B. estrogen.
   C. progesterone.
   D. ICSH.
   E. androgen.

8. During gamete production in the human female, the cell which undergoes the reduction divisions (meiosis) eventually produces _____ functional egg(s).

   A. 4
   B. around 300
   C. 8
   D. 1
   E. around 100

9. The sperm count of a normal 25-year-old male is:

   A. 1 million/ml.
   B. 100 million/ml.
   C. 100,000/ml.
   D. 4 million/ml.
   E. 10,000/ml.

10. Sperm utilize the substance _____ to penetrate the corona radiata of the egg in fertilization.

    A. spermatase
    B. chondroitin sulfatase
    C. hyaluronidase
    D. deoxyribonuclease
    E. ribonuclease

11. During the process of meiosis in the human male four functional sperms are produced, while in the female one functional egg and three _____ are the end result.

    A. zygotes

B. follicles
C. polar bodies (polocytes)
D. blastocysts
E. embryos

12. Conversion of a haploid cell into a diploid cell occurs during _____ in most animals.

A. fertilization
B. organogenesis
C. cleavage
D. blastulation
E. gastrulation

13. Ectoderm, mesoderm, and endoderm form as distinct layers during _____ in most animal embryos.

A. fertilization
B. organogenesis
C. cleavage
D. blastulation
E. gastrulation

14. The process of _____ converts the single-celled zygote into a multicellular structure in most animal embryos.

A. fertilization
B. organogenesis
C. cleavage
D. blastulation
E. gastrulation

15. Different cell types (muscle, brain, liver, etc.) within a single human body:

A. have genetically identical nuclei (contain the same genes) and express (transcribe) the same genes.
B. have genetically different nuclei (do not contain the same genes) but express (transcribe) the same genes.
C. have genetically identical nuclei (contain the same genes) but express (transcribe) different genes.
D. have genetically different nuclei (do not contain the same genes) and express (transcribe) different genes.

16. Gastrulation involves:

A. rapid cell division forming a multicellular embryo.
B. formation of ectoderm, mesoderm, and endoderm.
C. conversion of a larva into an adult.

D. formation of sperm and eggs.
E. fusion of haploid cells to form a zygote.

17. The process of embryonic development which most closely follows after fertilization is:

A. metamorphosis.
B. organogenesis.
C. cleavage.
D. blastulation.
E. gastrulation.

18. Gametogenesis involves:

A. rapid cell division forming a multicellular embryo.
B. formation of ectoderm, mesoderm, and endoderm.
C. conversion of a larva into an adult.
D. formation of sperm and eggs.
E. fusion of haploid cells to form a zygote.

19. Fertilization involves:

A. rapid cell division forming a multicellular embryo.
B. formation of ectoderm, mesoderm, and endoderm.
C. conversion of a larva into an adult.
D. formation of sperm and eggs.
E. fusion of haploid cells to form a zygote.

20. Cleavage involves:

A. rapid cell division forming a multicellular embryo.
B. formation of ectoderm, mesoderm, and endoderm.
C. conversion of a larva into an adult.
D. formation of sperm and eggs.
E. fusion of haploid cells to form a zygote.

21. The food reserves which will support the development of a human embryo are:

A. stored in the unfertilized egg or ovum.
B. stored in the sperm.
C. stored in both the unfertilized egg and the sperm.
D. transferred to the embryo by the epithelium of the female reproductive tract.
E. transferred to the embryo from maternal blood in the endometrium of the uterus.

Answers

1. **D.** Semen is a fluid secreted by the male accessory sex glands—namely, the prostate, seminal vesicles, and bulbo-urethral glands. Fructose is added by the prostate, as are acid phosphatase, citric acid, calcium, and fibrinolysin. The seminal vesicles add phosphorylcholine. The vas deferens is just a tube through which sperm are transported from the testes to the urethra.

2. **D.** Forty-four autosomal chromosomes are present in every diploid cell of the human body. Mature gametes, however, are haploid. The total chromosome number of the human being is 46 (male 44 plus X and Y; female 44 plus X and X).

3. **C.** The production of gametes, or sex cells—egg and sperm, is known as gametogenesis. Because an individual possesses an equal amount of genetic material from both parents and the same number of chromosomes as either parent, a reduction to one half that number must be accomplished in the development of the egg and sperm. The second meiotic division takes place between the secondary spermatocyte and spermatid.

4. **A.** A hermaphrodite possesses both male and female reproductive tissue.

5. **A.** Human sperm and ova are similar in the respect that they both carry a haploid chromosomal complement. After fertilization the diploid composition is again found.

6. **B.** Vasectomy involves an interruption of the vas deferens in the male.

7. **C.** While on the pill the female produces no new eggs and is kept in the progestational phase (second half) of the menstrual cycle.

8. **D.** During meiosis in the female one functional gamete (egg) and three polar bodies are produced.

9. **B.** Between 3 to 4 ml of semen comprise one ejaculate, which contains between 300–400 million sperm cells.

10. **C.** Hyaluronidase, an enzyme carried by sperm, is capable of hydrolysis of hyaluronic acid, promoting fertilization (penetration of sperm). Hyaluronidase is medically used to promote the diffusion and absorption of many injected medications.

11. **C.** In the human male four functional cells (sperms) are produced, while in the human female one functional cell (egg) and three polar bodies (polocytes) are produced during meiosis.

12. **A.** Fusion of the haploid sperm with the egg (which eventually becomes haploid) produces a diploid zygote.

13. **E.** Gastrulation completes formation of a three-layered embryo with ectoderm, endoderm, and mesoderm. In some animals, both endoderm and mesoderm form during gastrulation. In other animals, part of the endoderm may be in place at the beginning of gastrulation, so gastrulation completes endoderm formation and forms the mesoderm.

14. **C.** Cleavage converts the single-celled zygote into a multicellular embryo. Cleavage consists of rapid mitotic cell division.

15. **C.** Different cell types form by activation of different sets of genes. In most cases studied so far, no permanent changes occur in the genetic makeup of the different cells. The exceptions include lymphocytes, in which genetic rearrangements occur in the process of forming antibodies and T-cell receptors.

16. **B.** Gastrulation completes formation of a three-layered embryo with ectoderm, endoderm, and mesoderm. In some animals, both endoderm and mesoderm form during gastrulation. In other animals, part of the endoderm may be in place at the beginning of gastrulation, so gastrulation completes endoderm formation and forms the mesoderm.

17. **C.** Mitotic cell division (called cleavage) must occur after fertilization to produce a sufficient number of cells to form the parts of the embryo.

18. **D.** Gametogenesis is the process of converting body cells into sperm or eggs. In most animals, this process involves meiosis to convert diploid body cells into haploid cells and differentiation of body cells into the highly specialized cells called sperm and eggs.

19. **E.** Fertilization involves fusion of a sperm with an egg. The initial fusion typically activates

the egg to begin development; the fusion of the haploid nucleus from the sperm with a haploid nucleus in the egg forms the diploid nucleus of the embryo.

20. **A.** Cleavage converts the single-celled zygote into a multicellular embryo. Cleavage consists of rapid mitotic cell division. Mitotic cell division must occur after fertilization to produce a sufficient number of cells to form the parts of the embryo.

21. **E.** In humans and other mammals with deep implantation, some nutrients may be taken up from the lumen of the female reproductive tract prior to implantation, but most of the food reserves which support development are transferred from maternal blood (which forms a pool around the implanted embryo in the endometrium of the uterus) into the embryo. In the fully implanted embryo, this occurs in the placenta.

Defense Against Foreign Organisms and Abnormal Cells

Routine defense against foreign organisms which are not adapted to function as parasites is primarily due to *barrier layers* at body surfaces. *Clot formation* reduces foreign organism entry following mechanical damage to a barrier layer. *Innate defense mechanisms* destroy most nonpathogenic organisms which have passed barrier layers, destroy many types of abnormal host cells, and reduce the numbers of newly encountered pathogenic organisms until a specific immune defense can be established. *Specific immune responses* require time to develop following the initial exposure to a particular organism, but are capable of completely wiping out most infections under optimal conditions. The specific components of a foreign organism that are responded to by a specific immune response are called antigens.

Barrier Layers

Barrier layers protect all body surfaces that may be exposed to foreign organisms. These barrier layers include skin, respiratory system linings, digestive system linings, urinary system linings, and reproductive system linings. A typical barrier layer consists of a surface epithelium and an underlying connective tissue layer. The tight junctions between the cells in the epithelium prevent movement of organisms across the barrier through extracellular spaces. The connective tissue layers underlying the epithelium provide mechanical strength to the barrier.

Organs in which the barrier function is reduced as an adaptation to the requirements of the physiological processes occurring across the barrier are protected by mechanisms which reduce the chance of living foreign organisms reaching the organ. The lungs have a very thin lining to allow efficient gas exchange and are protected by the mucus layer in the nose, trachea, and bronci; the small intestine has a simple columnar to allow effective food absorption and is protected by the acidic environment in the stomach; and the uterus has a thin lining, which allows embryos to penetrate into the endometrium, and is protected by the mucus plug in the cervix. The cavities communicating with these organs are also populated with nonpathogenic microorganisms which compete with pathogens and reduce the chance of their successful entry.

As a result of the effectiveness of barrier layers, infections usually result from either mechanical damage to a barrier layer or penetration of a barrier layer through specific pathogenic mechanisms which evolved in the pathogens as ways to enter the host.

Clot Formation

A clot provides a temporary barrier when an epithelium (normal barrier) is damaged. Clot formation can be initiated by either blood vessel damage or tissue damage and involves a cascade of sequential clotting factor reactions which culminate in deposition of a fibrin clot blocking access to the damaged area.

Innate Defense Mechanisms

Purely innate or paraimmune mechanisms require no prior exposure to a particular foreign organism before the mechanisms can function at full efficiency. This is partly because innate mechanisms are directed at features shared by groups of foreign organisms and typically have less specificity than specific immune mechanisms.

Unfortunately, innate mechanisms are less capable of completely destroying an invading population of foreign organisms than are specific immune mechanisms. Therefore, innate mechanisms may destroy small invasions if the organisms lack effective mechanisms of avoiding destruction, but usually serve to hold larger, more pathogenic invasions in check until a specific immune response can develop. In other words, your innate mechanisms usually keep you alive long enough to generate a specific immune response to finish off the infection.

In addition, some innate mechanisms also serve as effectors for specific immune responses and may chemically enhance specific immune responses. In general, defense mechanisms are closely integrated.

Numerous innate mechanisms have been identified. A few typical examples are listed below.

1. *Neutrophils* are granular leukocytes which are intrinsically capable of phagocytosis of

some types of bacteria. This response is vastly increased by innate complement activation or by specific immune responses which deposit antibodies and complement on the bacteria.

    2.   *Macrophages* are monocyte-derived connective tissue cells which are intrinsically capable of phagocytosis of some types of bacteria. This response is vastly increased by innate complement activation or by specific immune responses which deposit antibodies and complement on the bacteria.

    3.   *Natural killer (NK)* cells are lymphocytes which are intrinsically capable of killing some types of cancer cells and some types of virus-infected cells. Additional types of abnormal or foreign cells are killed if the NK cells are activated by cytokines secreted by helper T lymphocytes or if the target cells are coated with antibodies produced by a specific immune reaction.

    4.   Some types of bacteria spontaneously activate *complement* proteins by the alternate pathway, resulting in killing the bacteria. Complement proteins are innate components of blood plasma and tissue fluid. Interaction between some innate inflammatory response proteins and some bacteria increases complement activation. Complement is also activated very efficiently by many of the classes of antibodies produced in specific immune responses.

    5.   Release of *interferon* by virus-infected cells is an innate response which makes surrounding cells more resistant to virus infection.

Specific Immune Mechanisms

Specific immune responses require prior exposure to the same or a very similar foreign organism to be fully effective because initial exposure to a foreign organism causes a primary immune response, which is much slower and less efficient than the secondary immune response which is triggered by subsequent exposure to the same organism. As a result, natural immunization against a pathogenic foreign organism will only occur if the infection is successfully held in check by innate mechanisms while the specific immune response develops.

This problem may be overcome by immunizing the host prior to the initial exposure to the pathogenic organism. Immunity may be clinically produced through two processes.

Passive immunization is achieved by transfer of antibodies directed against a foreign organism from one organism to another. This causes the recipient to immediately but temporarily become immune to the foreign material.

Passive immunization occurs naturally in mammals as a result of antibodies transferred from the mother to the fetus across the placenta and to the newborn in milk. Passive immunization is used clinically in cases in which a functional immune response is needed more quickly than it can be generated by active immunization; for example, in a patient who was bitten by a rabid animal and who did not begin active immunization soon enough to be sure that rabies shots would generate active immunity in time to prevent rabies.

Passive immunization can only be used with antibodies because transferred cell-mediated immune components could reject the body of the recipient. In addition, passive immunization is undesirable when it is not essential because the injected antibodies reduce the effectiveness of simultaneous active immunization.

Active immunization is achieved by exposure of the patient to a nonpathogenic form of a foreign organism or to isolated components of a foreign organism. This results in a primary immune response which produces immunity against the foreign organism after a delay of days or weeks. Subsequent exposure to the same foreign organism results in a secondary immune response which produces a rapid and effective response.

Patterns of Specific Immune Responses

The principal response mechanisms of the immune system are traditionally divided into cell-mediated responses and humoral or antibody-mediated responses. With the exception of a few situations, both of these responses require interactions with helper T lymphocytes.

TYPE OF SPECIFIC IMMUNE RESPONSE

	Cell-mediated Immunity	Antibody-mediated Immunity
Targets of response	Virus infected cells, cancer cells, transplanted cells	bacteria, viruses, foreign molecules
Lymphocytes involved	Activated cytotoxic T (T_c) lymphocytes	activated B lymphocytes which differentiate into plasma cells
Effector mechanisms	Cell-mediated killing of target cells and organisms	antibody-mediated killing of target cells and organisms

Both types of responses involve receptors (T cell receptors on T_c and antibodies on B lymphocytes) that are generated by random recombination of gene segments which code for the variable regions of the receptors. This generates an enormous number of receptor specificities. After the initial recombination during the development of the lymphocytes, the cells undergo positive selection for cells bearing functional receptors and negative selection against cells bearing receptors reactive against components of the organism's own body. Cells which fail either test die in the formative organ. The cells that pass both tests leave the formative organ as potentially functional lymphocytes which require activation to become fully functional. At this point, only a few lymphocytes will react effectively with any particular foreign component. Successful activation triggers proliferation of the cells whose receptors interact effectively with abnormal or foreign components, and some of the resulting cells remain as memory cells. As a result, a second exposure to the same components results in a much faster response because the process is beginning with many more cells.

Cytotoxic T Lymphocyte Responses

In a cell-mediated response, T_c lymphocytes recognize viral or abnormal peptides displayed on major histocompatibility complex class I (MHC I) molecules on the surface of body cells. T cell receptor molecules on the T_c cells specifically recognize the peptides and closely associated CD8 molecules on the T_c cells recognize the MHC I molecules. If a peptide is recognized by a T cell receptor on an activated T_c, the cell displaying the peptide on its MHC I is killed. Cell-mediated killing of target cells and organisms may involve secretion of perforins (pore-forming proteins) onto the target cells or may involve secretion of cytokines which stimulate receptors on the target cells and trigger programmed cell death through apoptosis.

Antibody Structure

A functional antibody contains a Y-shaped unit structure consisting of two heavy-chain–light-chain pairs joined by disulfide bonds and containing two antigen-binding sites. Each arm of the Y is formed by one of the light-heavy chain pairs. The base of the Y is formed by the parts of the two heavy chains which extend past the light chains.

Antibodies are subdivided into classes or isotypes based on the type of heavy chain found in the molecule as shown in the following table.

Immunoglobulin class	Subclass	Heavy chains	Light chains
IgA	IgA1	alpha1	kappa or lambda
	IgA2	alpha2	kappa or lambda
IgD		delta	kappa or lambda
IgE		epsilon	kappa or lambda
IgG	IgG1	gamma1	kappa or lambda
	IgG2	gamma2	kappa or lambda
	IgG3	gamma3	kappa or lambda
	IgG4	gamma4	kappa or lambda
IgM		mu	kappa or lambda

Each light and heavy chain has a variable region formed by rearrangement of DNA segments in the corresponding gene during the development of the B lymphocyte and a constant region characteristic of the category of polypeptide. An antigen binding pocket in an antibody is formed by the association of variable regions of a light plus a heavy chain. The large number of variable segments and the process of recombining them during B lymphocyte development results in an enormous number of antibody specificities in each individual.

Cell surface receptor forms of IgM and IgD and circulating forms of IgE and IgG consist of single fundamental units (two heavy chains plus two light chains). IgA occurs as single fundamental units and also occurs in a complex containing two of the fundamental units joined by a J polypeptide. IgA which has been transported across an epithelium contains an additional secretory polypeptide. Circulating IgM consists of an assembly of five antibody fundamental units plus a J polypeptide.

IgD exists only as a cell surface receptor in unstimulated B lymphocytes. IgM functions primarily within blood vessels. Because IgG can function within blood vessels and is easily moved across blood vessel walls in tissue fluid, it is the primary antibody in connective tissues. IgG is also moved across the placenta from the mother to the fetus during late pregnancy. IgA is transported across lining epithelia in the digestive and respiratory systems and functions on the mucosal surfaces. IgE also occurs on and below the same surfaces, and apparently evolved as a defense against parasitic worms. Its ability to trigger mast cell secretions unfortunately also results in allergies.

In an antibody-mediated response, foreign components bind to antibodies on the surfaces of B lymphocytes and stimulate the B lymphocytes to proliferate and differentiate into plasma cells which secrete antibodies of the same specificity as the antibody receptors which were triggered. The antibodies then bind specifically to proteins or carbohydrates on the surface of the target cells.

Antibody-mediated killing of target cells and organisms may involve activation of complement, resulting in pore formation in the plasma membranes of the target cells. Antibodies bound to target cells can also trigger killing of eukaryotic target cells by NK cells or macrophages through the process of antibody-dependent cellular cytotoxicity (ADCC) or can act alone or with activated complement to trigger phagocytosis followed by intracellular killing of bacteria by neutrophils and macrophages.

Helper T Lymphocytes

Helper T lymphocytes (T_h, CD4+) are essential to provide chemical stimuli to the responding cells in almost all cell-mediated and antibody-mediated responses. T_h lymphocytes function by secreting cytokines which stimulate T_c or B lymphocyte activation and function and which may also activate macrophages and NK cells.

T_h lymphocytes are activated by interaction with an antigen-presenting cell presenting a fragment of a molecule (an antigen) recognized by the receptors on the T_h lymphocyte. The antigen must be presented on a major histocompatibility class II (MHC II) molecule and the antigen-presenting cell must provide appropriate costimulation. Antigen presentation without costimulation appears to inactivate T_h lymphocytes.

Antigen-Presenting Cells

Antigen-presenting cells are essential in activation of T_h lymphocytes. Macrophages and B lymphocytes can act as antigen-presenting cells under some circumstances, but interdigitating dendritic cells appear to be the most important antigen-presenting cells for T_h activation in intact organisms. These cells take in foreign material by phagocytosis or pinocytosis and partially degrade the molecules, then bind fragments to MHC II molecules and present them on the cell surface. Antigen-presenting cells must also provide T_h lymphocytes with costimulation signals on the antigen-presenting cell surfaces, usually in the form of B7 molecules. Antigen-presenting cells are also involved in activation of T_c lymphocytes, but the process is not well understood.

A separate population of follicular dendritic cells appear to be critical in developing and maintaining B cell populations for antibody-mediated responses. Follicular dendritic cells apparently accumulate antigen complexed with antibody on their cell surfaces by binding to receptors for antibody and complement. This bound antigen is available for interaction with B cells, both during their development and during memory cell maintenance.

Development of T Lymphocytes

Bone marrow is where most unspecialized lymphocytes appear to be produced. Most T lymphocytes leave the bone marrow and differentiate in the thymus. While in the thymus, developing T lymphocytes rearrange DNA segments within their T cell receptor (TCR) genes to form a functional TCR. A functional TCR usually contains one alpha and one beta polypeptide complexed with a CD3 complex of additional polypeptides. A smaller number of T lymphocytes have TCR with gamma and delta polypeptides in place of the alpha and beta polypeptides. Each alpha, beta, gamma, and delta polypeptide has a variable region formed by rearrangement of DNA segments in the corresponding gene and a constant region characteristic of the category of polypeptide. An antigen-binding pocket in a TCR is formed by the association of variable regions of an alpha plus a beta polypeptide or by association of variable regions of a gamma plus a delta polypeptide.

Positive and Negative Selection of T Lymphocytes in the Thymus

As they begin to express TCR on their surfaces, developing T lymphocytes initially express both CD4 and CD8 on their surfaces as well. Developing T lymphocytes whose TCR fails to interact with either MHC I or MHC II die as a result of the initial positive selection for cells with minimally functional TCR. If the TCR interacts more effectively with MHC I, the T lymphocyte loses CD4, retains CD8, and becomes a T_c. If the TCR interacts more effectively with MHC II, the T lymphocyte loses CD8, retains CD4, and becomes a T_h. Subsequently, both T_c and T_h lymphocytes which interact too strongly with antigens presented on MHC I and MHC II in the thymus die in the process of negative selection. The components used in negative selection appear to include most of the normal body components which could easily be presented by MHC I or MHC II. As a result, the T_c and T_h lymphocytes leaving the thymus have functional TCR which do not react excessively with normal components from the organisms' own cells. The tendency of presentation of an antigen without appropriate costimulation to inactivate a T_c or T_h lymphocyte appears to protect most individuals adequately against any remaining T lymphocytes carrying TCR reactive with normal body components, but these selection processes clearly fail in cases of autoimmune responses.

Development of B Lymphocytes

B lymphocytes appear to complete their differentiation in the bone marrow where they are initially produced and emerge into the circulation as mature B lymphocytes with antigen specificity.

Development of a functional B lymphocyte requires genetic recombination in the genes which code for the amino acid sequence of the immunoglobulin light and heavy chains. Light chains are coded for by a kappa gene or a lambda gene, only one of which will be used in a particular B lymphocyte. Heavy chains are coded for by a single set of heavy chain genes, each of which contains a constant region segment for each of the classes or isotypes of antibodies.

Heavy chain recombination occurs initially, followed by light chain recombination. Failure to generate a functional antibody apparently results in cell death in a process similar to positive selection in the thymus, but the detailed interactions are not understood. In addition, developing B lymphocytes producing antibodies which are excessively reactive toward normal body components present in bone marrow are also eliminated in a process which is apparently similar to negative selection in the thymus. The antibodies at this point are present on the B lymphocyte cell surface as IgM and IgD molecules which serve as cell surface receptors.

Exposure to an antigen which reacts with cell surface IgM or IgD begins the process of activation of the B lymphocyte. With the exception of a few polymeric antigens, material which binds to the immunoglobulin receptors on a B lymphocyte is internalized, processed, and returned to the surface of the B lymphocyte on MHC II molecules. The B lymphocyte must then present the antigen on its MHC II molecules to a T_h lymphocyte and be stimulated by the cytokines secreted by the T_c before the B lymphocyte is activated.

Activation triggers proliferation of the B lymphocyte. Some of the progeny remain as memory B lymphocytes, but most of the progeny differentiate into plasma cells which secrete antibodies. During differentiation into plasma cells, the functional heavy chain gene is altered by deletion of at least the delta and mu segments, resulting in secretion of antibodies of IgA, IgE, or IgG classes. This process is called class or isotype switching. During the activation process, mutations also occur which result in small changes in amino acid composition of the antigen-binding site and the resulting cells compete for antigen, with cells carrying more effective receptors becoming more frequent and the secreted antibodies becoming more specific.

Reactive Lymphoid Organs

Reactive organs or secondary lymphoid organs are locations in which lymphocytes provide surveillance of body cavities connected to microbe-containing environments or surveillance of body fluids. All of these organs contain B lymphocyte-rich follicles or nodules and associated T lymphocyte-rich areas. Secondary lymphoid organs can be classified into two functional and organizational patterns.

1. *External cavity screening organs* are located in the walls of tubular organs which routinely contain microorganisms. *Diffuse lymphoid tissue* (populations of lymphocytes and innate response cells) in the subepithelial connective tissue in the walls of the digestive, respiratory, urinary, and reproductive systems is involved in surveillance of the contents of those organ lumens and walls. The *tonsils* in the wall of the posterior part of the pharynx are involved in surveillance of organisms in the oral cavity. *Peyer's patches* in the wall of the ileum are involved in surveillance of organisms in the lower small intestine. The *appendix* extending from the blind end of the large intestine is involved in surveillance of organisms in the large intestine.

2. *Fluid screening organs* are interposed in the circulatory system. *Lymph nodes* are expanded areas in lymphatic vessels which contain aggregates of lymphoid tissue. They are involved in surveillance of organisms in lymph. Because lymph is tissue fluid which has just left organs, its contents represent a sample of any organisms which have invaded the organs of the host organism. The *spleen* (along with some areas in bone marrow) is involved in surveillance of organisms in blood. The spleen receives blood from the systemic circulation. The blood is intimately exposed to lymphocytes and macrophages while in the spleen.

Quick Recall Test Questions and Answers

Choose the Best Answer

1. Antibodies are synthesized by:

   A. the liver.
   B. granulocytes.
   C. platelets.
   D. B lymphocytes and plasma cells.
   E. T lymphocytes.

2. B lymphocytes initially develop in:

   A. bone marrow.
   B. the thymus.
   C. the wall of the digestive tract.
   D. the wall of the reproductive tract.
   E. the wall of the urinary tract.

3. Most T lymphocytes develop their antigenic specificity in:

   A. bone marrow.
   B. the thymus.
   C. the wall of the digestive tract.
   D. the wall of the reproductive tract.
   E. the wall of the urinary tract.

4. Helper T lymphocytes may contribute to an immune response by:

   A. producing antibodies.
   B. stimulating the production or activity of cytotoxic T lymphocytes.
   C. killing virus-infected cells.
   D. releasing clotting factors to restore a barrier layer.

5. Cytotoxic T lymphocytes respond effectively to:

   A. bacteria.
   B. virus-infected cells.
   C. toxic food molecules.

6. The "non-specific immune" or paraimmune (early phase inflammatory) system in humans does not require prior exposure to most foreign organisms in order to mount a rapid response; the specific immune system responds only to an initial exposure to a foreign organism after a delay of approximately a week.

   A. TRUE
   B. FALSE

7. The "non-specific immune" (early phase inflammatory) system in humans does not involve cell-mediated responses; the specific immune system does use cell-mediated responses to some targets.

   A. TRUE
   B. FALSE

8. The initial mechanism that acts to prevent infection of a normal human body by most types of bacteria is:

   A. skin.
   B. blood clotting.
   C. inflammatory or paraimmune reactions.
   D. specific immune reactions.

9. For maximum effectiveness, _____ require previous exposure to the same (or a very closely related) foreign organism.

   A. skin barrier functions
   B. blood clotting reactions
   C. inflammatory or paraimmune reactions
   D. specific immune reactions

10. Lymph nodes respond to foreign organisms present in:

    A. the lumen of the digestive tract.
    B. the lumen of the respiratory tract.
    C. the lumen of the reproductive tract.
    D. tissue fluid draining from many organs and body regions.
    E. blood.

11. The spleen responds to foreign organisms present in:

    A. the lumen of the digestive tract.
    B. the lumen of the respiratory tract.
    C. the lumen of the reproductive tract.
    D. tissue fluid draining from many organs and body regions.
    E. blood.

12. Peyer's patches respond to foreign organisms present in:

    A. the lumen of the digestive tract.
    B. the lumen of the respiratory tract.

C. the lumen of the reproductive tract.

D. tissue fluid draining from many organs and body regions.

E. blood.

13. A foreign protein, when introduced into the body, is recognized and elicits an immunologic response; this substance is known as a(an):

A. antigen.

B. antibody.

C. complement.

D. vitamin.

E. enzyme.

Answers

1. **D.** Membrane-bound antibodies (IgM and IgD) are synthesized by B lymphocytes. After antigen stimulation, B lymphocytes proliferate and most of their progeny become plasma cells which secrete IgM, IgG, IgA, or IgE.

2. **A.** B lymphocytes primarily develop in bone marrow, then migrate to secondary lymphoid organs as naive B lymphocytes. Some B lymphocytes may develop in other locations.

3. **B.** Most developing T lymphocytes initially form their T cell receptors (TCR) while in the thymus. Some T lymphocytes may develop in the gut wall or in other locations.

4. **B.** Most helper T lymphocytes primarily either stimulate macrophage activity and stimulate proliferation and function of cytotoxic T lymphocytes or stimulate development of B lymphocytes. Some T lymphocytes with helper T lymphocyte surface markers may kill virus-infected cells.

5. **B.** Cytotoxic T lymphocytes respond most effectively to virus-infected cells.

6. **A.** Inflammatory or paraimmune responses use cells and molecular components which are produced routinely in the body, so the first exposure triggers an effective response. Specific immune components are present in very small numbers until they are stimulated to proliferate by exposure to a particular foreign organism. The requirement for proliferation before an effective response can occur results in a delay.

7. **B.** Both systems use cell-mediated responses. Inflammatory responses usually use macrophages and commonly use neutrophils against bacteria and natural killer cells against virus-infected cells. Specific immune responses almost always use helper T lymphocytes and use cytotoxic T lymphocytes against virus-infected cells.

8. **A.** Skin is the initial barrier against most bacteria. The other mechanisms come into play if the skin (or respiratory of gut lining) is penetrated.

9. **D.** Specific immune components are present in very small numbers until they are stimulated to proliferate by exposure to a particular foreign organism. The requirement for proliferation before an effective response can occur results in a delay. Prior exposure results in generation of memory T and B lymphocytes which allow a rapid, effective response.

10. **D.** Lymphatic fluid entering the lymph nodes originates from tissue fluid in the organs being drained by the lymphatic vessels. Any foreign organisms present in the tissue fluid are exposed to T and B lymphocytes in the lymph nodes.

11. **E.** Blood circulating through the spleen passes through sinuses, which allow exposure of any foreign materials in the blood to T and B lymphocytes in the spleen.

12. **A.** Peyer's patches contain specialized intestinal lining cells (M cells) which pass foreign materials from the intestinal lumen of the digestive tract to the T and B lymphocytes in the Peyer's patch.

13. **A.** Any substance that has the ability to elicit an immunological response, such as the production of antibody that is specific to that substance, is considered an antigen.

Genetics

Chromosomes within the nucleus of the cells are the source of DNA (deoxyribonucleic acid), the inheritable material; chromosomes contain specific units called genes which are arranged in linear order on the chromosomes. Genes are paired elements, held together in a specific linkage arrangement. One member of each pair of genes separates during germ cell production; therefore, each germ cell contains only one set. An allele is one of a pair of genes that occupies the same locus on homologous chromosomes. Genotype refers to the genetic make-up of the organism. The genotype is expressed via phenotypic characteristics that are visible and observable under normal circumstances.

Mendel is responsible for the discovery of several intriguing phenomena:

1. He showed that each member of a pair of genes will be found in a different gamete; they were contributed to that individual by his parents and underwent no change such as blending while they were associated. This is Mendel's first law (law of segregation) which affirms that *allelomorphs segregate*.

2. Mendel also documented that the distribution of members of one pair has absolutely no bearing on the distribution of another pair. For example, if an individual possesses one pair of alleles Y and y, and another pair Z and z, the individual will produce approximately equal numbers of gametes of the four possible chance combinations of one member from each pair (YZ; Yz; yZ; yz). This law is known as independent assortment; the law does not apply to linked genes but only to genes located on different chromosomes. Independent behavior of chromosomes during meiosis is essential.

Mendel also showed that certain characteristics mask other traits; this phenomenon is known as dominance.

Genetic phenomena are best explained and demonstrated by problem solving, and it will be attempted in this manner.

Mendelian Characteristics

Dominance: Dominance is expressed in terms of a pair of alleles. A gene which produces and expresses the same characteristic whether it is present alone (in the heterozygous state matched to a gene not possessing the same trait) or with a gene possessing the same trait (in the homozygous state) is said to be dominant to the allele with which it is paired. The allele which is ineffective in the expression of its trait in the heterozygote is said to be recessive to the dominant. Let us illustrate with the following example.

The trait of green eyes did not occur in the F_1 (offspring from parents) but made its appearance in the F_2 (offspring of F_1 or offspring of offspring from the parents) generation. We are dealing with a recessive trait that is being masked by a dominant one. AA (brown eyes) bred with aa (green eyes) results in all F_1, Aa (genotypically heterozygous but phenotypically A; all brown eyes). Breeding of the offspring Aa with Aa results in 1 AA 2 Aa 1 aa genotype and 3:1 phenotype. The above demonstrates a one factor cross.

Let us now demonstrate several typical two-factor crosses:

1. Crossing of two types of organisms yields the classical 9:3:3:1 ratio. The cross would be considered an expression of phenotypic ratio.

The example calls for a cross between individuals possessing a genetic makeup of RrSs × RrSs. Construct the Punnett square below and see the results in a 9:3:3:1 phenotypic ratio.

	RS	Rs	rS	rs
RS	RRSS	RRSs	RrSS	RrSs
Rs	RRSs	RRss	RrSs	Rrss
rS	RrSS	RrSs	rrSS	rrSs
rs	RrSs	Rrss	rrSs	rrss

R__S__ or RS = 9
R__ss or Rss = 3
rrS__ or rrS = 3
rrSS or rrss = 1

2. In rabbits, rough coat is dominant over smooth coat. Brown is dominant over gray fur color. A rough, brown male is mated to a couple of smooth, gray females. The offspring are counted as: 18 rough, brown; 21 rough, gray; 16 smooth, brown; 24 smooth; gray. If this male had been mated to a female of his own genotype, what proportion of the offspring would have exhibited rough, gray coats? The answer is 3 out of 16 and is obtained in the following manner.

Basic genetic knowledge is applied.

$$
\begin{array}{ll}
\text{rough} & = \text{(dominant)} \\
\text{smooth} & = \text{(recessive)} \\
\text{brown} & = \text{(dominant)} \\
\text{gray} & = \text{(recessive)}
\end{array}
$$

The male is crossed to several smooth gray females; they had to be homozygous recessive genotype. Because all four combinations appeared, we can assume that the male was genotypically heterozygous even though he appeared phenotypically dominant. If first we crossed this heterozygous male RrBb × rrbb, the result would be RrBb; Rrbb; rrBb; in other words, the four combinations given. Now let us cross the RrBb male × RrBb female; the following combinations would have to be considered in both male and female: RB; Rb; rB; rb. If these are crossed, we find 3 out of 16 possess rough gray coats (namely, RRbb; Rrbb and Rrbb).

Incomplete Dominance: Seeds from a self-pollinated gold flowering plant produce 56 charcoal, 130 gold and 61 beige flowering plants. The plant is heterozygous with incomplete dominance of its traits.

The phenomenon illustrated here is incomplete dominance (blending of two traits). Let us assume:

$$
\begin{array}{ll}
\text{charcoal} & C \\
\text{beige} & B \\
\text{gold} & BC
\end{array}
$$

Cross: → BC × BC
Result: 1 BB (beige)
2 BC (gold)
1 CC (charcoal)

Backcross: A backcross consists of crossing a dominant phenotype with a pure homozygous recessive. In this manner a breeder can determine if the phenotype is heterozygous or homozygous. The backcross is used, therefore, to determine if a line is genotypically pure.

Probability Ratios: Genetic ratios are probability ratios. If, for example, we mate (B = black dominant; b = gray recessive) two heterozygous black squirrels (Bb) and 4 offspring are produced, the ratio of 3 black and 1 gray should be probable. However, what are the chances of all black and all gray litters?

Many crosses of heterozygous (Bb) animals will result in a fairly close 3:1 ratio. We, therefore, can see that we have 3 chances out of 4 to produce an individual exhibiting the dominant trait, and 1 chance out of 4 to show the recessive trait.

Therefore, to produce black squirrels (BB or Bb, 3 out of 4) we multiply $\frac{3}{4} \times \frac{3}{4} \times \frac{3}{4} \times \frac{3}{4} = \frac{81}{256}$; to produce gray squirrels (bb, 1 out of 4) we multiply $\frac{1}{4} \times \frac{1}{4} \times \frac{1}{4} \times \frac{1}{4} = \frac{1}{256}$.

Polygenic Traits

In morning glories, genes C and P are necessary for pink flowers. In the absence of either (ccP__ or C__pp) or both (ccpp) of these genes, the flowers are blue. What will be the result of the following crosses as far as flower color of the offspring and proportion of the offspring are concerned? Cross a. Ccpp × ccPp = 1 pink: 3 blue; b. ccpp × CcPp = 1 pink: 3 blue.

In essence, the expression of pink requires C__P__, and all others will be blue. The offspring may be Cc or cc with equal probability (i.e., 50%); the same is true for Pp and pp (50%). If the chance of C__ is 0.5 and the chance of P__ is 0.5, then the chance of C__P__ is 0.5 × 0.5 = 0.25. Thus, ¼ will be pink and ¾ will be blue.

Sex Determination: A male carries an XY and a female an XX complement of chromosomes. If a male embryo were to result, the sperm that fertilizes an egg would have to possess a Y chromosome.

Sex-Linked Traits: Both sexes carry a complete complement of sex-linked genes. A female, however, with the XX arrangement will only exhibit a recessive gene if it has received it from both parents (a rare event if we are dealing with an uncommon gene of the population), while in the male with the XY arrangement the recessive gene cannot be masked since there is no partner X chromosome and, therefore, a larger number of recessive genes are expressed (examples are hemophilia and color blindness). A man receives his X chromosome from his mother and passes it on to his daughters, not his sons. His daughters in this respect are the carriers of his sex-linked traits and their sons will be the affected ones. Let us illustrate with an example. The normal czarinas of Russia produced sons suffering from hemophilia, a disease that is caused by a sex-linked recessive gene, h. The more dominant gene, H, produces normal blood clotting. Genotypically, these women must have carried Hh (X_H and X_h). A daughter, depending on the father (X_HY or X_hY), could have carried X_HX_h or X_HX_H while a son could have been born with either an X_HY or an X_hY (hemophilic) chromosal complement.

Another way of expressing a sex-linked or, strictly speaking, sex-limited phenomenon is shown in the example below.

A cattle breeder has in his herd a y-linked trait which produces white stockings. A calf sired by a white-stockinged bull is born. The breeder determines that the chances of white stockings by this inheritance are 50%. If the calf born had been a female, the chances of exhibiting the trait (or serving as a carrier) were zero. The explanation is that the male may contribute gametes containing either X or Y chromosomes, but the female can contribute only gametes containing X chromosomes. If the X chromosome is contributed by the male, an unaffected female offspring will result; if the Y chromosome is contributed by the male, an affected male offspring will result. These two possibilities are of equal probability (i.e., 50%). If the sex of the offspring is known, there is no doubt about whether it has the trait. All males (100%) and no females (0%) would have the trait. Females could not even be carriers for a Y-linked trait.

Mutation: A mutation may be thought of as a sudden change in the genetic makeup of the organism. It may be beneficial or harmful. It may occur spontaneously or may be experimentally produced with chemicals, X-ray, cosmic rays, and so forth. It may or may not be passed on to the next generation because, for example, it may be lethal or otherwise preclude reproduction.

Blood Types: The ABO blood grouping system is explained on the basis of a single triallelic system with genes A, B, and O operating at a single genetic locus. Phenotypic and genotypic characteristics may be expressed as follows:

Phenotype	Genotype
A	A/A; A/O
B	B/B; B/O
O	O/O
AB	A/B

The A and B genes appear to be codominant; they are dominant over O, which is recessive.

As can be seen from the above table, there are four major blood types and the explanation as to universal donor and recipient is based on the following:

Type	Agglutinogens on Cells	Agglutinins in Serum and Plasma
AB—can receive A, B, AB, or O (universal recipient)	A,B	none
A—can receive A, O	A	anti b
B—can receive B, O	B	anti a
O—can receive only O, but can give to all; therefore, O is the universal donor	O	anti ab

Rh Factor: Rhesus (Rh) agglutinogen is present in humans and is represented by a dominant gene R. The agglutinogen of an Rh positive fetus passes across the placenta, enters the maternal bloodstream, and elicits the production of an agglutinin (antibody) by the mother. The agglutinin passes into the circulation of the fetus and if present in sufficient concentration can produce agglutination, at times fatal to the developing fetus.

Mode of Inheritance of Some Common Human Traits: Among the human traits inherited as single-gene dominants are:

a) brachydactyly (short digits),
b) white forelock in the hair,
c) blue sclera (white of the eye),
d) Rh-positive blood.

Among the traits inherited as recessives:

a) albinism (lack of skin pigment),
b) alkaptonuria (urine turns black).

Sex-linked traits:

a) hemophilia,
b) colorblindness.

Crossing-Over: During the process of meiosis a recombination of genetic material is possible. One way this is effected is through crossing over. In crossing-over, comparable portions of chromatids are exchanged. Because crossing-over is more the rule than the exception, we shall illustrate it with two diagrams. These portions may differ in alleles but they do carry the same gene sites (loci) and control the same specific trait, as, for example, eye color.

Let us start with one pair of homologous chromosomes:

As illustrated, replication results during the first part of meiosis in four chromatids:

Of the four chromatids, two may exchange materials in a process known as crossing-over:

The configuration shown by the central two chromosomes is termed a chiasma, the region where crossing-over occurs. After separation in the second reduction division of meiosis, the resulting chromatids include two recombinants, having new combinations of genetic material.

We shall next illustrate crossover using two specific genes.

Two gametes unite and form a new hybrid individual (F_1).

Without crossover these four gametes are produced:

With crossing-over these four gametes are produced:

and the result is two new types of gametes with new combination of genes.

Crossing-over may occur anywhere along the chromosome; however, the recombination frequency is higher for genes separated by a greater distance than those that are close together. Crossing-over has provided the investigator with the tool to measure distances between genes and make chromosome maps.

Abnormalities in Chromosome Number: Chromosomes can be identified in somatic cells and a *karyotype,* a standardized display of an individual's chromosomes, can be constructed. Chromosomes vary in size and shape but the number is species specific. In humans the chromosome number is 46. A karyotype is helpful in the diagnosis of genetic abnormalities.

In humans some abnormalities of chromosome number are:

Down's syndrome (formerly called mongolism) This phenomenon is most often characterized by three, instead of two, chromosomes 21 in group G; a total number of 47 chromosomes are present in these individuals.

Turner's syndrome Females possess only one X chromosome (not the normal female XX). Total number of chromosomes present is 45.

Klinefelter's syndrome This syndrome is characterized by the presence of two X chromosomes and a Y, which results in 47 chromosomes being present.

Epistasis (or Gene Interaction): In morning glories, genes C and P are necessary for pink flowers. In the absence of either ($ccP\_\_$ or $C\_\_pp$) or both ($ccpp$) of these genes, the flowers are blue. What will be the result of the following crosses as far as flower color of the offspring and proportion of the offspring are concerned?

$$Ccpp \times ccPp = 1 \text{ pink} : 3 \text{ blue};$$
$$ccpp \times CcPp = 1 \text{ pink} : 3 \text{ blue}$$

In essence, the expression of pink requires $C\_\_P\_\_$, and all others will be blue. In this example, the epistasis is of the complementary interaction type. The offspring may be Cc or cc with equal probability (i.e., 50%); the same is true for Pp and pp (50%). If the chance of $C\_\_$ is 0.5 and the chance of $P\_\_$ is 0.5, then the chance of $C\_\_P\_\_$ is $0.5 \times 0.5 = 0.25$. Thus, ¼ will be pink and ¾ will be blue.

Polygenic Traits: Certain conditions are determined by genes at several loci. Each of the genes involved has a small effect which may be additive. Expression of this kind of trait is usually very sensitive to environmental influences.

Lethal Genes: Certain genes are lethal in the homozygous condition and cause the demise of the organism. An example is yellow coat in mice. If two hybrid yellow mice are mated, the typical 1:2:1 genotypic ratio results—namely, ¼ homozygous dominant (yellow dead embryos), ½ hybrid (yellow mice), and ¼ homozygous recessive (wild type or agouti mice), but the phenotypic ratio among the live born mice is 2 yellow : 1 gray.

Modifying Genes: These genes affect the performance of other genes but apparently exhibit no trait of their own. If, for instance, in mice the gene for black hair is present, the gene for agouti color will elicit a yellow banding. When it is absent there is no effect.

Paternity Exclusion and Reassignment of Misassigned Infants

1. Paternity will be excluded if the child
    a. has an antigen that is present in neither the mother nor the putative father;
    b. does not have an antigen that the putative father has and would have had to give to his progeny (for example, a type O child and a type AB putative father).
2. Correct reassignment of infants misassigned to parents in a hospital is often achieved by looking for any of the following kinds of incompatibilities between the infants and the couples and then assigning each infant to the couple with which only compatibilities exist:
    a. The child has an antigen present in neither spouse;
    b. The child lacks one or more antigens that either or both spouses would have had to give him/her.
3. Increased probability of exclusion of a falsely accused male or of correct parental reassignment of misassigned infants results if several kinds of blood groups, HLA, and some of the following kinds of other genetically determined proteins are also included in the studies: hemoglobins, serum proteins, red cell enzymes, and several other enzymes.

Quick Recall Test Questions and Answers

Choose the Best Answer

1. Alleles are genes which:

   A. arise during the cross-over process.
   B. are linked to one chromosome only.
   C. are always sex-linked and are transmitted from mothers to their sons.
   D. occupy corresponding positions on homologous chromosomes.
   E. are sex-linked and are transmitted from fathers to their daughters.

2. The ABO blood group is transmitted in humans as alleles A and B that are codominate, occurring at the same autosomal chromosome as a recessive allele O. In some cases it may be utilized to assist in determining paternity or in reuniting a lost child with his or her biological parents.

   A woman of blood type O claims a child of blood type AB, and alleges that the father is a man of blood type B. The most likely explanation is that:

   A. these are the biological parents.
   B. she is the mother but the man is not the father.
   C. neither is a possible parent of the child.
   D. she is not the mother but the man's blood type does not rule him out as the father.
   E. there is insufficient information to allow one to reach any conclusion as to the child's parentage.

3. Seeds from a self-pollinated gold flowering plant produce 56 charcoal, 130 gold, and 61 beige flowering plants. The plant is:

   A. unhealthy.
   B. heterozygous recessive.
   C. heterozygous with incomplete dominance.
   D. heterozygous with complete dominance.
   E. homozygous with incomplete dominance.

4. In ant lions the gene for dull teeth is dominant D. The recessive gene d produces sharp teeth. Another gene T, when homozygous, produces dark-brown coats. Its allele t, when homozygous, produces albino coats. The heterozygote Tt is chocolate colored.

   If a chocolate colored, dull tooth male whose father was sharp toothed is mated to a chocolate, sharp toothed female, what is the probability that an albino, sharp tooth offspring will be produced?

   A. $\frac{1}{16}$
   B. $\frac{2}{16}$

   C. $\frac{4}{16}$
   D. $\frac{12}{16}$
   E. $\frac{8}{16}$

5. A mink breeder finds that 50% of the offspring are aa. What genotype were their parents?

   A. aa × aa
   B. Aa × Aa
   C. AA × aa
   D. Aa × aa
   E. Aa × AA

6. During metaphase of mitosis:

   A. there is a dissolution of the chromosomal material.
   B. the centrioles with asters are at the opposite poles.
   C. the cell membrane starts to reappear.
   D. the nuclear membrane disappears.

7. A hog breeder would use a backcross to:

   A. produce a bigger and healthier strain.
   B. produce a larger number of offspring.
   C. maintain a pure line of desirable traits.
   D. determine if a particular hog is genotypically pure.
   E. eliminate chances of congenital malformations.

8. Rh-related hemolytic anemia of the newborn (erythroblastosis foetalis) may result when the:

   A. father, mother, and fetus are all Rh negative.
   B. father and mother are Rh positive, but the fetus is Rh negative.
   C. mother is Rh negative and the fetus is Rh positive.
   D. mother is Rh positive and the fetus is Rh negative.
   E. father, mother, and fetus are all Rh positive.

9. In rabbits, rough coat is dominant over smooth coat. Brown is dominant over gray fur color. A rough, brown male is mated to a couple of smooth, gray females. The offspring present the following ratios: 18 rough, brown, 21 rough, gray; 16 smooth, brown; 24 smooth, gray. If this male had been mated to a female of his own genotype, what proportion of the offspring would have exhibited rough, gray coats?

   A. 4 out of 16
   B. 3 out of 32

C. 3 out of 16

D. 12 out of 16

E. 1 out of 16

10. Twinning is an interesting biological phenomenon. Identical twins usually result from fertilization of:

   A. two eggs by one sperm.

   B. one egg by two sperms.

   C. one egg by one sperm and separation of cells during the early cleavage division.

   D. one egg and one polar body.

   E. two eggs by two sperms.

11. A man with blood cell genotype B/O marries a woman with type A/B. Their offspring could have:

   A. A/B, B/B, A/O, B/O.

   B. A/B and B/O only.

   C. A/O and B/B only.

   D. none of the combinations above.

12. Two people are planning to have a family. The woman has blood type A/A and the man B/B. Their children might have the following:

   A. A and B.

   B. B only.

   C. A/B only.

   D. A and B and A/B.

13. Alleles are genes which:

   A. arise during the cross-over process.

   B. are linked to one chromosome only.

   C. are always sex-linked and are transmitted from mothers to their sons.

   D. occupy corresponding positions on homologous chromosomes.

   E. are sex-linked and are transmitted from fathers to their daughters.

14. Phenotype may be defined as:

   A. genetic makeup of an individual.

   B. hidden traits of an individual.

   C. unrelated characteristics.

   D. visible expression of genotype.

   E. genetic material carried on the Y chromosome only.

15. The czarinas of Russia and the queens of England produced sons suffering from hemophilia, a disease that is caused by a sex-linked recessive gene, h. The more common dominant gene, H, produces normal blood clotting. Genotypically, these women must have carried:

   A. HH.

   B. Hh.

   C. hh.

   D. none of the above.

16. The hematology laboratory reports to the surgeon that his patient's blood clumped with both anti A and anti B serum. The patient's blood type is:

   A. AB.

   B. A.

   C. B.

   D. O.

   E. Rh⁺.

17. The hematology laboratory reports to the surgeon that his patient's blood clumped with both anti A and anti B serum. In this case, what percentage of the population would the surgeon expect to have the blood type of the patient?

   A. 47

   B. 41

   C. 9

   D. 15

   E. 3

18. The ABO blood grouping system is explained on the basis of a single triallelic system with genes A, B, and O operating at a single genetic locus. Phenotypic and genotypic characteristics may be expressed as follows:

Phenotype	Genotype
A	A/A; A/O
B	B/B; B/O
O	O/O
AB	A/B

The A and B genes appear to be codominant; they are dominant over O, which is recessive. Transfusions have become relatively safe under this system. The universal recipient is considered to be type:

   A. A.

   B. B.

   C. O.

   D. AB.

   E. Rh.

19. The ABO blood grouping system is explained on the basis of a single triallelic system with genes A,

B, and O operating at a single genetic locus. Phenotypic and genotypic characteristics may be expressed as follows:

Phenotype	Genotype
A	A/A; A/O
B	B/B; B/O
O	O/O
AB	A/B

The A and B genes appear to be codominant; they are dominant over O, which is recessive. Which of the following agglutinogens do these individuals carry on their red blood cells?

A. A
B. B
C. O
D. A,B
E. None

20. The ABO blood grouping system is explained on the basis of a single triallelic system with genes A, B, and O operating at a single genetic locus. Phenotypic and genotypic characteristics may be expressed as follows:

Phenotype	Genotype
A	A/A; A/O
B	B/B; B/O
O	O/O
AB	A/B

The A and B genes appear to be codominant; they are dominant over O, which is recessive. A person of blood type A can receive blood of type(s):

A. A.
B. B; A.
C. O.
D. A; O.
E. A; AB.

Answers

1. **D.** An allele is one of a pair of genes that occupies the same locus on homologous chromosomes.

2. **D.** This woman is not the mother. She can contribute only the O gene, and this child must receive an A gene from one parent and a B gene from the other parent. The man cannot be ruled out as the father with the limited information given, since he can contribute a B gene to a child.

3. **C.** The phenomenon illustrated here is incomplete dominance (blending of two traits). Let us assume:

    charcoal C
    beige B
    gold BC
    Cross: BC × BC
    Result: 1 BB (beige)
    2 BC (gold)
    1 CC (charcoal)

4. **B.** Basic genetic knowledge applies:
    dull teeth—D
    sharp teeth—d
    dark-brown—T
    albino—t
    chocolate—Tt

    The male is TtDd; the female Ttdd; want ttdd offspring; what proportion? The male provides us with the following TD, Td, tD, td. The female provides us with the following Td, Td, td, td. $\frac{2}{16}$ of the offspring will be ttdd.

5. **D.** Use your basic genetic knowledge.
    (1) 100% aa
    (2) 25% AA, 50% Aa, 25% aa
    (3) 100 Aa
    (4) 50% Aa, 50% aa

6. **B.** During metaphase of mitosis the centrioles with asters are at the opposite poles; the chromosomes move to the equator of the cell and duplicate.

7. **D.** A backcross consists of crossing a dominant phenotype with a pure homozygous recessive. In this manner the breeder determines if the phenotype is heterozygous or homozygous.

8. **C.** Multiple alleles determine the human blood types. The common blood types are A, B, AB, and O. Red blood cells of a person classified as Type A contain Agglutinogen A and their serum contains Agglutinin b. Type AB contains agglutinogens A and B but no agglutinins. Type O possesses no agglutinogens but the serum carries a + b agglutinins. Rhesus (Rh) agglutinogen is present in humans and is represented by a dominant gene R. The agglutinogen of an Rh positive fetus passes across the placenta, enters the maternal bloodstream, and elicits the production of an agglutinin (antibody) by the mother. The agglutinin passes into the circulation of the fetus, and if present in sufficient concentration can produce agglutination, at times fatal to the developing fetus.

9. **C.** Basic genetic knowledge applies:
rough—R (dominant)
smooth—r (recessive)
brown—B (dominant)
gray—b (recessive)

The male is crossed to several smooth gray females; the females had to be homozygous recessive genotype. Since all four combinations appeared, we can assume that the male was genotypically heterozytous even though he appeared phenotypically dominant. If first we crossed this heterozygous male RrBb × rrbb, the result would be RrBb, rrbb; rrbb; Rrbb—in other words, the four combinations given. Now let us cross the RrBb male × RrBb female; the following combinations would have to be considered in both male and female: RB, Rb; rB; rb. If these are crossed, we find that 3 out of 16 possess rough gray coats (namely, RRbb; Rrbb and Rrbb).

10. **C.** Identical twins arise from the same egg. One egg is fertilized by one sperm and a splitting (separation) occurs during the early cleavage divisions. Fraternal twins arise from the fertilization of two eggs, each by one sperm. Identical twins always are the same sex. Fraternal twins may be of either sex (50–50 proposition).

11. **C.** The ABO blood grouping system is explained on the basis of a single triallelic system with genes A, B, and O operating at a single genetic locus. Phenotypic and genotypic characteristics may be expressed as follows:

Phenotype	Genotype
A	A/A; A/O
B	B/B; B/O
O	O/O
AB	A/B

The A and B genes appear to be codominant; they are dominant over O, which is recessive.

12. **C.** The ABO blood grouping system is explained on the basis of a single triallelic system with genes A, B, and O operating at a single genetic locus. Phenotypic and genotypic characteristics may be expressed as follows:

Phenotype	Genotype
A	A/A; A/O
B	B/B; B/O
O	O/O
AB	A/B

The A and B genes appear to be codominant; they are dominant over O, which is recessive.

13. **D.** An allele is one of a pair of genes that occupies the same locus on homologous chromosomes.

14. **D.** Genotype refers to the genetic makeup of the organism. The genotype is expressed via phenotypic characteristics that are visible and observable under normal circumstances.

15. **B.** Hemophilia, a frequent disease of the royal houses of Europe, is a bleeding disorder transmitted through a sex-linked recessive gene. It results in abnormal coagulation; hemophilia A is the classical true hemophilia, resulting from a deficiency of factor VIII.

16. **A.** Four primary blood groups are found in humans: O (47%), A (41%), B (9%), and AB (3%). These blood groups are based on the presence or absence of antigens (agglutinogens) on red blood cells and antibodies (agglutinins) in the serum.

17. **E.** Four primary blood groups are found in humans: O (47%), A (41%), B (9%), and AB (3%). These blood groups are based on the presence or absence of antigens (agglutinogens) on red blood cells and antibodies (agglutinins) in the serum.

18, 19, and 20.

D. As can be seen from the table, there are four major blood types, and the explanation as to universal donor and recipient is based on the following:

Type	Agglutinogens on Cells	Agglutins in Serum and Plasma
AB—can receive A, B, AB, or O (universal recipient)	A, B	none
A—can receive A, O	A	anti b
B—can receive B, O	B	anti a
O—can receive only O, but can give to all; therefore, O is the universal donor	O	anti ab

The Animal Kingdom

Distribution of Living Organisms

Every living organism has a distinct yet interactive role, a place, and a mode of life, which are determined by that individual's structure and physiological makeup. The earth represents diverse *habitats* (places where one lives), which are characterized by conditions such as temperature, moisture, soil conditions, terrain, pressure, chemical cycles (gases and minerals), sunlight, seasonal variations, and others; organisms (species) must adapt and adjust their *life cycles* to the *climate* they live in. No species lives in a vacuum and is entirely independent; all are part of an integrated, systematically functioning, living (dynamic) *community* that includes many varieties of plants, animals, viruses, etc.

Although many populations of different species live together as a *community,* and although *turnover* is continuous, automatic, and self-adjusting, the result is an internally balanced community; there is a remarkable numerically steady state that is determined essentially by food supply, reproduction, and protection of the bonds of interdependency of community members.

Six factors are important to any habitat.

1. *Temperature* controls the speed of every reaction; raising the temperature by 10°C doubles the speed. While there exists a large range of temperature, most life exists in a narrow range; species have limits, and most are destroyed by excess at either end of the scale. Warm-blooded organisms (mammals and birds) possess internal regulation of body temperature, whereas cold-blooded animals (fishes, reptiles, amphibians, and invertebrates) do not and their function is directly related to their external environment. The oceans represent a fairly stable environment, and marine organisms are less prone to seasonal variations. Many land animals have adapted to seasonal changes by migration or hibernation.

2. *Moisture* (water) is critical to the existence of life since it is a solvent (minerals used by plants), a constituent of tissues, and the medium in which many species live and breed. The water cycle (evaporation, cloud formation, precipitation, drainage, and soil percolation) is dynamic and continuous (between sea, land, and air) and affects every particle of the universe. Also, water prevents rapid temperature fluctuations, a critical element in homeostasis.

3. *Soil conditions* are a crucial factor. The chemical makeup of the soil determines the presence or type of plants and, in some cases, the animals of the region. Texture and porosity play a role in moisture content, pH, and the presence or absence of burrowing animals. Slope affects drainage, while exposure to sunlight modulates absorption of heat.

4. *Pressure* varies with elevation (atmospheric pressure reflected in barometric reading) and with depth (water pressure: 15 pounds/10 meters equals one atmosphere of pressure). Availability of oxygen decreases with increasing altitude and depth. People living at high altitudes have higher red blood cell (erythrocyte) counts to compensate.

5. *Chemical interchange* occurs continuously in all habitats. Here are three good examples:
   a. Oxygen derived from air and water serves the oxidative machinery of life; after usage it returns to the life cycle in the form of carbon dioxide or, combined with hydrogen, as water. Carbon dioxide is used in the process of photosynthesis; some of the oxygen released is utilized by plants in respiration, but most is returned to the environment.
   b. Nitrogen is utilized directly by nitrogen-fixing bacteria to produce plant proteins; after utilization by animals these become animal proteins, and their eventual metabolic fate results in nitrogenous wastes. These wastes are converted by bacteria into nitrites and ammonia with release of nitrogen into the atmosphere; the nitrites are converted into nitrates, which again are utilized to make plant proteins.
   c. Carbon is the backbone of protoplasm; it is derived from carbon dioxide (via photosynthesis) and synthesized into carbohydrates, which, together with proteins and fats, comprise the tissues of all plants and animals. Metabolism returns carbon for recycling as carbon dioxide.

6. *Sunlight* provides all the energy utilized by most living organisms. Energy is transformed from one type to another, but it is neither created nor destroyed. Lavoisier (1743–1794)

showed that processes of organisms conform to the First Law of Thermodynamics—namely, the total amount of energy in a system is constant but is capable of transformation. Radiation from the sun includes heat, visible light, and ultraviolet radiation. Solar radiation, especially of the longer wavelengths, controls most climatic variations because of the effects of soil heating, water evaporation, and air expansion. Light controls the photoperiod responsible for the flowering of plants and the migration of animals.

Interrelationships of Animals

Competition for food, shelter, and mates is considerable; some organisms (termites, bees), however, have developed a cooperative society based on distinct roles (workers, protectors, reproducers, nurses, etc.). Plants (producers—autotrophs) commonly compete for sunlight (energy), minerals, and water. The passing of energy from one organism to another constitutes the *food chain* or pyramid; the small (more abundant) are eaten by the large (fewer in number). Plants are eaten by *herbivores* (primary consumers); these in turn are eaten by *carnivores* (secondary consumers); and as larger carnivores eat smaller ones the energy is passed along the chain. As the energy is transferred through the predator chain, the total declines progressively, and successive members are usually larger in size but fewer in number. Organisms eaten by a predator are called *prey;* an organism that consumes its own species is considered a *cannibal,* and one that devours dead material is a *scavenger*.

Factors such as disease control the number of organisms in the food chain; organisms such as viruses, rickettsias, bacteria, protozoans, parasitic worms, and arthropods which by themselves are populations also control the populations on/in which they live. The *parasite* obtains its food from its host, generally harming the host. *Ectoparasites* (lice) live *on* the host, while *endoparasites* (trichina worm) live *in* the host (gut or tissues). Some parasites such as the tick are intermediate hosts, as demonstrated in the transmission of Rocky Mountain spotted fever. Parasites that may destroy the host are called *pathogenic,* and are a considerable element in the regulation and control of the host population. All viruses are parasitic, and bacteria that lack photosynthetic abilities (are saprotrophic) are also parasitic.

The long-term relationship of two organisms of different species is commonly referred to as *symbiosis*. When one gains without harming the other, we speak of *commensalism* (barnacles on whales and epiphytes—plants—that grow on another host plant); in *mutualism* both parties are benefited (the flagellate in the termite digests the wood the termite eats, and the tick bird on the rhinoceros eats ticks, and cleans and warns the larger animal of danger).

Saprophytism is the obtaining of food from dead or decaying material (bacteria of decay and filamentous fungi are examples); the saprophytes essentially function to release chemicals back to the food chain. Without their role many essential elements would soon be unavailable, and the balance of energy transfer and transformation would be disturbed.

As previously emphasized, no organism can be successful in isolation because every specialized being depends on others for some product or process. The smallest congregation of like organisms is the *family;* a larger number comprises a *population*. The key element of a population is the fact that its members interbreed with one another; all populations are composed of *species*. Reproductive barriers exist between species. Speciation has many causes, such as separation by differences in climate, mountain ranges, rivers, or just distance. Only inheritable variations (e.g., skin color) controlled by genes are transmitted to new generations; acquired ones (e.g., muscle build) die with the individual. Individual variations of the members of a species are denoted as *polymorphism,* while the differences due only to sex are referred to as dimorphism.

All organisms live together in a dynamic state under the influence of environmental (chemical and physical) factors; not all are friendly since natural enemies exist for every species (they consume one another or compete for the same food source). Protective adaptation helps in survival. Many organisms blend well into their surroundings (polar bears are white), so that they are hard to see; some organisms such as the flounder can adapt readily to several backgrounds, and others (insects are good examples) mimic their surroundings (butterflies look like flowers and leaves).

Another process facilitating survival is *holotropism,* which denotes eating other living cells as a whole.

All the processes discussed so far are self-limiting. Parasitism, saprotrophism, and holotrophism (known collectively as heterotrophic forms of nutrition) merely affect distribution of foodstuff without adding resources.

In order for the evolutionary process to progress, a new way of synthesizing organic material was needed. Organisms evolved that could utilize external energy to produce organic compounds; we now speak of *autotrophs*. Two types evolved. Organisms that could utilize inorganic material, break the chemical bonds, and convert this energy into metabolic products (specifically, carbohydrates) appeared, and the process became known as *chemosynthesis* (carried out by chemosynthesizers).

The sun, however, came to the rescue as an energy source to solve the food problem. Light-trapping mechanisms evolved and the substance chlorophyll saved the day. The process of converting CO_2 and water into food is called *photosynthesis*.

Population Dynamics

According to their mode of mobility, organisms are classifed as *free-living* (the organism gets around by itself) or *sessile* (it is fixed to another structure). Among both groups there are *solitary* (independent) individuals and others that live in colonies (groups).

All organisms of one species that live in a definable area comprise a population that has distinct organizational features.

As part of the group dynamics of a population, certain factors must be considered:

1. *population density*—the number of organisms in a unit of area,
2. *birth rate*—the number of new organisms per unit of time,
3. *mortality rate*—the number of organisms dying per unit of time,
4. *reproductive or biotic potential*—the potential of a population to increase its numbers under optimal conditions.

Populations are usually considered in terms of the number per unit occupying a given area. As mentioned before, the number of larger organisms is considerably smaller. *Biotic potential* (maximum rate of increase) is continuously checked by *environmental resistance* (competition, disease, inclement climate, etc.). When a population settles in a new area, growth at first is slow (lack of mates), then increases rapidly (exponentially), and finally levels off as an equilibrium is reached because of limits of food supply, the settling of suitable habitats, and the increase of parasites and predators. Usually, as a population increases the environmental resistance, which initially was low, also increases as a result of population density.

A dynamic community of different plants and animals (interdependent) evolves to form an *ecosystem* with the physical environment. No situation is permanent; and while some changes occur rapidly, most are due to a sequential *succession* (lake-pond-swamp-grassland). No one species is present in every corner of the world; geography (geographical range) and environment (ecological range) are key elements. Physical (land and water), climatic (temperature and moisture), and biological (food and predators) barriers are limiting factors to the spread of populations.

Each species requires certain minimal elements for growth and reproduction; this fact led Liebig in 1840 to formulate the "law of the minimum," which states that the rate of growth of an organism is limited by the factor present in the scarcest amount. Too much of a certain factor, according to Shelford (1913), can be just as limiting since the well being of a species is determined by its *range of tolerance*. Organisms are usually more sensitive during development and early and late in life. The range varies greatly from factor to factor. *Stenothermic* organisms can tolerate only slight variations in temperature, while *eurythermic* organisms are able to survive a wide range.

Major Environments–Habitats

1. Water:

a. *Salt Water.* Over 70 percent of the earth is covered by salt water, and the environment, while varying widely overall, is quite stable in a specific region in regard to temperature (a range of 35°C), gas composition, and salinity (30–37 parts of salt per thousand). Ocean currents affect movements of marine organisms and the adjacent regional climate. Tidal fluctuations affect organisms in the shore region. Depth varies, pressure increases with depth, while light decreases with depth (about a 600-ft. limit).

b. *Fresh Water.* Freshwater bodies are scattered in their distribution, have less volume and depth, and exhibit great variability in temperature, gas composition, mineral content, light penetration, and mobility. Organisms living in fresh water, because of its low salinity (low osmotic pressure), have had to develop organs for effectively regulating the osmotic pressure. Unlike oceans, freshwater bodies are subject to periodic drying, changing flow rates, and high turbidity.

2. **Land or Terrestrial Habitat:** The greatest variability is present on land, when one considers minerals, topography, temperature, water content, air movement, and light. Temperature and moisture vary tremendously with the seasons, altitude, latitude, and with topography. Soil and air temperatures vary as much as 120°C.

Learning, Conditioning, Rhythms

1. **Learning:** Many definitions of learning exist, but the process of learning, simply defined, is a change in the behavior of an organism based on some experience or practice. Many organisms have been very successful without much learning; their inborn patterns or instincts allow them to compete for food, find shelter, mate, and live out their life spans. Familiar examples of instinctive behavior are spiders spinning webs (specific patterns), birds building nests and migrating and returning, and fish returning to spawning grounds thousands of miles away. More complex, but still instinctive, are societies of bees and ants where a definite division of labor exists. Humans, on the other hand, while high in the evolutionary scale, must learn from their interaction with the environment and use that knowledge to succeed; for many years a human child is quite dependent, while most animals from day 1 are quite independent. Changes in behavior are often hard to assess but might include:

a. a new pattern of the organism, and
b. a change in the response to a stimulus not previously exhibited.

2. **Conditioning:** Many of our actions seem automatic, and in most instances we cannot attribute definite reasons for them. These behaviors (responses) may be learned even though we have no recollection of the learning process. On the other hand, many actions are unlearned reflexes. An example of the latter is the fact that the autonomic nervous sytem (sympathetic and parasympathetic) allows an organism to adapt to certain phenomena. When we walk into bright sunlight the sphincter pupillae contracts, but if we enter a dark area the dilator opens the pupillary opening; the sphincter is under parasympathetic, and the dilater under sympathetic, control. For close vision (reading) convergence and change in the shape of the lens allow the eye to accommodate. Salivary secretion (parotid, submandibular, and sublingual glands) and tearing by the lacrimal gland of the eye are other superb examples of these homeostatic reflexes. Fright produces an increase in heart rate, blood pressure, and metabolic states to prepare an organism to cope; all this takes place at the subconscious level.

Classical Conditioning. Some actions, however, can be learned by a process called *classical conditioning,* that is, learning to associate two previously linked phenomena. First reported by Pavlov in 1927, it is exemplified by the responses of dogs to the introduction of food. When a dog sees or smells food, it is stimulated to begin a reflexive behavior—secretion of saliva. Pavlov restrained dogs in a harness and then simply used an auditory stimulus such as a bell. When the bell was rung, the dog did not secrete saliva. When food alone was provided, the expected salivary secretion occurred. If, thereafter, the two stimuli—bell and food—were presented for some time simultaneously, salivary secretion occurred. After many trials, the bell alone elicited the salivary response; the dog had learned to react to a different stimulus via conditioning. In 1920 Watson showed the same reaction in an 11-month-old baby, who was conditioned by a loud noise and the presentation of a furry object to eventually be frightened by fur alone. Many of the results of conditioning can be reversed through reconditioning the organism to a different association.

Pavlov identified five components of classical conditioning:

1. unconditioned stimulus—the food; it automatically stimulates salivation;
2. conditioned stimulus—the bell; it is neutral at the beginning but eventually effective and undistinguishable;
3. reinforcement—the pairing of two stimuli;
4. unconditioned response—salivation—the automatic response by the parasympathetic division of the autonomic nervous system;

5. conditioned response—the bell—the response as a result of learning by the central nervous system; the unconditioned and conditioned stimuli function as one.

Five other aspects of conditioning should be mentioned.

1. Extinction. The conditioned response can be reversed. Pavlov showed that, after an animal was conditioned, if for some time thereafter only the bell was rung without food being offered, the flow of saliva started to decrease and eventually stopped.
2. Spontaneous Recovery. In this set of experiments, Pavlov let a response achieve extinction and then gave the animal a long rest from the experimental protocol. After this rest the bell was rung and the response reappeared. This spontaneous recovery may explain phenomena we all experience, such as fears or preferences for certain things for which we have no conscious basis.
3. Stimulus Generalization. In these experiments, Pavlov was able to show that somewhat different but basically similar stimuli (e.g., different tones of music) may evoke the same response and effect. The more similar the new stimulus is to the familiar one, the stronger the response usually will be.
4. Stimulus Discrimination. In another set of experiments, food was offered to animals only at the sound of a specific bell, and salivation was elicited only when that particular bell was rung. The animal did not salivate at the ringing of a different bell; it had learned to discriminate between different stimuli.
5. Onset of Neurotic Behavior. In 1927 Pavlov also observed that, after an animal had learned stimulus discrimination and then the difference between the two stimuli was decreased to the point where the animal could not recognize it, the animal's behavior became unpredictable and aberrant.

In general, conditioning is best accomplished when a short interval between stimuli is used and when positive phenomena are elicited or are the end result. Conditioning is also enhanced when the stimulus is truly different (strong and novel) from many of the background stimuli.

Operant Conditioning. The results described above are due chiefly to the influence of the learning process on autonomic reflexes. However, other forms of behavior are also of consequence in reactions to stimuli. When, for instance, a cat is introduced into a new environment, the animal will react by exploring and marking its territory. In this case, the organism itself is acting on the environment, as Skinner demonstrated in the 1930s with the help of a box and a food bar to reward the animal for a certain action.

In 1938 Skinner observed that a rat placed in a box explored actively and even pressed a bar that released a pellet of food. At first the animal did not make an association but soon learned to connect the pressing of the food lever with the dispensing of food and a reward for the action of pressing. The key element in this situation is that reinforced operant behavior is repeated (the lever is pressed frequently), while nonreinforced activities are quickly abandoned. Extinction, spontaneous recovery, and stimulus generalization and discrimination are also part of operant behavior.

Instrumental Conditioning (Operant) and the Law of Effect. In 1898 Thorndike addressed similar issues and found that, when cats were placed in a box and had to learn to open the door in order to obtain food, the reward enhanced their conditioning. The law of effect essentially states that, when a stimulus is followed by a reward, the response is strong, consistent, and likely to be repeated by the experimental subject.

Certain factors called *reinforcers* have been identified by psychological researchers:

1. Primary—in animals, food and water.
2. Secondary—love and affection, shown, for example, by petting.
3. Immediate—a reward given on accomplishing a feat produces the most efficient learning.
4. Constant—repeated (short-interval) stimuli result in very efficient and rapid learning.
5. Partial—extinction is less apt to occur if there is at least partial reinforcement.

Operant Escape—Escape Learning. When an animal is exposed to an unpleasant stimulus (shock), it will quickly learn to leave the environment to avoid the experience.

Operant Avoidance—Active Avoidance Learning. If an animal is conditioned to a warning signal (bell) and knows that a shock will follow it will heed the warning and rapidly leave the hostile environment.

Aversive Conditioning. In this experimental setup the unconditioned stimulus is offensive and is of negative value to the organism. In this case the organism (e.g., after a shock is administered) not only exhibits a specific response such as muscular twitching but also develops a generalized "fear reaction," which results in modification of heart rate, respiratory activity, sweating, etc.

Primary Activities. Many activities occur as the organism goes through life, but some very organized ones are limited to early development. Human beings are fairly helpless, but other animals (e.g., rats) on day 1 can perform highly complex motor patterns independently. Two classical phenomena of rat behavior will serve as examples:

1. Suckling. Suckling involves some very complicated sensory input aspects, helps meet the nutritional needs of the organism, is an effective reinforcing activity leading to other skills, and provides thermal support and transport for the young. In order for suckling to occur, the mother's nipple must be coated by amniotic fluid, saliva, or both; the pup in utero swallows and excretes amniotic fluid during the last trimester and it is that familiarity with the substances that directs the pup's first act of suckling. Also, because the mother licks the pups and the nipples (milk-line), saliva is a behavioral stimulus. The key factor in this primary activity is that it is the animal's previous exposure to the stimulus that leads it to react to it (it has had gustatory and olfactory clues). Thereafter, however, the pup's saliva becomes the stimulus. Ability of the pup to adapt to its new environment is categorized as developmental plasticity.
2. Huddling. This activity is undertaken by neonates and is beneficial in temperature regulation, which results in less energy expenditure by the young (a homeostatic response). Huddling is not a self-serving mechanism; it benefits the whole brood. An animal starting at the periphery will eventually end up in the center, and so on; the shifting of places helps the group to survive and to adapt to and identify with littermates. Young animals that know their littermates will find their nest readily.

Conditioning and Biofeedback. Biofeedback manipulation is an attempt by the physician to let the individual know what his/her spontaenous functions—heart rate, blood pressure, respiratory activity, skin and internal body temperature, brain waves, peristaltic activity, muscular activity—are at a particular time and circumstance. Patients learn, for example, to recognize when their muscles are tense and may with conditioning be able to relax them to avoid spasms or relieve tension; in the same way vascular headaches may perhaps be avoided. In these procedures patients learn to manipulate and control nonconscious processes. Although results have been mixed, this arena has excited the imagination of researchers and is undergoing active analysis.

3. Rhythms—Biological Clocks: Interest has mainly focused on rhythms that appear in close approximation with natural periodicities such as day-night cycles; tidal rhythms; monthly, seasonal and annual phenomena; circadian rhythms (about 24 hours); and circatidal rhythms (12-hour cycles in marine organisms).

Rhythms are present from the cellular to the tissue-organ-system-organismal level, and from unicellular organisms to humans. Circadian rhythms persist even when the cues for the cycle are deleted. When cues are controlled, cycles are extremely constant and exact, but in the wild they tend to vary slightly. There is considerable evidence that endogenous and autonomic, genetically controlled mechanisms account for the persistence of rhythms.

Most living things, both animals and plants, show a circadian rhythm of activity and rest. It is well documented that humans perform differently on physiological and psychological tests at different periods of the day and night. Local time is not a critical factor, as has been well established by shift workers who work at night and sleep during the day; the shift worker's temperature is falling during the daytime, while in the rest of the population, which is working, temperatures are rising. The shift workers at the same time exhibits low levels of adrenal steroids, while in the rest of the population levels are high. These are relevant examples that the body's biological clock adjusts to the mechanical clock of society.

Characteristics of Rhythms. Rhythms are usually described in terms of four characteristics.

1. *Period*— the number of times required to complete the cycle; it is the time between peaks.
2. *Frequency*—the number of times that a peculiar event, such as sleeping occurs.
3. *Phase*—time location when a specific event occurs in a particular organism; the highs and lows of a substance are phase phenomena. Adrenal corticosteroid levels in day and night workers can be described as 180 degrees out of phase;
4. *Amplitude*—the extent (amount) of change that takes place (e.g., body temperature varies as much as 2° during one cycle).

Factors that Affect Rhythms. Among the commonly cited factors that influence rhythms are these six:

1. geomagnetic fields,
2. cosmic rays,
3. electric fields,
4. X-rays,
5. light and darkness,
6. atmospheric pressure.

Cycles can be disrupted by many factors; commonly cited ones are shift work, jet travel, and space flight.

Importance of Rhythms. As a consequence of our daily circadian rhythms we have a susceptibility or a resistance to drugs, stress, allergy, pain, infection, and many other factors. The responsiveness to different regimens, doses, and procedures have ramifications in therapeutic plans. The outcome of surgical procedures and the effect of anesthetic agents certainly are influenced by rhythms and the time they were performed and administered, respectively. Pain tolerance, for instance, shifts according to the time of day (more pain is experienced at night). What is just an annoyance at one time in the cycle is fatal at another point. Births and deaths mainly occur at night and in the early morning. Ulcers, allergies, and psychoses are more prevalent in the spring. Arctic hysteria is a winter phenomenon. In humans, deaths from arteriosclerotic disease peak in January and suicides in May.

To illustrate the importance of rhythms in every activity, here is a partial list of the factors they influence:

1. Body and skin temperature
2. Blood pressure
3. Pulse rate
4. Respiration
5. Blood sugar levels and glucose tolerance
6. Hemoglobin levels
7. Protein utilization and amino acid levels
8. Production and breakdown of ATP
9. Adrenal hormone levels
10. Urinary production, volume, and rate and urinary electrolytes
11. Mitosis
12. Enzyme activities
13. EEG rhythms
14. Stamina and physical vigor
15. Emotional state
16. Metabolic rate
17. Pancreatic enzymatic activity and insulin production

Quick Recall Test Questions and Answers

Choose the Best Answer

1. The relationship of two organisms living together for their mutual benefit is classified as:

   A. symbiosis.
   B. commensalism.
   C. saprophytism.
   D. parasitism.

2. The stimulus that induces migration in animals is:

   A. hydrotrophic.
   B. photoperiodic.
   C. geotrophic.
   D. hydroperiodic.

3. The functional role that an organism plays in a community is referred to as its:

   A. habitat.
   B. home range.
   C. niche.
   D. environment.

4. Some marine animals have unusual rhythms of behavior because:

   A. tides function as the external determinant.
   B. their eyes perceive only ultraviolet light.
   C. the moon hypnotizes them.
   D. circadian rhythms do not effect them.

5. If a new species were to develop, which of the following phenomena would have to be considered as having played a predominant determining role?

   A. geographical isolation
   B. migration every year
   C. extensive outbreeding
   D. extensive inbreeding

6. The ecological niche of an organism denotes:

   A. where the organism lives.
   B. on whom the organism feeds.
   C. the status of an organism within the ecosystem.
   D. the habits of the organism.

7. An ecosystem is composed of:

   A. producers.
   B. consumers.

   C. decomposers and nonliving components.
   D. all of the above.

8. Which of the following statements is not correct?

   A. Most life exists in a narrow range of temperature.
   B. Cold- and warm-blooded organisms possess internal regulation of body temperature.
   C. Water is a critical component of life.
   D. Texture and porosity of the soil play a role in moisture content.
   E. Availability of oxygen decreases with increasing altitude and depth.

9. As part of the group dynamics of a population, which of the following does not play a major role?

   A. population density
   B. birth rate
   C. mortality rate
   D. reproductive or biotic potential
   E. protective adaptation

10. Which of the following is not considered under the phenomenon of conditioning?

    A. stimulus
    B. response
    C. reinforcement
    D. phototropism
    E. neurotic behavior

Answers

1. **A.** Symbiosis is defined as association of organisms from which each member derives some advantage. Commensalism is defined as association of organisms which share the same food and so forth (one utilizing the leftovers from the other). Saprophytism is defined as organisms living on dead organisms or products of living ones; they bring about putrefaction or decay. Parasitism is defined as organisms that live in or on their hosts and feed on their tissues or their products.

2. **B.** Alternating periods of light and darkness and the proportion thereof is extremely important to the functioning (cycles) of plant and animal life observed.

3. **C.** A niche is defined as the position or status that an organism occupies with respect to the other organisms with which it associates.

4. **A.** Tides are important determinants for some marine animals.

5. **A.** Geographical isolation is a most important factor for the development of a new species.

6. **C.** An ecological niche defines the status of an organism within a particular community. An organism has a habitat which denotes where an organism lives. The niche places it in relation to the other organisms that live in the same surroundings (e.g., it will indicate who the organism feeds on and who feeds on it).

7. **A.** An ecosystem such as a pond may be divided into a nonliving part which is composed of the water, gases, inorganic salts, and many organic compounds and a living entity which is made up of:
   (1) producers—the green plants
   (2) consumers—insects, crustacea, fish, etc.
   (3) decomposers—bacteria and fungi

8. **B.** Cold-blooded organisms do not possess internal regulation of body temperature.

9. **E.** All organisms live together in a dynamic state under environmental influences which are not all friendly, since natural enemies exist for every species. Protective adaptation helps in survival.

10. **D.** Phototropism is a response to light by a plant.

Evolution

The cornerstone of evolution is the fact that species arise from preexisting species.

Key People and Concepts

Aristotle (384–332 B.C.) philosophized that living organisms represent a succession and progression of more suitable forms, rather than random creations.

Redi (1627–1697) showed by experiment that organisms do not arise spontaneously from nonliving material; he demonstrated that maggots did not appear in meat unless the meat was exposed to flies, which laid their eggs on it.

Spallanzani (1729–1799) repeated Redi's work and showed that no life appeared in solutions first boiled and then protected from air.

Lamarck (1744–1829) believed that simple animals and plants are spontaneously generated but that lineage presents a series of evolutionary forms and that there can be independent branching and development. However, his incorrect ideas of inherited characteristics and of use and disuse of parts overshadowed his correct ideas that individual variations are retained because of adaptive value and that these variations lead to the emergence of different species suited for particular environments.

John Ray (1627–1705) was the first to attempt to define a species and to point out the difference between constant and incidental features of organisms.

Louis Pasteur (1822–1895) showed that life cannot arise in a medium from which all living things are excluded.

Charles Darwin (1809–1882) and *Alfred Russel Wallace* (1823–1913) documented the fact that natural processes can bring about a gradual development of new types.

Alfred Russel Wallace sent a manuscript to Darwin that dealt with the tendency of organisms to depart from the original type. Wallace had observed the same things as Darwin had on his voyage on the *Beagle,* and Darwin, being the scholar and gentleman he was, forwarded Wallace's article for publication and included a short article on his own observations. The failure of the articles to arouse much interest gave Darwin the impetus to proceed with his own work, and in 1859 he published his *Origin of Species by Natural Selection*. He argued two main premises:

1. No two members of a species are exactly alike even if they have the same parents.
2. Some variations are advantages, giving the organism the chance to branch out into new environments and to enlarge its numbers, while others are detrimental and diminish its chances of survival.

These premises lead to the conclusion that a population is likely to change in the relative frequency of its various characteristics (i.e., it *evolves*), because of the *natural selection* of some characteristics over others. The environment was cited as a major cause of natural selection, because it weeds out organisms with unfavorable characteristics and strengthens those with favorable variations.

As one can gather, the modern theory of evolution is not the work of a single individual, but it was Darwin, via his careful documentation and voluminous writings, who marshaled the evidence.

Mechanisms of Evolution on a Small Scale (Microevolution)

Two conceptual frameworks have heavily influenced modern thinking about microevolution. These are not competing explanations, but represent two ways of describing the same pattern. Both conceptual frameworks view evolution as occurring in *populations,* which are groups of organisms of one species that occur in the same place at the same time.

Evolution by natural selection (as proposed by Darwin and Wallace) occurs because of the following patterns.

1. Organisms within a population vary in their characteristics.
2. At least some of the variations in a population are inheritable.
3. More organisms are produced in each generation than live to reproduce.
4. Organisms with some variations within a population (the best-adapted variations) are more likely to survive and reproduce than are other organisms.

Evolution may also be viewed as occurring as a result of failure of the genetic equilibrium described by Hardy and Weinberg. The Hardy-Weinberg Law in population genetics states that as long as 5 conditions are reasonably well met, gene frequencies in a population will be constant. In other words, no evolution will occur. Therefore, violations of these conditions could result in evolution. The 5 conditions for the Hardy-Weinberg Law to be valid are as follows:

1. The population must be large enough that random fluctuations in gene frequency are unimportant. This usually requires population sizes of hundreds or thousands of organisms.
2. Mating in the population must be random, or at least no mate selection based on phenotypes must occur.
3. No net gene flow (selective immigration or emigration of organisms or reproductive structures) may occur into or out of the population.
4. No net mutations may occur in the population. This requirement can be met if mutational equilibrium exists (if changes offset each other).
5. No natural selection (differential survival and/or reproduction based on phenotypes) may occur in the population.

Current views of mechanisms of microevolution incorporate multiple possible mechanisms of evolution. Evolution requires production of genetic variations in a population followed by selective removal of some of the variations, resulting in change in the genetic composition and the typical phenotypes in the population.

Genetically based variations in a population are created by three mechanisms:
1. *Mutation* of existing genes to form new alleles is the only process which can create new forms of genes. Most new forms of genes are less functional than the existing forms, but a few mutations do turn out to be beneficial. While mutation is the only process that can create new forms of genes, the rates at which mutations occur under normal conditions are very low (usually $\frac{1}{100,000}$ to $\frac{1}{1,000,000}$). Therefore, although mutations are essential in advance of most large-scale evolutionary changes, mutations do not usually contribute to the visible rate of evolutionary change.

2. *Gene flow* is movement of genetic information between populations, usually in the form of spores, seeds, or organisms but occasionally in the form of gametes (eggs or sperm) or pollen. Gene flow does not create new forms of genes, but gene flow can move a new form of a gene from a population in which it exists into a population in which it does not exist. The effect on the population into which the new form of the gene was moved is the same as if the new form of the gene was created in the population by mutation. Gene flow is usually slow in stable ecosystems with well-defined boundaries, but may be rapid in unstable ecosystems.

3. *Recombination of existing genes* into all possible combinations is the major mechanism increasing genetic variations in populations. *Crossing over* exchanges material between homologous chromosomes during prophase I of meiosis. *Independent assortment* of chromosomes at the transition from metaphase I to anaphase I of meiosis shuffles chromosomes so that the entire set of chromosomes from one parent is unlikely to be passed on to one offspring. *Fertilization* combines genetic information from two parents into a new individual. *Chromosomal rearrangements* (translocations, etc.) can produce new genetic combinations in some cases, but are much less frequent than recombination due to meiosis or fertilization. Recombination does not create new forms of genes, but instead "shuffles" existing genes into new combinations. Recombination therefore creates new combinations of genes, and the combination of genes is what determines the genetically controlled aspects of the phenotype of the organism.

Genetically based variations in a population are decreased by two mechanisms:
1. Selective loss of organisms due to *natural selection* will reduce genetic variation and may or may not result in evolutionary change. *Stabilizing natural selection* removes all extreme phenotypes equally. This decreases the variation in the population without changing the average or "typical" characteristics and therefore causes no apparent evolution. *Directional natural selection* differentially removes some extreme phenotypes but not others. This causes a change in the average characteristics of the population (i.e., evolution), with characteristics selected against becom-

ing less frequent. *Disruptive natural selection* favors extreme phenotypes over the average phenotype(s). This may eventually result in creating two or more distinct sets of characteristics or phenotypes (i.e., evolution). Under extreme conditions these phenotypes may evolve into separate species if they become too different to interbreed.

2. Nonselective changes in gene frequency due to *small population sizes* usually reduce genetic variations and may lead to evolution. *Founder effects* result from establishment of a new population by individuals which do not contain all of the alleles that are present in the original population. *Bottleneck effects* result from reduction of the original population to a small remnant population whose members do not contain all of the alleles present in the original population. *Genetic drift* refers to random fluctuations in gene frequency which occur in small populations owing to the small number of individuals in the population. Changes in gene frequency which result from small population sizes are by definition evolution, and these changes result in changes in the average characteristics of small populations. Unlike natural selection, changes due to small populations are random and therefore do not necessarily result in better-adapted organisms.

Mechanisms of Evolution on a Large Scale (Macroevolution)

Some scientists have argued that mechanisms of *microevolution* (changes in gene frequency in a population, usually resulting in small or gradual changes in the average phenotypes of the organisms) do not provide a satisfactory explanation for *macroevolution* (larger-scale changes in gene frequency and phenotype frequency, including changes resulting in formation of new species). In particular, some of these scientists have pointed out that many macroevolutionary changes appear to occur during brief periods separated by long periods in which little macroevolutionary change occurs. Other scientists have argued that macroevolution usually occurs by the same mechanisms which cause microevolution but requires longer time periods. The detailed mechanisms by which most large-scale evolutionary changes occur is still unresolved, but probably involves natural selection (and probably other causes of genetic change such as genetic drift) acting on the genetic and developmental equilibrium in organisms. Multiple mechanisms for major evolutionary changes are quite likely.

Speciation

Speciation is probably the most dramatic example of macroevolution. A *species* is "biologically" defined as the largest group of organisms which can successfully sexually reproduce with each other. In cases in which use of the biological definition is impractical, a species is defined as a group of organisms which resemble each other more than they resemble other organisms. The resemblances may be physical, chemical, or behavioral. *Speciation* (formation of new species) appears to occur by two major types of mechanisms (allopatric speciation, sympatric speciation) with intermediate mechanisms (parapatric speciation) possible.

Allopatric speciation involves reproductive isolation of two or more groups of organisms (derived from the same species) through mechanisms which require geographic isolation of the groups from each other followed by reproductive isolation.

Geographic isolation occurs whenever populations become spatially separated due to climatic changes, geological changes, migration, or other causes. While separated, different populations may undergo different changes in gene frequency and average phenotype, becoming progressively more different. If these differences become sufficiently large, allopatric speciation has occurred.

Reproductive isolation in most cases of allopatric speciation probably initially results from accumulated genetic differences, which result in no offspring or less fit offspring being produced if members of the isolated populations come in contact again. The inability to produce successful offspring is referred to as *postmating* or *postzygotic* reproductive isolation. If the different groups begin to come in contact frequently, they will probably evolve *premating* or *prezygotic* reproductive isolating mechanisms, simply because individuals which acquire those mechanisms through mutation or inheritance will not waste resources trying to mate with the "wrong" population and will therefore leave more offspring than will individuals which lack those mechanisms. Prezygotic isolating mechanisms could include temporal, behavioral, ecological, or mechanical isolation or inability of gametes to survive long enough after mating to allow fertilization. Postzygotic isolating mechanisms could include lethality, sterility, or low fitness in offspring.

Sympatric speciation involves reproductive isolation of two or more groups of organisms through mechanisms which do not require geographic isolation of the groups from each other. Sympatric speciation may occur through polyploidy, through disruptive natural selection, or through some types of mutations, and may occur through other as yet unknown mechanisms.

Polyploidy can result in sympatric speciation in organisms which can reproduce asexually and in which polyploidy (extra sets of chromosomes) is not lethal. Many plants and some animals appear to have formed new species by polyploidy without any geographic isolation. In the simplest case, one or both parents form gametes (sex cells) without doing meiosis to reduce the number of chromosomes. When these sex cells are involved in fertilization, the new offspring will have one or more extra sets of chromosomes, making it a polyploid. Alternatively, polyploidy may occur if the first cleavage division in the embryo is incomplete, resulting in chromosome duplication without cell division. Since a polyploid organism cannot produce fertile offspring when mated with a diploid organism because the chromosomes do not pair properly in the offspring, the polyploid organism is immediately reproductively isolated. Since polyploidy would not interfere with asexual reproduction, asexual reproduction could produce new individuals until enough organisms existed to begin sexually reproducing with each other. Polyploidy is also frequently involved in formation of new species after hybridization (interbreeding) between two existing species.

Other mechanisms such as *disruptive natural selection* may also be involved in sympatric speciation, since examples of apparent sympatric speciation without polyploidy have been described, but the detailed mechanisms have not been worked out. One suggested mechanism involves developmental timing mutations. Developmental timing mutations involving small changes in DNA sequence may result in large changes in phenotype. Mutations which alter the early stages in the formation of a structure usually result in a structure which is so abnormal that the change is lethal, but mutations which alter later stages in the development of the structure can result in altered but functional phenotypes. As an example, the developmental stages during which the body is being formed in vertebrate animals are relatively similar even though the adults are as different as fish and humans. In more closely related groups such as chimpanzees and humans, the embryos and the infants are very similar and the DNA sequence is at least 98% identical, but the growth patterns from infancy to adulthood are very different and result in distinctly different adult morphology. A human can be viewed as retaining many juvenile features (skull and head shape, lack of body hair) which are altered in adult chimps. Since the protein-coding parts of most genes in humans and chimpanzees are almost identical, the genetic changes which caused the differences between humans and chimpanzees probably occurred in genetic control elements which influence developmental timing.

Parapatric speciation involves reproductive isolation of two or more groups of organisms through mechanisms which create partial geographic isolation of the groups from each other. Species which occupy large geographic ranges frequently vary in their features at different points in their range and form multiple subspecies. A series of organisms of this type is frequently called a *cline*. As long as all of the subspecies are present, the organisms are still considered one species because all adjacent subspecies can interbreed, allowing gene flow among all of the populations. However, if some of the connecting subspecies become extinct because of climate changes or competition with other organisms, the subspecies at the extremes of the series of subspecies may have already become so different that they cannot interbreed successfully with each other. If this happens, the former subspecies are now different true species.

Other Patterns of Macroevolution

Scientists who study macroevolution use several terms to describe patterns seen in the fossil record.

Phyletic evolution indicates change in the average characteristics of a group (population or species) over time. This probably is nothing more than microevolution viewed over a much longer time frame. Rates of phyletic evolution vary from one group of organisms to another and within the same group at different times. Sometimes organisms appear unchanged (at least as far as the fossils indicate) over long periods while sometimes changes appear to be relatively rapid.

Adaptive radiation refers to the rapid fragmentation of a group (usually a species) of organisms into multiple groups, usually occurring as a result of geographic isolation or immigration of the organisms into an area with numerous unoccupied ecological niches. This is basically a spectacular case of speciation, either allopatric or sympatric.

Extinction refers to the loss of a species from the fossil record or from the modern earth. Most species which can be identified from the fossil record no longer exist on the modern earth and are therefore extinct. Some of those species may have gradually changed into different species by phyletic evolution, but most apparently disappeared abruptly from the fossil record. In addition to loss of individual species, the fossil record indicates that periodic *mass extinctions* have occurred in which numerous species disappeared at the same time. Some of these mass extinctions may have resulted from climate changes such as ice ages, but some may have resulted from asteroid impacts with the earth or other rare catastrophic events.

Terms describing relative or interactive patterns of evolution include *divergent evolution, parallel evolution, convergent evolution*, and *co-evolution*.

Divergent evolution describes a pattern in which two or more groups from a single population or species become isolated from each other and become progressively less similar through accumulation of different changes. Speciation occurs when divergent evolution has progressed to the point that successful interbreeding is no longer possible. Structures which arose from a common ancestral structure are referred to as *homologous structures* even if they take on very different functions as a result of divergent evolution. The wing of a bird and the arm of a human are homologous structures.

Parallel evolution describes two groups which begin as a single species or population and which continue to evolve similar adaptations independently after they are separated.

Convergent evolution describes two groups which do not originate from a common group, but which evolve similar adaptations, usually as a result of exposure to similar environments. Structures which are derived from unrelated ancestral structures but which acquire similar features and functions through convergent evolution are referred to as *analogous structures*. The wing of a bird and the wing of a butterfly would be analogous structures.

Co-evolution describes the interlocking evolutionary changes occurring in two populations which interact through herbivory, predation, parasitism, commensalism, or mutualism.

The recent capability to analyze genetic and biochemical similarities/differences has greatly increased our ability to decipher evolutionary phenomena. All organisms use their DNA as the carrier for genetic material and all use ATP as the energy carrier. Amino acid sequence elucidation has confirmed a relation between all organisms to an extent. The amino acid sequences correspond closely to the evolutionary scheme worked out by comparative anatomists. An example is the closeness of chromosomes between the chimpanzee and the human being.

The Concept of Species

Modern biologists have abandoned the idea that there is a constant struggle and only the fit survive in the sense that Darwin envisioned. Rather, a species becomes established because it is well adapted to its given environment and therefore survives and through increased reproduction inhabits the area in greater numbers than less well-adapted forms. Reproductive success is the key element from fertilization to reaching the age to reproduce in kind. A species is an interbreeding population that has a common thread but also individual variation. There is free mating and production of fertile offspring. The group is reproductively isolated from others. Even though geographically-isolated subspecies may exist, the potential for interbreeding is a communality.

Reproductive Isolation

Isolation may be based on geography, ecology, or biology. Geographic isolation may lead to the evolvement of differences. Ecological phenomena such as climate, light duration, and intensity may result in the decrease of interbreeding. Biological factors such as differences in breeding habits, (nocturnal) season, and anatomical differences of reproductive organs are factors in speciation. Any condition that results in a decrease of reproduction thus must be considered an isolating and segregating mechanism.

The Rate of Evolution

Evolution certainly does not proceed at a given and constant rate as well documented by the fossil record of a group. At times in relation to the earth's history, evolution has been slow or rapid; the fossil record of the horse definitely shows different rates. The horse started in stature resembling a fox terrier. Each period from (Eohippus, Mesohippus, Merichuppus, Pliochippus to Equus) is thought to have occupied about 7.5 million years, for example.

Artificial Selection

The best example in the literature is the domestic dog, which descended from a wolf (even today the two species are capable of cross-breeding), and the dog was specifically bred to achieve quite radical differences (Chihuahua vs. German Shepherd).

The Hardy-Weinberg Law of Equilibrium

In 1908, Hardy and Weinberg defined an equilibrium population as one in which neither the allele frequencies nor the distribution of genotype changes with new generations. Since there is no change in allele frequencies, evolution is at a standstill. The conditions for this to occur are a large population which undergoes no mutation, migration, or natural selection and if there is random mating, the frequencies of alleles will not change. If these conditions change, the evolutionary process occurs.

Mutations

Mutations due to radiation, chemical damage, or genetic mistakes which are fairly rare (once in 10,000 to 1,000,000 genes/generation/individual) are not a major force in evolution. However, new inheritable material is provided for evolution; it is only a potential which might or might not lead to a change.

Migration

In evolution, migration refers to the transmission of genetic material between populations. Certain animals (e.g., baboons) live in specific groups. When one animal leaves this group, it carries genes to the gene pool of another group. The effects are spreading of advantageous alleles throughout the species, maintaining the species which occupies a large area, and in that respect preventing substantial differences between groups.

Factors in Reproductive Isolation Between Species

1. Premating isolation—no compatability
2. Postmating isolation—no viable offspring
3. Geographic isolation—barriers
4. Ecological isolation—different living habitat
5. Temporal isolation—different breeding seasons
6. Behavioral isolation—courtship differences

Quick Recall Test Questions and Answers

Choose the Best Answer

1. Darwin's theory of evolution by means of natural selection proposes that:

   A. organisms within a population vary in their characteristics and the most advantageous variations occur more frequently in the next generation.
   B. organisms within a population vary in their characteristics, but these variations occur at the same frequency in subsequent generations.
   C. all organisms within the population are very similar, so naturally occurring variations are not involved in evolution.

2. Natural selection may cause:

   A. evolution of a population.
   B. a change in gene frequency in a population.
   C. differential survival and reproduction of different phenotypes in a population.
   D. adaptation of the population to the prevailing conditions.
   E. all of the above are correct.

3. Natural selection will typically _____ the genetic diversity in a population.

   A. increase
   B. decrease
   C. maintain (without increasing or decreasing)
   D. have no effect on

4. Sexual reproduction will typically _____ the genetic diversity in a population.

   A. increase
   B. decrease
   C. maintain (without increasing or decreasing)
   D. have no effect on

5. Mutations will typically _____ the genetic diversity in a population.

   A. increase greatly
   B. increase slightly
   C. maintain (without increasing or decreasing)
   D. have no effect on
   E. decrease

6. Natural selection would cause the most rapid adaptation in a population containing _____ phenotypes in each generation.

A. many similar
B. many different
C. a few similar

7. Adaptive radiation involves:

   A. a slow change in group characteristics so that one species is gradually transformed into a new species.
   B. formation of many new species from a single ancestral species, usually through adaptation to unoccupied ecological niches.
   C. movement of a single species into an area to which it is already well adapted, so that little change in the species occurs.

8. Evolutionary _____ describes a pattern of evolution in which two or more groups of organisms which originated from a common ancestor gradually become more different from each other.

   A. convergence
   B. divergence
   C. analogy
   D. homology
   E. extinction

9. Evolutionary _____ describes a pattern of evolution in which two or more groups of organisms which did not originate from a recent common ancestor and which were initially quite different from each other, gradually become more similar to each other.

   A. convergence
   B. divergence
   C. analogy
   D. homology
   E. extinction

Answers

1. **A.** Darwin believed that existing variations were selected among by natural selection, and the most advantageous variations became more frequent in subsequent generations.

2. **E.** As described by Darwin and Wallace, natural selection may cause evolution. Modern biologists define evolution as a change in gene frequency in a population. Natural selection acts by causing differences in the chance of survival of organisms with different characteristics (dif-

ferential survival of different phenotypes) and results in adaptation of the population to the current conditions. Therefore A, B, C, and D are all true.

3. **B.** Natural selection will always decrease the genetic diversity in a population because it results in elimination of less advantageous phenotypes (and the genes responsible for them).

4. **A.** Sexual reproduction creates new combinations of existing alleles (forms of genes) by combining genetic information from two parents at fertilization and reshuffling the genetic material in each parent through crossing over and independent assortment of homologous chromosomes during the first division of meiosis.

5. **B.** Mutation increases genetic diversity by creating new alleles (forms of genes), but mutation is so infrequent (typically 1 mutation per million replications of a gene) that its quantitative effect is very small. However,

mutation is the only mechanism which creates new alleles, so it is essential to the process of evolution.

6. **B.** The most rapid evolutionary change should occur in a population containing many different phenotypes for natural selection to act upon.

7. **B.** Adaptive radiation involves the splitting of one species into multiple species. This typically occurs most rapidly if vacant ecological niches (sets of ecological resources) are available to the organisms so that new variations do not have to compete with well-adapted organisms which are already using the ecological resources (occupying the niche).

8. **B.** Divergence is the pattern in which related organisms become more different from each other.

9. **A.** Convergence describes the pattern in which unrelated organisms become more similar.

CHEMISTRY

General Chemistry

The Atom

John Dalton's theories—still accepted
   a.   An element is composed of atoms. All atoms of an element possess the same chemical properties.
   b.   Atoms of different elements have different properties.
   c.   During a chemical reaction (nuclear reactions excepted, of course) atoms and elements are not created nor do they disappear.
   d.   Atoms of more than one element may react to form compounds. In a pure compound the number of atoms of each element is constant.

Components of the Atom

   1.   **Nucleus:** The nucleus—found at the center of an atom—contains neutrons and protons.
      a.   Neutrons—no charge—mass of about 1 dalton
      b.   Protons—charge of +1—mass of about 1 dalton. Number of protons in an atom determines the atomic number and the identity of the element.

   2.   **Electrons:** Electrons—charge of −1—mass of about 0.0005 dalton. Number of electrons circling the nucleus is equal to the number of protons in the nucleus.

Placement of Electrons—Energy Levels

1. **Quantum numbers:**

   a. Principal quantum number, n, determines the shell. It may be 1, 2, 3, 4, etc., in increasing distance from the nucleus and increasing energy. The K shell has a principal quantum number of 1.

   b. Angular momentum quantum number, l, determines the subshell. $l = 0, 1, 2, \ldots, (n-1)$.

   c. Magnetic quantum number, m_l, determines the orbital: $m_l = l, l-1, \ldots, 0, \ldots, 1-l, -l$. The energies are virtually identical.

   d. Spin quantum number, m_s, describes the spin of an electron. Allowed values are $+\frac{1}{2}$ and $-\frac{1}{2}$.

2. **Pauli exclusion principle:** No two electrons in an atom may have exactly the same quantum number (i.e., all four).

3. **Total number of electrons in a shell:** The total number of electrons in a shell is $2n^2$.

4. **Order of filling orbitals:** Orbitals are filled from lower to higher energy levels. They may be designated in shorthand form. For example, the following oxygen atom may be designated as $1s^2 2s^2 2p^4$. Within the $2p$ orbitals, it is possible for an electron to be in $2p_x$, $2p_y$, or $2p_z$. Hund's rule states that one electron of parallel spin will go into each of these until each has one electron; additional electrons of antiparallel spin will then be added as necessary until all are filled.

			2p	
1s	2s	$2p_x$	$2p_y$	$2p_z$
Oxygen (↑↓)	(↑↓)	(↑↓)	(↑)	(↑)

5. **The excited state:** The situation described above is that of the ground state. By input of energy it is possible to raise electrons to higher energy levels. When electrons drop back from these higher energy levels (excited state) to the levels required by the ground state, there is an emission of radiation (emission spectrum).

Periodic Table

The Periodic Table arranges the elements from left to right in order of increasing atomic number. The Periodic Law states that: The properties of the elements are periodic functions of their atomic numbers.

1. **Groups:** Vertical columns are called groups. All elements in the same group have the same number of valence electrons and, therefore, related chemical properties. For example, Group IA elements have only one electron in their outermost principal energy level. They tend to lose this electron readily to form +1 ions. Group VIIA elements have seven valence electrons. They tend to gain one electron to form −1 ions. At the extreme right of the table is the group known as the noble gases. These elements have complete outer shells and are essentially nonreactive. Properties of elements in other groups are now known to be related to placement of their electrons.

2. **Periods:** Horizontal rows of the table are called periods. Elements in the same period have the same number of principal energy levels. From left to right across a period, many properties exhibit periodicity (change with changes in atomic structure). For example, from left to right, atomic radii and metallic characteristics decrease while ionization energy and electronegativity increase.

3. **Applications:** Just as an element in group IA loses a single electron in its outer shell to become a cation with a charge of +1, an element in group IIA can lose two electrons to become a cation with a charge of +2. Just as an element in group VIIA can lose one electron in its outer shell to become an anion with a charge of −1, an element in group VIA can lose two electrons to become an anion with a charge of −2.

Within any period, an increase in first ionization energy is seen with an increase in atomic number. Thus, the group IA elements (Li, Na, K, Rb, etc.) have a lower first ionization energy than group VIIA elements such as F, Cl, Br, etc. (The first ionization energy referred to here is for the removal of an electron from the outermost shell.) Although VIIA elements tend to form ions, they ordinarily do so by gaining an electron. The noble gases of Group O have the highest first ionization energies. (This includes Ne, Ar, Kr, etc.)

Note also that group IA elements are the most metallic (Li, Na, K, etc.) and that the elements become less metallic toward the right side of the table. The elements in group IIIA (F, Cl, Br, etc.) are not metallic, and group O (Ne, Ar, Kr, etc.) elements are virtually inert.

Gases

1. **Ideal gas law:** Although early laws were formulated by Boyle, by Charles, and by Gay-Lussac to explain parts of the interrelationships between temperature, pressure, and volume of a gas, one simple formula sums it up:

$$\frac{P_1 V_1}{T_1} = \frac{P_2 V_2}{T_2} = nR$$

where P = pressure in atmospheres or torr
V = volume
T = absolute temperature in convenient units
n = moles of the gas
R = universal gas constant in appropriate units

Real gas behavior deviates from the ideal gas law at low temperature and high pressure.

2. **Partial pressures:**

$$P_T = P_1 + P_2 + \ldots + P_n$$

(i.e., the total pressure of a mixture of gases is equal to the sum of the partial pressures)

3. **Diffusion—Graham's Law:** Rate of diffusion is inversely proportional to the square root of the molecular weight.

$$\frac{v_1}{v_2} = \sqrt{\frac{m_2}{m_1}}$$

where v = velocity
m = molecular weight

Thus, a gas of twice the molecular weight will diffuse 0.71 as fast.

Liquids and Solids

Ideal gases are assumed to have negligible intermolecular interactions. Within a homologous series of organic compounds, the boiling point increases with increasing molecular weight. The same relationship may be seen within the halogens.

There are, however, forces in some compounds that cause them to be liquids or even solids at temperatures at which their molecular weights would suggest that they should be gases.

1. **Dipole forces:** In certain asymmetrical molecules the electrons become unevenly distributed between regions, and there results a partial positive charge in one region (and a partial negative charge in another). Molecules become arranged so that there is electrostatic attraction between adjacent molecules.

2. **Hydrogen bonds:** Hydrogen in one molecule may bond to oxygen, nitrogen, or fluorine in another molecule. The energy required to break this bond is about 10 kcal.

3. **London-van der Waals dispersion forces:** These forces involve interaction between molecules on the basis of their polarizability. They may be important in nonpolar compounds.

4. **Ionic forces:** Oppositely charged ions exhibit coulomibic attraction.

Phase Changes

1. **Nature of the solid, liquid, and gaseous phases:**

   where *A* is melting or fusion
   B is freezing
   C is vaporization or boiling
   D is condensation

$$\text{Solid} \underset{B}{\overset{A}{\rightleftharpoons}} \text{Liquid} \underset{D}{\overset{C}{\rightleftharpoons}} \text{Gas}$$

2. **Energy of phase transition:**

   a. The energy involved in conversion from the solid to the liquid phase is H_f.
   b. The energy involved in conversion from the liquid to the gaseous phase is H_v.
   c. All molecules in one phase do not have the same energy—there is a range. A liquid at a temperature below its boiling point is subject to some of its molecules being vaporized by virtue of the fact that some molecules are sufficiently energetic to be converted into the gaseous state. The temperature of the liquid, however, is a measure of the average kinetic energy.

3. **Phase diagram:** The phase diagram allows the visualization of possible phases at particular temperatures and pressures.

Note that the lines between phases in the phase diagram represent those conditions of pressure and temperature at which the phases indicated on the two sides of the lines may coexist. The point of intersection of the three lines is designated as *the triple point*; at this temperature and pressure all three phases may coexist.

Chemical Compounds

1. **Percent Weight and Empirical Formula:** Chemical compounds are pure substances that may be broken into two or more elements. A molecule is the smallest unit of a compound that still retains the properties of the compound; an atom is the smallest unit of an element.

A particular chemical compound will always have the same percentage composition by weight. Considering the compound iron (III) oxide, it is found to consist of:

$$Fe = 69.94\%$$

$$O = 30.06\%$$

Since it is agreed that a molecule of a compound is made up of whole atoms of elements, we will try to find the lowest multiple(s) of whole numbers. We may do this in two steps:

(1) Divide each percentage by the atomic weight of that element.

$$Fe = \frac{69.94}{55.85} = 1.252$$

$$O = \frac{30.06}{16.00} = 1.879$$

(2) Convert these numbers to the lowest whole multiple(s).

$$\frac{1.879}{1.252} = 1.501$$

This would indicate 1.5 atoms of oxygen for each atom of iron. Since it is agreed that whole atoms are involved, the simplest formula would be Fe_2O_3. This is known as the empirical formula.

2.   Molecular Formula: In some cases, however, the molecular weight of a compound does not agree with its empirical formula. (This is often true of organic compounds and sometimes true of inorganic ones.) The organic compound glucose may be used as an example. Its elemental composition would give an empirical formula of CH_2O. From molecular weight determination, however, we can show that the molecular formula is $C_6H_{12}O_6$.

3.   Mole and Avogadro's Number: If the molecular weight is known, we may weigh that many grams of the compound and we will have a mole. A mole of any compound contains 6.023×10^{23} molecules of that compound. This is known as Avogadro's number.

Balanced Chemical Equations

Chemical equations may be written in unbalanced or balanced form.

1.   Inorganic Chemistry:

$$H_2 + O_2 \rightarrow H_2O$$

This equation tells us that diatomic molecules of hydrogen and oxygen react to form water. Inspection indicates, however, that there are 2 atoms of oxygen on the left side but there is only 1 atom of oxygen on the right side. This does not agree with what we know about conservation of matter.

We could increase the atoms of oxygen on the right side by placing the coefficient 2 before H_2O, thus indicating 2 molecules of H_2O. This unbalances the hydrogen, however, with 2 atoms of hydrogen on the left and 4 on the right. We can correct this by placing the coefficient 2 before the H_2:

$$2H_2 + O_2 \rightarrow 2H_2O$$

Inspection indicates that there are now 4 atoms of hydrogen on each side and 2 atoms of oxygen on each side.

This is now a balanced equation. The coefficients tell us that 2 diatomic molecules of hydrogen will react with 1 diatomic molecule of oxygen to form 2 molecules of water. Since the same number of molecules (i.e., Avogadro's number) are required for a mole of any material, we can also say that 2 moles of hydrogen react with 1 mole of oxygen to produce 2 moles of water.

2.   Organic Chemistry: The equation

$$C_3H_8 + O_2 \rightarrow CO_2 + H_2O$$

is not balanced. Since there are 3 atoms of carbon on the left and 1 atom on the right, we need to multiply carbon dioxide by 3. Similarly, we need to multiply water by 4 to balance the hydrogen. Then, however, there will be too few oxygens on the left. We need to multiply O_2 by 5. Our balanced equation is then:

$$C_3H_8 + 5O_2 \rightarrow 3CO_2 + 4H_2O$$

Check to see that this equation is balanced. It tells us that 1 mole of propane reacts with 5 moles of oxygen to produce 3 moles of carbon dioxide and 4 moles of water.

Solutions

1.   Concentration units:
   a.   Molarity

moles/liter = grams/molecular weight/liters of solution

    b.   Molality = moles of solute/kilograms of solvent
    c.   Normality = equivalents of solute/liters of solution
    d.   Equivalents = grams/equivalent weight

   2. **Colligative properties:** Based on the number of dissolved particles, without regard to their nature.

      a.   Boiling point elevation

           Boiling point elevation = $K_b m$

                where K_b is a constant for the specific solvent and m = molality of solute.

Note, however, that a 1 molal solution of NaCl would have twice the calculated effect since it would be 1 molal each in Na^+ and Cl^- (i.e., 2 molal total).

      b.   Freezing point depression

           Freezing point depression = $K_f m$

                where K_f is a constant for the specific solvent and m = molality of solute particles (see comment above in 2.a. regarding ionizable solutes).

      c.   Osmotic pressure. When an aqueous solution is placed on one side of a semi-permeable membrane and pure water on the other side, there is net movement of water across the membrane. The applied pressure required to produce a net movement of zero is called the osmotic pressure.

$$\pi V = nRT$$

where π = osmotic pressure
     V = volume
     n = moles of particles in solution
     R = the universal gas constant
     T = the temperature, kelvin units (K)

   3. **Solubility:** A comparatively insoluble inorganic compound in water is in equilibrium with its soluble ions.

$$Al(OH)_3 \downarrow \rightleftharpoons Al^{3+} + 3OH^-$$

The solubility product constant is K_{sp}.

$$K_{sp} = 5 \times 10^{-33} = [Al^{3+}][OH^-]^3$$

Thus, in the specific case of $Al(OH)_3$, if the product of the molar concentration of OH^- raised to the third power and Al^{3+} exceeds 5×10^{-33}, precipitation will occur.

Acids and Bases, pH, and Buffers

   1. **Acids:**
      a.   Brönsted-Lowry acid—a material that donates a proton:

$$HCl + H_2O \longrightarrow H_3O^+ + Cl^-$$
               (acid)

      b.   Lewis acid—a material that accepts an electron pair

   2. **Base:**
      a.   Brönsted-Lowry base—a material that accepts a proton:

$$H_3O^+ + NaOH \rightleftharpoons 2H_2O + Na^+$$
               (base)

      b.   Lewis base—a material that donates an electron pair

   3. **Strength of acids and bases:**
      a.   Strong acids and bases. A strong acid or base is assumed to be completely ionized. Therefore, the concentration of acid is equal to the concentration of hydrogen ions (or hydronium ions).

$$HCl + H_2O \longrightarrow H_3O^+ + Cl^- \quad or \quad HCl \longrightarrow H^+ + Cl^-$$

b. Weak acids and bases
(1) $HF \rightleftharpoons H^+ + F^-$

$$K_a = \frac{[H^+][F^-]}{[HF]} = 7 \times 10^{-4} \text{ (in this specific case)}$$

Consider a $1M$ solution of HF for example:
$[H^+] = [F^-]$
So, $K_a[HF] = [H^+][F^-] = [H^+]^2$
and $[H^+] = \sqrt{K_a[HF]} = \sqrt{7 \times 10^{-4}} = 2.6 \times 10^{-2}$
In this example HF is called a conjugate acid, capable of releasing a proton. F^- is called a conjugate base, capable of combining with a proton.

(2) Bases
$NH_3 + H_2O \rightleftharpoons NH_4^+ + OH^-$
$K_b[NH_3] = [NH_4^+][OH^-]$
$K_b = 1.8 \times 10^{-5}$ for this particular base.
Computation similar to that for acid would allow one to determine the $[OH^-]$ for a 1 molar NH_3 solution. H_2O is not included in the equilibrium expression.

4. **pH, pOH, and pK_w:**
a. $pH = -\log[H^+]$
The pH of pure water is 7.
b. $pOH = -\log[OH^-]$
The pOH of pure water is 7.
c. $pK_w = pH + pOH = 14$
d. Changes in pH and hydrogen ions. Remember that pH is a logarithmic scale. A decrease of one unit in pH (e.g., from 7 to 6) indicates an increase in hydrogen ions by a factor of 10.

5. **Solution of salts:**
a. A solution of the salt of a strong acid and a strong base is highly ionized and neutral.
b. A solution of the salt of a strong acid and a weak base is acidic.
c. A solution of the salt of a weak acid and a strong base is basic.

6. **Buffers:** A buffer is a solution containing a weak acid or a weak base *and* a salt of that weak acid or weak base.
a. The ionization of a weak acid, HA, may be shown as

$$HA \rightleftharpoons H^+ + A^-$$

b. The ionization constant is defined as

$$K_a = \frac{[H^+][A^-]}{HA}$$

c. The negative logarithm of K_a is defined as pK_a. It is then possible to define a useful relationship called the Henderson-Hasselbalch equation:

$$pH = pK_a + \log\frac{[\text{conjugate base}]}{[\text{conjugate acid}]}$$

In the example we have already considered, of course, A^- would be the conjugate base and HA would be the conjugate acid in the buffer pair.

Although the conjugate acid is weakly ionized, it is assumed that the salt that produces the conjugate base is strongly ionized. Thus, the mixture of 500 ml each of $0.1M$ acetic acid and $0.1M$ sodium acetate would produce 1 liter of a solution that contains $0.05M$ acetic acid and $0.05M$ acetate ion. The Henderson-Hasselbalch equation would provide us with

$$pH = pK_a + \log\frac{(0.05)}{(0.05)} = pK_a + \log 1 = pK_a$$

Thus, a mixture of equal concentrations of the conjugate base and the conjugate acid will produce a pH equal to the pK_a. From a practical standpoint it is usually considered that a buffer system is useful in the restraint of changes of pH only over the range of $pK_a \pm 1$ pH unit.

7. **Volumetric calculations with acids and bases:**
   a. Molarity = grams acid or base/molecular weight/liters
   b. Normality = grams acid or base/equivalent weight/liters

For a monoprotic acid such as HCl, the normality equals the molarity. For a diprotic acid such as H_2SO_4, the normality is twice the molarity.

   c. Number of equivalents in neutralization:

$$L_{acid} \times N_{acid} = L_{base} \times N_{base} = \text{number of equivalents}$$

   d. Neutralizations may be done using the experimental technique of titration.

Electrochemistry

The electrolytic cell uses the flow of electrical current to cause a chemical reaction to occur. This type of chemical reaction is an oxidation-reduction (otherwise known as redox). In the electrolysis of molten NaCl, there is production of both Na and Cl_2. The half reactions involved are:

$$Na^+ + e^- \rightarrow Na^0 \quad \text{(reduction)}$$
$$2Cl^- \rightarrow Cl_2^0 + 2e^- \quad \text{(oxidation)}$$

In balancing these half reactions, we must first balance one half reaction against the other to obtain the same number of electrons in each:

$$2[Na^+ + e^- \rightarrow Na^0] = 2Na^+ + 2e^- \rightarrow 2Na^0$$
$$1[2Cl^- \rightarrow Cl_2^0 + 2e^-] = 2Cl^- \rightarrow Cl_2^0 + 2e^-$$

When these balanced half reactions are added together, the electrons drop out to give a balanced equation for the net reaction:

$$2Na^+ + 2Cl^- \rightarrow 2Na^0 + Cl_2^0$$

or

$$2NaCl \rightarrow 2Na^0 + Cl_2^0$$

Thermodynamics

1. **Laws:**
   a. *First law*. Energy can neither be created nor destroyed.
   b. *Second law*. The spontaneous flow of heat is always unidirectional from the higher to the lower temperature.
   c. *Third law*. The entropy of all pure crystalline solids may be taken as zero at the absolute zero of temperature.

2. **Change in enthalpy:** The change in enthalpy is ΔH. A negative ΔH for a reaction indicates that the products have a lower heat content than the reactants; therefore, heat is evolved. Since enthalpy is independent of the route of a reaction, it is possible to algebraically add reactions.

$Pb(s) + O_2(g) \longrightarrow PbO_2(s)$		$\Delta H = -66.1$
$2H_2O(g) \longrightarrow 2H_2(g) + O_2(g)$		$\Delta H = +115.6$
Sum $\quad Pb(s) + 2H_2O(g) \longrightarrow PbO_2(s) + 2H_2(g)$		$\Delta H = +49.5$

In this example the overall reaction would require input of heat.

3. **Change in entropy:** The change in entropy is ΔS. Entropy may be described as the degree of disorder of a system. It is also seen as unrecoverable energy. Without the addition of energy to a system, entropy increases to a maximum.

4. Changes in Gibbs free energy: Changes in Gibbs free energy are ΔG. Some of the energy of a reaction is unavailable for useful work. The term ΔG indicates the energy that is available for useful work.

$$\Delta G = \Delta H - T\Delta S$$

where T = absolute temperature, K°

A negative ΔG indicates a spontaneous reaction. A positive ΔG indicates a reaction that would be spontaneous in the reverse direction. When $\Delta G = 0$, the system is at equilibrium.

Rate Processes in Chemical Reactions

1. Rate-Controlling Step: Although we sometimes write an equation in a simple way such as

$$A + B \rightarrow X + Z$$

it is not always so simple. There may be many intermediates in the process. For example, a product C could be formed, and then converted to D, etc. Somewhere along such a series of steps there would be a slowest or rate-controlling step. In spite of the other series of reactions, as the name implies, this step would control or determine the rate of the overall reaction.

2. Activation Energy, Catalysts, Enzymes: Although a reaction is thermodynamically favorable, it will often require a certain activation energy.

A catalyst or an enzyme (essentially a biological catalyst) may substantially increase the rate of a reaction by decreasing the activation energy that is required.

3. Equilibrium Constant: Consider a reversible reaction:

$$A + B \rightleftharpoons C + D$$

We may calculate an *equilibrium constant*:

$$K_{eq} = \frac{[C][D]}{[A][B]}$$

4. Le Chatelier's Principle: Le Chatelier's principle states that when a system is at equilibrium, it will shift to relieve any stress placed on it. Thus, in the above example, addition of more C to the system would bring about the consumption of D and the production of more A and B (without changing the equilibrium constant).

General Principles

Characteristics of Mixtures and Compounds

	Mixture	Compound
1.	Physical union	Chemical union
2.	No new substances are formed	New substances are formed
3.	Can be separated by physical means	Can be separated by chemical means
4.	Elements form no definite proportions	Elements form definite proportions

Reactions

1. Single Replacement Reaction: In a single replacement reaction a more active element reacts with a compound to replace a less active one. A new element and a new compound are the result.

$$\text{Examples: } Fe + CuSO_4 \longrightarrow FeSO_4 + Cu$$

$$Zn + CuSO_4 \longrightarrow ZnSO_4 + Cu$$

2. Double Replacement Reaction: Double replacement reactions involve a double exchange; compounds react chemically to form two new compounds.

$$\text{Examples: } NaCl + AgNO_3 \longrightarrow NaNo_3 + AgCl$$

$$HCl + NaOH \longrightarrow NaCl + H_2O$$

In the first example a precipitate ($AgCl$) is formed and in the second example a weakly ionized compound (H_2O) is formed. In the other cases (e.g., $NaCl + KNO_3$) a double replacement reaction could be written, but the equilibrium would involve all possible combinations of cations and anions since neither a precipitate, nor a gas, nor a weakly ionized compound is formed.

3. Synthesis Reaction: In a synthesis reaction two or more elements or compounds can unite to form a single compound.

$$\text{Examples: } Fe + S \xrightarrow{\Delta} FeS$$

$$CO_2 + H_2O \longrightarrow H_2CO_3$$

4. Decomposition Reaction: In a decomposition reaction a compound is broken down into simpler compounds or into its elements.

$$\text{Examples: } 2KClO_3 \longrightarrow 2KCl + 3O_2$$

$$2HgO \longrightarrow 2Hg + O_2$$

Role of Enzymes in a Reaction

Consider the following reaction:

$$A + B + C \xrightarrow{\text{E (enzyme)}} ABCE \longrightarrow D + F + E$$
$$1 \qquad\qquad 2 \qquad\qquad 3 \qquad\quad 4 \quad 2$$

Substrate(s) or reactant(s) (1) react(s) with the enzyme (2) to form an enzyme-substrate complex (3). This complex breaks down into product(s) (4), and free enzyme (2) ready for the formation of a new enzyme-substrate complex is available again.

An enzyme speeds up the rate of the reaction but is not used up itself in the reaction.

Temperature Conversion Factors

On the Celsius scale (°C) the freezing point of water is 0°, and the boiling point is 100°. On the Fahrenheit scale (°F) they are respectively 32° and 212°.

The absolute Kelvin scale lists as absolute zero a temperature of −273°C, and therefore, the Kelvin and Celsius scales differ only in the choice of point zero. Kelvin temperature is, therefore, 273 plus the Celsius temperature. Let us illustrate and work two examples:

1. 104°F is what temperature on the Kelvin scale? The answer is 313 K and is obtained in the following manner:

First we must convert Fahrenheit to Celsius by using the following formulas:

$$\text{Celsius equals } \frac{5}{9} \times (\text{Fahrenheit} - 32)$$

$$\text{Fahrenheit equals } \frac{5}{9}C + 32$$

$$\text{Celsius} = \frac{5}{9} \times (104 - 32)$$

$$C = \frac{5}{9} \times 72$$

$$C = 40°$$

Now we take 273°, add 40°, and obtain a Kelvin temperature of 313 K.

2. 45°C will equal how many degrees F?
We utilize the conversion factors:

$$F = \frac{9}{5}C + 32$$

or

$$C = \frac{9}{5}(F - 32)$$

$$F = \frac{9}{5}(45) + 32$$

$$F = 81 + 32$$

$$F = 113°$$

Formulas and Laws

1. Specific Gravity: Specific gravity is usually expressed as the weight of an object in air divided by the loss of weight when weighed in water.

Example: A ball of steel weighs 300 grams in air and 250 grams when submerged in water; its specific gravity is 6.

$$\text{Specific Gravity} = \frac{\text{Weight in Air}}{\text{Loss of Weight}}$$

$$\text{Specific Gravity} = \frac{300}{50} = 6$$

2. Density: Density is expressed as $\frac{M(\text{mass})}{V(\text{volume})}$

Example: A piece of iron 60 inches long, 12 inches wide and 2 inches high has a mass of 2000 lb. The density of this piece is 1.39 lb/in³ and was obtained as follows:

$$D = \frac{M}{V} = \frac{2000\,\text{lb}}{60\,\text{in.} \times 12\,\text{in.} \times 2\,\text{in.}}$$

$$D = \frac{2000\,\text{lb}}{1440\,\text{in}^3} = 1.39\,\text{lb/in}^3$$

Organic Chemistry

It is not possible to present a course in organic chemistry in the limited space we have allotted. All we can hope to do is to help you review some of the high points.

General Considerations

1. Definition: Organic chemistry is the chemistry of compounds of carbon. Historically, it has been the study of chemical compounds from living or dead organisms. Until 1828, it was believed that these compounds could not be synthesized from "inorganic" compounds outside living organisms. This theory was first breached by Friedrich Wöhler in 1828; he was successful in synthesizing urea from the inorganic compound, ammonium cyanate.

2.   Bonds: In general, the bonds in the stable organic compounds are covalent bonds, formed by the sharing of electrons between atoms. If the electrons are shared unequally between two atoms, the bond is said to be a polar bond (e.g., C—Br or C—O).

Such a polar bond is a dipole, and the molecule possesses a dipole moment. The dipole moment is calculated by multiplying the charge by the distance of separation. Thus, methane (CH_4) has a dipole moment of zero. By comparison, CH_3Cl has a dipole moment of 1.87.

3.   Electronic Configuration of the Carbon Atom: It is generally true that the orbital electrons in the outer unfilled shell are the most important in predicting the metal/nonmetal character of the compound as well as the expected valence. The carbon atom has two electrons in the K shell and four in the L shell ($1s^2 2s^2 2p_x^1 2p_y^1$). It might be expected to lose four electrons to produce the electronic configuration of the noble element helium, or gain four electrons to produce the electronic configuration of the noble element neon. For the most part it shares electrons to complete the L shell. Thus, it may be said to have a valence of 4 (see below).

4.   Bond Hybridization: The orbital electrons of the carbon atom consist of two electrons in the $1s$ orbital, two electrons in the $2s$ orbital, and one electron each in the $2p_x$ and $2p_y$ orbital (This may be written as $1s^2 2s^2 2p_x^1 2p_y^1$.) It exhibits a valence of 4. In simple compounds such as methane, four equivalent covalent bonds are formed. This may be considered to occur by raising one of the $2s$ orbital electrons to the $2p_z$ orbital and then forming four hybridized orbitals from the three $2p$ orbitals and the one remaining $2s$ orbital. These hybridized orbitals are sp^3 orbitals. The four covalent bonds in methane are the result of overlap of the one orbital electron of each of four hydrogen atoms with one sp^3 hybridized orbital electron of the carbon atom. These four bonds are called sigma bonds.

In a compound such as ethylene (ethene), however, there are pi as well as sigma bonds. Two of the three $2p$ orbital electrons are hybridized with the remaining $2s$ orbital electron. Thus, there are three equivalent sp^2 hybridized orbital electrons for each carbon atom. These participate in the covalent sigma bond between the two carbon atoms and in the covalent sigma bonds between the carbon atom and the hydrogen atoms. The remaining $2p$ orbital electron in each carbon atom participates in the weaker second bond between the two carbon atoms (a pi bond).

Compounds such as acetylene (ethyne) have a triple bond, consisting of one sigma bond and two pi bonds. In each carbon atom participating in a triple bond, there is contribution of two hybridized sp orbital electrons to produce two pi bonds. The stronger sigma bond between the carbon atoms is produced by the contribution of one $2p$ electron from each carbon atom. In acetylene itself there is another sigma bond between the carbon atom and a hydrogen atom; this bond is produced by the overlap of a $2p$ orbital from the carbon atom and the sole electron from the hydrogen atom.

5.   Stereochemistry: Chemical compounds with the same molecular formula but different structural formulas are termed *isomers*. Those having atoms joined in a different order are *structural isomers* (e.g., 2-propanol and 1-propanol). Those having their atoms joined in the same order are termed *stereoisomers*. Stereoisomers that are mirror images of each other are termed *enantiomers*. Stereoisomers that are not enantiomers are called *diastereomers*.

$$
\begin{array}{ccc}
\text{H—C=O} & \text{H—C=O} & \text{H—C=O} \\
| & | & | \\
\text{H—C—OH} & \text{H—C—OH} & \text{HO—C—H} \\
| & | & | \\
\text{HO—C—H} & \text{HO—C—H} & \text{H—C—OH} \\
| & | & | \\
\text{H—C—OH} & \text{HO—C—H} & \text{H—C—OH} \\
| & | & | \\
\text{H—C—OH} & \text{H—C—OH} & \text{HO—C—H} \\
| & | & | \\
\text{CH}_2\text{OH} & \text{CH}_2\text{OH} & \text{CH}_2\text{OH} \\
\text{D-glucose} & \text{D-galactose} & \text{L-galactose}
\end{array}
$$

D-Glucose and D-galactose are diastereomers. D-galactose and L-galactose are enantiomers.

To possess optical activity a compound must have a chiral center. A *chiral center* is a carbon atom that is attached to four different substituents. A compound possessing a chiral center may still not possess optical activity if there is a plane of symmetry in the molecule.

Light ordinarily oscillates in all planes. If it is passed through a polarizer, its oscillation is reduced to only one plane. If this plane-polarized light is allowed to pass through a solution of an optically active compound, the plane of the light will be rotated. If it is rotated to the right, the rotation is termed dextrorotatory or (+). If it is rotated to the left, the rotation is termed levorotatory or (−). The specific rotation [α] is characteristic of an optically active compound:

$$[\alpha] = \frac{\alpha}{(c)(l)}$$

where α = observed degrees of rotation

c = concentration, grams per milliliter

l = length of light path, decimeters

For comparison in the literature, the D line of sodium as the incident light and a temperature of 25°C have been agreed upon as standard.

A mixture of equal amounts of two enantiomers (called a *racemic* mixture) will have a rotation of zero. The rotations are opposite in sign and equal in numerical value, canceling each other.

The Alkanes

Alkanes are saturated noncyclic compounds of carbon and hydrogen. If carbon atoms are arranged in a straight chain sequence

$$\text{C—C—C—C}$$

and hydrogen atoms are added to account for each carbon atom's valence of four, we produce a compound like this:

$$
\begin{array}{cccc}
\text{H} & \text{H} & \text{H} & \text{H} \\
| & | & | & | \\
\text{HC—} & \text{C—} & \text{C—} & \text{CH} \\
| & | & | & | \\
\text{H} & \text{H} & \text{H} & \text{H}
\end{array}
$$

This compound is *n*-butane. The *n* designates the straight chain character. Another compound with the same numbers of carbon and hydrogen atoms is isobutane (or 2-methyl-propane).

$$
\begin{array}{c}
\text{H}_3\text{C—CH—CH}_3 \\
| \\
\text{CH}_3
\end{array}
$$

It is useful to learn the names of many of the alkanes. With modification these names are an integral part of the names of the derivatives of alkanes.

Chain Length	Name	Chain Length	Name
1	Methane	11	Undecane
2	Ethane	12	Dodecane
3	Propane	13	Tridecane
4	Butane	14	Tetradecane
5	Pentane	15	Pentadecane
6	Hexane	16	Hexadecane
7	Heptane	17	Heptadecane
8	Octane	18	Octadecane
9	Nonane	19	Nonadecane
10	Decane	20	Eicosane

The IUPAC rules for nomenclature require that a compound that is not a straight chain be named on the basis of its longest chain. Thus, the following compound is 2-methyl-4-ethyl-heptane:

$$H_3C—CH—CH_2—CH—CH_2—CH_2—CH_3$$
$$\qquad\quad | \qquad\qquad\quad |$$
$$\qquad\quad CH_3 \qquad\qquad CH_2$$
$$\qquad\qquad\qquad\qquad\qquad |$$
$$\qquad\qquad\qquad\qquad\qquad CH_3$$

1. **Synthesis—Wurtz Reaction:**

$$2RBr + 2Na \longrightarrow RR + 2NaBr$$

(R will often be used to refer to an unspecified alkyl group.) More specifically:

$$2CH_3Br + 2Na \longrightarrow CH_3 - CH_3 + 2NaBr$$

If a mixture of two alkyl bromides is used, a mixture of three possible products is expected.

2. **Reactions:**

The alkanes are not very reactive, but they will undergo some reactions.

  a. *Halogenation*

$$\qquad\quad H\quad H \qquad\qquad H\quad H$$
$$\qquad\quad |\qquad | \qquad\qquad\ |\qquad |$$
$$Cl_2 + HC—CH \xrightarrow[\text{u.v.} \\ \text{light}]{\text{heat}} HC—C—Cl + HCl$$
$$\qquad\quad |\qquad | \qquad\qquad\ |\qquad |$$
$$\qquad\quad H\quad H \qquad\qquad H\quad H$$

Reaction may continue and produce a more highly chlorinated product.

  b. *Oxidation*

Alkanes may be oxidized to produce CO_2, water, and energy.

The Cycloalkanes

The small ring cycloalkanes (cyclopropane and cyclobutane) are strained and are more reactive. Cyclopropane is planar, and the bond angles must be 60°. The normal bond angle is 109° 28′. Five- and six-membered rings are not appreciably strained. Larger rings were once thought to be unstable because of the strain (Baeyer), but puckering allows relative freedom from strain.

Example:

$$CH_2$$
$$\diagup\diagdown$$
$$CH_2\text{---}CH_2$$
cyclopropane

The Alkenes

The alkenes may be considered as alkanes from which hydrogen has been removed, producing a carbon-to-carbon double bond. The simplest example of this series is ethene (ethylene).

$$H_2C\text{==}CH_2$$ ethene

$$H_2C\text{==}CH\text{---}CH_2\text{---}CH_3$$ 1-butene

$$\begin{array}{c} H \\ | \\ H_3C\text{---}C\text{==}C\text{---}CH_3 \\ | \\ H \end{array}$$ *trans*-2-butene

$$\begin{array}{c} H \quad H \\ | \quad | \\ H_3C\text{---}C\text{==}C\text{---}CH_3 \end{array}$$ *cis*-2-butene

1. **Synthesis:**
   a. *Dehydrohalogenation*

   $$H_3C\text{---}CH_2Br + \text{alcoholic KOH} \longrightarrow H_2C{=}CH_2 + H_2O + KBr$$

   b. *Dehydration*

   $$H_3C\text{---}CH_2OH \xrightarrow[H_2SO_4]{\text{heat}} H_2C{=}CH_2 + H_2O$$

   c. *Dehalogenation*

   $$Br\text{---}CH_2\text{---}CH_2\text{---}Br + Zn \longrightarrow H_2C{=}CH_2 + ZnBr_2$$

   d. *Cracking* (relatively nonspecific decomposition reactions)

   $$H_3C\text{---}(CH_2)_4\text{---}CH_3 \xrightarrow[\text{cracking}]{\text{heat}} H_2C{=}CH_2 + H_3C\text{---}CH_2CH_2\text{---}CH_3$$

2. **Reactions:**
   a. *Addition of HX to the double bond*

   $$H_3C\text{---}CH{=}CH_2 + HBr \longrightarrow H_3C\text{---}\overset{\displaystyle H}{\underset{\displaystyle Br}{\overset{|}{\underset{|}{C}}}}\text{---}CH_3$$

The Markownikoff Rule says that in the addition of an acid across a double bond, the double-bonded carbon having the most hydrogen will receive the H of HX. The above is true for ionic addition, but in the presence of peroxides we see a free radical anti-Markownikoff addition:

$$H_3C\text{---}CH{=}CH_2 + HBr \xrightarrow{\text{peroxide}} H_3C\text{---}CH_2\text{---}CH_2Br$$

   b. *Hydrogenation* (catalyst such as Pt, Pd, or Ni):

   $$H_2C{=}CH_2 + H_2 \xrightarrow{Pt} H_3C\text{---}CH_3$$

   $$3H_2C{=}CH\text{---}CH{=}CH_2 + 4H_2 \xrightarrow{Pt} H_3C\text{---}CH{=}CH\text{---}CH_3$$
   $$+ H_2C{=}CH\text{---}CH_2\text{---}CH_3$$
   $$+ H_3C\text{---}CH_2\text{---}CH_2\text{---}CH_3$$

c. $H_2C=CH_2 + Br2 \longrightarrow BrCH_2-CH_2Br$

d. $H_2C=CH_2 \xrightarrow{\text{catalyst}}$ polymer (polyethylene in this case)

The Alkynes (derivatives of acetylene)

$HC\equiv CH$ acetylene or ethyne

1. **Synthesis:**
   a. $CaC_2 + H_2O \longrightarrow C_2H_2 + CaO$

   b. *Dehydrohalogenation*

   $$H_3C-CHBr_2 + \text{alcoholic } 2KOH \longrightarrow HC\equiv CH + 2H_2O + 2KBr$$

   c. *Dehalogenation*

   $$HCBr_2-CBr_2H + 2Zn \longrightarrow HC\equiv CH + 2ZnBr_2$$

2. **Reactions:**
   a. *Hydrogenation*

   $$HC\equiv CH + H_2 \xrightarrow{Pt} H_2C=CH_2 + H_2 \xrightarrow{Pt} CH_3-CH_3$$

   b. *Hydrohalogenation*—see reactions of alkenes

   c. *Halogenation*—see reactions of alkenes

   d. *Reaction of active hydrogen*

   $$H_3C-C\equiv CH + Ag^+ \longrightarrow H_3C-C\equiv CAg + H^+$$
   $$H_3C-C\equiv CH + NaNH_2 \longrightarrow H_3C-C\equiv CNa + NH_3$$
   $$H_3C-C\equiv CNa + CH_3Br \longrightarrow H_3C-C\equiv C-CH_3 + NaBr$$

Aromatic Compounds

Aromatic compounds consist of benzene and compounds whose chemical reactions are similar to those of benzene. Almost all aromatic compounds that you would be expected to recognize as such are derivatives of benzene; there are other unrelated aromatic compounds.

1. **Nature of Benzene—Resonance:** Although we may draw benzene as having three discrete double bonds and three discrete single bonds in conjugation, this does not adequately describe its structure. It may be shown as two structures in resonance.
In reality, however, it appears that each carbon atom has three discrete covalent bonds, and the fourth bonding electron of each carbon atom is delocalized in electron clouds around the ring.

2. **Synthesis of the Aromatic Ring:** This is unusual; in general one will only be interested in reactions of compounds containing the benzene ring rather than in the synthesis of the aromatic ring.

3. **Reactions:** (ϕ is sometimes used as a shorthand designation for the phenyl group. Thus, benzene could be indicated as ϕ-H.)

   a. *Monosubstitution*

   $$\phi\text{-H} + HNO_3 \longrightarrow \phi-NO_2 + H_2O$$
   $$\phi\text{-H} + H_2SO_4 \longrightarrow \phi-SO_3H + H_2O$$
   $$\phi\text{-H} + Br_2 \xrightarrow{Fe} \phi-Br + HBr$$

b. *Friedel-Crafts reaction*

$$\phi\text{-H} + RCl \xrightarrow{AlCl_3} \phi\text{—R} + HCl$$

$$\phi\text{-H} + R\text{—}\overset{\displaystyle O}{\overset{\|}{C}}\text{—Cl} \xrightarrow{AlCl} \phi\text{—}\overset{\displaystyle O}{\overset{\|}{C}}\text{—R} + HCl$$

c. *Substitution in a benzene ring that already has one substituent*

ortho   para
isomer   isomer

The placement of the second substituent is ordained by the first substituent. The OH substituent, as shown above, is an ortho, para-directing group. Other ortho, para-directing substituents include the CH_3 group and the halogens. The halogens deactivate the ring and also direct ortho, para. Many electrophilic substituents are said to be meta-directing: NO_2, CN, SO_3H, COOH, and so forth.

meta
isomer

The above meta-directing substituents also deactivate the ring.

Note that the reactions above *do* balance. In many cases below, we will write organic reactions that do not balance. This is done for the sake of simplicity and to emphasize the desired products.

d. *Diazotization of amines*

$$\phi\text{—}NH_2 + HNO_2 \longrightarrow \phi\text{—}N_2{}^+$$

e. *Reactions of diazonium salts* (see above)

$$\phi\text{—}N_2{}^+ + CuBr \longrightarrow \phi\text{—Br}$$

$$\phi\text{—}N_2{}^+ + CuCN \longrightarrow \phi\text{—CN}$$

$$\phi\text{—}N_2{}^+ + H_2O \xrightarrow{H+} \phi\text{—OH}$$

$$\phi\text{—}N_2{}^+ + \phi\text{—OH} \longrightarrow \phi\text{—N}{=}\text{N—}\phi\text{—OH (Coupling)}$$

$$\phi\text{—}N_2{}^+ + H_2 \xrightarrow{Pt} \phi\overset{\displaystyle H}{\overset{|}{N}}\text{—}NH_2$$

4. Acidity and Basicity:

a. *Acidity.* Phenol will ionize as an acid with a K_a of about 1×10^{-10}. A methyl substituent in the ortho position will lower the K_a (and the acidity) to about 6×10^{-11}. The electron-releasing methyl substituent contributes electrons to the ring and depresses release of H^+. A nitro substituent in the ortho position, conversely, increases the acidity (K_a about 7×10^{-8}) by withdrawing electrons from the ring.

   b.   *Basicity*. Aniline (aminobenzene or phenylamine) has a K_a of about 4×10^{-10}. The introduction of an electron-releasing methyl group in the para position (i.e., *p*-methylaniline) increases basicity (K_b about 1×10^{-9}). The introduction of the electron-withdrawing nitro group into the para position (i.e., *p*-nitroaniline) decreases basicity (K_b about 1×10^{-13}). The methyl substituent releases electrons into the ring, and the nitro substituent withdraws electrons from the ring. An electron-rich ring coincides with an electron-rich N in the NH_2 substituent. This will add stability to the NH_3^+ substituent which is formed by reaction of the NH_2 substituent with a proton, and the tendency of the NH_3^+ group to ionize by releasing the proton is decreased.

The Grignard Reagent

   The Grignard reagent is one of the most important and versatile in organic chemistry. We will try to outline only a few of its reactions.

   1.   Synthesis: The Grignard reagent is synthesized by the reaction of an alkyl halide with elemental magnesium in the presence of anhydrous ether.

   Example:

$$H_3C-CH_2Br + Mg \xrightarrow[\text{ether}]{\text{anhydrous}} H_3C-CH_2MgBr$$

   or

$$RBr + Mg \xrightarrow[\text{ether}]{\text{anhydrous}} RMgBr$$

   2.   Reactions:
   a.   *Reaction with active hydrogen*. A Grignard reagent will react with any compound having active hydrogen (e.g., H_2O, an alcohol, an acid, or a l-alkyne) to form a hydrocarbon.

$$RMgBr + H_2O \longrightarrow RH + MgBrOH$$

   b.   *Reaction with aldehydes and ketones*

$$RMgBr + HCHO \xrightarrow[\text{ether}]{\text{anhydrous}} R-CH_2OMgBr \xrightarrow{H^+} RCH_2OH \text{ (primary alcohol)}$$

$$RMgBr + R'CHO \xrightarrow[\text{ether}]{\text{anhydrous}} RC\overset{\displaystyle R'}{\underset{\displaystyle H}{-}}OMgBr \xrightarrow{H^+} RC\overset{\displaystyle R'}{\underset{\displaystyle H}{-}}OH$$

(secondary alcohol)

$$RMgBr + R'-\overset{\displaystyle R''}{C}=O \xrightarrow[\text{ether}]{\text{anhydrous}} R'-\overset{\displaystyle R''}{\underset{\displaystyle R}{C}}-OMgBr \xrightarrow{H^+} R'-\overset{\displaystyle R''}{\underset{\displaystyle R}{C}}-OH$$

(tertiary alcohol)

   c.   *Reaction with CO_2*

$$RMgBr + CO_2 \xrightarrow[\text{ether}]{\text{anhydrous}} R-\overset{\displaystyle O}{\overset{\displaystyle \|}{C}}-OMgBr \xrightarrow{H^+} RCOOH$$

d. *Reaction with an ester or an acyl halide*

$$RMgBr + R'COOR'' \xrightarrow[\text{ether}]{\text{anhydrous}} R'\overset{\displaystyle O}{\overset{\displaystyle \|}{-C-}}R$$

$$RMgBr + R'COBr \xrightarrow[\text{ether}]{\text{anhydrous}} R'\overset{\displaystyle O}{\overset{\displaystyle \|}{-C-}}R$$

Alcohols

Alcohols may be designated as ROH. The simplest alcohol is CH_3OH and is named methanol (i.e., methan-ol) as a derivative of the one-carbon hydrocarbon, methane. Other alcohols are similarly named as derivatives of hydrocarbons. The compound below is named 2-pentanol or 2-hydroxypentane.

$$H_3C-CH_2-CH_2-\underset{\underset{\displaystyle OH}{|}}{CH}-CH_3$$

The alcohols are very weak acids, even weaker than water. Polarity and hydrogen bonding cause short chain alcohols to be soluble in water.

1. **Synthesis:**
   a. *Hydration of alkenes*

$$H_2C=CH_2 + H_2O \underset{}{\overset{H^+}{\rightleftharpoons}} H_3C-CH_2OH$$

   b. *Using Grignard reagents–discussed elsewhere*
   c. *Hydrolysis of alkyl halides*

$$R-I + H_2O \underset{}{\overset{KOH}{\rightleftharpoons}} ROH + I^-$$

   d. *Reduction of aldehydes and ketones*

$$R-CHO + NaBH_4 \xrightarrow{H_2O} R-CH_2OH$$

2. **Reactions:**
   a. *Oxidation to form aldehydes or ketones*

$$R-CH_2OH + K_2Cr_2O_7 \xrightarrow{H^+} R-CHO$$

This is useful only if the aldehyde may be removed (sometimes by distillation) before further oxidation to the carboxylic acid. A ketone may not be easily oxidized further, but chain rupture is possible.

   b. *Dehydration to form alkenes–discussed elsewhere*
   c. *Formation of esters*

$$R-COOH + R-CH_2OH \underset{}{\overset{H^+}{\rightleftharpoons}} R-COOCH_2-R$$

   d. *Conversion to halides*

$$ROH + HI \rightleftharpoons RI + H_2O$$

Amines

Amines have the structure $R-NH_2$. The simplest example is methylamine (or aminomethane):

$$H_3CNH_2$$

1. **Synthesis:**
   a. $RX + NH_3 \longrightarrow R\text{—}NH_2$
   b. $RCN + LiAlH_4 \longrightarrow R\text{—}CH_2\text{—}NH_2$
   c. *Hofmann degradation*

$$R\text{—}CONH_2 \xrightarrow{\text{Br}_2,\ \text{NaOH}} RNH_2$$

2. **Reactions:**

   a. $R\text{—}NH_2 + HONO \xrightarrow{\text{H}_2\text{O}} ROH + N_2$
   (This is the reaction for a primary alkyl amine)
   b. $R\text{—}NH_2 + HONO \longrightarrow RN_2^+$
   (This is the reaction for a primary aromatic amine. The diazonium salt is stable at the temperatures of ice water. It is capable of numerous further reactions under appropriate conditions.)
   c. $R\text{—}NH_2 + R'\text{—}COOH + \text{dicyclohexylcarbodiimide} \longrightarrow R\text{—}NH\text{—}COR'$
   (an amide)

Amides

Amides have the structure R—NH—COR.
A simple example is acetanilide, ϕ—NH—CO—CH$_3$.

1. **Synthesis:**

   a. $R\text{—}NH_2 + R'\text{—}COCl$ (an acyl chloride) $\longrightarrow R\text{—}NH\overset{\displaystyle O}{\overset{\displaystyle \|}{\text{—}C}}\text{—}R'$

   b. $R\text{—}NH_2 + (R'\text{—}CO)_2O$ (an anhydride) $\longrightarrow R\text{—}NH\overset{\displaystyle O}{\overset{\displaystyle \|}{\text{—}C}}\text{—}R'$

   c. $R\text{—}NH_2 + R'\text{—}COOH + \text{dicyclohexylcarbodiimide} \longrightarrow R\text{—}NH\overset{\displaystyle O}{\overset{\displaystyle \|}{\text{—}C}}\text{—}R'$

(Primary amines are shown, but secondary amines may also be used.)

2. **Reaction:**

$$R\text{—}NH\text{—}COR' + H_2O \xrightarrow{\text{H+}} R\text{—}NH_3^+ + R'\text{—}COOH$$

(The reaction may also be accomplished in an aqueous base.)

Aldehydes and Ketones

1. **Synthesis:**
   a. *Reaction of a Grignard reagent with a carboxylic ester or an acyl halide to form a ketone* (outlined on page 237 under "Grignard Reagent")
   b. *Mild oxidation of an alcohol* (often feasible in the synthesis of ketones and sometimes in the synthesis of aldehydes)

$$RCH_2OH \xrightarrow{\text{Cu},\ \triangle} R\text{—}CHO \text{ (aldehyde)}$$

$$R\text{—}\underset{\displaystyle H}{\overset{\displaystyle R'}{\underset{|}{\overset{|}{C}}}}OH \xrightarrow{\text{Cu},\ \triangle} > R\text{—}\overset{\displaystyle R'}{\overset{|}{C}}{=}O \text{ (ketone)}$$

c. *Friedel-Crafts acylation to produce aromatic ketones* (see "Aromatic Compounds," page 235)

d. *Decarboxylation of acids to produce ketones*

$$2RCOOH \xrightarrow{ThO_2, \triangle} R\text{---}\overset{\displaystyle O}{\overset{\|}{C}}\text{---}R + CO_2$$

e. *Oxidation of diols to form aldehydes*

$$R\text{---}\underset{\overset{\displaystyle |}{OH}}{CH}\text{---}\underset{\overset{\displaystyle |}{OH}}{CH}\text{---}R' \xrightarrow{HIO_4 \text{ or } Pb(OAc)_4} R\text{---}CHO + R'\text{---}CHO$$

$$R\text{---}\underset{\overset{\displaystyle |}{OH}}{CH}\text{---}\underset{\overset{\displaystyle |}{OH}}{CH}\text{---}\underset{\overset{\displaystyle |}{OH}}{CH}\text{---}R' \xrightarrow{HIO_4 \text{ or } Pb(OAc)_4} R\text{---}CHO + R'\text{---}CHO + HCOOH$$

$$R\text{---}\underset{\overset{\displaystyle |}{OH}}{CH}\text{---}CH_2\text{---}\underset{\overset{\displaystyle |}{OH}}{CH}\text{---}R' \xrightarrow{HIO_4 \text{ or } Pb(OAc)_4} \text{No reaction}$$

2. **Reactions:**

a. *Reaction with Grignard reagents*

$$R\text{---}\overset{\displaystyle O}{\overset{\|}{C}}\text{---}R' + R''MgBr \xrightarrow[\text{ether}]{\text{anhydrous}} R\text{---}\underset{\overset{\displaystyle |}{R''}}{\overset{\overset{\displaystyle OMgBr}{|}}{C}}\text{---}R' \xrightarrow{H_2O} R\text{---}\underset{\overset{\displaystyle |}{R''}}{\overset{\overset{\displaystyle OH}{|}}{C}}\text{---}R'$$

$$R\text{---}CHO + R'MgBr \xrightarrow[\text{ether}]{\text{anhydrous}} R\text{---}\underset{\overset{\displaystyle |}{H}}{\overset{\overset{\displaystyle OMgBr}{|}}{C}}\text{H---}R' \xrightarrow{H_2O} R\text{---}\overset{\overset{\displaystyle OH}{|}}{C}H\text{---}R'$$

$$HCHO + RMgBr \xrightarrow[\text{ether}]{\text{anhydrous}} R\text{---}CH_2\text{---}OMgBr \xrightarrow{H_2O} R\text{---}CH_2OH$$

b. *Reaction of aldehydes or ketones with HCN*

$$R\text{---}CHO + HCN \longrightarrow R\text{---}\underset{\overset{\displaystyle |}{H}}{\overset{\overset{\displaystyle OH}{|}}{C}}\text{---}CN \xrightarrow{H_2O, H^+} R\text{---}\underset{\overset{\displaystyle |}{H}}{\overset{\overset{\displaystyle OH}{|}}{C}}\text{---}COOH$$

c. *Reaction of aldehydes or methyl ketones with NaHSO₃*

$$R\text{---}CHO + NaHSO_3 \longrightarrow R\text{---}\underset{\overset{\displaystyle |}{H}}{\overset{\overset{\displaystyle OH}{|}}{C}} - SO_3^-Na^+$$

d. *Reaction with alcohols*

$$R\text{---}CHO + R'\text{---}OH \xrightarrow{H^+} R\text{---}\underset{\overset{\displaystyle |}{H}}{\overset{\overset{\displaystyle OH}{|}}{C}}\text{---}OR' \xrightarrow{R'OH, H^+} R\text{---}\underset{\overset{\displaystyle |}{H}}{\overset{\overset{\displaystyle OR'}{|}}{C}}\text{---}OR'$$

$$\text{(a hemiacetal)} \qquad\qquad\qquad \text{(an acetal)}$$

$$R-\overset{\overset{\displaystyle O}{\|}}{C}-R' + R''OH \xrightarrow{H^+} R-\overset{\overset{\displaystyle OH}{|}}{\underset{\underset{\displaystyle OR''}{|}}{C}}-R' \xrightarrow{R''OH,\ H^+} R-\overset{\overset{\displaystyle OR''}{|}}{\underset{\underset{\displaystyle OR''}{|}}{C}}-R'$$

(a hemiketal)　　　　　　(a ketal)

e. *Reaction of ketones and aldehydes with hydroxylamine*

$$R-CHO + NH_2OH \xrightarrow{H^+} R-\overset{\overset{\displaystyle H}{|}}{C}=NOH$$

(an oxime)

f. *Reaction of ketones and aldehydes with hydrazine or hydrazine derivatives*

$$R-CHO + NH_2NH_2 \xrightarrow{H^+} R-\overset{\overset{\displaystyle H}{|}}{C}=N-NH_2$$

(a hydrazone)

g. *Oxidation of aldehydes*

$$R-CHO + Ag(NH_3)_2{}^+ \xrightarrow{OH^-} R-\overset{\overset{\displaystyle O}{\|}}{C}-O^- + Ag$$

(Tollens' reagent)　　　　(silver mirror)

$$R-CHO + Cu^{++} \xrightarrow{OH^-,\ citrate} R-\overset{\overset{\displaystyle O}{\|}}{C}-O^- + Cu_2O$$

(Benedict's reagent)　　　　(red ppt.)

h. *Haloform reaction with acetaldehyde or methyl ketones*

$$R-\overset{\overset{\displaystyle O}{\|}}{C}-CH_3 \xrightarrow{IO^-} RCO^- + CHI_3$$

i. *Aldol condensation* (requires alpha-hydrogen). Further reaction can also lead to polymers.

$$2CH_3-CHO \xrightarrow{OH^-} H_3C-\overset{\overset{\displaystyle OH}{|}}{\underset{\underset{\displaystyle H}{|}}{C}}-CH_2-CHO$$

j. *Cannizzaro reaction* (for aldehydes having no alpha-hydrogen)

$$2\phi-CHO \xrightarrow{OH^-} \phi-CH_2OH + \phi-\overset{\overset{\displaystyle O}{\|}}{C}-O^-$$

Carboxylic Acids

The carboxylic acids are organic compounds that ionize to produce free protons and carboxylate anions. The simplest example is formic acid, $H-\overset{\overset{\displaystyle O}{\|}}{C}-OH$

1. **Synthesis:**
   a. *Addition of carbon dioxide to a Grignard reagent*

$$R\ MgBr + CO_2 \longrightarrow R-\overset{\overset{\displaystyle O}{\|}}{C}-OMgBr \xrightarrow{H^+} R-\overset{\overset{\displaystyle O}{\|}}{C}-OH$$

b. *Oxidation of alkene*

$$R-\overset{\overset{\displaystyle H}{|}}{C}=\overset{\overset{\displaystyle H}{|}}{C}-R' + KMnO_4 \longrightarrow R-\underset{\underset{\displaystyle OH}{|}}{\overset{\overset{\displaystyle H}{|}}{C}}-\underset{\underset{\displaystyle OH}{|}}{\overset{\overset{\displaystyle H}{|}}{C}}-R'$$

$$R-\underset{\underset{\displaystyle OH}{|}}{\overset{\overset{\displaystyle H}{|}}{C}}-\underset{\underset{\displaystyle OH}{|}}{\overset{\overset{\displaystyle H}{|}}{C}}-R' + KMnO_4 \longrightarrow RCOOH + R'COOH$$

c. *Oxidation of primary alcohol*

$$R-CH_2OH + KMnO_4 \longrightarrow RCOOH$$

d. *Hydrolysis of nitrile*

$$RCN \xrightarrow{H_2O,\ H^+} RCOOH$$

e. *Hydrolysis of esters*

$$R-\overset{\overset{\displaystyle O}{\|}}{C}-O-R' + H_2O \underset{}{\overset{H^+}{\rightleftharpoons}} R-COOH + R'OH$$

f. *Saponification of esters*

$$R-\overset{\overset{\displaystyle O}{\|}}{C}-O-R' + NaOH \rightleftharpoons R'OH + R-\overset{\overset{\displaystyle O}{\|}}{C}-ONa \xrightarrow{H^+} R-COOH$$

2. Reactions:

a. *Neutralization of base*

$$RCOOH + NaOH \longrightarrow R\overset{\overset{\displaystyle O}{\|}}{C}-O^- + Na^+ + H_2O$$

b. *Esterification*

$$RCOOH + R'OH \underset{}{\overset{H^+}{\rightleftharpoons}} R-\overset{\overset{\displaystyle O}{\|}}{C}-OR' + H_2O$$

c. *Formation of acylhalide*

$$RCOOH \xrightarrow{PBr_3} R\overset{\overset{\displaystyle O}{\|}}{C}-Br$$

d. *Formation of anhydride*

$$2RCOOH \longrightarrow R-\overset{\overset{\displaystyle O}{\|}}{C}-O-\overset{\overset{\displaystyle O}{\|}}{C}-R + H_2O$$

e. *High-temperature decomposition*

$$2RCOOH \xrightarrow{ThO_2, \Delta} R-\overset{\overset{\displaystyle O}{\|}}{C}-R + CO_2 + H_2O$$

Esters

Esters may be formed from the reaction between an acid and an alcohol. Upon hydrolysis the products are an acid and an alcohol. We often think first of carboxylic acid esters, but they are not the only ones known. Phosphate esters are common in biochemistry.

The simplest carboxylic acid ester is methyl formate:

$$H-\overset{\overset{\displaystyle O}{\|}}{C}-O-CH_3$$

1. **Synthesis:**

a. $R-COCl + R'-OH \longrightarrow R-\overset{\overset{\displaystyle O}{\|}}{C}-OR'$

b. $(R-\overset{\overset{\displaystyle O}{\|}}{C})_2O + R'-OH \longrightarrow R-\overset{\overset{\displaystyle O}{\|}}{C}-OR'$

c. $R-COOH + R'-OH \underset{}{\overset{H^+}{\rightleftharpoons}} R-\overset{\overset{\displaystyle O}{\|}}{C}-OR' + H_2O$

An equilibrium will be established. Removal of water by an appropriate method such as azeotropic separation will produce good yields. High yields based on one reactant can also be achieved by adding large quantities of the other reactant.

2. **Reactions:**

a. *Acid hydrolysis*

$$R-COOR' + H_2O \xrightarrow{H^+} R-COOH + R'OH$$

b. *Saponification*

$$R-COOR' + H_2O \xrightarrow{OH^-} R-COO^- + R'OH$$

Ethers

1. **Synthesis:**

a. *Dehydration. (Remember that the choice of conditions determines whether the ether or the unsaturated hydrocarbon, in this case ethylene, is the major product.)*

$$2CH_3-CH_2OH \xrightarrow{H_2SO_4, \Delta} CH_3-CH_2-O-CH_2CH_3$$

b. *Williamson synthesis.* Much more useful than the dehydration method if an unsymmetrical ether is desired.

$$RONa + R'Br \longrightarrow ROR'$$

2. **Reactions:** Ethers are generally unreactive compounds. They are often useful as solvents in organic reactions because of their unreactive nature. They may be cleaved by heated halogen acids:

$$ROR + HI \xrightarrow{heat} RI + ROH$$

The ROH which is formed may react with HI to form an additional RI.

Final Remarks

As stated earlier, you cannot learn organic chemistry from a brief presentation such as this. We recognize that we have been able to present only some of the more important points. It is our intent that you use this material (and the questions and answers in the practice tests) to review the organic chemistry you have learned in your coursework. If you find areas of weakness in your preparation, we would recommend that you study those areas in your organic chemistry textbook.

Biochemistry

Biochemistry or biological chemistry may be seen as an attempt to better understand life by studying the chemicals that are important in living cells and organisms. One must consider the amounts and identities of a variety of chemicals, as well as the ways in which they are transformed during different life processes. Perhaps it should not be surprising that biochemistry calls upon the background of other areas of chemistry, including organic chemistry, analytical chemistry, inorganic chemistry, and physical chemistry.

In these few pages we can only touch lightly on a few concepts in biochemistry. Those of you who continue in the life sciences, such as medicine, dentistry, or pharmacy, will be taught a great deal more about this fascinating area. Here we can only begin to delineate the forest, leaving you to study the trees at a later time. For those who have had little or no exposure to biochemistry, this brief introduction will help to prepare you for the Medical College Admission Test and will also lay the groundwork for your course in professional school. For those who have already taken a course in biochemistry, this material will assist in consolidating the information you already possess.

Areas of Biochemistry

Although there are a number of ways of subdividing biochemistry, there are substantial similarities among them. The subdivision is done according to similarities in the properties of the compounds within each subdivision. A biochemist usually specializes in the study of one of these subdivisions:

    I.   pH and Buffers
   II.   Amino Acids, Peptides, and Proteins
        A.   Amino Acids
        B.   Peptides and Proteins
  III.   Enzymes
        A.   Nomenclature
        B.   Cofactors
        C.   Energy
        D.   Velocity and Inhibition
  IV.   Carbohydrates
        A.   Chemistry
        B.   Functions
        C.   Metabolism
            1.   Glycolysis
            2.   Krebs Cycle
            3.   Hexose Monophosphate Shunt
   V.   Lipids
        A.   Chemistry
        B.   Metabolism
            1.   Hydrolysis to Produce Fatty Acids
            2.   Oxidation of Fatty Acids in the Mitochondria

3. Synthesis of Fatty Acids
4. Synthesis of Glycerides
VI. Nucleotides and Nucleic Acids; Biosynthesis of Nucleic Acids and Proteins
A. Nucleotides
B. Nucleic Acids
C. Biosynthesis of Nucleic Acids and Proteins

pH and Buffers

The concepts of pH and buffers presented on pages 225–227 under acids and bases are used also in biochemistry. The biochemist applies these principles in the context of the human body.

The human body (and other animal bodies) requires that the pH be maintained over a rather small range. The pH of human blood is ordinarily maintained from 7.36 to 7.42. Buffers prevent greater fluctuation, which could occur in response to loss or gain of acid or base.

The buffer pairs used in human blood include HCO_3^-/H_2CO_3; base/acid species of oxygenated hemoglobin; and base/acid species of deoxygenated hemoglobin. The phosphate pair $HPO_4^{2-}/H_2PO_4^-$ would offer a possible buffer, but little is present in the blood.

Amino Acids, Peptides, and Proteins

Amino Acids: The naturally occurring amino acids are primarily α-amino acids of the general structure

$$
\begin{array}{c}
NH_2 \\
| \\
R-C-COOH \\
| \\
H
\end{array}
$$

If R does not represent H, then it will be noted that an asymmetric center exists, allowing for L and D isomers. The ones commonly found in nature, especially in higher animals, are usually of the L series. (The amino acid having no asymmetric center, and thus devoid of optical activity, is glycine.)

Although approximately 300 amino acids are found in nature, some are relatively rare. About 20 amino acids occur in all organisms. Amino acids can serve as biological active compounds in their own right (e.g., neurotransmitters), but we tend to think of them most often as the monomers of which the polymeric peptides and higher molecular weight proteins are composed.

Subdivisions of Amino Acids. It is possible to subdivide the amino acids based on their R groups. This is useful in predicting such things as the folding of a protein in a lipoprotein membrane; it is also helpful in remembering the different amino acids. Thus, they may be subdivided into aliphatic, hydroxy, sulfur, aromatic, dicarboxy (or dicarboxy with one carboxyl as an amide), diamino, and imino on the basis of the R groups.

They may also be subdivided into acidic, basic, and neutral. Those having a second amino function are basic (two basic functional groups and only one carboxyl). Those having a second proton-releasing functional group are acidic. (This second group could be a carboxyl. It could also be the more weakly ionized phenolic or sulfhydryl group.) The neutral amino acids contain only a single acidic and a single basic group, thus canceling each other.

Essential Amino Acids. Although many amino acids may be synthesized in the animal body, certain animals are unable to synthesize sufficient quantities of particular amino acids, called *essential amino acids*. (The term indicates no judgment of the importance of these amino acids compared to that of the other amino acids. It simply indicates that for optimal health these amino acids must be supplied in the diet.) In humans, ten amino acids are usually called essential: phenylalanine, valine, tryptophan, threonine, isoleucine, methionine, histidine, arginine, leucine, and lysine. Of these, histidine and arginine may be required in the diet only of infants or under special circumstances.

Forms of an Amino Acid. A simple amino acid such as glycine can exist in three forms. At a low pH such as 1, the amino group is protonated (and carrying a charge of +1); the carboxyl is not ionized or charged; and the net charge is +1. At an intermediate pH such as 7, the amino function and the carboxyl function carry equal and opposite charges of +1 and −1, and the net is a charge of zero. At a still higher pH such as 12, the carboxyl is ionized and the amino not ionized, resulting in a net of −1. The mean of the pK_a of these two ionizable groups is the pH at which the amino has no net charge and will not move in an electrical field. This pH is defined as the *isoionic point* and designated as pI.

Peptides and Proteins: Peptides are linear chains of amino acids with the carboxyl group of one amino acid attached in amide (specifically peptide) linkage to the amino group of the next amino acid.

$$H_3N^+ \!-\! \underset{\underset{H}{|}}{\overset{\overset{R_3}{|}}{C}} \!-\! \overset{\overset{O}{\|}}{C} \!-\! \overset{\overset{H}{|}}{N} \!-\! \underset{\underset{H}{|}}{\overset{\overset{R_2}{|}}{C}} \!-\! \overset{\overset{O}{\|}}{C} \!-\! \overset{\overset{H}{|}}{N} \!-\! \underset{\underset{H}{|}}{\overset{\overset{R}{|}}{C}} \!-\! COO^-$$

Proteins are larger assemblies of amino acids. The linear sequence of amino acids in a chain is called the *primary structure*. The orientation of the peptide chain (e.g., the alpha helix) is called the *secondary structure*. The relationship of portions of the polypeptide chains to one another is called the *tertiary structure*. In some cases there are dimers, trimers, tetramers, etc., of the polypeptide chains. This is called the *quaternary structure*. Sometimes the units are identical, sometimes not. In the enzyme lactate dehydrogenase, two different monomers are assembled into an active tetramer. Five different active lactate dehydrogenase tetramers are possible and are separable by electrophoresis.

The primary structure of a peptide or protein may be determined by a combination of procedures. The carboxy terminal amino acid may be determined by its enzymatic release by carboxypeptidases. The rate of release allows determination of the sequence of a small number of amino acids at the carboxy terminal end. Another method, the Edman degradation, utilizes reaction of the amino terminus with phenylisothiocyanate, hydrolysis of the derivative of this amino acid from the peptide chain, and identification of the amino acid derivative. This Edman degradation allows determination of a number of amino acids in sequence at the amino terminal end.

Determination of a number of amino acids at each end of a peptide chain would not allow determination of the sequence of a long peptide chain. Fortunately there are also other enzymes (endopeptidases) that perform internal cleavage with a high degree of specificity. The smaller peptides thus formed may be separated and sequenced. By utilizing different endopeptidases, it is possible to prepare a series of overlapping peptides. When they are sequenced, it is possible to determine the sequence of the intact peptide.

By other methodology it is also possible to synthesize peptides. This procedure, referred to as the Merrifield synthesis, utilizes a solid material with a functional group to which the peptide chain is attached.

Enzymes

In 1926 Sumner isolated the enzyme urease from jack beans and claimed the enzyme to be a protein. Few believed this initially, and the claim was not accepted until about 1935.

Now, over 2600 enzymes have been isolated. Although biological in origin and protein in nature, enzymes are simply catalysts, serving to increase the rate of reactions in which they are involved.

Nomenclature: Some enzymes are given trivial names, such as the proteolytic enzymes trypsin or pepsin, names that provide no information unless one is familiar with these specific enzymes. Others have names that identify the substrate and type of reaction; examples are histidine decarboxylase (decarboxylating histidine to produce CO_2 and histamine), urease (breaking down urea to produce CO_2 and NH_3), and alcohol dehydrogenase (removing hydrogen and electrons from an alcohol to produce a reduced coenzyme and an aldehyde).

Since about 1965 (with a revision in 1972), there has been an attempt to confer more systematic nomenclature and classification on enzymes. An enzyme commission (EC) number is given as four numbers separated by periods. The first of these numbers indicates the main class.

1. Oxidoreductases—oxidation-reduction reactions
2. Transferases—transfer intact groups of atoms from donors to acceptors
3. Hydrolases—cleave by hydrolysis
4. Lyases—cleave C—C, C—O, C—N, and other bonds without hydrolysis or oxidation. (Hydration and dehydration reactions are included in this class.)
5. Isomerases—interconvert isomers, such as cis → *trans*; D—→L
6. Ligases—form bonds as a result of condensation of two different substances with energy provided by ATP.

An example of EC nomenclature and numbering is alcohol: NAD^+ oxidoreductase (EC1.1.1.1). The first number identifies it as an oxidoreductase; the second number identifies its subclass; the third number identifies its sub-subclass; and the final number is a serial listing within the sub-subclass. EC1.1.1.1 is more commonly known as alcohol dehydrogenase.

Cofactors: In addition to the protein portion, many enzymes need cofactors or coenzymes. The protein enzyme without cofactor is known as an *apoenzyme*; the complete enzyme with cofactor or coenzyme is called a *holoenzyme*. The term coenzyme is usually given to an organic cofactor. A cofactor may serve by altering the three-dimensional structure of the enzyme and/or the bound substrate, or it may participate effectively as a second substrate. Thus, the enzyme lactate dehydrogenase catalyzes the oxidation of lactate to pyruvate as the coenzyme NAD^+ is reduced to $NADH + H^+$.

Energy: Enzymes are often looked upon as defying or contradicting the laws of chemistry. This is not true, of course. The free energy of the substrate initially must be higher than the free energy of the products or the reaction will not occur (without net input of energy). In this case we say that the reaction is thermodynamically unfavorable. Indeed, in this case, the reverse reaction would be thermodynamically favorable.

In the case of a thermodynamically favorable reaction, however, input of energy may still be necessary. This energy input, called the *energy of activation*, will be released again as the energy of the system proceeds to the lower energy level of the final products. (This is sometimes compared to a large stone being rolled from one valley into a valley of lower elevation. The energy expended in rolling the stone to the crest of the intervening hill will be released as the stone proceeds downhill. In addition to the release of energy equal to the input of energy to reach the crest, there is also release of energy related to the difference in elevation of the starting and the ending positions.) The role of the enzyme or of other catalysts is seen as lowering the activation energy of the reaction, thus increasing the rate.

Velocity and Inhibition: In the study of enzymes several relationships must be considered: (1) the rate of the reaction will increase with temperature until there is partial denaturation of the enzyme; (2) rates of reactions of enzymes are affected by pH and will ordinarily exhibit a pH range over which maximal activity is seen; (3) reaction rates ordinarily increase linearly with substrate concentration up to the point of maximum velocity, where it is considered that all enzyme molecules have substrate bound at the same time; (4) reaction rates ordinarily increase linearly with enzyme concentration.

The determination of maximum velocity is somewhat difficult because a plot of velocity versus substrate only approaches the maximum velocity with a reasonable substrate concentration. A more accurate method for determining maximum velocity involves a double reciprocal plot:

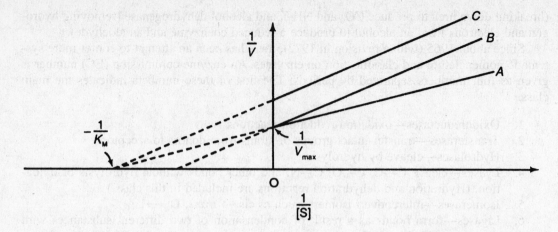

In this graph *A* is a plot of an uninhibited enzyme; *B* is a plot of the same enzyme in the presence of a competitive inhibitor; *C* is a plot of the enzyme in the presence of a noncompetitive inhibitor; *v* represents velocity and [S] represents substrate concentration. Note that the y-intercept is the reciprocal of maximal velocity, and the x-intercept is the negative of the reciprocal of the Michaelis constant, K_M, a characteristic of the individual enzyme. Note that the maximal velocity in the presence of a competitive inhibitor is the same as for the uninhibited enzyme. The maximal velocity in the presence of a noncompetitive inhibitor is lower (as noted by the fact that the reciprocal is higher).

Carbohydrates

Chemistry: Carbohydrates are a group of polyhydroxy aldehydes, polyhydroxy ketones, and closely related compounds. They may exist as monomers (monosaccharides), dimers (disaccharides), or polymers (polysaccharides).

D-glucose and D-fructose are two of the most common monosaccharides found in the human body. They are shown on the previous page in straight-chain form and in ring form (as they are usually found in solution). Note that in the ring structure a hemiacetal or a hemiketal has been formed.

Disaccharides such as sucrose and lactose are formed by reaction of monosaccharides. Sucrose hydrolysis will produce equal quantities of D-glucose and D-fructose. Lactose hydrolysis will produce equal quantities of D-galactose and D-glucose.

Polysaccharides are polymers of ring-form monomers. Animal glycogen and plant starch are polymers of α-D-glucopyranose. Cellulose is a polymer of β-D-glucopyranose.

Functions: Carbohydrates play a number of roles in nature. For example, they are metabolized for energy (4 kcal/g), metabolized for production of other required compounds such as certain amino acids, serve as components of nucleic acids (ribose in RNA and deoxyribose in DNA), serve as a structural element (cellulose of plants and cell walls of bacteria), serve as components of lubricants of bone joints, serve as cellular antigens, and are components of heparin.

Metabolism: Many pathways of carbohydrate metabolism could be considered here. We will confine ourselves to comments about glycolysis, the Krebs cycle (also known as the citric acid cycle or the tricarboxylic acid cycle), and the hexose monophosphate shunt (also known as the pentose phosphate pathway).

The complete metabolism of a molecule of glucose proceeds in a series of linked reactions, as shown on page 251. Energy associated with the bonds of glucose is eventually transferred to bonds of adenosine triphosphate (ATP) molecules, which are the molecules used most often to release this energy for work in the cell. Several of the steps shown in the diagram produce ATP directly; however, most ATPs made in the cell carry energy brought to them via "carrier" molecules, either NADH (reduced nicotinamide adenine dinucleotide) or $FADH_2$ (reduced flavin adenine dinucleotide), both of which are made in the reactions shown on page 251. Glycolysis occurs in the cytoplasm; the Krebs cycle, in the mitochondria.

Glycolysis. Glycolysis, in a series of reactions, converts glucose to pyruvic acid (or to lactic acid under conditions of oxygen deficiency). Thus, there is a net formation of 2 moles of ATP from the anaerobic glycolysis of 1 mole of glucose.

Krebs Cycle. Pyruvic acid may be converted to acetyl coenzyme A, producing 3 moles of ATP for each mole of pyruvate. The Krebs cycle may then metabolize the acetyl CoA through a series of reactions to produce 12 moles of ATP for each mole of acetyl CoA. Since the Krebs cycle is often studied with carbohydrate metabolism, many people unconsciously associate them. It should be recognized, however, that acetyl CoA is produced in metabolism of fatty acids and amino acids as well. Acetyl CoA from these other sources is also metabolized in the Krebs cycle.

The Krebs cycle, unlike glycolysis, cannot operate under anaerobic conditions. Oxygen and a functioning electron transport system are required for regeneration of oxidized FAD and NAD^+ (from reduced $FADH_2$ and NADH), but they are also required to produce and capture most of the energy that is realized from the Krebs cycle.

Hexose Monophosphate Shunt. The hexose monophosphate shunt is a series of reactions that serve primarily to produce NADPH and the pentoses (D-ribose and D-deoxyribose). NADPH is important in numerous biosynthetic reactions, including those for biosynthesis of fatty acids and cholesterol. As noted earlier, the pentoses are required for biosynthesis of the nucleic acids (DNA and RNA).

Lipids

Chemistry: Lipids are defined as compounds that may be extracted from biological materials with nonpolar solvents and that are insoluble in aqueous polar solvents. This includes the neutral glycerides (largely triglycerides), the phosphoglycerides, the sphingolipids, the steroids, the eicosanoids (particularly the prostaglandins), free fatty acids, and the lipidsoluble vitamins (A, D. E, and K).

Fatty acids are components of many lipids, thus suggesting the need for a discussion of their structure. Fatty acids are generally long, unbranched hydrocarbons with a carboxyl group at one terminus. In the simplest case there are no carbon-to-carbon double bonds, but unsaturation (presence of double bonds) is common. When double bonds are present, they are usually in a *cis*-configuration and in a methylene-interrupted sequence (if more than one double bond is present).

Neutral Glycerides. Neutral glycerides, or acylglycerols, are simply glycerol in ester linkage with one to three fatty acid molecules. Esterification with one fatty acid molecule produces a monoglyceride (monoacylglycerol); esterification with two fatty acid molecules produces a diglyceride (diacylglycerol); and esterification with three molecules of fatty acid produces a triglyceride (triacylglycerol). As previously stated, the triglycerides represent the principal form of storage of excess food. This appears to be a wise arrangement because triglyceride produces 9 kcal/g during metabolism, compared to 4 kcal/g for either carbohydrate or protein, and triglyceride is stored in a substantially water-free state, compared to the hydrated carbohydrates and proteins.

$$
\begin{array}{c}
O \\
\parallel \\
O \quad H_2C-O-C-R_1 \\
\parallel \quad | \\
R_2-C-O-C-H \quad O \\
| \quad \parallel \\
H_2C-O-C-R_3
\end{array}
\qquad
H_3C-(CH_2)_4-\overset{H}{\underset{|}{C}}=\overset{H}{\underset{|}{C}}-CH_2-\overset{H}{\underset{|}{C}}=\overset{H}{\underset{|}{C}}-(CH_2)_7-COOH
$$

triglyceride   a fatty acid (linoleic acid)

Phosphoglycerides. The phosphoglycerides are similar to the neutral glycerides, but a phosphate group is substituted for the fatty acid that would be found in the 3-position in a triglyceride. Various substituents may be attached to the phosphate group, thus forming other phosphoglycerides. Attachment of choline, for example, produces phosphatidylcholine; ethanolamine → phosphatidylethanolamine; serine → phosphatidylserine; inositol → phosphatidylinositol; and glycerol produces phosphatidylglycerol.

$$
\begin{array}{c}
O \\
\parallel \\
O \quad H_2C-O-C-R_1 \\
\parallel \quad | \\
R_2-C-O-C-H \quad O \\
| \quad \parallel \\
H_2C-O-P-O^- \\
| \\
O^-
\end{array}
$$

phosphatidic acid

Sphingolipids. The sphingolipids are based on a long-chain amino alcohol, sphingosine, rather than on glycerol.

$$
H_3C-(CH_2)_{12}-\overset{H}{\underset{|}{C}}=\overset{OH}{\underset{|}{\underset{H}{C}}}-\overset{NH_2}{\underset{|}{\underset{H}{C}}}-\overset{}{\underset{|}{\underset{H}{C}}}-CH_2OH
\qquad
R-\overset{OH}{\underset{|}{\underset{N}{C}}}-\overset{H}{\underset{|}{\underset{NH}{C}}}-CH_2-O-X
$$

sphingosine
$$
\begin{array}{c}
| \\
C=O \\
| \\
R'
\end{array}
$$

a sphingolipid

Some Major Steps in Glycolysis and the Citric Acid Cycle*

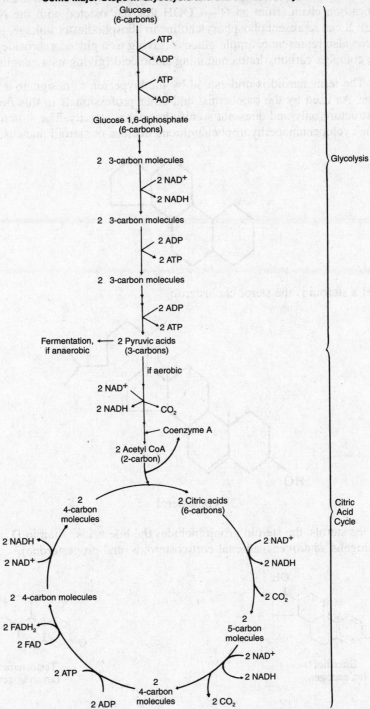

*Reprinted with permission from Barron's *How to Prepare for the Graduate Record Examination in Biology, Third Edition,* © 1989.

In the preceding formula, R represents an unsaturated hydrocarbon chain, R′ represents another hydrocarbon chain (from an R′—COOH that has reacted with the NH_2 to form an amide linkage). X can represent phosphorylcholine in phosphodiester linkage, giving us sphingomyelin. It can also represent a simple glucose (giving us a glucocerebroside), or it can represent a more complex carbohydrate containing sialic acid (giving us a ganglioside).

Steroids. The term steroid is understood by the layperson to designate a natural or synthetic hormone. As used by the biochemist and other professionals in this field, however, it refers to the structure only and does not signify hormonal activity. The structure of a steroid is based on the cyclopentanoperhydrophenanthrene nucleus or steroid nucleus:

An example of a steroid is the sterol cholesterol:

HO

cholesterol

In addition to the sterols, the steroid group includes the bile acids, vitamin D, and the steroid hormones (estrogens, androgens, adrenal corticosteroids, and progesterone).

OH

HO

Estradiol
(an estrogen)

OH

O

Testosterone
(an androgen)

CH_2OH
|
C = O
‖---OH

HO

O

Cortisol
(an adrenal corticosteroid)

CH_3
|
C = O

O

Progesterone
(the progestational agent
of the corpus luteum)

Cholic Acid
(a bile acid)

Vitamin D₃

Note that all of these compounds are derivatives of the steroid nucleus. Although we have shown only one representative of each class, some generalizations may be made if larger numbers of compounds are considered:

1. Total number of carbon atoms
   a. Sterols (e.g., cholesterol)—27–29
   b. Estrogens—18
   c. Androgens—19
   d. Adrenal corticosteroids—21
   e. Progesterone—21
   f. Bile acids—24
   g. Vitamin D₃—27

2. Other structured characteristics
   a. Sterols—β-hydroxyl in the A ring, ring double bond only in the B ring
   b. Estrogens—aromatic A ring, phenolic hydroxyl in the A ring
   c. Androgens—ketone in the A ring, ring double bond only in the A ring
   d. Adrenal corticosteroids—ketone in the A ring, ring double bond only in the A ring
   e. Progesterone—ketone in the A ring, ring double bond only in the A ring
   f. Bile acids—no double bonds in the ring system, only α-hydroxyls are attached to the rings, carboxyl group is present at the end of sidechain
   g. Vitamin D₃—incomplete B ring, double bonds in conjugation in "ring" B, methene group rather than methyl at the point that is usually the junction of rings A and B, β-hydroxyl in the A ring

Eicosanoids. Some fatty acids, including linoleic acid, are very important to mammalian health, but cannot be synthesized in the body. These are therefore called *essential fatty acids.* Among the products of linoleic acid are the prostaglandins, 20-carbon fatty acids that include a 5-carbon ring. Prostaglandins are active in a variety of physiologically important ways and are sometimes used pharmacologically.

prostaglandin E₁
(PGE₁)

Two other important classes of eicosanoids are the leukotrienes and thromboxanes. Linoleic acid may be converted to arachidonic acid in the animal body (including humans). Arachidonic acid is a 20-carbon fatty acid with four *cis* double bonds. Arachidonic acid is stored in the 2-position of phosphoglycerides in membranes. The fatty acid in the 2-position is released by the enzyme phospholipase A_2. If it has the appropriate structure (such as arachidionic acid), it can be converted into prostaglandin, leukotriene, or thromboxane by appropriate enzymes.

Activity of phospholipase A_2 may be inhibited by aspirin and other nonsteroidal anti-inflammatory drugs (NSAIDs), leading to release of less polyunsaturated fatty acid from the membrane and ultimately less production of prostaglandins, leukotrienes, and thromboxanes. Inhibition of cyclooxygenase, however, by anti-inflammatory steroids leads to diminished production of prostaglandins but has no effect on leukotriene or thromboxane production.

Free Fatty Acids. Free fatty acids may sometimes be found in small amounts in various tissues. Fatty acids are also found in unesterified form in blood plasma, but in this case they are ordinarily bound noncovalently to plasma proteins, particularly albumin.

Lipid-soluble Vitamins. The lipid-soluble vitamins A, D, E, and K may also be classified as lipids, based on their solubility. They are stored in the body, and, in contrast to water-soluble vitamins, *steady* dietary intake of these vitamins is not vitally important.

Arachidonate — Cyclooxygenase / $2O_2$ / 5-Lipoxygenase →

Thromboxane A_2 — Various Prostaglandins Including PGE_2, $PGF_{2\alpha}$, and $PGF_{2\beta}$ — Leukotriene A_4

Metabolism:

Hydrolysis to Produce Fatty Acids. Neutral glycerides may be hydrolyzed by lipases such as pancreatic lipase or hormone-sensitive lipase, thus releasing free fatty acids. Fatty acids may also be released from phosphoglycerides by hydrolysis that is catalyzed by phospholipase A_1 and phsopholipase A_2.

Oxidation to Fatty Acids in the Mitochondria. Fatty acids may then be oxidized via β-oxidation to produce acetyl CoA+ reduced flavin adenine dinucleotide ($FADH_2$) and reduced nicotinamide adenine dinucleotide ($NADH + H^+$). Thus, a molecule of fatty acid 16:0 would produce 8 molecules of acetyl CoA, 7 molecules of $FADH_2$, and 7 molecules of $NADH + H^+$. Each molecule of acetyl CoA can be metabolized in the Krebs cycle to produce 12 molecules of ATP. Each molecule of $FADH_2$ can produce 2 molecules of ATP when it is oxidized in the electron transport chain, and each molecule of $NADH + H^+$ can produce 3 molecules of ATP when oxidized in the electron transport chain.

Synthesis of Fatty Acids. Synthesis of fatty acids occurs in the nonparticulate cytoplasm. The pathway is not simply a reversal of β-oxidation; it requires biotin and carbon dioxide in addition to acetyl CoA. The carbon dioxide, however, is not incorporated into the fatty acid. Also the reducing equivalents required for the synthesis are derived from $NADPH + H^+$.

Synthesis of Glycerides. The neutral glycerides require L-3-glycerol phosphate in their biosynthesis. This glycerol phosphate may be formed by the enzymatic phosphorylation of glycerol or by the enzymatic reduction of dihydroxyacetone phosphate, which is produced in glycolysis.

Nucleotides and Nucleic Acids; Biosynthesis of Nucleic Acids and Proteins

Nucleotides: Both deoxyribonucleic acid (DNA) and ribonucleic acid (RNA) are polymers of nucleotides. A nucleotide consists of a nitrogen base (either a purine or a pyrimidine), a pentose (ribose or 2-deoyxribose), and a phosphate group. Deoxyribose is found in DNA; ribose, in RNA.

The nitrogen bases include the purines (adenine and guanine) in both DNA and RNA. The pyrimidines include cytosine and thymine in DNA; cytosine and uracil are present in RNA. Other nitrogen bases are found in small quantities. Some synthetic nitrogen bases are used in the treatment of cancer and certain viral infections.

Nucleic Acids: As mentioned above, DNA and RNA are polymers of appropriate nucleotides. The attachment between nucleotides is phosphate–pentose-phosphate-pentose–, etc. This leaves the nitrogen base as an appendage from the linear chain. In double-stranded DNA there are two strands that are paired and linked (noncovalently) through their nitrogen bases. Adenine pairs with thymine, and cytosine pairs with guanine. Methods are available to allow determination of the primary structures of both DNA and RNA.

Biosynthesis of Nucleic Acids and Proteins: It is recognized that DNA codes for its own duplication, as well as for RNA synthesis. Messenger RNA, in turn, codes for the biosynthesis of polypeptide chains. Since there is a triplet code without commas, there are $4 \times 4 \times 4 = 64$ possibilities and sequences for specification of a single amino acid. Only about 21 amino acids, however, are known to have codes. It turns out that some codes give other instructions (e.g., initiation or termination of a peptide chain biosynthesis) and some amino acids have more than one code for their placement. Arginine, for example, has six different codons that can specify its placement.

Mutations in the DNA chain can occur, of course, as a result of errors in duplication, spontaneous changes in DNA, or changes resulting from radiation or mutagenic chemicals. A point mutation results in the presence of a different nitrogen base. This may, in turn, cause problems, or it may be a silent mutation. It would be silent if the base change resulted in no difference in the amino acid or if it resulted in the substitution of a very similar amino acid.

A frame shift mutation is likely to be more serious. Consider that insertion or deletion of a nitrogen base will change the sequence of bases following it in the chain. (Remember that there are no commas.) This may be a lethal mutation.

Mutations can be repaired by a number of mechanisms. For example, sometimes an affected area is removed and replaced by a strand that is duplicated again from the complementary DNA strand. Specific cellular enzymes exist to aid in identifying and repairing mutations.

Separation and Quantitation Techniques

1. **Chromatography:** One of the most important techniques for separation of compounds in biochemistry is *chromatography*. Although it may also be used in inorganic and organic chemistry, the usually smaller quantities involved in biochemistry make it even more popular and useful there.

Chromatography may be considered to be a separation process in which a mobile phase passes across a stationary phase. Molecules that are in the mobile phase 100% of the time will elute from the chromatograph very quickly; those that are in the stationary phase 100% of the time will never elute. Those spending intermediate percentages of time in each phase will elute at intermediate times.

Different phases are used in various kinds of chromatography. Probably the most important ones are *gas-solid*, *gas-liquid*, *liquid-liquid*, and *liquid-solid*. (In the previous examples the first phase is the mobile one.)

The reason for the time spent in the mobile versus the stationary phase is influenced by properties such as size, charge, solubility, and volatility.

Gas-solid chromatography involves the passage of a mobile phase (gas) over a stationary phase (solid). Movement is increased (and elution time decreased) by high volatility and low affinity for the stationary phase.

Gas-liquid chromatography involves the passage of a mobile phase (gas) over a stationary phase (liquid). The stationary liquid phase needs to be stable at the temperature used for the chromatography. The compounds eluted most rapidly are those that are volatile and show little or no affinity for the stationary liquid phase.

Liquid-liquid chromatography involves the passage of a mobile phase (liquid) over a stationary phase (also liquid). The stationary phase must be bound to a surface and the two liquids must be essentially immiscible. The faster-eluting compounds are those that are quite soluble in the mobile phase and less soluble in the stationary phase.

Liquid-solid chromatography uses solid as the stationary phase. The faster-moving compounds are those that are quite soluble in the liquid phase and show little or no affinity for the solid phase.

One specialized form of liquid-solid chromatography is *affinity chromatography*. In this chromatography a specific compound is attached to the solid phase. This attached compound is one to which at least one component in a mixture has great affinity.

We will use the example of separation of enzymes by this method. Subjecting a mixture of enzymes to affinity chromatography allows one enzyme to be retarded or even stopped. (The solid has an attached compound for which one of the enzymes in the mixture has greater affinity. It could even be an antibody.) Then the retarded or bound enzyme (separated) can be eluted by a stronger salt solution.

2. **Spectrophotometry:** Spectrophotometry or colorimetry is an analytical tool that is used in the identification and quantification of light-absorbing compounds. Identification is based on the fact that different compounds absorb light to a greater or lesser extent at different wavelengths. Thus, identification of compounds may often be made by a plot of light absorption against wavelength.

Compounds may often be quantified without actually being separated. Either the compound itself or an appropriate derivative may absorb light at a characteristic wavelength. In that case, the absorbance at that wavelength may be used to measure the amount of the compound.

As an example, both NAD^+ and NADH absorb light at a peak of 260 nm. However, NADH (and not NAD^+) has another absorption peak at 340 nm. Thus the enzymatic conversion of NAD^+ to NADH may be followed by the increase in absorbance at 340 nm.

Spectrophotometry and colorimetry are terms that are often used synonymously. Actually, it is preferable to use colorimetry to refer to absorbance of light that is selected by a filter. The filter will usually produce light that is only somewhat pure (a range of wavelengths). A spectophotometer usually refers to a device in which the light of a particular wavelength is obtained from a prism or a diffraction grating.

If the transmitted light (I) is divided by the incident light striking a sample (I_0), the fraction I/I_0 is called transmittance (T). The Beer-Lambert equation is given as

$$-\log_{10} T = \varepsilon c l$$

where ε is the absorption coefficient, c is the concentration, and l is the path length.

PHYSICS

Test-taking Suggestions for the Physics Portion of the MCAT

The MCAT physics problems are somewhat different from problems that you may have found on college physics tests. The physics questions are alternated with inorganic chemistry questions on the Physical Sciences test, instead of all being grouped together. A sometimes lengthy reading passage will contain information that you need in order to work the 6 to 8 problems that follow the passage. All of the information needed will not always be in the reading passage. Generally, you must understand the *concepts* of physics and the "conservation laws." Topics will encompass nearly all of physics: mechanics, simple harmonic motion, wave motion, heat and gas laws, electricity and magnetism, light and optics, modern physics, and nuclear physics, including radioactive decay. Memorizing hundreds of formulas will be of little benefit. You must practice making simple sketches, especially for problems in mechanics. Many are nearly impossible to work without a sketch to help you understand relationships. In addition to problems associated with specific passages, the test will have "independent" questions unrelated to any passage. The latter may be similar to end-of-chapter problems that you worked in your introductory physics classes. MCAT physics questions may be based on passages that seem to be "nonphysics." One recent set of test questions, involving novae composed of white dwarf stars and an ordinary star, required some understanding of gravitation. Another section included a passage about colliding continents and radioactive dating of rocks with questions on conservation of momentum and Newton's Third Law.

Look for *key words* in the questions. Words like "work," "potential energy," and "kinetic energy," especially when connected with the word "initial" or "final," might require you to use the conservation of mechanical energy principle. If you see the word "collide" or "collision," you will undoubtedly use the conservation of momentum principle and/or Newton's Third Law.

Because calculators are not permitted, you should practice problems like those in this book. Get practice in moving the decimal place in order to make the calculation easier. For example:

$$400 \text{ N} \times 0.35 \text{ millisec} = 0.4 \times 10^3 \text{ N} \times 0.35 \times 10^{-3} \text{ sec} = 0.4 \times 0.35 \text{ N sec}$$

You will probably benefit from using a college physics text to prepare. Your college or university library will have several on the shelves. Note: The words "University Physics" or "for Science and Engineering Students in a title," refer to textbooks that use the calculus. Good luck!

Frequently Encountered Physics Problems and Their Answers

Accelerated Motion

Example: A boat accelerates uniformly from 7 m/sec to 20 m/sec in 10 sec.

1. Calculate acceleration.

$$a = \frac{v_2 - v_1}{t}$$

a = acceleration
v_1 = initial speed *or* velocity
v_2 = final speed *or* velocity
t = time

$$a = \frac{20 \text{ m/sec} - 7 \text{ m/sec}}{10 \text{ sec}} = \frac{13 \text{ m/sec}}{10 \text{ sec}} = 1.3 \text{ m/sec}^2$$

2. Calculate average speed.

$$v = \frac{v_1 + v_2}{2} \qquad v = \text{average velocity}$$

$$v = \frac{7 \text{ m/sec} + 20 \text{ m/sec}}{2} = 13.5 \text{ m/sec}$$

3. Distance covered?

$$s = \text{distance covered}$$
$$s = vt$$
$$s = 13.5 \text{ m/sec} \times 10 \text{ sec} = 135 \text{ m}$$
$$\text{distance covered} = 13.5 \text{ m/sec} \times 10 \text{ sec} = 135 \text{ m}$$

Example: An object is accelerated from rest to 100 km/hr in 30 sec; the object has been subjected to an acceleration of 0.93 m/sec².

A convenient unit for acceleration is meters per second squared (m/sec²). First, convert the velocity units:

$$\frac{100 \text{ km}}{\text{hr}} \times \frac{1000 \text{ m}}{\text{km}} \times \frac{1 \text{ hr}}{3600 \text{ sec}} = 27.8 \text{ m/sec}$$

Then

$$a = \frac{v}{t}$$

$$a = \frac{27.8 \text{ m/sec}}{30 \text{ sec}} = 0.93 \text{ m/sec}^2$$

Another way of expressing this type of phenomenon is to solve a problem as follows:

Example: A car is traveling at a speed of 50 km/hr and accelerates for 10 sec to reach a speed of 65 km/hr. Its rate of acceleration was 1.5 (km/hr)/sec. Mathematically expressed:

$$a = \frac{\text{Final Velocity} - \text{Initial Velocity}}{\text{Time}}$$

$$a = \frac{65 \text{ km/hr} - 50 \text{ km/hr}}{10 \text{ sec}}$$

$$a = \frac{15 \text{ km/hr}}{10 \text{ sec}} = \frac{1.5 \text{ km/hr}}{\text{sec}}$$

Falling Objects—Gravity Acceleration

Recall: $g = 32 \text{ ft/sec}^2$ or 9.8 m/sec^2

Example: An object in free fall travels for 1 sec.

1. Calculate speed (velocity) obtained, when the body is released from rest.

$$v_2 = v_1 + at \qquad\qquad v_1 = \text{initial speed} = 0$$
$$v_2 = 0 + (32 \text{ ft/sec}^2)(1 \text{ sec}) \qquad v_2 = \text{final speed}$$
$$v_2 = 32 \text{ ft/sec} \qquad\qquad a = \text{acceleration}$$
$$\qquad\qquad\qquad\qquad\qquad t = \text{time}$$

2. The above body started from rest; the distance covered in the time was?

$$s = v_1 t + \frac{1}{2} at^2 \qquad\qquad v_1 = \text{initial speed} = 0$$
$$\qquad\qquad\qquad\qquad\qquad t = \text{time}$$
$$s = 0 + \frac{1}{2}(32 \text{ ft/sec}^2)(1 \text{ sec})^2 \qquad s = \text{distance traversed}$$
$$s = 16 \text{ ft} \qquad\qquad\qquad a = \text{acceleration}$$

Example: A rocket traveling upward is going 60 m/sec when its fuel is exhausted.
Then:

1. The distance covered after an additional 1 sec is?

$$s = v_1 t + \frac{1}{2}at^2$$

$$v_1 = 60 \text{ m/sec}$$
$$a = -9.8 \text{ m/sec}^2$$
$$t = 1 \text{ sec}$$

$$s = (60 \text{ m/sec})(1 \text{ sec}) + \frac{1}{2}(-9.8 \text{ m/sec}^2)(1 \text{ sec})^2$$

$$s = 55.1 \text{ m}$$

2. Calculate the speed obtained after 1 sec.

$$v_2 = v_1 + at$$

$$v_2 = 60 \text{ m/sec} + (-9.8 \text{ ft/sec}^2)(1 \text{ sec})$$

$$v_2 = 50.2 \text{ m/sec}$$

v_1 = initial velocity

v_2 = final velocity

a = acceleration

t = time

Example: a. At the end of 1 sec a falling object will attain a velocity of 10 m/sec.

$$v_f = at = 10 \text{ m/sec}^2 \times 1 \text{ sec} = 10 \text{ m/sec} \qquad v_f = \text{final velocity}$$

(using $g = 10 \text{ m/sec}^2$ rather than 9.8 m/sec^2).

b. During this 1 sec of falling, however, an object previously at rest will have covered a distance of 5 m.

$$s = v_0 t + \frac{at^2}{2}$$

$$s = (0 \text{ ft})(1 \text{ sec})$$

$$+ \frac{(10 \text{ m/sec}^2)(1 \text{ sec})^2}{2} = 5 \text{ m}$$

s = distance traversed

v_0 = velocity at rest

= initial velocity = 0

t = time

Uniform Velocity

Example: A car travels with a constant velocity of 30 mi/hr for 40 mi. What time is needed to travel this distance?

$$t = \frac{s}{v}$$

$$t = \frac{40 \text{ mi}}{30 \text{ mi/ hr}}$$

$$t = 1.33 \text{ hr}$$

v = velocity = 30 mi/hr

s = distance traversed = 40 mi

t = time

Nonuniform Motion

Example: A rocket with an initial velocity of 25 m/sec is accelerated at 75 m/sec^2 for 10 sec.

1. The rocket covers a distance of how many meters during the period of acceleration?

$$s = v_0 t + \frac{1}{2}at^2$$

s = distance traversed

$$s = (25 \text{ m/sec})(10 \text{ sec}) + \frac{1}{2}(75 \text{ m/sec}^2)(10 \text{ sec})^2$$

$$s = 250 \text{ m} + \frac{7500 \text{ m}}{2}$$

$$s = 250 \text{ m} + 3750 \text{ m}$$

$$s = 4000 \text{ m}$$

2. How far would the rocket travel if it started from rest?

$$x = \frac{1}{2}(75 \text{ m/sec}^2)(10 \text{ sec})^2$$

$$x = 3750 \text{ m}$$

Uniform Deceleration

Example: A train travels at 70 km/hr; the brakes are applied for 2 sec. and it decelerates at a rate of 30 km/hr/sec. Calculate its final velocity.

$v = v_0 - at$

$v = 70 \text{ km/hr} - 30 \text{ km/hr/sec} \times 2 \text{ sec}$

$v = 10 \text{ km/hr}$

Free Fall

Example: A construction worker drops a brick while working at a height of 300 m.

$$v_0 = 0$$
$$g = 10 \text{ m/sec}^2$$
$$t = 3 \text{ sec}$$
$$y = \text{distance traversed}$$

1. What distance does the brick cover in 3 sec?

$$s = v_0 t + \frac{1}{2} g t^2$$

$$s = \frac{1}{2} g t^2$$

$$s = \frac{1}{2}(10 \text{ m/sec}^2)(3 \text{ sec})^2$$

$$s = 45 \text{ m}$$

2. How long does it take for the brick to land on the ground?

$$s = \frac{1}{2} g t^2$$

$$t = \left(\frac{2s}{g}\right)^{1/2}$$

$$t = \left(\frac{(2)(300 \text{ m})}{10 \text{ m/sec}^2}\right)^{1/2}$$

$$t = (60 \text{ sec}^2)^{1/2}$$

$$t = 7.75 \text{ sec}$$

3. What is the velocity of the brick at 2 sec of travel?

$$v = gt$$

$$v = 10 \text{ m/sec}^2 \times 2$$

$$v = 20 \text{ m/sec}$$

Forces and Motion

Forces and Acceleration

Newton's Second Law: Force = Mass × Acceleration or $f = ma$

Newton's Third Law: For every acting force there exists a reacting force of equal magnitude but in the opposite direction, that is, $F(\text{action}) = F(\text{reaction})$.

$$F = \text{force}$$

$$m = \text{mass}$$

$$a = \text{acceleration}$$

Recall: A unit of force applied is the *newton*; 1 newton is the force that will impart to a 1 kg mass an acceleration of 1 m/sec^2, that is, $1 \text{ N} = 1 \dfrac{\text{kg} \cdot \text{m}}{\text{sec}^2}$

Example: A force of 2000 N is applied to a mass of 250 kg. Calculate the acceleration obtained.

$$a = \frac{F}{m}$$

$$a = \frac{2000 \text{ N}}{250 \text{ kg}}$$

$$a = \frac{2000 \text{ kg m/sec}^2}{250 \text{ kg}} = 8 \text{ m/sec}^2$$

$$a = 8 \text{ m/sec}^2$$

Example: What is the force exerted on the surface of an asteroid by a man of 70-kg mass if the acceleration due to gravity of the asteroid is 2.5 m/s^2?

$$F = mg$$

$$F = 70 \text{ kg} \times 2.5 \text{ m/sec}^2 = 175 \text{ N}$$

(A newton, abbreviated as N, is a unit of force expressed in kilograms × meter/second^2.)

Weight and Acceleration

$$F = \frac{w}{g}a \quad \text{OR} \quad F = ma$$

$$w = mg$$

$F = \text{force}$

$a = \text{acceleration}$

$w = \text{weight}$

$m = \text{mass}$

$g = \text{acceleration due to gravity}$

Example: A force of 130 N is applied to a mass of 20 kg. Calculate the acceleration produced.

$$F = ma$$

$$a = \frac{F}{m} = \frac{130 \text{ N}}{20 \text{ kg}}$$

$$a = \frac{130 \text{ kg m}}{20 \text{ kg sec}^2} = 6.5 \text{ m/sec}^2$$

Example: A 75 kg astronaut is accelerated upward by his rocket at 25 m/sec^2. Calculate the force that the seat exerts on him.

$$F = ma$$

$$F = (75 \text{ kg})(25 \text{ m/sec}^2)$$

$$F = 1875 \text{ N}$$

This is the net accelerating force. The seat is also supporting his weight, so the total force is

$$F = 1875 \text{ N} + mg = 1875 + 75 \ (9.8 \text{ m/sec}^2) = 2610 \text{ N}$$

Example: A 20-kg mass located on a frictionless table is acted upon by a horizontal force of 240 N.

1. Calculate the acceleration of the object.

$$F = ma$$

$$a = \frac{F}{m}$$

$$a = \frac{240 \text{ N}}{20 \text{ kg}}$$

$$a = 12 \text{ m/sec}^2$$

2. Calculate the distance the mass will travel in 10 sec.

$$s = v_0 t + \frac{1}{2} at^2$$

$$s = 0 + \frac{1}{2}(12 \text{ m/sec}^2)(10 \text{ sec})^2$$

$$s = \frac{1200 \text{ m}}{2}$$

$$s = 600 \text{ m}$$

Negative Acceleration

Example: A test vehicle of mass 2000 kg travels at 108 km/hr (30 m/sec). Its stopping distance is 100 m.

1. Calculate the negative acceleration.

$$v^2 = v_0^2 + 2ax$$

$$a = \frac{v^2 - v_0^2}{2x}$$

$$a = \frac{0 - (30 \text{ m/sec})^2}{2(100 \text{ m})}$$

$$a = 4.5 \text{ m/sec}^2$$

2. What force is required to stop the vehicle?

$$F = ma$$

$$F = (2000 \text{ kg}) \times (-4.5 \text{ m/sec})$$

$$F = -9000 \text{ N}$$

Example: A crane is lowering a 5000 kg air conditioning unit, and the tension in the cable is 40,000 N as the unit *begins* to go downward.

1. Net force on the unit?
The weight of the unit is

$$w = mg = (5000 \text{ kg})\left(\frac{9.8 \text{ m}}{s^2}\right) = 49,000 \text{ N}$$

So the net downward force is

$$49,000 \text{ N} - 40,000 \text{ N} = 9000 \text{ N}$$

2. Acceleration of unit?

$$a = \frac{F}{m} = \frac{9000 \text{ N}}{5000 \text{ kg}} = 1.8 \text{ m/sec}^2$$

3. How long will it take the unit to reach a speed of 4 m/sec?

$$t = \frac{v}{a} = \frac{4 \text{ m/sec}}{1.8 \text{ m/sec}^2} = 2.2 \text{ sec}$$

Resultant Forces

a. Forces Acting Upon Each Other at Right Angles.

Example: If a force of 3 N and a force of 4 N acted upon each other at right angles, the resultant would be 5 N. The answer is obtained by utilizing the formula:

$$R = \sqrt{(\text{Force 1})^2 + (\text{Force 2})^2}$$

Thus,

$$R = \sqrt{(3 \text{ N})^2 + (4 \text{ N})^2}$$
$$R = \sqrt{25 \text{ N}^2}$$
$$R = 5 \text{ N}$$

b. Forces Acting in the Same Direction.

Example: The resultant of two forces of 3 N and 10 N acting in the same direction is 13 N. Any combination of forces acting upon the same object in the same direction will result in an addition of the forces and the result will be equal to the sum of the forces.

Equilibrium States

An object is in equilibrium when all forces on it add to zero.

Example: An instrument weighing 35 N is placed in a stream, suspended by a rope that makes an angle of 40° with the vertical. A scale inserted in the rope reads 28 N. Find the force of buoyancy and the force exerted on the instrument by the current.

1. Determine the vertical and horizontal components of the tension in the rope.

$$T_{\text{vert}} = (28 \text{ N})(\cos 40°) = 21 \text{ N}$$
$$T_{\text{hor}} = (28 \text{ N})(\sin 40°) = 18 \text{ N}$$

2. Set all upward forces equal to all downward forces.

$$\text{Weight} = \text{Buoyancy } (B) + \text{Upward Component}$$
$$B = 35 \text{ N} - 21 \text{ N} = 14 \text{ N}$$

3. Set upstream forces equal to downstream forces.

$$\text{Horizontal Component} = \text{Current Force } (C)$$
$$C = 18 \text{ N}$$

Example: A 28-kg packing case is on a ramp inclined at 25° to the horizontal, and is pulled uphill at constant speed with a force of 160 N. Determine the coefficient of friction.

1. Determine the weight of the case.

$$w = mg = (28 \text{ kg})(9.8 \text{ m/sec}^2) = 247 \text{ N}$$

2. Find the components of the weight parallel and perpendicular to the ramp.

$$W_{\text{par}} = (274 \text{ N})(\sin 25°) = 116 \text{ N}$$
$$W_{\text{perp}} = (274 \text{ N})(\cos 25°) = 248 \text{ N}$$

3. Find the friction by setting uphill forces equal to downhill forces.

$$160 \text{ N} = 116 \text{ N} + F$$
$$F = 44 \text{ N}$$

4. Find the coefficient of friction.

$$\mu = \frac{\text{friction}}{\text{normal force}} = \frac{44 \text{ N}}{248 \text{ N}} = 0.18$$

Projectile Motion

$$v = \text{initial velocity}$$
$$\theta = \text{angle with horizontal}$$
$$v_h = \text{horizontal component of path} = v \cos \theta$$
$$v_v = \text{vertical component of path} = v \sin \theta$$

Example: A cannonball with initial speed of 60 m/sec with a 30° horizontal projection.

1. Determine the height the ball reaches. Look up the sine and cosine in a standard table or use a scientific calculator.

$$\sin 30° = 0.5; \quad v_v = v \sin \theta = (60 \text{ m/sec})(\sin 30°) = 30 \text{ m/sec}$$
$$\cos 30° = 0.866; \quad v_h = v \cos \theta = (60 \text{ m/sec})(\cos 30°) = 52 \text{ m/sec}$$

Utilize the equation for the vertical motion:

$$v_f^2 - v_i^2 = 2as \qquad v_i = 30 \text{ m/sec}$$
$$v_f = 0$$
$$a = -9.8 \text{ m/sec}$$

Thus we have:

$$0 - (30 \text{ m/sec})^2 = 2(-9.8 \text{ m/sec}^2)s$$
$$s = \frac{900 \text{ m/sec}^2}{19.6 \text{ m/sec}^2}$$
$$s = 46 \text{ m}$$

2. Calculate the time necessary to reach maximum height.

$$v_f - v_i = at$$
$$0 - 30 \text{ m/sec} = (-9.8 \text{ m/sec}^2)t$$
$$t = \frac{30 \text{ m/sec}}{9.8 \text{ m/sec}^2} = 3.1 \text{ sec}$$

3. The ball will return to the earth in what time? If 3.06 sec are used for ascending, $2t$ should be required. The answer is 6.12 sec.

4. Determine the horizontal range (R) of the ball.

$$R = v_h t$$
$$R = (52 \text{ m/sec})(6.12 \text{ sec})$$
$$R = 318 \text{ m}$$

Friction

$$\text{Formula } \mu = \frac{F}{N_p} \qquad \mu = \text{coefficient of friction}$$
$$F = \text{frictional force}$$
$$N_p = \text{normal or perpendicular force}$$

Example: A 10,000 N force draws a 130,000 N railroad car at constant speed on level terrain.

1. Determine the coefficient of friction.

$$\mu = \frac{F}{N_p}$$
$$\mu = \frac{10,000 \text{ N}}{130,000 \text{ N}} = 0.077$$

(The coefficient of friction is the ratio of the frictional force to the perpendicular force N_p pressing the two surfaces together.)

2. The railroad car is pulled on a horizontal track at constant speed by a steel cable that makes a 30° angle above the horizontal. The tension in the cable is 1400 N. Determine the coefficient of friction.

$$F \text{ (parallel frictional force)} = F = 1400 \text{ N} \times \cos 30°$$
$$= 1400 \text{ N} \times 0.866$$
$$= 1212 \text{ N}$$

The normal force N—which is the weight of the car—is 130,000 N. However, the vertical component of tension must be subtracted from it.

$$N = 130,000 - 1400 \times \sin 30°$$
$$= 130,000 \text{ N} - 700 \text{ N}$$
$$= 129,300 \text{ N}$$
$$\mu = \frac{F}{N}$$
$$\mu = \frac{1212 \text{ N}}{129,300 \text{ N}}$$
$$\mu = 0.009$$

Work and Power

Work (W) equals the force (F) times the displacement (d) in the direction of the force, that is, $W = Fd$.

Example: A machine is pushed 30 m on a level floor. The frictional force is determined as 10,000 N. Calculate the work performed.

$$W = Fd$$
$$W = (10,000 \text{ N})(30 \text{ m})$$
$$W = 300,000 \text{ N} \cdot \text{m}$$
$$= 300,000 \text{ J}$$

Recall: The work-energy unit, Joule is: $1 \text{ J} = 1 \text{ N} \cdot \text{m}$

Example: Instead of being pushed, the above machine is dragged via a steel cable at an angle of 30° with the floor and with a force on the cable of 10,000 N. The work performed is?

$$W = (F \cos 30°)d$$
$$W = 10,000 \text{ N} \times 0.866 \times 30 \text{ m}$$
$$W = 259,800 \text{ J}$$

Work and Energy

Example: A man pushes his snowblower with a constant force of 50 lb. The shaft makes an angle of 45° with the horizontal. The work done by the man in 150 ft is?

$$W = Fd \cos 45°$$
$$W = (50 \text{ lb})(150 \text{ ft})(0.707)$$
$$W = 5300 \text{ ft-lb}$$

Power and Power Units

$$\text{Power} = \frac{\text{Work}}{\text{Time}} \text{ or } P = \frac{W}{t}$$

Units: 1 watt $= 10^7$ ergs/sec $= 1$ Joule/sec

1 horsepower (hp) $= 500$ ft-lb/sec $= 746$ watts

1 kilowatt $= 1000$ watts $= 1.34$ hp

Example: By means of its steel pulleys, a crane raises a machine weighing 2200 N to a height of 30 m in 200 sec. The average horsepower necessary is?

$$P = \frac{W}{t}$$

$$P = \frac{\text{Force} \times \text{Distance}}{\text{Time}}$$

$$P = \frac{(2200 \text{ N})(30 \text{ m})}{200s} = 330 \text{ J/sec}$$

$$P = 330 \text{ watts}$$

$$P = 330 \text{ watts} \times \frac{1 \text{ hp}}{746 \text{ watts}}$$

$$P = 0.44 \text{ hp}$$

Example: A man of mass 80 kg is taking a stress test. The test equals the activity of climbing stairs a vertical distance of 10 m in 5 sec. Calculate the horsepower he develops.

$$P = \frac{W}{t} = \frac{(mg)y}{t} = \frac{(80 \text{ kg})(9.8 \text{ m/sec}^2)(10 \text{ m})}{5 \text{ sec}}$$

$$P = 1568 \text{ kg} \cdot \frac{m^2}{\text{sec}}$$

$$P = 1568 \text{ watts}$$

$$P = 1568 \text{ watts} \times \frac{1 \text{ hp}}{746 \text{ watts}}$$

$$P = 2.1 \text{ hp}$$

Example: To take the MCAT examination you must climb stairs to a height of 60 ft, and you weigh 180 lb. The work you do against the force of gravity is 10,800 ft-lb.

$$W = F \times D$$

$$W = 180 \text{ lb} \times 60 \text{ ft} = 10,800 \text{ ft-lb}$$

Energy

Potential Energy

Potential energy (*PE*)—or energy of position—is the product of the weight (*w*) of an object and the height (*h*) to which the object is elevated, or the work done in elevating it: $PE = wh$.

Example: A machine weighing 23,000 N is raised onto the roof of a building 50 m high. Calculate the increase in potential energy or the work done in lifting the machine.

$$PE = wh$$

$$PE = (23,000 \text{ N})(50 \text{ m})$$

$$PE = 1,150,000 \text{ J}$$

Kinetic Energy

Kinetic energy = energy of motion.

Formulas: 1. $KE = \dfrac{1}{2} mu^2$ $\qquad$ $KE = J$

2. $KE = \dfrac{1}{2} mv^2$

Example: Determine the kinetic energy of a locomotive with mass of 110,000 kg and traveling at a speed of 50 km/hr (13.9 m/sec).

$$KE = \dfrac{1}{2} mu^2$$

$$KE = \dfrac{1}{2}(110,000 \text{ kg})(13.9 \text{ m/sec})^2$$

$$KE = 10,723,000 \text{ J}$$

Recall: The joule (J) is a unit of energy. It is a N · m, the work done by a force of 1 N through a distance of 1 m. It is the heat produced by an ampere flowing against an ohm for one second. One joule is equal to 10^7 ergs, and 4.185 J are equal to one calorie.

Example: A rocket with a mass of 2000 kg is fired vertically upward with an initial velocity of 100 m/s.
1. Calculate the change in kinetic energy at maximum height reached.

$$\Delta K = K - K_0 \qquad\qquad K = \text{kinetic energy at maximum}$$
$$\text{height} = 0$$

$$-K_0 = -\dfrac{1}{2} mv_0^2 \qquad\qquad K_0 = \text{initial kinetic energy}$$
$$V_0 = \text{initial velocity}$$

$$-K_0 = -\dfrac{1}{2}(2000 \text{ kg})(100 \text{ m/sec})^2$$

$$\Delta K = -K_0 = -10,000,000 \text{ J}$$

Answer: At maximum height reached, the rocket has lost 10,000,000 J of kinetic energy.

2. Calculate the potential energy at maximum height, and the change in kinetic energy upon return to lift-off point.

a. $\quad v^2 = v_0^2 - 2gy$ $\qquad\qquad v_0 = \text{initial velocity}$

$$y = \dfrac{v_0^2}{2g} \qquad\qquad\qquad y = \text{maximum height}$$

$$g = \text{gravitational acceleration}$$

$$y = \dfrac{(100 \text{ m/sec})^2}{2(9.8 \text{ m/sec}^2)}$$

$$y = \dfrac{10,000 \text{ m}^2/\text{sec}^2}{19.6 \text{ m/sec}^2}$$

$$y = 510 \text{ m}$$

b. $PE = mgh$

$PE = (2000 \text{ kg})(9.8 \text{ m/sec}^2)(510 \text{ m})$

$PE = 10,000,000 \text{ J}$

The increase in potential energy, then, is 10,000,000 J, and one can deduce that the rocket returns to its lift-off point with the same velocity it had at the beginning. The rocket had lost 10,000,000 J of kinetic energy on the original flight, but gained this amount in potential energy and, therefore, the total change in energy was zero. The KE and PE balance each other and are constant; the principle of conservation of energy is demonstrated.

Momentum

Momentum is the product of the mass and velocity of an object:

$$p = mv \qquad p = \text{momentum}$$
$$m = \text{mass}$$
$$v = \text{velocity}$$

The change of momentum is equal to the force applied times time.

Example: A 80 kg man is shot out of a cannon at the speed of 10 m/sec. What is his momentum?

$$p = mv$$
$$p = (80 \text{ kg})(10 \text{ m/sec})$$
$$p = 800 \text{ kg} \cdot \text{m/sec}$$

Example: On landing, a plane is traveling at 100 km/hr. Brakes are applied, and the plane comes to a stop in 10 sec. Assuming the average mass to be 70 kg, what is the force of the seat belts on each passenger? (100 km/hr = 28 m/sec)

Step 1. Calculate the change in momentum.

$$p = -mv_0$$
$$p = -70 \text{ kg} (28 \text{ m/sec})$$
$$p = -1960 \text{ kg} \cdot \text{m/sec}$$

Step 2. Now calculate the force applied by the seat belt on a passenger.

$$F = \frac{p}{t}$$
$$F = -\frac{1960 \text{ kg m}}{(10 \text{ sec}) \text{ sec}}$$
$$F = -\frac{196 \text{ kgm}}{\text{sec}^2}$$
$$= -196 \text{ N}$$

Uniform Circular Motion

Centripetal Acceleration

Example: A subway car traveling at a speed of 50 km/hr (14 m/sec) negotiates a curve whose radius is 200 m. What is its acceleration?

$$a = \frac{v^2}{r} \qquad \begin{aligned} a &= \text{acceleration} \\ v &= \text{velocity} \\ r &= \text{radius} \end{aligned}$$

$$a = \frac{(14 \text{ m/sec})^2}{200 \text{ m}}$$
$$a = \frac{196 \text{ m}^2/\text{sec}^2}{200 \text{ m}}$$
$$a = 0.98 \text{ m/sec}^2$$

Circular Motion

Recall: $\dfrac{360°}{2\pi} = 1 \text{ rad} = 57.3°$

$360° = 2\pi \text{ rad}; \ 180° = \pi \text{ rad}; \ 90° = \dfrac{\pi}{2}\text{rad}$

The radian is a unit of measurement equal to the angle obtained at the center of a circle making an arc equal to the length of the radius.

Example: An airplane has its automatic pilot fly a circular route at a constant speed of 100 km/hr. The route has a diameter of 3000 m.

1. Calculate the plane's angular speed.

$$\omega = \frac{v}{r}$$

$$\omega = \frac{27.8 \text{ m/sec}}{1500 \text{ m}}$$

$$\omega = 0.0186 \text{ rad/sec}$$

ω = angular speed

v = velocity = 100 km/hr = 27.8 m/sec

d = diameter = 3000 m

r = radius = $\dfrac{d}{2}$ = 1500 m

2. Calculate the angular distance and the arc length flown in 45 sec.

$$\text{Angular distance } \theta = wt$$

$$\theta = (0.0186 \text{ rad/sec})(45 \text{ sec})$$

$$\theta = 0.837 \text{ rad}$$

$$\text{Arc length } s = r\theta$$

$$s = (1500 \text{ m})(0.837)$$

$$s = 1256 \text{ m}$$

OR

$$s = vt$$

$$s = (27.8 \text{ m/sec})(45 \text{ sec})$$

$$s = 1251 \text{ m}$$

Centripetal Force

Centripetal force may be expressed as mass times velocity squared divided by the radius, that is, $F_c = \dfrac{mv^2}{r}$.

Example: The previously cited subway car has a mass of 130,000 kg, travels at 50 km/hr, (14 m/sec) and rounds the above radius of 200 m. Its centripetal force is?

$$F_c = \frac{mv^2}{r}$$

v = 14 m/sec

r = 200 m

$$F_c = 130,000 \text{ kg} \times \frac{(14 \text{ m/sec})^2}{200 \text{ m}}$$

$$F_c = 127,400 \text{ N}$$

Example: A satellite is in circular orbit at an altitude of 5.0×10^2 km. One complete revolution takes 95 minutes.

1. Calculate the tangential velocity.

Radius of earth = 6400 m

Radius of orbit, $r = 6400$ km $+ 500$ km $= 6900$ km, or 6.9×10^6 m

$$v = \frac{s}{t} = \frac{2\pi r}{t} = \frac{2\pi(6.9 \times 10^6 \text{ m})}{5700 \text{ s}} = 7600 \text{ m/s}$$

2. Calculate the angular speed

$$\omega = \frac{\theta}{t} = \frac{2\pi}{5700 \text{ s}} = 1.10 \times 10^{-3} \text{ rad/s}$$

To get the tangential speed from this:

$$v = r\omega = (6.9 \times 10^6 \text{ m})(1.10 \times 10^{-3} \text{ rad/s}) = 7600 \text{ m/s}$$

3. Calculate the centripetal acceleration, due to gravity:

$$a_c = \frac{v^2}{r} = \frac{(7600 \text{ m/sec})^2}{6.9 \times 10^6 \text{ m}} = 8.4 \text{ m/sec}^2$$

Example: An astronaut with a mass of 75 kg is being spun in a centrifuge with a radius of 40 m at a speed of 26 m/sec. What is the centripetal force on the astronaut?

$$F_c = \frac{mv^2}{r}$$

$$F = \frac{(75 \text{ kg})(26 \text{ m/sec})^2}{40 \text{ m}}$$

$$F = 1268 \text{ N}$$

(Astronaut weights 735 N)

Centrifugal Force

$$F_r = \frac{mv^2}{r}$$

Example: A 0.5-kg object is traveling in a circular orbit 20 m in diameter at a speed of 2 m/sec. The cord is subjected to a force of 0.2 N. What is the centrifugal force *on the cord*?

$$F_r = \frac{mv^2}{r} = \frac{(0.5 \text{ kg})(2 \text{ m/sec})^2}{10 \text{ m}} = 0.2 \text{ N}$$

Since the mass is expressed in kilograms, velocity in meters per second, and distance in meters, the unit of force will be the newton. Note that the diameter of the circle was given, but the radius is required in the equation.

Fluids at Rest

Pressure

$$P = \frac{F}{A}$$

P = Pressure
F = Force
A = Area

Example: The end of a pillar of a building has an area of 400 in². The air hammer applies a force of 600 lb as the pillar is driven into the ground. What is the pressure under the pillar?

$$P = \frac{F}{A}$$

$$P = \frac{600 \text{ lb}}{400 \text{ in}^2}$$

$$P = 1.5 \text{ lb/in}^2$$

Example: A man has a mass of 75 kg; his shoes have a surface area of 84 cm^2 (84×10^{-4} m^2), and therefore, the pressure exerted because of his weight. The formula to be employed is:

$$P = \frac{mg}{A} = \frac{(75 \text{ kg})(9.8 \text{ m/sec}^2)}{84 \times 10^{-4} \text{ m}^2}$$

$$P = 87,500 \frac{\text{N}}{\text{m}^2}$$

Density

Density is the mass per unit volume of a substance.

$P = hdg$ $P =$ pressure

$h =$ height

$d =$ density

$g =$ acceleration due to gravity

Example: A tank $10 \times 10 \times 10$ ft is filled with gasoline (weight-density 42 lb/ft^3). Weight density $d_w = dg$.

1. Calculate the pressure at the bottom of the tank in lb/ft^2 and lb/in^2.

$$P = hd_w$$
$$P = 10 \text{ ft} \times 42 \text{ lb/ft}^3$$
$$P = 420 \text{ lb/ft}^2$$
$$P = \frac{420 \text{ lb/ft}^2}{144 \text{ in}^2/\text{ft}^2}$$
$$P = 2.92 \text{ lb/in}^2$$

2. Calculate the force at the bottom of the tank.

$$P = \frac{F}{A}$$
$$F = PA$$
$$F = (420 \text{ lb/ft}^2)(100 \text{ ft}^2)$$
$$F = 42,000 \text{ lb}$$

Example: Find the pressure due to a column of mercury 100 cm high.

$P = hdg$ $h = 100$ cm $= 1.0$ m

$P = (1.0 \text{ m})(13,600 \text{ kg/m}^3)(9.8 \text{ m/sec}^2)$ $d = 13.6$ g/cm^3 (given) $= 13,600$ kg/m^3

$P = 133,280 \dfrac{\text{Newtons}}{\text{m}^2}$ $g = 9.8 \dfrac{\text{m}}{\text{sec}^2}$

Specific Gravity

$$\text{Specific Gravity} = \frac{d}{d_?}$$

$d =$ density of a substance

$d_? =$ density of standard substance, usually water (d_w)

Example: A metal bar is suspended from a spring scale that reads 900 gm in air and 600 gm when submerged in water.

1. Calculate the specific gravity.

$$\text{Specific Gravity} = \frac{\text{Weight in Air}}{\text{Weight Lost in Water}} = \frac{900 \text{ gm}}{900 - 600 \text{ gm}}$$

$$\text{Specific Gravity} = \frac{900}{300} = 3$$

Specific Gravity = 3

2. Calculate the density of the metal.

$$d_w = \frac{1 \text{ gm}}{\text{cm}^3}$$

$$d = \text{Specific Gravity} \times d_w$$

$$d = 3\left(1\frac{\text{gm}}{\text{cm}^3}\right)$$

$$d = 3\frac{\text{gm}}{\text{cm}^3} = 3000\frac{\text{kg}}{\text{m}^3}$$

Buoyancy

Example: A balloon on a transatlantic flight is operating where the density of air is 0.8 kg/m³. It weighs 1300 N, has a volume of 225 m³, and is filled with helium, with a d of 0.176 kg/m³. What load can it support?

Step 1. $w = Vdg$ $w = \text{weight} = mg$

$V = \text{volume}$

$d = \text{density}$

Weight of Air Displaced = 225 m³ × 0.8 kg/m³ × 9.8 m/sec² = 1764 N

Weight of Helium = 225 m³ × 0.176 kg/m³ × 9.8 m/sec² = 388 N

Weight of Balloon = 1300 N

Step 2. $L = w_a - w_h - w_b$ L = load balloon can support

$L = 1764 \text{ N} - 388 \text{ N} - 1300 \text{ N}$ w_a = weight of air displaced

$L = 76 \text{ N}$ w_h = weight of helium

w_b = weight of balloon

The load the balloon can support is 76 N.

Gravity

All objects in the universe attract each other with a force equal to

$$F_{\text{grav}} = \frac{Gm_1m_2}{r^2}$$

where m_1 and m_2 are the two masses, r is the distance between them, and G is the universal constant of gravitation, equal to 6.67×10^{-11} N · m²/kg².

Example: What is the force of attraction between a 10-metric-ton wrecking ball and a 50-kg man if they are 6 m apart?

$$F = \frac{(6.67 \times 10^{-11} \text{ N} \cdot \text{m}^2/\text{kg}^2)(10 \times 10^3 \text{ kg})(50 \text{ kg})}{(6 \text{ m})^2} = 9 \times 10^{-7} \text{ N}$$

Example: What is the mass of the earth? The force on 1 kg at the surface (6400 km from the center) is 9.8 N.

$$m_2 = \frac{Fr^2}{Gm_1} = \frac{(9.8 \text{ N})(6.4 \times 10^6 \text{ M})^2}{(6.67 \times 10^{-11} \text{ N} \cdot \text{m}^2/\text{kg})(1 \text{ kg})} = 6.0 \times 10^{24} \text{ kg}$$

Temperature Calculations and Measurement

Recall:

	Freezing Point	Boiling Point of Water
Celsius	0°	100°
Fahrenheit	32°	212°
Kelvin	273	373

Formulas: $\quad C = \dfrac{5}{9} \times (F - 32°)$

$$F = \frac{9}{5}C + 32°$$

Example: A Celsius thermometer records a temperature of 37°C in a patient. What is the temperature on the Fahrenheit scale?

$$F = \frac{9}{5} \times 37° + 32°$$

$$F = 66.6° + 32°$$

$$F = 98.6°F$$

Example: An indoor arena is kept at a temperature of 72°F. What is the corresponding reading on the Celsius scale?

$$C = \frac{5}{9} \times (72° - 32°)$$

$$C = \frac{5}{9} \times 40°$$

$$C = 22°C$$

Absolute Scale: Absolute zero (0 on the Kelvin scale) is the theoretical temperature at which all molecular motion ceases. The Kelvin scale, therefore, has no negative degrees. Celsius temperatures can be expressed on the Kelvin scale ($K = 273 + C$).

Example: 40°C and −40°C can be expressed on the Kelvin scale as follows:

    a. $K = 273 + 40$

         $K = 313$ K

    b. $K = 273 + (-40)$

         $K = 233$ K

Heat

Heat is expressed in Joules, calories, or British thermal units. One British thermal unit is the heat required to raise the temperature of one pound of water one Fahrenheit degree. One calorie (cal) is the heat necessary to raise the temperature of one gram of water one Celsius degree. However, it requires 4186 J of heat to raise the temperature of 1 kg of water one Celsius degree. The "big" Calorie used in nutrition is a *kilocalorie*. (1 Cal = 4186 J and 1 "little" cal = 4.186 J.)

Specific Heat

Example: How much heat is required to raise the temperature of 5 kg of ethylene glycol (2200 J/Kg·°C) from 20 to 60°C?

$$H = ms\Delta t \qquad\qquad \text{where } m = \text{mass}$$
$$s = \text{specific heat}$$
$$\Delta t = \text{temperature change}$$

$$H = (5 \text{ kg})(2000 \text{ J/kg} \cdot {}^\circ\text{C})(60^\circ - 20^\circ \text{C})$$
$$= (5 \text{ kg})(2000 \text{ J/kg} \cdot {}^\circ\text{C})(40^\circ \text{C})$$
$$= 440,000 \text{ J}$$

Heat Lost = Heat Gained

Example: 15 kg of steel at 150°C are cooled in 22 kg of water at 40°C. The final temperature obtained in the water is 47°C. Calculate the specific heat of steel. (Remember that the heat lost by the steel equals the heat gained by the water.)

M_B = mass of first object (steel)
S_B = specific heat of first object
Δt_B = initial temperature of first of object − final temperature of first object
M_W = mass of second object (water)
S_W = specific heat of second object (4186 J/kg·°C)
Δt_W = final temperature of second object − initial temperature of second object

$$M_B S_B \Delta t_B = M_W S_W \Delta t_W$$
$$(15 \text{ kg}) S_B (150^\circ\text{C} - 47^\circ\text{C}) = (22 \text{ kg})(4186 \text{ J/kg} \cdot {}^\circ\text{C})(47^\circ - 40^\circ\text{C})$$
$$S_B = (22 \text{ kg})(4186 \text{ J/kg} \cdot {}^\circ\text{C})(7^\circ\text{C})/(15 \text{ kg})(103^\circ\text{C})$$
$$= 420 \text{ J/kg} \cdot {}^\circ\text{C}$$

Heat of Vaporization

Example: How much heat is necessary to change 200 gm of ice at −12°C to steam at 100°C? The specific heat of ice = 0.51 cal/gm · °C; the heat of fusion of ice = 80 cal/gm; specific heat of water = 1.0 cal/gm · °C; and heat of vaporization of water = 540 cal/gm.

Step 1. Heat required to raise the temperature of ice to the melting point

$$= M_i s_i (0^\circ\text{C} - 12 \,{}^\circ\text{C})$$
$$= 200 \text{ gm } (0.51 \text{ cal/gm} \cdot {}^\circ\text{C})(12^\circ\text{C})$$
$$= 1224 \text{ cal}$$

Step 2. Heat required to melt ice

$$= 200 \text{ gm } (80 \text{ cal/gm})$$
$$= 16,000 \text{ cal}$$

Step 3. Heat required to bring water to its boiling point

$$= (200 \text{ gm})\left(1 \frac{\text{cal}}{\text{gm} \, {}^\circ\text{C}}\right)(100 - \text{C}^\circ)$$
$$= 20,000 \text{ calories}$$

Step 4. Heat required to vaporize water

$$= 200 \text{ gm } (540 \text{ cal/gm})$$
$$= 108,000 \text{ cal}$$

Step 5. Total heat required:

$$1,224 \text{ cal}$$
$$16,000 \text{ cal}$$
$$20,000 \text{ cal}$$
$$\underline{108,000 \text{ cal}}$$
$$146,448 \text{ cal}$$

Thermodynamics

Work and Heat

The following conversion values of mechanical energy to heat should be utilized:

$$4.18 \text{ J equals 1 cal}$$
$$1 \text{ J equals 0.239 cal}$$
$$778 \text{ ft-lb equals 1 Btu}$$
$$1055 \text{ J equals 1 Btu}$$

$$W = J \text{ (constant) } H \qquad W = \text{work}$$
$$J = \text{constant}$$
$$H = \text{heat}$$

Example: Water drops 90 m over the horseshoe falls at Niagara. Calculate the rise in temperature of the water if its potential energy were converted into heat.

Step 1. Energy transformed per kg of water

$$w = mgh$$
$$= (1 \text{ kg})(9.8 \text{ m/sec}^2)(90 \text{ m})$$
$$= 882 \text{ J}$$

Step 2. Heat produced

$$= 882 \text{ J}$$

Step 3. Rise in temperature:

Δt = rise (change) in temperature

H = heat change in material

M = mass (1 kg of water)

S = energy or units of work (Btu), or the specific heat of a substance

(heat /unit mass -degree change in temperature)

$$= 4186 \frac{J}{kg \cdot °C}$$

$$= \Delta t = \frac{H}{MS}$$

$$= \Delta t = \frac{882 \text{ J}}{(1 \text{ kg})\left(4186 \dfrac{J}{kg \cdot °C} \right)}$$

$$\Delta t = 0.21°C$$

Example: A compressed gas at a constant pressure of 75 lb/in^2 enters a cylinder 2 in diameter and pushes a piston 5 in. The work done by the gas is?

$$W = P\Delta V \qquad\qquad P = 75 \text{ lb/in}^2$$
$$W = (75 \text{ lb/in}^2)(5\pi \text{ in}^3) \qquad \Delta V = \pi r^2 s$$
$$W = 1200 \text{ in-lb} \qquad\qquad = \pi(1.0 \text{ in})^2 \times 5 \text{ in}$$
$$W = 100 \text{ ft-lb} \qquad\qquad = 5\pi \text{ in}^3$$

Efficiency of a Boiler

Recall: The maximum efficiency of a heat engine supplied with heat at temperature T_1 and delivering heat to a reservoir at temperature T_2 can be calculated as follows:

$$E = \frac{T_1 - T_2}{T_1} = 1 - \frac{T_2}{T_1}$$

Example: An engine driven by a boiler receives steam at 300°C. Its exhaust temperature is 100°C. Its efficiency is?

$$E = \frac{T_1 - T_2}{T_1}$$
$$E = \frac{(300 + 273)\text{K} - (100 + 273)\text{K}}{(300 + 273)\text{K}}$$
$$E = \frac{573 \text{ K} - 373 \text{ K}}{573 \text{ K}}$$
$$E = 0.349$$
$$E = 34.9\%$$

Example: A heat engine removes 6000 J per cycle of heat energy from the heat chamber and exhausts 1000 J to a cold chamber.

1. What is the thermal efficiency of the engine?

$$E = 1 - \frac{T_{cold}}{T_{hot}} \text{ or } \frac{Q_{cold}}{Q_{hot}}$$
$$E = 1 - \frac{1000 \text{ J}}{6000 \text{ J}}$$
$$E = 1 - 0.17$$
$$E = 83\%$$

2. What is the work done by the engine?

$$W = Q_{hot} - Q_{cold}$$
$$W = 6000 \text{ J} - 1000 \text{ J}$$
$$W = 5000 \text{ J}$$

Electrostatics

The Electric Force

A positive and a negative charge attract each other; two similar charges repel each other. The force is given by Coulomb's Law:

$$F_{elec} = \frac{kq_1q_2}{r^2}$$

where q_1 and q_2 are electric charges in coulombs (C), r is the distance between them, and k is the electric constant of free space, equal to $9.0 \times 10^9 \text{ N} \cdot \text{m}^2/\text{C}^2$.

Example: What is the electric force between two plastic spheres, carrying charges of 20 nC and 12 nC, respectively, if they are 15 cm apart? (1 nC $= 10^{-9}$ C)

$$F = \frac{(9.0 \times 10^9 \text{N} \cdot \text{m}^2/\text{C}^2)(20 \times 10^{-9}\text{C})(12 \times 10^{-9}\text{C})}{(0.15 \text{ m})^2} = 9.6 \times 10^{-5} \text{ N}$$

Since the charges are alike, the force is a force of repulsion.

The Quantum of Charge

All electric charges are integral multiples of the charge on an electron, 1.60×10^{-19} C. Example: How many electrons are there in a charge of 12 nC?

$$\frac{12 \times 10^{-9}\text{C}}{1.60 \times 10^{-19}\text{C}} = 7.5 \times 10^{10}$$

Electric Field

A positive charge in an electric field experiences a force in the direction of the field; a negative charge gets a force in the opposite direction. The magnitude of the force is

$$F_{\text{elec}} = \mathscr{E}q$$

where $\mathscr{E}$ is the electric field in newtons per coulomb.

Example: How strong an electric field will exert a force of 2.0×10^{-16} N on the electron?

$$\mathscr{E} = \frac{F_{\text{elec}}}{q} = \frac{2.0 \times 10^{-16} \text{ N}}{1.60 \times 10^{-19} \text{ C}} = 1250 \text{ N/C}$$

Example: How strong is the field at a distance of 3 cm from a point charge of 20 μC? The field is the force per coulomb of charge in the field. From Coulomb's law

$$\frac{F}{q} = \frac{kq_1}{r^2} = \frac{(9.0 \times 10^9 \text{ N} \cdot \text{m}^2/\text{C}^2)(20 \times 10^{-6}\text{C})}{(0.03 \text{ m})^2} = 20 \times 10^6 \text{N/C}$$

which is the electric field strength.

Electric Potential Difference

The electric potential difference between two points in an electric field is the energy change in moving a unit charge from one point to the other. The unit is the joule per coulomb, called a volt (V).

$$V = \frac{E_{\text{elec}}}{q}$$

Example: The potential difference between the terminals of an automobile battery is 12 V. If the battery is charged using 1800 J of energy, how much charge is transferred from one terminal to the other?

$$q = \frac{E_{\text{elec}}}{V} = \frac{1800 \text{ J}}{12 \text{ V}} = 150 \text{ C}$$

Example: In a uniform electric field of 650 N/C, what is the potential difference between two points that are 20 cm apart in the direction of the field?

1. Determine the force on a coulomb in the field.

$$F = \mathscr{E}q = (650 \text{ N/C})(1 \text{ C}) = 650 \text{ N}$$

2. Determine the work done in moving the charge.

$$W = Fs = (650 \text{ N})(0.20 \text{ m}) = 130 \text{ J}$$

This is the electric energy difference between the points.

3. Determine the potential difference.

$$V = \frac{E_{elec}}{q} = \frac{130 \text{ J}}{1 \text{ C}} = 130 \text{ V}$$

Electricity

Ohm's Law

In a metal conductor at constant temperature, the ratio of the voltage to the current is a constant, that is,

$$R(\text{a constant}) = \frac{V}{I}$$

The constant is called resistance, measured in ohms = volts per ampere.

Example: The difference in potential between two terminals is 10 volts. A current of 5 A passes; calculate the resistance.

$$R = \frac{V}{I}$$

$$R = \frac{10 \text{ volts}}{5 \text{ A}}$$

$$R = 2 \text{ ohms}$$

Example: Increase the difference of the above potential to 20 volts. Calculate the current that passes. Remember that according to Ohm's Law, the resistance (R) will remain the same when the voltage is increased—it is constant.

$$R = \frac{V}{R}$$

$$I = \frac{20 \text{ volts}}{2 \text{ ohms}}$$

$$I = 10 \text{ A}$$

Example: A motor needs a current of 8 A and has a resistance of 40 ohms. What voltage is necessary for the operation?

$$V = IR$$

$$V = 8 \text{ A} \times 40 \text{ ohms}$$

$$V = 320 \text{ volts}$$

Example: A 150-watt bulb operates on a potential difference of 110 volts.

1. Calculate the current drawn.

$$P = IV$$

$$I = \frac{P}{V}$$

$$I = \frac{150 \text{ watts}}{110 \text{ volts}}$$

$$I = 1.36 \text{ A}$$

2. Calculate the resistance.

$$V = IR$$

$$R = \frac{V}{I}$$

$$R = \frac{110 \text{ volts}}{1.36 \text{ A}}$$

$$R = 81. \text{ ohms}$$

Example: A current of 10 A flows through a wire for 45 min. The charge that passes through a cross section of the wire may be calculated as follows:

$$I = \frac{q}{t}$$

$$q = It$$

$$q = (10 \text{ A})(2700 \text{ sec})$$

$$q = 27,000 \text{ A} \cdot \text{sec or coulombs}$$

Electric Circuits

Electromotive Force (emf) and Internal Resistance

$$V = E - Ir \qquad V = \text{terminal potential difference}$$

$$E = \text{no-load potential difference or emf}$$

$$r = \text{internal resistance}$$

$$I = \text{current}$$

Example: A battery powering a portable television has an emf of 10 volts and an internal resistance of 0.20 ohm. It supplies a current of 6 A. Calculate the terminal potential difference.

$$V = E - IR$$

$$V = 10 \text{ volts} - (6 \text{ A} \times 0.20 \text{ ohm})$$

$$V = 10 \text{ volts} - 1.2 \text{ volts}$$

$$V = 8.8 \text{ volts}$$

Resistors in Series

Example: A direct-current circuit is wired with resistances of 3 ohms, 6 ohms, and 2 ohms in series. These resistances could be replaced by one resistor of 11 ohms to produce equivalent resistance.

Example: Three lamps are connected in series and exhibit a resistance of 15, 10, and 5 ohms, respectively. How much current is produced by a potential difference of 100 volts across its terminals?

1. Determine the current in the lamp.

$$R = (15 + 10 + 5) \text{ ohms}$$

$$R = 30 \text{ ohms}$$

$$I = \frac{V}{R}$$

$$I = \frac{100 \text{ volts}}{30 \text{ ohms}}$$

$$I = 3.33 \text{ A}$$

2. Determine the voltage across each lamp; it is the product of its resistance and the current.

$$V_1 = (3.33 \text{ A})(15 \text{ ohms}) = 50 \text{ volts}$$

$$V_2 = (3.33 \text{ A})(10 \text{ ohms}) = 33 \text{ volts}$$

$$V_3 = (3.33 \text{ A})(5 \text{ ohms}) = 17 \text{ volts}$$

Resistors in Parallel

$$\frac{1}{R} = \frac{1}{R_1} + \frac{1}{R_2} + \frac{1}{R_3}$$

Recall that addition to a circuit of resistors in series increases the resistance while addition to a circuit of resistors in parallel decreases the resistance.

Example: Using the example of 3, 6, and 2 ohms, the equivalent resistance can be calculated as follows:

$$\frac{1}{R_{eq}} = \frac{1}{R_1} + \frac{1}{R_2} + \frac{1}{R_3}$$

$$\frac{1}{R_{eq}} = \frac{1}{3 \text{ ohms}} + \frac{1}{6 \text{ ohms}} + \frac{1}{2 \text{ ohms}}$$

$$= \frac{2}{6 \text{ ohms}} + \frac{1}{6 \text{ ohms}} + \frac{3}{6 \text{ ohms}} = \frac{6}{6 \text{ ohms}}$$

$$\frac{1}{R_{eq}} = 1 \text{ ohm}, \text{ OR, } R_{eq} = 1 \text{ ohm}$$

Example: A circuit has resistances of 15, 10, and 5 ohms. If these are wired in parallel what is their combined resistance?

$$\frac{1}{R} = \frac{1}{R_1} + \frac{1}{R_2} + \frac{1}{R_3}$$

$$\frac{1}{R} = \frac{1}{15 \text{ ohms}} + \frac{1}{10 \text{ ohms}} + \frac{1}{5 \text{ ohms}}$$

$$\frac{1}{R} = (0.07 + 0.1 + 0.2) \text{ ohm}$$

$$\frac{1}{R} = 0.37 \text{ ohm}$$

$$R = \frac{1}{0.37} \text{ ohm}$$

$$R = 2.7 \text{ ohms}$$

Example: Find the current in a series circuit with two energy sources ($E_1 = 12$ volts, $E_2 = -4$ volt) and two resistors ($R_1 = 15$ ohms, $R_2 = 10$ ohms).

$$E_1 + E_2 = I_1(R_1 + R_2) \text{ or } V_1 + V_2 = I_1(R_1 + R_2)$$

$$I_1 = \frac{E_1 + E_2}{R_1 + R_2} \text{ or } \frac{V_1 + V_2}{R_1 + R_2}$$

$$I_1 \frac{(12 - 4) \text{ volts}}{(15 + 10) \text{ ohms}}$$

$$I_1 = \frac{8 \text{ volts}}{25 \text{ ohms}} = 0.32 \text{ A}$$

Example: A circuit has three resistors—of 2 ohms, 4 ohms, and 8 ohms.

1. What is the resistance of these three resistors when connected in series?

$$R_s = R_1 + R_2 + R_3$$
$$R_s = (2 + 4 + 8) \text{ ohms}$$
$$R_s = 14 \text{ ohms}$$

2. What is their resistance when connected in parallel?

$$\frac{1}{R_p} = \frac{1}{R_1} + \frac{1}{R_2} + \frac{1}{R_3}$$
$$\frac{1}{R_p} = \frac{1}{2 \text{ ohms}} + \frac{1}{4 \text{ ohms}} + \frac{1}{8 \text{ ohms}}$$
$$\frac{1}{R_p} = \frac{4}{8 \text{ ohms}} + \frac{2}{8 \text{ ohms}} + \frac{1}{8 \text{ ohms}}$$
$$\frac{1}{R_p} = \frac{7}{8 \text{ ohms}}$$
$$R_p = \frac{8}{7} \text{ ohms}$$

3. How much current would be drawn from a 12-volt battery?

SERIES

$$I = \frac{V}{R_s} = \frac{12 \text{ volts}}{14 \text{ ohms}} = 0.857 \text{ A}$$

Potential drop in each resistor:

$$V_1 = IR_1 = (0.857 \text{ A})(2 \text{ ohms})$$
$$= 1.7 \text{ volts}$$
$$V_2 = IR_2 = (0.857 \text{ A})(4 \text{ ohms})$$
$$= 3.4 \text{ volts}$$
$$V_3 = IR_3 = (0.857 \text{ A})(8 \text{ ohms})$$
$$= 6.9 \text{ volts}$$

The drop equals the voltage rise in the battery:

$$V_i = V_1 + V_2 + V_3$$
$$V_i = 12 \text{ volts}$$

PARALLEL

$$I = \frac{V}{R_p} = \frac{12 \text{ ohms}}{8/7 \text{ ohms}} = 10.5 \text{ A}$$

Current in each resistor:

$$I_1 = \frac{V}{R_1} = \frac{12 \text{ volts}}{2 \text{ ohms}} = 6 \text{ A}$$
$$I_2 = \frac{V}{R_2} = \frac{12 \text{ volts}}{4 \text{ ohms}} = 3 \text{ A}$$
$$I_3 = \frac{V}{R_3} = \frac{12 \text{ volts}}{8 \text{ ohms}} = 1.5 \text{ A}$$
$$I_i \text{ and } I_1 + I_2 + I_3 = 10.5 \text{ A}$$

Cells in Series

Example: Three cells are connected in series; each has an emf of 10 volts and a resistance of 2 ohms. Calculate the current after the combination is connected to an external resistance of 20 ohms.

$$\text{Total emf} = 10 \text{ volts} + 10 \text{ volts} + 10 \text{ volts}$$
$$= 30 \text{ volts}$$
$$\text{Total Resistance } (R) = 2 \text{ ohms} + 2 \text{ ohms} + 2 \text{ ohms} + 20 \text{ ohms}$$
$$= 26 \text{ ohms}$$
$$\text{Total Current} = \frac{\text{Total emf}}{\text{Total Resistance}}$$
$$\text{Total Current} = \frac{30 \text{ volts}}{26 \text{ ohms}}$$
$$\text{Total Current} = 1.15 \text{ A}$$

Cells in Parallel

Example: Consider the following three arrangements:

    a. A single cell
    b. Two cells in series
    c. Two cells in parallel

Compare the currents maintained in a 5-ohm resistor under each condition. Each cell has an emf of 3 volts and negligible internal resistance. The emf of (a) is 3 volts, of (b) 6 volts, and of (c) 3 volts.

$$(a): I_{\text{total}} = \frac{E_{\text{total}}}{R_{\text{total}}}$$

$$I_a = \frac{3 \text{ volts}}{5 \text{ ohms}}$$

$$I_a = 0.6 \text{ A}$$

$$(b): \quad I_b = \frac{6 \text{ volts}}{5 \text{ ohms}}$$

$$I_b = 1.2 \text{ A}$$

$$(c): \quad I_c = \frac{3 \text{ volts}}{5 \text{ ohms}}$$

$$I_c = 0.6 \text{ A}$$

In each cell, however, the current is 0.3 A (in part c).

Electric Energy

Joule's Law

$$\text{Voltage} = \frac{\text{Energy}}{\text{Charge}} \qquad V = \text{volts}$$

$$V = \frac{W}{Q} \qquad W = \text{usually in joules}$$

$$\text{OR } VIt = I^2 Rt \qquad Q = \text{usually in coulombs}$$

Rewriting $W = VQ$, we can make the substitutions $Q = It$ and $V = IR$. Then, the basic equation for electric energy may be $W = VQ = VIt = I^2 Rt$. This equation indicates that one joule must be expended in maintaining for one second a current of one ampere in a circuit of one-ohm resistance.

Example: A motor is used for 45 min to drive a conveyor belt. It uses 35 A at 110 volts. Calculate the electric energy used.

$$W = VIt$$

$$W = (110 \text{ volts})(35 \text{ A})(2700 \text{ sec})$$

$$W = 10,395,000 \text{ J}$$

$$W = 10.4 \times 10^6 \text{ J}$$

Example: How many calories are produced in a central electric resistance heating system in 5 min as it draws 30 A connected to a 220-volt line?

Recall: 1 cal = 4.18 J

$$H = \frac{VIt}{J} \text{ or } H = \frac{W}{J}$$

$$H = \frac{(220 \text{ volts})(30 \text{ A})(300 \text{ sec})}{4.18 \text{ J/cal}}$$

$$H = \frac{1,980,000}{4.18 \text{ J/cal}}$$

$$H = 470,000 \text{ cal}$$

Power and Resistance

Example: The above furnace operating at 220 volts requires 2 hp. What are the current and the resistance of the unit?

1. Current

$$P = 2\text{hp} \times 746 \frac{\text{watts}}{\text{hp}}$$

$$P = 1492 \text{ watts}$$

$$P = VI$$

$$1492 \text{ watts} = 220 \text{ volts} \times I$$

$$I = 6.78 \text{ A}$$

2. Resistance

$$R = \frac{V}{I}$$

$$R = \frac{220 \text{ volts}}{6.78 \text{ A}}$$

$$R = 32 \text{ ohms}$$

Alternating Current

Effective Values

In a sine-wave varying current, the average power is half the maximum power. The average power is $I_{rms}^2 R$, where I_{rms} is the root-mean-square, or effective, value of the current.

Example: A sine-wave alternating current with a peak current of 60 A is passing through a resistance of 2.0 Ω. Find the peak power, average power, effective current, and effective potential difference.

1. The peak power is $I_{max}^2 R$:

$$P_{max} = (60 \text{ A})^2 (2.0 \text{ Ω}) = 7200 \text{ W}$$

2. The average power is half the maximum, 3600 W.

3. The effective current produces the average power:

$$I_{rms}^2 R = 3600 \text{ W}$$

$$I_{rms} = \sqrt{\frac{3600 \text{ W}}{2.0 \ \Omega}} = 42 \text{ A}$$

4. Effective potential difference:

$$V_{rms} = I_{rms} R = (42 \text{ A})(2.0 \ \Omega) = 84 \text{ V}$$

Example: An effective potential difference of 120 V supplies a resistance of 40 Ω. Find the maximum potential difference and current.

1. Maximum is RMS value times the square root of 2:

$$V_{max} = (120 \text{ V})\sqrt{2} = 170 \text{ V}$$

2. Effective current is

$$I_{rms} = \frac{V_{rms}}{R} \ \frac{120 \text{ V}}{40 \ \Omega} = 3.0 \text{ A}$$

3. Maximum current is

$$(3.0 \text{ A})\sqrt{2} = 4.2 \text{ A}$$

Machines and Mechanical Advantage

Actual Mechanical Advantage (AMA) = F_o/F_i,

where F_o = output force and F_i = input force.

Theoretical Mechanical Advantage (TMA) = d_i/d_o,

$$Efficiency(E) = \frac{F_o/F_i}{d_i/d_o} = \frac{AMA}{TMA} = \frac{\text{Output Work}}{\text{Input Work}}$$

Example: A man pushing down with a force of 200 N lifts a 800 N crate by utilizing a lever system. The lever arms are 2 m and 40 cm respectively.

1. Calculate the AMA.

$$AMA = \frac{F_o}{F_i}$$

$$AMA = \frac{800 \text{ N}}{200 \text{ N}}$$

$$AMA = 4$$

2. Calculate the TMA.

$$TMA = \frac{d_i}{d_o}$$

$$TMA = \frac{2 \text{ m}}{0.4 \text{ m}}$$

$$TMA = 5$$

3. What is the efficiency?

$$E = \frac{AMA}{TMA}$$

$$E = \frac{4}{5}(100\%)$$

$$E = 80\%$$

Example: A car with a mass of 680 kg (weight = 6664 N) is pushed up a 30 m ramp exhibiting an incline of 30°. A parallel force of 4400 N is used to accomplish this task.

1. What is the AMA?

$$AMA = \frac{F_o}{F_i} = \frac{6664 \text{ N}}{4400} = 1.51$$

2. What is the efficiency of the system?

$$TMA = \frac{30 \text{ m}}{30 \sin 30°}$$

$$= \frac{1}{0.5} = 2$$

$$E = \frac{AMA}{TMA} = \frac{1.51}{2}$$

$$E = 76\%$$

Simple Harmonic Motion

Period and Frequency

The motion of an oscillating object is described by its:

displacement—distance from central position
amplitude—maximum displacement
period (T)—time for one full cycle
frequency (f)—cycles per unit time. One cycle per second is called a hertz (Hz)

Frequency is the reciprocal of period.

Example: What is the frequency of a vibrating rod that completes each cycle in 1/20 sec?

$$f = \frac{1}{T} \frac{1}{1/20 \text{ sec}} = 20/\text{sec} = 20 \text{ Hz}$$

Phase

Phase is the time difference, in fractions of a cycle, between two objects oscillating with the same frequency. One cycle is 360°.

Example: What is the phase difference between two identical pendulums with periods of 1.5 sec if one reaches its maximum displacement 0.2 sec before the other?

$$\text{Phase differnece } = \left(\frac{0.2 \text{ sec}}{1.5 \text{ sec}}\right)(360°) = 48°$$

Waves

A wave is a system of oscillating particles or fields, in which each point transmits energy to the next point in turn. The next point follows with a slight time delay, so the phase varies continuously.

crest—a point of maximum displacement that appears to travel through the medium
trough—a traveling point of negative maximum displacement
wave velocity—speed of travel of crests and troughs
wavelength (λ, Greek lambda)—distance between successive points in phase

Frequency, Wavelength, and Phase

Wavelength depends on frequency and velocity:

$$v = \lambda f$$

Example: If a wave in a rope travels at 4.6 m/sec and the rope is shaken at one end with a frequency of 2.0 Hz, what is the wavelength of the wave in the rope?

$$\lambda = \frac{v}{f} = \frac{4.6 \text{ m/sec}}{2.0/\text{sec}} = 2.3 \text{ m}$$

Example: If a 120-Hz wave of vibration in a steel rail travels at 840 m/sec, how far apart are two points that are 90° out of phase?

1. Find the wavelength.

$$\lambda = \frac{v}{f} = \frac{840 \text{ m/sec}}{120/\text{sec}} = 7.0 \text{ m}$$

2. Each phase cycle corresponds to a wavelength, so

$$\frac{90°}{360°} \times 7.0 \text{ m} = 1.75 \text{ m}$$

Interference

When two identical waves arrive simultaneously at a point, their displacements add. If they arrive out of phase, the interference is *destructive*, and a *node*, a point of no vibration, is formed. If they arrive in phase, the interference is *constructive*, and an *antinode*, a point of maximum vibration, develops.

Standing Waves

A standing wave in a string has alternate nodes and antinodes, spaced ¼ wavelength apart.

Example: In the fundamental mode, a string vibrates with a node at each end and an antinode in the middle. What is the frequency of vibration if the string is 25 cm long and the wave in it travels at 390 m/sec?

1. Find the wavelength. Since there is a node at each end, the string is a half-wavelength long.

$$\lambda = 2 \times 25 \text{ cm} = 0.50 \text{ m}$$

2. Now find the frequency.

$$f = \frac{v}{\lambda} = \frac{390 \text{ m/sec}}{0.50 \text{ m}} = 780 \text{ Hz}$$

Example: At a higher mode, there are 5 antinodes in the string of the preceding problem. What is the frequency at this mode?

1. Find the wavelength. Since there are 2 antinodes in each wavelength, there are $2^{1}/_{2}$ wavelengths in the string.

$$\lambda = \frac{25 \text{ cm}}{2.5} = 10 \text{ cm}$$

2. Find the frequency.

$$f = \frac{v}{\lambda} = \frac{390 \text{ m/sec}}{0.10 \text{ m}} = 3900 \text{ Hz}$$

Sound Waves

A vibrating object sets the adjacent air into vibration. This starts a longitudinal wave traveling through the air, a sound wave.

Pitch and Frequency

The *pitch* of the sound is its apparent tonal level, as defined by musical scales. An increase of 1 octave represents doubling the frequency.

Example: When the oboe sounds 440-A, what is the frequency of the tuba, sounding A two octaves lower? One octave lower is 220 Hz, the next octave below is 110 Hz.

In the equal-tempered chromatic scale, each increase of a half tone represents a frequency increase by a factor of $2^{1/12} = 1.05946$.

Example: What is the frequency of high C, which is 3 halftones above A?

$$\text{Frequency} = 440 \text{ Hz} \times 1.05946^3 = 523.2 \text{ Hz}$$

Intensity

The intensity, or loudness, of a sound in bels is the order of magnitude of its energy as compared with the softest audible sound. Thus, 3 bels (B), or 30 decibels (dB), has 10^3 times the zero level.

Example: If a rock band produces sound at 80 dB, how does the intensity of this sound compare with that of the softest audible sound?
The value of 80 dB is 8 B, so the loudest sound has 10^8 times the intensity of 0 B.

Speed of Sound

The speed of a sound wave depends on the nature of the medium in which it travels. It travels faster in liquids than in gases, and much faster in elastic solids. In air, the speed of sound depends on the temperature and can be calculated from the following formula:

$$v_{air} = 331 \frac{m}{sec} + 0.6 \, T \frac{m}{s \cdot {}^\circ C}$$

Example: How far away is a wall if an echo is received from it 3.9 sec after the sound is produced when the temperature is 26°C?

1. Find the speed of sound.

$$v_{air} = 331 \frac{m}{sec} + \left(0.6 \frac{m}{s \cdot {}^\circ C} \right)(26 {}^\circ C) = 346.6 \text{ m/sec}$$

2. Calculate the distance the sound traveled:

$$s = vt = (346.6 \text{ m/sec})(3.9 \text{ sec}) = 1352 \text{ m}$$

3. Since the sound had to travel both ways, the distance of the wall is half this distance, or 676 m.

Beats

Two sound waves of different frequencies arriving at a point will interfere, alternating constructive and destructive interference. The beat frequency is the difference between the frequencies of the two sounds.

Example: As an orchestra tunes up, the oboe sounds 440-A. If the clarinetist hears 3 beats per second when he plays A, what is the frequency of the clarinet's A?

It could be either 443 Hz or 437 Hz.

Doppler Effect

If a sound source is moving away from an observer, the frequency heard is lower than the frequency emitted, and conversely.

$$f = f_s \frac{v}{v + v_s}$$

where f is the observed frequency, f_s is the frequency of the source, v is the speed of sound, and v_s is the speed of the source as it moves away from the observer.

Example: With the temperature at $-10°C$, a train moving toward the observer at 32 m/sec sounds its horn at 380 Hz. What frequency does the observer hear?

1. Find the speed of sound.

$$v = 331 \frac{m}{sec} + \left(0.6 \frac{m}{s \cdot °C} \right)(-10°C) = 325 \text{ m/sec}$$

2. Apply the formula; v_s is negative because the source is moving toward the observer:

$$f = (380 \text{ Hz}) \frac{325 \text{ m/sec}}{(325 - 32)\text{m/sec}} = 421 \text{ Hz}$$

Light Rays

Light travels in straight lines (rays) unless deflected by reflection or refraction.

Reflection

In specular reflection, the angle of reflection is equal to angle of incidence. Angles are measured with respect to the perpendicular to the surface (the normal).

Example: If a light ray strikes a mirror at an angle of incidence of 22°, what is the angle between the incident and reflected rays?

Since the angles are measured from the normal, there are 44° between the incident and reflected rays.

Refraction

When a light ray goes from one medium into another, it will bend. The speeds of light in the two media are proportional to the sines of the angles the rays make with the normal.

Example: A light ray in air enters a piece of glass, in which light travels at 2.20×10^6 m/sec. If the angle of incidence is 25°, which is the angle of refraction?

$$\frac{\sin \theta_{glass}}{\sin 25°} = \frac{2.20 \times 10^8 \text{ m/sec}}{3.00 \times 10^8 \text{ m/sec}}$$

$$\theta_{glass} = 18°$$

Index of Refraction

The index of refraction (n) of a medium is the ratio between the speed of light in vacuum and the speed in the medium.

Example: What is the index of refraction of the glass in the preceding example?

$$n_{glass} = \frac{c}{v_{glass}} = \frac{3.00 \times 10^8 \text{ m/sec}}{2.20 \times 10^8 \text{ m/sec}} = 1.36$$

Refraction between Two Media

If light passes from medium A to B, or vice versa,

$$\frac{\sin \theta_A}{\sin \theta_B} = \frac{n_B}{n_A}$$

Example: A ray of light passes from crown glass ($n = 1.62$) into water ($n = 1.33$), making an angle of incidence of $40°$. What is the angle of refraction?

$$\frac{\sin \theta_{glass}}{\sin \theta_{water}} = \frac{n_{water}}{n_{glass}}$$

$$\sin \theta_{water} = \sin 40° \left(\frac{1.62}{1.33}\right)$$

$$\theta_{water} = 52°$$

Total Internal Reflection

If a ray passes into a medium of higher index of refraction, the calculated angle of refraction may exceed $90°$. Then the ray is totally reflected.

Example: What is the largest angle of incidence (the critical angle) at which a ray of light can pass from crown glass into water (constants given above)?

$$\frac{\sin i_c}{\sin 90°} = \frac{n_{water}}{n_{glass}} = \frac{1.33}{1.62}$$

$$i_c = 55°$$

Mirrors

Plane Mirrors

In a plane mirror, the image is virtual, erect, the same size as the object, and just as far behind the mirror as the object is in front of it.

Example: The image in a plane mirror of a book is 25 cm high when the book is 50 cm from the mirror. How high is the image if the book is moved to 150 cm?

The answer is 25 cm; the size of the image is always the same as the size of the object.

Convex Mirrors

In a convex mirror, the focal length is half the radius of curvature and the image distance obeys the rule

$$\frac{1}{f} = \frac{1}{D_o} + \frac{1}{D_i}$$

where f is focal length, D_o is object distance, and D_i is image distance. The focal length is negative. The image is always erect, virtual, smaller than the object, and behind the mirror.

Example: A convex mirror has a radius of curvature of 60 cm. Where is the image of a lamp that is 180 cm from the mirror?

1. Find the focal length; it is half the radius of curvature, 30 cm, and is negative.
2. Use the formula to find the image distance.

$$\frac{1}{-30 \text{ cm}} = \frac{1}{180 \text{ cm}} + \frac{1}{D_i}$$

$$\frac{1}{D_i} = \frac{-180 \text{ cm} - 30 \text{ cm}}{(180 \text{ cm})(30 \text{ cm})}$$

$$D_i = -26 \text{ cm}$$

A negative sign indicates that the image is behind the lens. The sizes of the object (S_o) and of the image (S_i) are in the same ratio as the respective distances.

Example: If the lamp in the preceding example is 40 cm tall, how tall is the image?

$$S_i = S_o\left(\frac{-D_i}{D_o}\right) = 40 \text{ cm}\left(\frac{+26 \text{ cm}}{180 \text{ cm}}\right) = +5.8 \text{ cm}$$

The image is virtual.

Concave Mirrors

Focal length is half the radius of curvature and positive. Image is either real, inverted, and in front of the lens, or virtual, erect, and behind the lens.

Example: (Object distance greater than focal length) A concave mirror has a radius of curvature of 80 cm. Find the size and location of the image of a lamp that is 60 cm high and 180 cm from the mirror.

1. Find the focal length; it is half the radius of curvature, +40 cm.
2. Apply the formula to find the image distance.

$$\frac{1}{D_i} = \frac{1}{f} - \frac{1}{D_o} = +\left(\frac{1}{40 \text{ cm}}\right) - \frac{1}{180 \text{ cm}}$$

$$D_i = +\left(\frac{(40 \text{ cm})(180 \text{ cm})}{180 \text{ cm} + 40 \text{ cm}}\right) = +33 \text{ cm}$$

3. Set the sizes proportional to the distances.

$$S_i = (60 \text{ cm})\left(\frac{33 \text{ cm}}{180 \text{ cm}}\right) = 11 \text{ cm}$$

Example: (Object distance less than focal length) A can 15 cm high is placed 25 cm in front of the same mirror as above. Find the size and location of the image.

1. Find the image distance.

$$\frac{1}{D_i} = \frac{1}{f} - \frac{1}{D_o} = \left(\frac{1}{40 \text{ cm}}\right) - \frac{1}{25 \text{ cm}}$$

$$D_i = -\left(\frac{(25 \text{ cm})(40 \text{ cm})}{25 \text{ cm} + 40 \text{ cm}}\right) = -66.7 \text{ cm}$$

The image is behind the mirror.

2. Solve for the size.

$$S_i = (15 \text{ cm})\left(\frac{66.7 \text{ cm}}{25 \text{ cm}}\right) = 40 \text{ cm}$$

The image is virtual.

Lenses

Concave Lenses

Lenses that are thinner in the middle than at the edges form the same kinds of images as convex mirrors. They obey the same equations, and the focal length is negative.

Example: Find the size and location of the image formed in a lens of focal length −40 cm of a book 25 cm high placed 30 cm from the lens.

1. Find the image distance:

$$\frac{1}{D_i} = \frac{1}{f} - \frac{1}{D_o} = \frac{1}{-40 \text{ cm}} - \frac{1}{30 \text{ cm}}$$

$$D_i = \frac{(-40 \text{ cm})(30 \text{ cm})}{(30 \text{ cm}) - (-40 \text{ cm})} = -17 \text{ cm}$$

The negative sign shows that the image is behind the mirror.

2. Find the image size.

$$S_i = S_o\left(\frac{-D_i}{D_o}\right) = (25 \text{ cm})\left(\frac{17 \text{ cm}}{30 \text{ cm}}\right) = 14 \text{ cm}$$

The image is virtual.

Convex Lenses

Lenses that are thicker in the middle than at the edges form the same kinds of images as concave mirrors. They obey the same equations, and the focal length is positive.

Example: (Object distance less than focal length) Find the size and position of the image formed in a +12.0-cm lens of a postage stamp 2.4 cm high placed 10.0 cm from the lens.

1. Find the image position.

$$\frac{1}{D_i} = \frac{1}{f} - \frac{1}{D_o} = \frac{1}{12.0 \text{ cm}} - \frac{1}{10.0 \text{ cm}}$$

$$D_i = \frac{(10.0 \text{ cm})(12.0 \text{ cm})}{(10.0 \text{ cm}) - (12.0 \text{ cm})} = -60 \text{ cm}$$

The negative sign shows that the image is in front of the lens.

2. Find the image size.

$$S_i = S_o\left(\frac{-D_i}{D_o}\right) = 2.4 \text{ cm}\left(\frac{60 \text{ cm}}{10.0 \text{ cm}}\right) = 14 \text{ cm}$$

The image is enlarged and virtual.

Example: (Object distance greater than focal length) What focal-length lens is needed to form a real image 35 mm high of a man 2.0 m tall when the man is 1.7 m from the lens?

1. Find the image distance in centimeters.

$$D_i = D_o\left(\frac{S_i}{S_o}\right) = 170 \text{ cm}\left(\frac{3.5 \text{ cm}}{200 \text{ cm}}\right) = 3.0 \text{ cm}$$

The image is real.

2. Find the focal length.

$$\frac{1}{f} = \frac{1}{D_o} + \frac{1}{D_i} = \frac{1}{170 \text{ cm}} + \frac{1}{3.0 \text{ cm}}$$

$$f = \frac{(170 \text{ cm})(3.0 \text{ cm})}{170 \text{ cm} + 3.0 \text{ cm}} = 2.9 \text{ cm}$$

The image is real and small.

Combinations of Lenses

The power of a lens, in diopters, is the reciprocal of its focal length in meters. When lenses are combined, their powers add.

Example: What is the focal length of a combination of a +50-cm convex lens and a −20-cm concave lens?

1. Find the powers of the two lenses.

$$\frac{1}{+0.50 \text{ cm}} = +2.0 \text{ diopters}, \qquad \frac{1}{-0.20 \text{ m}} = -5.0 \text{ diopters}$$

2. Add the powers.

$$2.0 - 5.0 = -3.0 \text{ diopter}$$

3. Find the focal length.

$$\frac{1}{-3.0 \text{ diopter}} = -0.33 \text{ m, or } -33 \text{ cm}$$

Any number of lenses can be combined in this way.

Composition of the Atom

Subatomic Particles

Recall that the nucleus of an atom is composed of neutrons (no charge) and protons (positive electric charge). The total number of particles equals the mass number; the number of protons equals the atomic number. In an atom, the number of protons equals the number of electrons. The number of neutrons can be found by subtracting the atomic number from the mass number.

Example: How many particles of each type are there in an atom of $^{35}_{17}\text{Cl}$?
The atomic number is 17, so the element is chlorine (Cl). There are 17 protons in the nucleus and 17 electrons outside it. The number of neutrons in the nucleus is $(35 - 17) = 18$.

Isotopes

Isotopes of the same element have the same atomic number, but different mass numbers (because of different numbers of neutrons).

Example: Of the following, which are isotopes of the same element?

$$^{65}_{29}\text{Cu} \qquad ^{65}_{30}\text{Zn} \qquad ^{60}_{29}\text{Cu} \qquad ^{60}_{28}\text{Ni}$$

There are two isotopes of copper (Cu), both with atomic number 29.

Nuclear Reactions

In any nuclear reaction, the mass numbers and the electric charges must be the same on both sides of the equation.

Example: When aluminum atoms are bombarded with helium nuclei, which isotope is produced along with a neutron?

$$^{27}_{13}\text{Al} + ^{4}_{2}\text{He} \rightarrow ^{30}_{15}\text{P} + ^{1}_{0}\text{n}$$

An isotope of phosphorus is produced along with the neutron. The mass numbers are $27 + 4 = 30 + 1$. The electric charge (on the protons) is $13 + 2 = 15 + 0$.

Radioactivity

Large nuclei are unstable and break down, releasing particles and energy. There are two kinds of radioactivity in nature: alpha and beta.

Alpha Decay

In alpha decay, the nucleus releases an alpha particle, which is a nucleus of helium, ^4_2He.

Example: What nucleus results from the alpha decay of a nucleus of radon-210?

$$^{210}_{86}\text{Rn} \rightarrow \, ^4_2\text{He} + \, ^{206}_{84}\text{Po} + \gamma$$

The γ (gamma ray) is a high-energy photon, which always accompanies alpha decay. The mass numbers agree: $210 = 4 + 206$. The electric charges agree: $86 = 2 + 84$.

Beta Decay

In beta decay, a neutron emits an electron, turning into a proton. It also produces a charge-less, massless particle called a neutrino.

Example: What is the result of the beta decay of radium-227?

$$^{277}_{88}\text{Ra} \rightarrow \, ^{227}_{89}\text{Ac} + \, ^{0}_{-1}\text{e} + \nu$$

Because the electron and the neutrino have negligible mass, there is no change in the mass number; $227 = 227 + 0$. The atomic number increases by 1, and the electric charge balance is $88 = 89 - 1$.

Half-life

The half-life of a nucleus is the time required for half of any given sample to undergo radioactive decay.

Example: The half-life of radon-214 is 2.5 sec. If a sample of this gas contains 200 g, how much will be left at the end of 10 sec?

Ten seconds is 4 half-lives, so the mass drops to half 4 times. The amount left will be

$$(200 \text{ g})(0.5)^4 = 13 \text{ g}$$

Example: What is the half-life of a radioactive nucleus if it takes 4 billion years for 40 g to decay down to 10 g?

The mass of the sample has dropped to half twice, so the half-life is 2 billion years.

Nuclear Energy

The mass of a nucleus is less than the sum of the masses of the protons and neutrons that compose it. The difference is called the mass defect of the nucleus, which corresponds to the binding energy ($E = mc^2$).

Units of Measure

The mass of nuclei is measured in unified mass units, or u.

$$1 \text{ u} = 1.66 \times 10^{-27} \text{ kg}$$
$$1 \text{ kg} = 6.02 \times 10^{26} \text{ u}$$
$$1 \text{ u} \leftrightarrow 931 \text{ MeV}$$

Example: If the mass defect of a nucleus is 0.0067 u, how much energy will be needed to separate it into protons and neutrons?

$$0.0067 \text{ u} \times \frac{931 \text{ MeV}}{\text{u}} = 6.2 \text{ MeV}$$

Example: If a nuclear reaction yields 6.5×10^{12} J of energy, how much mass disappears?

$$m = \frac{E}{c^2} = \frac{6.5 \times 10^{12} \text{ J}}{(3.0 \times 10^8 \text{ m/sec})^2} = 7.2 \times 10^{-5} \text{ kg, or 72 mg}$$

Fusion Reactions

When two small nuclei combine, their binding energy must be released.

Example: How much energy is released when lithium-6 combines with deuterium to form two helium nuclei (deuterium is hydrogen-2)?

1. Write the equation.

$$^{6}_{3}\text{Li} + ^{2}_{1}\text{H} \rightarrow 2^{4}_{2}\text{He}$$

The mass numbers are $6 + 2 = 2 \times 4$. The electric charge numbers are $3 + 1 = 2 \times 2$.

2. Add the nuclear masses on each side of the equation to find the mass deficit.

$$
\begin{array}{ll}
\text{Li - 6:} & 6.01512 \text{ u} \\
\text{H - 2:} & \underline{2.0140 \text{ u}} \\
 & 8.02912 \text{ u} \\
\text{He - 4:} & 2 \times 4.00260 \text{ u} = 8.00520 \text{ u}
\end{array}
$$

The mass deficit is $8.0912 - 8.00520 = 0.0239$ u.

3. Determine the energy equivalent of the mass deficit:

$$0.0239 \text{ u} \left(\frac{930 \text{ MeV}}{\text{u}} \right) = 22 \text{ MeV}$$

Nuclear Fission

When a very large nucleus splits into two medium-sized nuclei, the combined mass of the two fragments is less than the mass of the original nucleus. Thus, energy is released.

Example: When Uranium-235 is split by impact with a slow neutron, how many neutrons are produced?

$$^{235}_{92}\text{U} + ^{1}_{0}\text{n} \rightarrow ^{92}_{36}\text{Kr} + ^{141}_{56}\text{Ba} + ?^{1}_{0}\text{n}$$

Barium and krypton result. To balance the mass numbers, three neutrons must be produced. These neutrons can split additional uranium nuclei, producing a chain reaction.

Photons

Light has a dual nature; it can be described as a wave or a stream of particles (photons).

Wave Property of Light

As a wave, light obeys the equation

$$c = \lambda f$$

where c is the speed of the wave (3.00×10^8 m/sec); λ (lambda) is the wavelength, and f (nu) is the frequency.

Example: What is the frequency of yellow light of wavelength 570 nm (nanometers)?

$$f = \frac{c}{\lambda} = \frac{3.00 \times 10^8 \text{ m/sec}}{570 \times 10^{-9} \text{ m}} = 5.26 \times 10^{14} \text{/sec} = 5.26 \times 10^{14} \text{ Hz}$$

Photon Energy

The energy of a photon obeys the equation

$$E = hf = \frac{hc}{\lambda}$$

where h is Planck's constant, 4.14×10^{-15} eV·s.

Example: What is the energy of a photon of red light with wavelength 730 nm?

$$E = \frac{hc}{\lambda} = \frac{(4.14 \times 10^{-15} \text{ eV} \cdot \text{sec})(3.00 \times 10^8 \text{ m/sec})}{730 \times 10^{-9} \text{ m}} = 1.70 \text{ eV}$$

Photoelectric Effect

A photon may release an electron from a metal surface. The energy of the electron is equal to the energy of the photon minus the work function of the metal.

Example: What is the maximum energy of an electron emitted by a metal whose work function is 2.60 eV if the incident light is ultraviolet with a wavelength of 370 nm?

1. Find the energy of the photon.

$$E = hf = h\frac{c}{\lambda} = \frac{(4.14 \times 10^{-15} \text{eV} \cdot \text{sec})(3.00 \times 10^8 \text{m/sec})}{370 \times 10^{-9} \text{ m}} = 3.36 \text{ eV}$$

2. Subtract the work function of the metal.

$$3.36 \text{ eV} - 2.60 \text{ eV} = 0.76 \text{ eV}$$

Example: What is the longest wavelength of light that will release an electron from a metal whose work function is 3.61 eV?

The minimum energy of the photon is the work function of the metal, so

$$\lambda = \frac{hc}{E} = \frac{(4.14 \times 10^{-15} \text{ ev} \cdot \text{sec})(3.00 \times 10^8 \text{ m/sec})}{3.61 \text{ eV}} = 3.4 \times 10^{-7} \text{ m}$$

or 340 nm, in the ultraviolet.

Atomic Energy Levels

The electrons in the outer shells of an atom can be raised from ground state to excited states in quantized steps.

Spectra

When an electron falls to a lower energy state, it loses a definite amount of energy by emitting a photon having that energy. The spectrum of the light emitted by a substance contains only photons of certain definite energies.

Example: What is the wavelength of the light emitted when an electron drops from a 4.70-eV excited state to a 3.22-eV state?

1. The energy of the photon is 4.70 eV − 3.22 eV = 1.48 eV.

2. The wavelength of the photon is

$$\lambda = \frac{hc}{E} = \frac{(4.14 \times 10^{-15} \text{ ev} \cdot \text{sec})(3.00 \times 10^8 \text{m/sec})}{1.48 \text{ eV}} = 8.39 \times 10^{-7} \text{ m}$$

which is the wavelength of an infrared photon, at 839 nm.

Spectrum of Atomic Hydrogen

The single electron of a hydrogen atom occupies quantum states which can be represented by the expression -13.6 eV$/n^2$, where n is any whole number.

Example: What is the wavelength of a photon that is emitted when a hydrogen electron drops from the fifth to the second state?

1. Find the energy levels of the two states:

$$\frac{-13.6 \text{ eV}}{2^2} = -3.40 \text{ eV} \qquad \frac{-13.6 \text{ eV}}{5^2} = -0.54 \text{ eV}$$

2. Subtract to get the energy of the photon:

$$-0.54 \text{ eV} - (-3.40 \text{ eV}) = 2.86 \text{ eV}$$

3. Find the wavelength of the photon:

$$\lambda = \frac{hc}{E} = \frac{(4.14 \times 10^{-15} \text{ eV} \cdot \text{sec})(3 \times 10^8 \text{ m/sec})}{2.86 \text{ eV}} = 4.34 \times 10^{-7} \text{ m or } 434 \text{ nm}$$

Example: What is the wavelength of a photon that will ionize a hydrogen atom in its ground state?

1. The energy needed is enough to raise the total energy level to zero:

$$0 - \frac{(-13.6 \text{ eV})}{1^2} = 13.6 \text{ eV}$$

2. Calculate the wavelength of this photon:

$$\lambda = \frac{hc}{E} = \frac{(4.14 \times 10^{-15} \text{ eV} \cdot \text{sec})(3.00 \times 10^8 \text{ m/sec})}{13.6 \text{ eV}} = 9.1 \times 10^{-8} \text{ m or } 91 \text{ nm}$$

MATHEMATICS REVIEW

An understanding of basic mathematical skills is essential for the science and quantitative skills test questions. This section reviews the most important mathematical concepts that may be present in these tests. This presentation does not attempt to cover all areas in great depth. Rather, it should be used in conjunction with texts so that the student will be prepared for mathematically-oriented test questions.

ARITHMETIC

Operations on Numbers

Whole numbers are the counting numbers, 1, 2, 3, 4, 5, . . . *Integers* are the positive and negative whole numbers and zero: . . . , −3, −2, −1, 0, 1, 2, 3, . . . A *mixed number* consists of an integer combined with a fraction, for example, $3\frac{1}{8}$. Many questions call for rounding off an answer "to the nearest integer." To round off a mixed number to the nearest integer, drop the fraction part of the number; if the fraction part is $\frac{1}{2}$ or more than $\frac{1}{2}$, increase the integer by 1; if the fraction part is less than $\frac{1}{2}$, keep the original integer. For example, $4\frac{7}{8}$ rounded off to the nearest integer is 5, but $3\frac{1}{3}$ rounded off to the nearest integer is 3.

Questions often require that decimal answers be rounded off to some specified degree of precision, for example, to the nearest tenth, or the nearest hundredth, or to the nearest thousandth. To answer such a question, drop all digits in the decimal which are to the right of the specified digit; if the first digit dropped is 5 or more, increase the last digit retained by 1; if the first digit dropped is less than 5, keep the last digit retained at its present value. As examples, 81.698 rounded to the nearest tenth is 81.7; 81.698 rounded to the nearest hundredth is 81.70 (note that the zero is retained to show a hundredths place); 45.639 rounded to the nearest tenth is 45.6.

The rules for rounding off decimals also apply to rounding off whole numbers to a specified degree of precision. For example, 102,681 rounded off to the nearest thousand is 103,000; 102,681 rounded off to the nearest hundred is 102,700; 49,294 rounded off to the nearest thousand is 49,000.

Precision and Significant Digits

All measurements are approximate. Consider a measurement said to be 43 grams to the nearest gram. The unit of measure is the smallest unit indicated by the number and is the unit which was applied in the measurement. In the illustration, the unit is the gram and the maximum possible error is one-half that unit. Thus, 43 grams to the nearest gram means the true measure is between 43 ± 0.5 grams. A measure of $28\frac{1}{2}$ feet means that the unit of measure is $\frac{1}{2}$ foot and the maximum error is therefore $\frac{1}{4}$ foot. A measure of $28\frac{1}{2}$ feet could represent a true measure of anywhere between $28\frac{1}{4}$ feet and $28\frac{3}{4}$ feet. A measurement of 2.05 inches means that the unit of measure is 0.01 inch (that is, $\frac{1}{100}$ of an inch), and the 2.05 may represent a true measure anywhere between 2.045 and 2.055 inches.

If an approximate number is multiplied by some number greater than 1, the precision of the result is reduced since the maximum error is also multiplied by that number. If the approximate measure of $28\frac{1}{2}$ feet, which has a maximum error of $\frac{1}{4}$ foot, is multiplied by 5, the result is $5 \times 28\frac{1}{2}$ or $142\frac{1}{2}$ feet with a maximum error of $5 \times \frac{1}{4}$ or $1\frac{1}{4}$ feet. Thus, the $142\frac{1}{2}$ foot approximation really represents a measure anywhere between $141\frac{1}{4}$ feet and $143\frac{3}{4}$ feet.

If an approximate number is represented as a decimal, every digit starting from the left-most non-zero digit and extending through the digit which represents the unit of measure is a *significant digit*. Thus, 2345 has 4 significant digits, 23.45 also has 4 significant digits, 0.00023 has 2 significant digits, and 2300 may have either 2, 3 or 4 significant digits depending on whether the two zeroes represent accurate measures in the tenths and units places or are merely used as "fillers" to locate the decimal point. Note that the position of the decimal point has nothing to do with the number of significant digits. The speed of light is 186,272 mi/sec; this figure has 6 significant digits; if we talk about the speed of light being 186,000 mi/sec., the figure has only 3 significant digits.

Performing mathematical operations on approximate numbers cannot increase the number of significant digits. If two approximate numbers are multiplied together or divided, you should carry out the multiplication or division and then round off your answer to the number of sig-nificant digits in the number with the *fewest* significant digits. Note that in the case of multi-plication and division, the position of the decimal point has nothing to do with the number of significant digits in the answer. The situation in addition and subtraction is very different. If 231.2 is added to 15.623, the sum becomes 246.823, but digits beyond 246.8 are not signifi-cant since 231.2 was accurate to the nearest tenth only. Thus, in adding or subtracting approxi-mate numbers, you should first carry out the operation and then round the answer to the first place where the *last* significant digit of any of the numbers is found. Note also that if 231.2 had been added to 15.673, the sum would first be 246.873, which would be rounded off to 246.9.

Percent and Percentage

Problems involving percent actually involve three quantities: the base, the percent (or rate), and the percentage. The *percent* (expressed as a decimal such as .20 or as a part of 100 such as 20%) is the ratio of one quantity (the percentage) to another (the base). The number of which the percent is taken is the *base*; the result after the percent of the base is taken is the *percentage*. For example, if we say that 40% of the 2000 bacteria in a certain culture are spiro-chetes, then there are 800 spirochetes present in the culture. 40% or .40 is the percent or rate, 2000 is the base, and 800 is the percentage. The best way to solve any problem involving percent or percentage is with an equation based on the formula $p = br$, that is, percentage equals base times rate. Thus, if asked to find what percent of the 2000 bacteria in a culture is represented by the 800 spirochetes, the equation $800 = 2000r$ is solved. If asked to find the number of bacteria in a culture in which 800 spirochetes are known to represent 40%, the equation $800 = b(.40)$ is solved. If asked to find how many spirochetes there are in a culture containing 2000 bacteria of which 400% are spirochetes, the equation $p = 2000(.40)$ is used.

ALGEBRA

Ratio and Proportion

Ratio: A comparison of two values that are expressed in the same units. It may be expressed as an indicated division or as two numbers separated by a colon.

Example: A comparison of the length of two insects might be expressed as 2 cm : 3 cm, that is, as 2:3 or as $\frac{2 \text{ cm}}{3 \text{ cm}}$, that is, as $\frac{2}{3}$. Note that in each case, the name of the units cancels and the ratio consists of two pure numbers, 2:3 or $\frac{2}{3}$. The units involved must be the same, however; the ratio of 3 inches to 2 yards is not 3:2, but 3 inches to 72 inches, that is 3:72 or $\frac{3}{72}$ or $\frac{1}{24}$.

Proportion: A statement that two ratios are equal. For example, $1:2 = 4:8$ or $\frac{1}{2} = \frac{4}{8}$ represents a proportion.

The first and last terms of a proportion are called the *extremes* and the second and third terms of a proportion are called the *means*. In the proportion $\frac{1}{2} = \frac{4}{8}$, 1 and 8 are the extremes and 2 and 4 are the means. A most important relation used to solve problems involving proportions is this: In any proportion, the product of the means equals the product of the extremes.

Example: If two substances, A and B, are to be mixed in the ratio of 2 parts of A to 3 parts of B, how many milliliters of A must be mixed with 15 milliliters of B to make the proper mixture?

Let x = the number of milliliters of A.

Since the ratio of A to B equals the ratio $2:3$, a proportion is formed:

$$\frac{x}{15} = \frac{2}{3}$$

In a proportion, the product of the means equals the product of the extremes (cross multiply):

$$3x = 2(15)$$
$$3x = 30$$
$$x = 10$$

If the means in a proportion are equal, either of the means is called the *mean proportional* between the two extremes. Thus, in the proportion $\frac{1}{3} = \frac{3}{9}$, 3 is the mean proportional between 1 and 9.

Example: Find the mean proportional between 4 and 16.

If x is the mean proportional, then:

$$\frac{4}{x} = \frac{x}{16}$$

In a proportion, the product of the means equals the product of the extremes (cross multiply):

$$x^2 = 4(16)$$
$$x^2 = 64$$

Take the square root of both sides of the equation: $x = \pm 8$.

Note that every positive number has two square roots, one positive and one negative. In a practical problem, one of the roots (usually the negative one) may have to be rejected as meaningless (for example, if x represents a length).

Equations

Equations Containing Fractions: These are solved by multiplying all terms on both sides of the equation by the Least Common Denominator of all the fractions.

Example: Find a if $\frac{a}{4} - \frac{a}{6} = \frac{1}{2}$.

The least common denominator for 4, 6, and 2 is 12. Multiply all terms on both sides of the equation by 12:

$$12\left(\frac{a}{4}\right) - 12\left(\frac{a}{6}\right) = 12\left(\frac{1}{2}\right)$$
$$3a - 2a = 6$$
$$a = 6$$

Quadratic Equations: Second-degree equations may often be solved by factoring.

Example: Solve $2x^2 + 5x = 3$.

Rewrite the equation so that all terms are on one side in descending order of exponents, equal to 0:

$$2x^2 + 5x - 3 = 0$$

The quadratic trinomial on the left factors into two binomials. The factors of the first term, $2x^2$, become the first terms of the binomials:

$$(2x \quad)(x \quad) = 0$$

The factors of the last terms, -3, become the second terms of the binomials, but they must be chosen in such a way that the product of the inner terms added to the product of the outer terms equals the middle term of the original trinomial, $+5x$. Try -1 and $+3$ as the factors of -3:

$$-x = \text{inner product}$$
$$(2x - 1)(x + 3) = 0$$
$$6x = \text{outer product}$$

Since $(-x) + (6x) = +5x$, these are the correct factors:

$$(2x - 1)(x + 3) = 0$$

Set each factor equal to zero:

$$2x - 1 = 0 \quad \text{OR} \quad x + 3 = 0$$
$$2x = 1 \qquad\qquad x = -3$$
$$x = \frac{1}{2}$$

The solution is $x = \frac{1}{2}$ or -3.

If a quadratic equation cannot be solved by factoring, the *quadratic formula* may be used: In a quadratic equation of the form $ax^2 + bx + c = 0$,

$$x = \frac{-b \pm \sqrt{b^2 - 4ac}}{2a}$$

Example: Solve $x^2 - 4x - 3 = 0$
Here $a = 1$, $b = -4$ and $c = -3$:

$$x = \frac{-(-4) \pm \sqrt{(-4)^2 - 4(1)(-3)}}{2(1)}$$
$$x = \frac{4 \pm \sqrt{16 + 12}}{2}$$
$$x = \frac{4 \pm \sqrt{28}}{2}$$
$$x = \frac{4 \pm \sqrt{(4)(7)}}{2}$$
$$x = \frac{4 \pm 2\sqrt{7}}{2}$$
$$x = 2 \pm \sqrt{7}$$

Radical Equations: Equations in which the variable appears under a radical sign. They may be solved by isolating the radical on one side of the equation and then squaring both sides.

Example: Solve $\sqrt{x^2 - 8} - x = 4$

Isolate the radical on one side of the equation:

$$\sqrt{x^2 - 8} = x + 4$$

Square both sides of the equation:

$$x^2 - 8 = (x + 4)^2$$
$$x^2 - 8 = x^2 + 8x + 16$$
$$-8 - 16 = 8x$$
$$-24 = 8x$$
$$-3 = x$$

The process of squaring may introduce an *extraneous root*; therefore, radical equations solved by squaring must always have the solution(s) checked to see if any are extraneous; checking must be done by substituting in the *original* equation:

$$\sqrt{(-3)^2 - 8} - (-3) \stackrel{?}{=} 4$$
$$\sqrt{9 - 8} + 3 \stackrel{?}{=} 4$$
$$1 + 3 \stackrel{?}{=} 4$$
$$4 \stackrel{?}{=} 4 \ \sqrt{}$$

−3 is a true root.

Equations Containing Decimals: Such equations are best solved by removing all decimals by multiplying each term in the equation by the highest power of 10 that will remove all the decimals:

Example: Solve $153 + 0.085x = 0.85x$
Multiply each term by 1000:

$$153,000 + 85x = 850x$$
$$153,000 = 850x - 85x$$
$$153,000 = 765x$$
$$200 = x$$

Formulas

Questions may be asked requiring you to transform a given formula so that it is solved for a specified variable in terms of the others. This is accomplished in the same manner as the solution of a literal equation; the specified variable must be isolated on one side of the equation with all terms not containing this variable on the other side.

Example: The formula for obtaining the Fahrenheit temperature, F, when the Celsius temperature, C, is known is $F = \frac{9}{5}C + 32$. Find an expression for C in terms of F.

To solve for C, first multiply both sides by 5:

$$5F = 9C + 160$$

Isolate the term containing C on the right side:

$$5F - 160 = 9C$$

Divide both sides by 9:

$$\frac{5F - 160}{9} = C$$

Factor out a 5 in the numerator:

$$\frac{5(F-32)}{9} = C$$

In another form:

$$C = \frac{5}{9}(F-32)$$

Scientific Notation

Scientific notation is a method of writing a number as the product of a power of 10 and a decimal number whose whole number part is between 1 and 10. For example, 3.6903×10^4 is in scientific notation. Scientific notation is a convenient method for designating very large or very small numbers. It is particularly useful when only a small number of significant digits are used in the number. For example, the speed of light is said to be 186,000 mi/sec. The only significant digits are "186" since the three zeros are merely used to indicate the placement of the decimal point. The speed of light is expressed more meaningfully in scientific notation as 1.86×10^5 mi/sec. Scientific notation makes the number easier to handle and also makes it clear that the zeros are not significant digits.

Questions may involve conversion from scientific notation to ordinary notation or vice versa. Since multiplication by 10 results in moving the decimal point one digit to the right, the number 1.25×10^4 becomes 12,500 in ordinary notation (the decimal point is moved 4 places to the right). Similarly, 10 raised to a negative exponent indicates division by 10 that many times. Division by 10 results in moving the decimal point to the left one place. Thus, 1.25×10^{-2} is equivalent to 0.0125 in ordinary notation. 81,250 in ordinary notation becomes 8.125×10^4 in scientific notation, and 0.002728 becomes 2.728×10^{-3}.

Exponents and Logarithms

Positive Exponents: A positive exponent is a number which indicates the number of times a quantity is to be used as a factor in a power. For example, 2^4 means $(2)(2)(2)(2)$ or 16.

Zero Exponents: By definition $x^0 = 1$ for all values of x except $x = 0$, which is undefined. Thus, $5^0 = 1$ and $(-3)^0 = 1$.

Negative Exponents: By definition, $x^{-n} = \frac{1}{x^n}$ provided $x \neq 0$. Thus, $3^{-2} = \frac{1}{3^2} = \frac{1}{9}$.

Fractional Exponents: By definition $x^{m/n} = \sqrt[n]{x^m}$ or $(\sqrt[n]{x})^m$ provided $n \neq 0$. Thus, $x^{1/2} = \sqrt{x}$, and $8^{2/3} = (\sqrt[3]{8})^2 = 2^2 = 4$.

Law of Exponents:

For multiplication: $(x^a)(x^b) = x^{a+b}$ Example: $y^3 \cdot y^4 = y^7$

For division: $x^a \div x^b = x^{a-b}$ Example: $y^6 \div y^2 = y^4$

For powers: $(x^a)^b = x^{ab}$ Example: $(y^2)^3 = y^6$

For roots: $\sqrt[b]{x^a} = x^{a/b}$ Example: $\sqrt{y^6} = y^3$

Exponential Equations: An exponential equation is an equation in which the variable appears in an exponent. Simple exponential equations may be solved by expressing both sides of the equation as powers of the same base.

Example: Solve $3^{x-1} = 9$

Express both sides of the equation as powers of the same base, in this case, 3:

$$3^{x-1} = 3^2$$

Since the bases are the same, the exponents must be equal:

$$x - 1 = 2$$
$$x = 2 + 1$$
$$x = 3$$

If it is impossible to express both sides of the equation as powers of the same base, logarithms must be used to solve an exponential equation (see next section).

Logarithms: The logarithm of a number is the exponent to which a given base must be raised to produce the number. The given base for *common logarithms* is 10.

Thus, $\log_{10} 100 = 2$ since $10^2 = 100$
$\log_{10} 10,000 = 4$ since $10^4 = 10,000$
$\log_{10} 50 = 1.6990$ since $10^{1.6990} = 50$
$\log_{10} 10 = 1$ since $10^1 = 10$

In writing common logarithms, the base, 10, is generally omitted. Thus, we say $\log 100 = 2$, $\log 10,000 = 4$, $\log 50 = 1.6990$, and $\log 10 = 1$.

Of course, $\log 50 = 1.6990$ cannot be found readily. Like all common logarithms, it consists of two parts. The whole number part, or *characteristic*, is positive and is 1 less than the number of digits before the decimal point if the number is 1 or greater. Thus, the characteristic for $\log 839$ would be 2. If the number is a positive number less than 1, the characteristic is negative and its absolute value is 1 more than the number of zeroes between the decimal point and the first significant digit. Thus, the characteristic for $\log 0.0072$ would be -3.

The *mantissa*, or decimal part of the logarithm, is found in the Table of Common Logarithms. The mantissa is always positive and is the same for the same sequence of significant digits. Thus, the mantissas for 365, 36.5, and 0.0365 are the same. The mantissa for $\log 50$ is found by looking for the sequence of digits, 500; the table shows the mantissa for this sequence to be .6990. The characteristic for $\log 50$ is 1, so $\log 50 = 1.6990$. Since the mantissa is always positive and the characteristic may be negative, the log for a number such as 0.00372 must be written as $7.5705 - 10$.

Interpolation: If we have a Table of Common Logarithms that provides entries for numbers with a sequence of only 3 digits, we must interpolate to find a mantissa of a number having 4 significant digits. To find the mantissa for $\log 183.6$, we look for the mantissa for the sequence 183 (it is .2625) and for the mantissa for the sequence 184 (it is .2648). Since 1836 lies between 1830 and 1840, its mantissa will lie at a proportionate distance between their mantissas.

$$\frac{6}{10} = \frac{x}{.0023}$$

The product of the means equals the product of the extremes (cross multiply):

$$10x = 6(.0023)$$
$$10x = .0138$$
$$x = .00138 \text{ or } .0014$$

Mantissa for $\log 1836$ is $.2625 + .0014 = .2639$
Log 183.6 is 2.2639 since the characteristic for 183.6 is 2.

Laws of Logarithms: Since logarithms are exponents, they obey the same laws of exponents:

For multiplication: $\log(ab) = \log a + \log b$
   Example: $\log 8 = \log (4 \cdot 2) = \log 4 + \log 2$

For division: $\log\left(\dfrac{a}{b}\right) = \log a - \log b$

   Example: $\log\left(\dfrac{12}{4}\right) = \log 12 - \log 4$

For powers: $\log a^n = n \log a$
   Example: $\log 2^3 = 3 \log 2$

For roots: $\log \sqrt[n]{a} = \dfrac{1}{n} \log a$

   Example: $\log \sqrt{5} = \dfrac{1}{2} \log 5$

Solving Exponential Equations by Logarithms:

Example: Solve for x: $3^x = 17$.

Since both sides cannot be written as powers of the same base, take logarithms of both sides of the equation:

$$x \log 3 = \log 17$$
$$x(0.4771) = 1.2304$$
$$x = \frac{1.2304}{0.4771}$$

The solution is completed by dividing 1.2304 by 0.4771.

Natural or Naperian Logarithms: Common logarithms use the base 10. In more advanced mathematics and in many scientific applications, it is more effective to use logarithms with a base called the natural number and represented by e; e is approximately 2.718. Logarithms using the base e are called natural or Naperian logarithms and are designated by ln. Thus, ln 100 = 4.605 since $e^{4.605} = 100$

$$\ln 100{,}000 = 9.210 \quad \text{since } e^{9.210} = 10{,}000$$
$$\ln e = 1.000 \quad \text{since } e^1 = e$$
$$\ln 1 = 0 \quad \text{since } e^0 = 1$$

Using either base 10 or base e, a negative logarithm indicates a number between 0 and 1. There are no logarithms for negative numbers.

Natural logarithms obey the same laws as common logarithms since both are exponents. For example, $\ln 65 = \ln(5 \cdot 13) = \ln 5 + \ln 13$.

Variation

Direct Variation: Many physical variables are so related that an increase in one will produce an increase in the other. For example, the pressure of a confined gas will increase as the temperature of the gas is increased. If the values of two variables bear a constant ratio to each other, they are said to be in direct variation; sometimes it is said that "y varies as x" or "y varies directly with x." Direct variation can be expressed in symbols as $\dfrac{y}{x} = k$ or $y = kx$, where k is called the constant of variation.

Example: If the work done, y, by a constant force varies directly as the distance, d, through which the force acts, and if $y = 16$ when $x = 3$, find y when $x = 9$.

Use the formula $y = kx$. Substitute 16 for y and 3 for x:

$$16 = 3k$$

Solve for k, the constant of variation:

$$\frac{16}{3} = k$$

Since k is a constant, substitute the new value of x in $y = \frac{16}{3}x$:

$$y = \frac{16}{3}(9)$$

$$y = 48$$

Inverse Variation: In many sciences, two variables are related so that their product is constant; when one gets larger, the other gets smaller. In an electrical circuit of constant voltage, for example, the product of the current and the resistance is constant. Current and resistance are said to vary inversely. Inverse variation involves a relationship of the form $xy = k$ or $y = \frac{k}{x}$, where k is the constant of variation.

Example: The volume, y, of a gas at a constant temperature is inversely proportional to the pressure, x. If $y = 30$ when $x = 2$, find y when $x = 12$.
Substitute in $xy = k$ to find the constant, k:

$$(2)(30) = k$$

$$60 = k$$

Since k is a constant and equal to 60, now substitute 12 for x in $xy = 60$:

$$12y = 50$$

$$y = 5$$

Joint Variation: Some physical phenomena involve the variation of more than two variables. If y varies directly with both x and z, then the basic relationship may be expressed as $y = kxz$. If y varies directly with x but inversely as the square of z, then the basic relationship may be expressed as $y = \frac{kx}{z^2}$.

TRIGONOMETRY AND THE RIGHT TRIANGLE

The Pythagorean Theorem

Many problems involving right triangles can be solved by use of the Pythagorean Theorem, which states that in any right triangle, the square of the length of the hypotenuse equals the sum of the squares of the lengths of the legs. In the diagram shown, where a and b are the lengths of the legs and c is the length of the hypotenuse, $a^2 + b^2 = c^2$. Thus, if the lengths of any two sides of a right triangle are known, the length of the third side can be found.

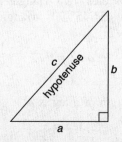

Example: If the hypotenuse of a right triangle is 7 feet, and the length of one leg is 4 feet, find the length of the other leg.

If b is the length of the other leg, apply the Pythagorean Theorem:

$$4^2 + b^2 = 72$$
$$16 + b^2 = 49$$
$$b^2 = 49 - 16$$
$$b^2 = 33$$

Take the square root of both sides of the equation:

$$b = \pm\sqrt{33}$$

Reject the negative value as meaningless for a length:

$$b = \sqrt{33}$$

Pythagorean Triples

Certain special cases result in right triangles in which the ratio of the lengths of the sides can be represented by integers. They are the 3-4-5, 5-12-13, and 8-15-17 right triangles. Note that in every case the largest number in the triple represents the hypotenuse; the other two represent the legs. These triples should be committed to memory as they make the solutions of many right triangles extremely easy.

Example: Find the remaining leg of a right triangle whose hypotenuse is 15 and one of the whose legs is 12.

The hypotenuse, 15, is equal to 3 times 5 and the leg, 12, is equal to three times 4. Hence the triangle is a 3-4-5 right triangle with all the values multiplied by 3. The remaining leg is three times 3 or 9.

45°-45°-90° and 30°-60°-90° Triangles

The MCAT includes questions that may require knowledge of the relationships among the sides of two special right triangles, the 45°-45°-90° triangle and the 30°-60°-90° triangle. The relationships can all be determined by use of the Pythagorean Theorem and certain facts from plane geometry, but it is recommended that the student commit to memory the two diagrams below and use the values shown as formulas to apply in solving either of these special triangles.

Example: Find the leg of an isosceles right triangle whose hypotenuse is $5\sqrt{2}$.

An isosceles right triangle is a 45°-45°-90° triangle. Applying the formulas from the diagram above, the hypotenuse is $a\sqrt{2}$:

$$a\sqrt{2} = 5\sqrt{2}$$
$$a = 5$$

From the diagram above, the length of a leg is a:

$$\text{leg} = 5$$

Example: If the hypotenuse of a 30°-60°-90° triangle is 6, find the length of the leg opposite the 30° angle and the length of the leg opposite the 60° angle.

The formula for the hypotenuse of a 30°-60°-90° triangle is $2a$:

$$2a = 6$$
$$a = 3$$

The formula for the leg opposite 30° is a:

$$a = 3$$

The formula for the leg opposite 60° is $a\sqrt{3}$:

$$a\sqrt{3} = 3\sqrt{3}$$

Trigonometric Functions

The three basic trigonometric functions are defined for acute angles from ratios in a right triangle:

$$\sin A = \frac{\text{opposite side}}{\text{hypotenuse}} = \frac{a}{c}$$

$$\cos A = \frac{\text{adjacent side}}{\text{hypotenuse}} = \frac{b}{c}$$

$$\tan A = \frac{\text{opposite side}}{\text{adjacent side}} = \frac{a}{b}$$

A convenient way to remember these definitions is by memorizing the mnemonic *soh-cahtoa*. Split into three parts, *soh,cah,toa*, where "*s*" stands for sine, "*o*" for opposite, "*h*" for hypotenuse, etc., the mnemonic gives all three definitions. Note that sin is an abbreviation for sine, cos for cosine, and tan for tangent. When any 2 parts from among the two acute angles and the three sides of a right triangle are known, any of the other parts can be found.

Example: In the right triangle shown, find the length of side $\overline{EG}$.

$\overline{EG}$ is the side adjacent to the 40° angle and 20 is the hypotenuse. Hence the cosine is used:

$$\cos 40° = \frac{\text{adjacent leg}}{\text{hypotenuse}}$$

From the Table of the Values of Trigonometric Functions, $\cos 40° = 0.7660$:

$$0.7660 = \frac{x}{20}$$

Multiply both sides of the equation by 20:

$$20(0.7660) = x$$
$$15.32 = x$$

A student taking the MCAT will be expected to know the sines and cosines of 0°, 90°, and 180°. These are shown in tabular form on the next page:

	0°	90°	180°
sin	0	1	0
cos	1	0	−1
tan	0	∞	0

The sines, cosines, and tangents of 0° and 90° are deduced from consideration of what happens as angle A in the diagram of $\triangle ABC$ collapses toward 0°. $\overline{BC}$ will approach 0, and thus the $\sin 0°$ and the $\tan 0°$ will both be 0. As angle A collapses, the hypotenuse $\overline{AB}$ will approach $\overline{AC}$, and hence $\dfrac{AB}{AC}$ will equal 1 at 0°, or $\cos 0° = 1$. The values for 90° are deduced in a similar manner; those for 180° are the result of an extension of the definitions of the trigonometric functions to values beyond the acute angles found in a right triangle.

MCAT candidates are also expected to know the sines, cosines, and tangents of 30°, 45°, and 60°. If the candidate commits to memory the formulas for the sides as recommended in the section of this book on the 45°-45°-90° triangle and the 30°-60°-90° triangle, these values need not be memorized since they can be obtained by applying the definition of the sine, cosine, or tangent to the expressions in the formulas. For example, $\sin 45° = \dfrac{\text{opposite side}}{\text{hypotenuse}} = \dfrac{a}{a\sqrt{2}} = \dfrac{1}{\sqrt{2}}$. The value $\dfrac{1}{\sqrt{2}}$ can be used for $\sin 45°$ or it can be changed to $\dfrac{1}{2}\sqrt{2}$, obtained by multiplying the numerator and denominator by $\sqrt{2}$. As another example, $\cos 60° = \dfrac{a}{2a} = \dfrac{1}{2}$. For the convenience of those candidates who would prefer to memorize the values of the sine, cosine, and tangent of 30°, 45°, and 60°, a table of these values is also given here:

	30°	45°	60°
sin	$\dfrac{1}{2}$	$\dfrac{1}{2}\sqrt{2}$	$\dfrac{1}{2}\sqrt{3}$
cos	$\dfrac{1}{2}\sqrt{3}$	$\dfrac{1}{2}\sqrt{2}$	$\dfrac{1}{2}$
tan	$\dfrac{1}{3}\sqrt{3}$	1	$\sqrt{3}$

SYSTEMS OF MEASUREMENT

The MCAT candidate will be expected to understand and operate in either the metric system of measurement or in the system of common British units. It may be required to perform conversions from one system to the other, but in all such cases, the conversion factor will be supplied with the question.

The Common British System

The following equivalences and abbreviations should be known:

> 1 yard (yd) = 3 feet (ft) = 36 inches (in)
>
> 1 foot = 12 inches
>
> 1 mile (mi) = 5280 feet = 1760 yards
>
> 1 pound (1b) = 16 ounces (oz)
>
> 1 ton (T) = 2000 pounds
>
> 1 gallon (gal) = 4 quarts (qt) = 8 pints (pt)
>
> 1 quart = 2 pints
>
> 1 pint = 16 fluid ounces (oz)

This table of equivalences permits conversions within the British system.

Example: How many ounces are there in 3 tons?

$$3 \text{ tons} \times \frac{2000 \text{ lbs}}{\text{ton}} \times \frac{16 \text{ oz}}{\text{lb}}$$

$$3 \times 2000 \times 16 \text{ oz} = 96,000 \text{ oz}$$

Note that names of units which appear once in a numerator and a denominator are cancelled. For example, tons ÷ tons = 1 and lbs ÷ lbs = 1. This leaves only the name of the units in which the answer is denoted.

Balancing Equations Containing Physical Units: The preceding comment on cancelling the names of units in an equation points up the importance of balancing the names of units on both sides of an equation that deals with physical units.

Example: Given that the distance, d, that a body falls if dropped from rest is $\frac{1}{2}$ the acceleration due to gravity, a, times the time, squared, t^2, find the distance in meters that a body will drop in 3 minutes.

The given equation is:

$$d = \frac{1}{2}at^2$$

We cannot substitute 16 ft/sec^2 for a, or 3 min for t and expect to get a distance in meters because the units involved will not balance:

$$d(\text{meters}) \neq \frac{1}{2} \cdot \frac{16 \text{ ft}}{\text{sec}^2} (3 \text{ min})^2$$

Since $1 \text{ min} = 60 \text{ sec}$, we can replace $(3 \text{ min})^2$ by $(3 \times 60)^2 (\text{sec})^2$, and since $1 \text{ ft} = 0.3 \text{ meter}$, we can replace 16 ft by $16(0.3 \text{ meter})$:

$$d(\text{meters}) = \frac{1}{2} \cdot \frac{16 \,(0.3 \text{ meter})}{\text{sec}^2} (3 \times 60)^2 (\text{sec})^2$$

Cancelling names of units wherever possible shows that both sides of the equation are in meters only:

$$d(\text{meters}) = \frac{1}{2} \cdot \frac{16 \,(0.3 \text{ meter})}{\text{sec}^2} (3 \times 60)^2 (\text{sec})^2$$

If the units in an equation cannot be balanced in this way, it is an indication that there is an error somewhere in the equation.

The Metric System

The basic units for the metric system are:

> For length: meters (abbreviated m)
> For volume: liters (abbreviated l or L)
> For mass: grams (abbreviated g)

The following prefixes are attached to the names of the basic units to denote other units whose size equals the basic unit multiplied or divided by a power of 10:

$$\text{pico (p)} = 10^{-12}$$
$$\text{nano (n)} = 10^{-9}$$
$$\text{micro } (\mu) = 10^{-6}$$
$$\text{milli (m)} = 10^{-3}$$
$$\text{centi (c)} = 10^{-2}$$
$$\text{deci (d)} = 10^{-1}$$
$$\text{deka (da)} = 10$$
$$\text{hecto (h)} = 10^{2}$$
$$\text{kilo (k)} = 10^{3}$$
$$\text{mega (M)} = 10^{6}$$

Thus, a kilometer (km) is 10^3 or 1000 times as large as a meter. A centimeter (cm) is 10^{-2} times a meter or $\dfrac{1}{100}$ the size of a meter. A milligram (mg) is 10^{-3} times the size of a gram or $\dfrac{1}{1000}$ the size of a gram.

Conversions may be made within the metric system simply by moving the decimal point. Thus, $53\,\text{cm} = 0.53\,\text{m}$ (since a meter is 10^2 centimeters). Similarly, $8.3\,\text{kg} = 8300\,\text{g}$ (since a kilogram is 10^3 grams).

ELEMENTARY PROBABILITY

$$\text{The probability of an event occurring} = \frac{\text{the number of favorable cases}}{\text{the total possible number of cases}}.$$

For example, the chance of a tossed coin landing heads up is $\dfrac{1}{2}$ or 0.5, since there is 1 favorable case, heads, out of a total possible number of 2 cases, either heads or tails. The probability of drawing a king on a single draw from a pack of 52 cards is $\dfrac{1}{13}$. The number of favorable cases is 4 (there are 4 kings) and the total possible number of cases is 52; $\dfrac{4}{52} = \dfrac{1}{13}$.

The probability of two or more independent events occurring is the product of their separate probabilities. Thus, the probability of tossing 3 coins and having them all land heads up is $\left(\dfrac{1}{2}\right)\left(\dfrac{1}{2}\right)\left(\dfrac{1}{2}\right) = \left(\dfrac{1}{2}\right)^3 = \dfrac{1}{8}$ or 0.125.

If a coin has been tossed 3 times and has landed heads up each time, what is the probability that a fourth toss will result in a head? The answer is still $\dfrac{1}{2}$ since the fourth result is not affected by the three previous cases (it is said that "coins and cards have no memory"). The probability that all of four tossed coins will land heads up is $\left(\frac{1}{2}\right)\left(\frac{1}{2}\right)\left(\frac{1}{2}\right)\left(\frac{1}{2}\right) = \left(\frac{1}{2}\right)^4 = \frac{1}{1} = 0.0625$.

In a medical situation, suppose that a patient requires ear surgery for which the success rate is 90%. Note that this is equivalent to saying that the probability of success is $\frac{9}{10}$ or 0.9. If the patient requires surgery on both ears, what is the probability of a successful outcome for both?

$$(0.9)(0.9) = 0.81 = 81\%$$

Note that in these calculations, the assumption has been made that the events are independent, that is, that one event does not influence another. Thus, it is assumed that the surgical patient is a normal patient and that success of surgery on one ear does not make success on the other ear more or less probable.

In a compound probability situation, be sure to examine the number of favorable cases and the total possible number of cases for each of the separate situations.

Example: What is the probability of drawing 2 blue marbles from a bag containing 4 red and 6 blue marbles if the first marble is not replaced before the second one is drawn?

The probability of drawing a blue marble on the first draw is $\frac{6}{10}$. But since this first blue marble is not replaced, there are now only 5 blue marbles in the bag out of a total of only 9 marbles. Therefore, the probability of drawing a blue marble on the second draw is $\frac{5}{9}$. The probability of the two events occurring one after the others is $\frac{6}{10} \times \frac{5}{9}$ or $\frac{30}{90}$ or $\frac{1}{3}$.

STATISTICS

Some Measures of Central Tendency

Suppose you are asked to examine the fasting blood glucose concentrations of several patients in a hospital and obtain the results in mg/dl as 100, 80, 100, 90, 100, 120, and 125.

The *range* (the distance between the extreme values) is from 80 to 125, or 45.

The *mode* (the most common value in the series) is 100.

The *arithmetic mean* or *average* is the sum of all the values divided by the number of values:

$$\frac{100 + 80 + 100 + 90 + 100 + 120 + 125}{7} = 102.1$$

The *median* (the middle value when they are arranged in order of size) is 100 since arrangement in order of size gives 80, 90, 100, 100, 100, 120, 125, and the middle number is 100. If there were an even number of items in the series, there would be no single middle number; in such a case, the median is taken as the value halfway between the two middle values.

The Standard Deviation

The standard deviation is a statistical measure that indicates the dispersion or spread of the values in a set of data. You will not be expected to calculate it on the MCAT, but you must be able to interpret it. In the previous illustration, the standard deviation is 15.8. You should know that in a normal distribution, 68% of the values will fall within the arithmetic mean ± 1 standard deviation and 96% of the values will fall within the arithmetic mean ± 2 standard deviations. Thus, in the example shown, 68% of the values would be expected to lie between

102.1 − 15.8 or 86.3, and 102.1 + 15.8 or 117.9. The fact that only 4 out of the 7 values fall in this range $\left(\frac{4}{7} = 57.1\%\right)$ is due to the sample being so small. 96% of the values would be expected to fall between 102.1 − 31.6 or 70.5, and 102.1 + 31.6 or 133.7. Actually, all 7, that is 100% of them, do so.

Correlation

Suppose two variables change at random. The *coefficient of correlation* is a statistical measure of the degree to which the variation in one imitates the variation in the other. On the MCAT, you will not be expected to calculate a coefficient of correlation, but you will be expected to understand the nature of this measure.

The coefficient of correlation may have values between −1 and +1 inclusive; for example, values of +.86 or −.23 are typical. A correlation of +1 is a perfect positive correlation; the two variables involved move up and down together although they may be measured in different units and the moves may be of different magnitudes. A correlation of −1 is a perfect negative correlation; the variables involved move at the same times and to the same degree but in opposite directions (one decreases when the other increases). A correlation of 0 means that there is no relation between the variations in the two.

The output of a factory and its direct costs would tend to move together to some degree; hence the correlation between these two could be expected to be positive although not nearly as great as +1. It is usually true that the higher the price, the lower the sales; if there is a price increase, sales tend to drop; hence price and sales can be expected to be negatively correlated.

The three graphs below represent "scatter diagrams" obtained by plotting random readings of two variables, x and y. Graph A shows no association between x and y and hence the correlation would probably be close to 0. Graph B shows a generally negative correlation (y decreases when x increases), and Graph C shows a positive correlation.

GRAPH A   GRAPH B   GRAPH C

GRAPHIC REPRESENTATION OF DATA AND FUNCTIONS

Medical and other scientific publications use graphic representation of data and of algebraic functions to make relationships clear and also to deduce other information from such a representation.

The Rectangular or Cartesian Coordinate System

This system permits the location of any point on a plane with reference to two perpendicular axes whose point of intersection is called the *origin*. The horizontal axis is the x-axis, and the vertical axis is the y-axis. The position of a point is specified by an ordered pair of numbers in parentheses, for example, (4,3), which are called the *coordinates* of the point. The *x*-coordinate, also called the *abscissa*, is always written first, and the *y*-coordinate, also called the *ordinate*, is second. The abscissa is the distance measured horizontally from the *y*-axis and the ordinate is the distance measured vertically from the *x*-axis to the point. In the diagram, *P* is the point (4,3), *Q* is the point (−2,5), and *R* is the point (−3,−6).

A first degree equation in two variables has an infinite number of pairs of values of *x* and *y* which satisfy it. These points may be plotted on a graph to represent the equation. A first degree equation always has a graph which is a straight line.

Example: Draw the graph of $x + 4y = 8$.
Solve the equation for *y* in terms of *x*:

$$4y = -x + 8$$
$$y = -\frac{1}{4}x + 2$$

Choose some convenient values for *x* and calculate the corresponding values of *y* from the equation:

x	−4	0	8
y	3	2	0

Plot the points (−4,3), (0,2), and (8,0) and draw a straight line through them. This line is the graph of $x + 4y = 8$.

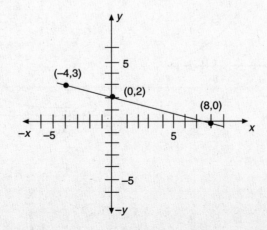

Slope of a Line: If Δy represents the change in the y-values from one point to another and Δx represents the change in the x-values of these two points, then the slope, m, of the line joining the two points is defined as $m = \dfrac{\Delta y}{\Delta x}$. If the coordinates of the two points are represented by (x_1, y_1) and (x_2, y_2), then the slope may also be defined as $m = \dfrac{y_2 - y_1}{x_2 - x_1}$. The slope is the rate of change of y with respect to x.

Example: Find the slope of the first two points plotted to draw the graph of the line $x + 4y = 8$ in the section preceding this. These are the points $(-4,3)$ and $(0,2)$.

Let $(-4,3)$ be (x_1, y_1) and $(0,2)$ be (x_2, y_2). Then $y_2 - y_1$ or Δy is $2 - 3$ or -1, and $x_2 - x_1$ or Δ_x is $0 - (-4)$ or 4. $m = \dfrac{-1}{4}$: The slope is $-\dfrac{1}{4}$.

The Slpope-Intercept Form of a Straight Line: In the last example, notice that the slope of the line is $-\dfrac{1}{4}$ and that $-\dfrac{1}{4}$ (or m) is also the coefficient of x in the equation

$$y = -\frac{1}{4}x + 2$$

The constant term $+2$, which we denote by b, is the y-intercept, that is, the value of y where the graph crosses the y-axis. By solving the equation of a line for y, we can put it in the form $y = mx + b$, which tells us immediately the slope and y-intercept of the line. For example, the line $y = \dfrac{2}{3}x - 4$ has a slope of $\dfrac{2}{3}$ and a y-intercept of -4. This information can be used to draw the graph of the equation instead of plotting points. Begin with the y-intercept (at the point $[0,-4]$), and move 3 units to the right and 2 units up to locate the next point on the line; continue this process for more points on the line.

Graphs of equations other than first degree do not appear as straight lines. The graphs of such equations may be drawn by preparing a table of corresponding values of x and y (obtained by substitution in the equation). These values are used to plot points whose coordinates they are; joining the points with a smooth curve produces the graph representing the equation. Figure 1 shows the graph of the equation $xy = 12$. An equation of the form $xy = k$ where k is a constant is a relationship between two variables that are *inversely proportional*; this type of relationship and its characteristic graph is common to many natural physical phenomena. Figure 2 illustrates the graph of $y = 2^x$ which is an *exponential function*; an exponential function and its

FIG. 1

FIG. 2

characteristic graph is common in many medical and scientific areas, such as the growth of bacteria in a culture or the decay of a radioactive substance. The graphs in both Figures 1 and 2 approach certain lines but never actually reach them; such lines are called *asymptotes*. In Figure 1, both the x- and y-axes are asymptotes; in Figure 2, the x-axis is an asymptote.

Finding the Equation from a Graph

Suppose that readings from experiments are taken on two variables, say blood clotting time and the quantity administered of a certain anti-clotting substance. If these data are used as coordinates of points plotted on a rectangular coordinate chart, and if the points turn out to lie in a straight line, then we know that we can represent the relationship between the two variables by a first degree algebraic equation. In fact, we can write the equation; all we need do is read the value of the y-intercept, b, from the graph and figure the slope, m, by noting the Δy and the Δx between two of the points; substituting the values of m and b in the slope-intercept form, $y = mx + b$, gives the equation.

But suppose that points plotted from experimental data readings do not lie in a straight line. Then the equation of the graph is not a first degree equation. To find out what it is, we use other types of coordinate systems. Two of those that are especially useful with the types of equations and graphs common in medicine and other sciences are the semi-log scale and the log-log scale.

Semi-log Graphs: The rectangular coordinate system uses scales on the x- and y-axes that are arithmetic, that is, the distances on the scale from 0 to 1, from 1 to 2, from 2 to 3, etc., are always the same. The semi-log coordinate system uses an x-axis that has an arithmetic scale, but the distances from the origin along the y-axis represent the values of the logarithms of the numbers instead of the numbers themselves. Thus, the y-axis scale begins at 1 (since log 1 = 0). Since log 10 = 1 and log 100 = 2, the distance on the scale from 1 to 10 is the same as the distance from 10 to 100. It is also the same as the distance from 100 to 1000, etc.

Now suppose that experimental data readings are plotted as points on a semi-log chart, and they turn out to lie in a straight line. Reading the slope, m, and the y-intercept, b, from the graph will enable us to write an equation, but the variable represented on the vertical scale will be log y instead of y and the intercept, b, will actually be log b. Note that log b is some constant. The equation will than be log $y = mx + \log b$. Since the common logarithm is defined as the exponent to which 10 must be raised to give the number, we can write $y = 10^{mx + \log b}$. Thus, we have found an exponential function from the data plotted on a graph.

Example: The graph above, drawn on semi-log coordinate paper, shows a line obtained by plotting a scattering of points from experimental data. Find the equation of the line.

Read the y-intercept, b, from the graph: $b = \log 10 = 1$. Calculate the slope, m:

$$m = \frac{\Delta y}{\Delta x} = \frac{\log 1000 - \log 10}{3 - 0} = \frac{3 - 1}{3} = \frac{2}{3}$$

Using the slope-intercept form of the straight line, $y = mx + b$:

$$\log y = \frac{2}{3}x + 1$$

Since log y is the exponent to which 10 must be raised to equal y:

$$y = 10^{2/3x+1}$$

Note that although for simplicity this discussion involves a y-axis scale which is for common logs (base 10), semi-log scales used in medicine could be scaled for natural logarithms (base e).

Log-log Graphs: In semi-log graphs, the x-axis has an arithmetic scale and the y-axis has a scale that is logarithmic. In log-log graphs, both the x-axis and y-axis have scales that are logarithmic.

Suppose we plot points from experimental data and find that they lie in a straight line on a log-log chart. As before, we can read the slope, m, and the y-intercept, b, and use them in the $y = mx + b$ form of the straight line to write the equation. However, the variables are now log y and log x instead of y and x, and the value we read for the y-intercept is actually log b. Thus, we can write an equation, $\log y = m \log x + \log b$. Making use of the laws of logarithms, $m \log x = \log x^m$, and $\log x^m + \log b = \log (bx^m)$. Thus, our equation becomes $\log y = \log (bx^m)$. Since we have the logs of two expressions equal, the expressions themselves are equal. Thus, our equation is $y = bx^m$. Since m may be any positive or negative integer or even a fraction, we have a powerful tool for converting data readings into complicated equations of degree greater than 1.

A first degree equation in two variables can always be rewritten in the form $y = mx + b$, and its graph is *always* a straight line on rectangular coordinate graph paper. The MCAT candidate should know that one type of exponential equation is of the form $y = a^{bx+c}$, where a, b, and c are constants, and that its graph is *always* a straight line when drawn on semi-log coordinate paper. In scientific work the "a" of $y = a^{bx+c}$ is frequently equal to e, the natural number, and c is frequently equal to 0, so that the most common form of an exponential equation in medicine or other sciences is $y = e^{bx}$.

MCAT candidates should also know that an equation of the form $y = ax^n$ where a and n are constants and n may be positive, negative, or a fraction, is known as a power law; its graph is *always* a straight line when drawn on log-log coordinate paper.

VECTOR ADDITION AND SUBTRACTION

Vectors

Most quantities are *scalar* quantities, that is, they have magnitude only. The length of a line, the number of pages in this book, or your bank balance are all scalar quantities. Some quantities have both a magnitude and a direction. They are called *vector* quantities. Examples are a wind velocity of 15 mph in an easterly direction, a downward (vertical) water pressure of 20 lb/in², or the motion of a ship sailing northeast at 23 knots. A directed line segment called a *vector* is used to represent such quantities; its length represents the magnitude of the quantity and its orientation represents the direction.

Vector Addition

Suppose that two forces, one of 20 lb and one of 25 lb act simultaneously on a body at an angle of 60° to each other. We may represent the 20 lb force by vector $\overrightarrow{OA}$ and the 25 lb force by the vector $\overrightarrow{OB}$. Complete the parallelogram of which $\overrightarrow{OA}$ and $\overrightarrow{OB}$ are two sides. The diagonal of the parallelogram, $\overrightarrow{OC}$, is a vector which is called the sum of the vectors $\overrightarrow{OA}$ and $\overrightarrow{OB}$. $\overrightarrow{OC}$ is also called the *resultant* of the two vectors, $\overrightarrow{OA}$ and $\overrightarrow{OB}$, and $\overrightarrow{OA}$ and $\overrightarrow{OB}$ are the *components* of the force represented by $\overrightarrow{OC}$. If the object on which forces $\overrightarrow{OA}$ and $\overrightarrow{OB}$ are acting is free-moving, the object will move in the direction represented by $\overrightarrow{OC}$ and with a force whose magnitude is represented by the length of $\overrightarrow{OC}$.

If it is desired to compute the magnitude of $\overrightarrow{OC}$ in the above example, $\triangle OBC$ must be solved. Since $AOBC$ is a parallelogram, $BC = OA = 20$, and $\angle B \triangleq 120°$. By the Law of Cosines, $(OC)^2 = (OB)^2 + (BC)^2 - 2(OB)(BC)\cos \angle B$. All the quantities on the right side of the equation are known, so $(OC)^2$, and hence $\overrightarrow{OC}$, can be calculated.

Questions on the MCAT involving vector addition could involve simpler cases than the above, usually those in which the two component forces are at right angles to each other.

Example: Find the resultant force and the angle it makes with the larger component, if two component forces, one of 10 lb and one of 20 lb, act at 90° to each other.

Draw vectors representing the two forces and complete the parallelogram of which they are sides. The diagonal of this parallelogram, which comes from their common origin, is the resultant or sum of the two forces. Vector $\overrightarrow{OC}$ is the resultant. In right $\triangle OBC$, $OB = 20$ and $CB = OA = 10$. By the Pythagorean Theorem, $(OC)^2 = 20^2 + 10^2$ or $(OC)^2 = 400 + 100$; since $(OC)^2 = 500$, $OC = \sqrt{500}$ or $10\sqrt{5}$. In right triangle OBC, $\tan \angle 1 = \dfrac{\text{opposite leg}}{\text{adjacent leg}} = \dfrac{10}{20} = \dfrac{1}{2} = 0.5000$. From the Tables of Trigonometric Functions, the angle whose tangent is 0.5000 is 27° to the nearest degree, so the resultant makes a 27° angle with the larger component.

Vectors may also be added by representing them as complex numbers. The vector represented by the complex number $3 + 2i$ is the vector which extends from the origin to the point representing $3 + 2i$ graphically. Suppose we wish to add the vector represented by $3 + 2i$ to the vector represented by $1 - 3i$. As before, the resultant can be drawn as the diagonal of the parallelogram formed by using the two given vectors as sides. The complex number which is the end point of the resultant can be read from the graph; it represents the resultant vector. However, the sum can be obtained more simply by adding the two complex numbers algebraically:

$$\begin{array}{r} 3 + 2i \\ 1 - 3i \\ \hline 4 - i \end{array}$$

The resultant is $4 - i$.

Subtraction of Vectors

To subtract one vector from another, we simply add the additive inverse of the vector to be subtracted. If the complex number representation of the vectors is used, this simply means that the signs of the vector being subtracted are changed and the resulting complex number is then added to the other vector. If the parallelogram method is used, the vector being subtracted is replaced by a vector of the same magnitude but extending in the opposite direction. This new vector is then added to the other vector by forming a parallelogram and finding the diagonal which is the resultant (see diagram).

SUBTRACTING $\vec{OB}$ FROM $\vec{OA}$

$\vec{OA} - \vec{OB} =$
$\vec{OA} + \vec{OB'}$ (where $\vec{OB'} = -\vec{OB}$)
Thus $\vec{OA} - \vec{OB} = \vec{OC}$

VERBAL REASONING—
TEST-TAKING STRATEGIES

This portion of the book will focus on various techniques to help you get the most out of reading.

You can learn to read efficiently and effectively, and the more you read the better you will read. People who do not like to read generally do not read well, and most people who do not read well read too slowly. They read almost word by word and must consequently backtrack to capture the main idea. You should read as fast as you can think without the loss of comprehension, misreading, or losing facts or ideas.

Learning to read rapidly takes effort, willpower, and a plan. Success depends on your interest and the effectiveness of the techniques and habits you acquire. Find the time for the activities that are necessary for academic success: first things first!

A great deal of your success depends on your frame of mind. You must develop confidence in your own ability. Believe in yourself. You have been successful in the past, and will be successful in the future. Confidence comes with knowledge, experience, and practice.

In the MCAT Examination, reading skill or verbal reasoning is assessed by presenting to the examinee one or more paragraphs of material. The selection is followed by a variable number of questions pertaining to it. Subjects from a wide variety of areas are used to test the student's ability to analyze data accurately. The information necessary to answer the questions is in the selection, and no prior knowledge is necessary to arrive at a correct answer.

APPROACH TO THE READING QUESTIONS

There is no one correct way to handle this section. Some people routinely read the selection first, and some read the questions first. With either approach, rapid processing of information and maximum retention are key elements. The techniques of underlining (described later in this chapter) are useful here.

If you prefer to read the selection first, use the underlining technique to highlight the details. When you finish the selection, you should immediately move on to the questions and answer them one by one while the information is still fresh in your mind.

Some people read the questions first since they feel that they have better attention to details when they know what to expect. If you choose this approach, you read the passage with specific questions in mind. Then you can either answer the questions as a group when you have finished the passage, or answer the questions as the answers appear in the selection. Whichever way you proceed, we still advocate the underlining method. If you have to go back later, the material is already grouped and easier to work with. This will make backtracking more efficient.

Do not, however, leave questions blank in the hope of returning to them later. This could be costly since rereading the entire passage may require a great deal of time. (In the knowledge sections of the examination this is not a problem because the questions are units in themselves and not based on paragraphs.) Answer all questions as best you can, marking those you are not certain of for checking if you have time at the end. Please remember that you must base your answers on the material presented in the passage, not on your own knowledge or experience.

Quantitative questions should be approached in the same way as Reading questions. The only difference is that the information is presented in tables, graphs, charts, maps, and other quantitative forms instead of straight prose. The student's ability to read and analyze the material is tested by the questions. There is no single perfect approach to this type of material. However, it is important to be sure you know what each number, axis, line, or graph means before proceeding to answer the questions. Make sure that you are aware what information has been presented, what the limitations of the data are and what reasonable conclusions may be drawn from it. Do not base your answer on information that isn't there.

Ways and Means

Reading experts seem to agree that the rapid reader's comprehension is usually excellent, and the slow reader's comprehension is usually poor. This does not mean that the rapid reader never slows down for difficult material. It does mean that the rapid reader is able to find the right speed for the material, while the slow reader habitually reads more slowly than the occasion or subject matter demands.

Word-by-Word Reading: Word-by-word reading does not improve comprehension and makes concentration more difficult. Understanding and comprehension demand that you read groups of words, or ideas. As you read, you must analyze, think, group ideas and topics, spot relationships, and see similarities and differences in the passage. The word-by-word reader sees only the trees and misses the forest.

Backtracking: Most readers backtrack occasionally. This technique is not only acceptable but also part of efficient reading. All of us look back and reread a word or several words now and then. The good reader, however, does it less frequently than the poor reader. The efficient reader basically looks back only when he needs to, while the slow reader does it mechanically and out of habit. The inefficient reader usually reads most words, phrases, sentences, and paragraphs more than once since he often misses the central idea or meaning the first time. The first time through, he has merely read the words and must therefore reread the selection to see how they are connected. The habit of reading single words rather than groups usually keeps you from grasping the central theme. Grouping words, sentences, and paragraphs as you go along allows you to make sense of the material and to focus on the theme and idea.

Pausing and Stopping: Inefficient readers usually allow long and frequent pauses as they proceed. This not only hinders concentration but also makes it difficult to absorb the ideas presented. If you pause after reading only a few sentences, you lose track of the author's train of thought. You may remember certain details, but the connections get lost.

Quick Skimming to Elicit the General Theme: This technique involves reading rapidly and concentrating on the key words and phrases that develop and support the theme. One might think that in this approach, the main point could be missed; however, nothing could be further from the truth. This is purposeful reading for comprehension, since its object is to grasp the central point and carefully note the key elements that support that point.

Key Words That Announce Conditions and Should Be Kept in Focus!

1. again, also, accordingly, just as
2. therefore, thus, hence, henceforth
3. for example, for instance, in other words
4. nevertheless, however, notice, but
5. always, at all times, under all circumstances, every time
6. finally, in conclusion, in brief, at last
7. never, not, no, none
8. only, specifically, significantly, importantly, decidedly
9. first, another, and, likewise, as well as, besides
10. despite, although, regardless

How is Material Usually Organized?

1. Most selections have a *central subject* (main idea) which could be used as the *title*. In many instances, the first sentence of a paragraph will tell you this main idea.
2. The material is usually presented in a fashion that answers a question, poses one, gives a solution, or gives a noncommittal statement of fact.
3. Key words and facts should substantiate and solidify the main idea of the reading. These are the details. Always look for key words. If you go back and read the key words, you should be able to get the essence of the passage.
4. The details are usually of two types. The main details are directly related to the central theme, and are used to develop it. The subordinate details break down and clarify the main details, to further develop the theme. Breaking the material down this way can help you to understand it.
5. Read in a questioning manner. This will ensure that you are actively involved. Ask *who*, *what*, *when*, and *where* to elicit key elements. Ask *how* and *why* to determine reasons.

Suggested Method for Efficient Analysis of Reading Material

1. Identify the topic or main theme and underline it with a <u>straight</u> line.
2. Find the main details about the topic and underline the key words or phrases with a curved line.
3. As you read the subordinate details about the details bracket them with (curved brackets).
4. Extraneous elements or qualifiers should be bracketed with [square brackets] as they are encountered.

Don't go overboard! Focus on key elements only. This simple method will allow you to backtrack if needed, and will help you answer the questions at the end of a selection. Your information is now arranged to highlight the interrelationships of facts. While you have read, you have been forced to think and organize the material. You have formed associations that will foster recall.

A PLAN FOR SELF-IMPROVEMENT

1. Set aside a time and place specifically for reading every day even if it is only 10 minutes. You know the conditions under which you function best. No one can set them for you.
2. Develop the habit of reading for ideas. After you have read a passage, ask yourself what the central theme was and verbalize it. The verbalization will quickly synthesize the material and draw upon relationships (similarities, differences) in the passage. The central idea will not only be highlighted but also be substantiated and amplified. Picture yourself as a critic who is writing a review that will evaluate the material for a potential reader.
3. Read different material; become a versatile reader.
4. Keep a record of your progress and be optimistic. A positive attitude is half the battle. Don't be discouraged by plateaus; they are common.

The Do's and Don'ts

1. Even though *scientific* reading, unlike pleasure reading, often involves word-by-word reading, you should coordinate speed and thought processes, and you should read as fast as you think. Backtracking usually interferes with efficient assimilation and processing of information.

2. Even though close, word-by-word reading is slower and more tedious, eliminate irrelevant thoughts. You don't want them to intrude just because you believe you must have something to think about. Irrelevant thoughts make concentration impossible.

3. Usually, poor concentration will lead to poor comprehension, and unnecessarily slow reading can lead to poor concentration and poor comprehension. Read as rapidly as you can without losing comprehension. Adapt speed as necessary.

4. Don't hold back your thinking processes by unnecessarily slow reading. Do not create a gap between reading and thinking. In the same vein, do not stop and pause frequently since this also will allow gaps in your thinking to occur.

5. Remember, it's a poor reader who stops too often and pauses too long at each stop.

6. Apply the same concentration whether a selection is long or short.

7. Look for a general impression, main thoughts, and implications so that you may draw inferences. Read ideas rather than words. Identify your topics, the details about them, and the details about the details. Above all, don't fail to note the important ideas.

8. Whether you are the original writer or the reader of a selection, you must approach it with the thought of a distinct design and technique to present a specific subject matter and topic. Look for special effects and results.

9. You can usually identify the main topic of a paragraph by key words or phrases that could serve as possible titles. Concentrate on why certain words are used and how they are used. By concentrating on why and how, you can establish and follow the main idea. During your reading, you should realize that the paragraph is merely a sum of its parts. In turn, look at paragraphs as key elements in the development of the ideas of the passage. Don't let minor details or sentences overshadow paragraphs or the whole selection. Where there are paragraph headings, these usually lead you to main ideas.

10. Central thoughts are usually found in the lead sentence or in the summary sentence, but they may be located in other places and may, at times, be implied rather than stated. Read to understand by focusing on central ideas and units of thought.

11. Exhibit versatility, and adjust to the material. Don't use the same technique for all material; be pliable, adapt, use common sense.

12. Most of the material you confront will be familiar and understandable to you. Don't stick too closely to the particular selection; always associate present material with previous material. Nothing is ever completely new. In this context, you must focus on detail and read for specific comprehension and specific meanings to see what is new. Whether you read for general or specific ideas, use your previous knowledge. Read for meaning. Try to determine the meaning of unfamiliar words as you reason through a selection. Don't let an unfamiliar word stump you and worry you unduly; the context will often help you determine the meaning.

13. Do not decrease speed because of fear that you might miss something, and do not fall into the trap of reading each sentence twice before you proceed. Don't reread material unless necessary, but if you need to reread, do not hesitate to spend the time to clarify meaning.

14. Do not read each sentence as a distinct unit, but use each unit to build the paragraph and the selection to create the whole.

15. As you read a selection composed of several paragraphs, reflect whether succeeding paragraphs amplify the ideas or points raised in the preceding paragraphs or whether they provide an example or illustration of them. Is a qualifier of a point introduced, or is another aspect of the same subject considered?

16. Before you answer the whole battery of questions, quickly review your underlinings to make sure you understood the point.

17. Under no circumstances should you get yourself involved more deeply than necessary with the reading selection and with the task. Don't read more into it than is there; answer the questions on the basis of only what is presented.

18. Be critical when you read; extract the important facts and see relationships and associations. Visualize descriptions accurately. Avoid misreading.

19. Avoid superficiality when you consider the selection. Don't come to a conclusion before you have read the whole passage and without sufficient thought. Don't jump to a conclusion.

PRACTICE READING EXERCISES

Exercise I

Identify the central theme or topic, details, and details about details.

DIRECTIONS: Read the sample and underline the topic, the details about the topic, and bracket (the details about the details).

Example: Following the work of Chalmers and others, 831 geriatric and orthopedic patients in West London were reviewed for osteomalacia.

(a) The topic deals with osteomalacia.
(b) Details or key words are geriatric and orthopedic patients.
(c) Details about details are (831 patients) and (West London).

DIRECTIONS: Read the sample paragraph and underline the topic, the details about the topic, and bracket (the details about the details). Use square brackets for [extraneous material].

Example: Following the work of Chalmers and others, 831 geriatric and orthopedic patients in West London were reviewed for osteomalacia. History, relevant blood tests (calcium, phosphate, alkaline phosphatase, 24-hour urinary calcium) and radiology were assessed. Thirty-eight bone biopsies were performed. Thirty-three were positive (32 female, 1 male). Average age was 73.4 years. None had a history of gastric surgery. Twenty-eight were widows living alone. Three were sisters (spinsters) living together. Twenty-two lived on their own property. Average weekly income was $25.00. Average weekly food bill, $9.00 (mostly bread, canned meat, and canned fruit). The minimum for a balanced diet was thought to be $18.00. Average milk consumption was one pint per week. None of the patients cooked regularly. Twenty-six never cooked at all. None had sought the assistance of any of the welfare organizations, through either pride, ignorance, or apathy. All showed subjective and objective improvement following calcium and Vitamin D supplementation and dietary improvement.

Method: Following the work of Chalmers and others, (831) geriatric and orthopedic patients in [West London] were reviewed for osteomalacia. History, relevant blood tests (calcium, phosphate, alkaline phosphatase, 24-hour urinary calcium) and radiology were assessed. Twenty-eight bone biopsies were performed. (Thirty-three were positive) ([32 female], 1 male). Average age was (73.4) years. [None] had a history of [gastric surgery]. (Twenty-eight) were (widows) living alone. Three were sisters (spinsters) living together. [Twenty-two] lived on their [own property]. Average weekly income was $25.00. Average weekly food bill, $9.00 (mostly bread, canned meat, and canned fruit). The minimum for a balanced diet was thought to be $18.00. Average milk consumption (one pint) per week. None of the patients cooked regularly (Twenty-six never) cooked at all. None had sought the assistance of any of the welfare organizations, through either pride, ignorance, or apathy. All showed subjective and objective improvement following calcium and Vitamin D supplementation and dietary improvement.

Method in Outline Form

(a) The topic: osteomalacia
(b) Details or key words:
1. geriatric, orthopedic patients
2. history, blood tests, radiology, bone biopsies
3. age, milk consumption, week
4. none cooked regularly, none assistance
5. improvement, calcium, Vitamin D, dietary

(c) Details about details:
   1. (831)
   2. (33 positive)
   3. (73.4 years)
   4. (twenty-eight widows)
   5. (one pint)
   6. (twenty-six never)
(d) Extraneous material:
   1. [West London]
   2. [32 female]
   3. [None gastric surgery]
   4. [Twenty-two own property]

Having used the underlining technique, let us use this information to answer the type of questions used in the examination.

DIRECTIONS: Choose the best answer.

1. Osteomalacia:

   A. has a predilection for males.
   B. occurs more frequently in females.
   C. can only be diagnosed by bone biopsy.
   D. has a predilection for apartment dwellers.

2. The average weekly income did not allow these people to buy more food.

   A. True
   B. False
   C. They needed to save for their old age.
   D. They spend their money on the little luxuries of life.

3. From these data we may conclude that:

   A. homeowners are more likely to develop osteomalacia than are renters.
   B. spinsters will not develop osteomalacia if they live alone.
   C. consumption of bread is a consistent factor in the development of osteo-malacia.
   D. there seems to be a correlation between an unbalanced diet, irregular meal consumption, and osteomalacia.

4. Given a greater income, these individuals would have:

   A. eaten more nutritious meals.
   B. cooked at least two meals a day.
   C. spent a greater percentage of their income on food.
   D. the passage does not give enough information to answer this question.

5. This study:

   A. indicated that dietary supplementation is beneficial.
   B. utilized every technique available.
   C. utilized a great variety of patients.
   D. showed that at least ten percent of the elderly suffer from osteomalacia.

Answers

1. Answer **B**
   Statement A: The numbers (32:1) clearly show that males are not prone to osteomalacia.
   Statement B: Explained above.
   Statement C: History, relevant blood tests, and radiological examination can be used to diagnose osteomalacia, as well as a bone biopsy.
   Statement D: Living in an apartment is not mentioned; however, the paragraph does mention that 22 of 33 lived on their own property.

2. Answer **B**
   Statement A: The average weekly income is stated as $25.00 and a minimum considered necessary for a balanced diet was $18.00.
   Statement B: Explained above.
   Statement C: These were elderly individuals and the issue of saving is not addressed.
   Statement D: The passage does not comment on the luxuries of life.

3. Answer **D**
   Statement A: There is no discussion of homeowners vs. renters in the passage as far as disease is concerned.
   Statement B: The paragraph does not differentiate between spinsters living alone or imply that widows are more prone to the disease because they might live alone.
   Statement C: Although bread was a high intake item, no relationship to the disease was implied.
   Statement D: An unbalanced diet and the irregular consumption of food are definite contributory factors.

4. Answer **D**
   Statement A: Income ($25.00) exceeded expenditures ($18.00) for a necessary balanced diet.
   Statement B: The passage states that most did not cook at all.
   Statement C: There is no issue of income and expenditure; income was adequate to live on a balanced diet.
   Statement D: This is the best answer since the passage truly does not discuss the issue of greater income and a person's spending habits.

5. Answer **A**
   Statement A: Improvement was noted after dietary supplementation.
   Statement B: Only three techniques were mentioned and no reference was made to limitations of techniques.
   Statement C: Only registered, orthopedic patients of West London were used; this is certainly not a great variety.
   Statement D: Of the 831 patients, 33 were diagnosed to have osteomalacia; this figure is not even 5 percent.

Exercise 2

Identify the central theme or topic, details, and details about details.

DIRECTIONS: Read the sample and underline the topic, the details about the topic, and bracket (the details about the details).

Example: James Berlin ends his discussion of "the New Rhetoric" with a list of four attitudes that work against social change.

(a) The topic deals with <u>attitudes that work against social change</u>.
(b) Details or key words are <u>James Berlin</u>, "<u>the New Rhetoric</u>."
(c) Details about details are (four).

Example: James Berlin ends his discussion of "the New Rhetoric" with a list of four attitudes that work against social change. Reification occurs when the system is fortified by the attitude that nothing can ever be changed. Prescientific thinking trusts in luck or good fortune to bring about the needed social change, no action is necessary. Acceleration refers to the increasingly fast-paced, data-saturated lifestyle that keeps people from critically examining the world around them as they slip into a consumerist trance. Finally, mystification refers to responses to social ills based on racism, sexism, nationalism, or any form of bigotry. These four mentalities are roadblocks to progressive change, but they are roadblocks that can be dismantled with the dialectic of New Rhetoric.

Students are told everywhere of the superior freedom that Americans enjoy yet they are ceaselessly faced with arbitrary authoritarian hierarchies which they must be empowered to examine and challenge. Berlin's "liberatory classroom" encourages self-autonomy and self-fulfillment in the students as they examine power structures and resist social influences that alienate and disempower. The development of this critical thinking process is worked out on paper in a nonhierarchical classroom where both student and teacher create the course together. The primary goal of this environment is to help students grow from being manipulated pawns to active, critical builders of an improving society. The best way to do this is to help them develop their rhetorical skills by examining these issues in writing.

Method: <u>James Berlin</u> ends his discussion of "the <u>New Rhetoric</u>" with a list of (four) <u>attitudes that work against social change</u>. <u>Reification</u> occurs when the system is fortified by the (attitude that nothing can ever be changed). <u>Prescientific thinking</u> trusts in (luck or good fortune) to bring about the (needed social change); no action is necessary. <u>Acceleration</u> refers to the increasingly (fast-paced, data-saturated lifestyle) that (keeps people from critically examining the world) around them as they slip into a consumerist trance. Finally, <u>mystification</u> refers to (responses to social ills) based on racism, sexism, nationalism, or any form of bigotry. These four mentalities are roadblocks to progressive change, but they are <u>roadblocks</u> that <u>can be dismantled</u> with the <u>dialectic of New Rhetoric</u>.

<u>Students</u> are <u>told</u> everywhere of the superior <u>freedom</u> that <u>Americans</u> enjoy yet they are ceaselessly <u>faced</u> with arbitrary <u>authoritarian hierarchies</u> which they <u>must</u> be empowered to <u>examine</u> and <u>challenge</u>. (<u>Berlin's</u>) "<u>liberatory classroom</u>" encourages self-autonomy and <u>self-fulfillment</u> in the students as they <u>examine</u> power structures and <u>resist social influences</u> that (<u>alienate and disempower</u>). The development of this <u>critical thinking process</u> is worked out <u>on paper in</u> a <u>nonhierarchical classroom</u> where both <u>student and teacher create</u> the <u>course together</u>. The primary <u>goal</u> of this environment is <u>to help students grow</u> (from <u>being manipulated pawns</u>) <u>to active, critical builders</u> of an improving society. The best way to do this is to help them <u>develop</u> their <u>rhetorical skills by examining</u> these issues <u>in writing</u>.

Method in Outline Form

(a) The topic: <u>attitudes that work against social change</u>
(b) Details or key words:
  1. <u>James Berlin, the "New Rhetoric"</u>
  2. <u>Reification</u>
  3. <u>Prescientific thinking</u>
  4. <u>Acceleration</u>
  5. <u>Mystification</u>
  6. <u>roadblocks can be dismantled with dialectic of New Rhetoric</u>
  7. <u>Students told of superior freedom Americans enjoy yet faced with arbitrary authoritarian hierarchies they must examine and challenge</u>

8. "liberatory classroom" encourages self-autonomy and self-fulfillment, examine power structures and resist social influences
9. critical thinking process on paper in nonhierarchical classroom, student and teacher create the course together
10. goal to help students grow to active, critical builders of improving society
11. develop rhetorical skills by examining issues in writing

(c) Details about details:
1. (four)
2. (attitude that nothing can ever be changed)
3. (luck or good fortune), (needed social change)
4. (fast-paced, data-saturated lifestyle keeps people from critically examining the world)
5. (responses to social ills)
6. (Berlin's)
7. (alienate and disempower)
8. (from being manipulated pawns)

Having read the passage and used the underlining technique, let us use this information to answer the type of questions used in the examination.

DIRECTIONS: Choose the best answer.

1. Which of the following statements is neither supported nor contradicted by the information in the passage?

   A. Students are told that Americans enjoy superior freedom.
   B. The "liberatory classroom" is a nonhierarchical one in which the student and teacher create the course together.
   C. An important component of the nonhierarchical classroom is the social hour in which members share ideas after the class is over.
   D. The four attitudes that are roadblocks to social change can be dismantled by the dialectic of New Rhetoric.

2. According to the passage, which of the following concerning the four attitudes that work against social change is/are correct?

   A. Prescientific thinking trusts that luck will bring about needed social change.
   B. An increasingly fast-paced, data-saturated lifestyle keeps people from critically examining their world.
   C. Both A and B are correct.
   D. Neither A nor B is correct.

3. Concerning the creation of the nonhierarchical classroom, which of the following comes closest, according to the passage, to describing its purpose?

   A. It allows students to see the teacher as a role model.
   B. It is designed to help students grow into active members of a society that they are helping to improve.
   C. It provides an environment where students can learn large amounts of information.
   D. It will prepare students to become effective classroom teachers.

4. Concerning the role of the "New Rhetoric" regarding social change, which of the following is neither supported nor contradicted by the passage?

   A. According to the passage, the "New Rhetoric" can dismantle the roadblocks to progressive change.

B. Part of the process involved in the "New Rhetoric," the passage implies, is to make students more socially aware, a process that involves the examining of issues and writing about them.

C. The passage indicates that the "New Rhetoric" approaches writing by having students revise drafts of their work-in-progress.

D. The "liberatory classroom," the passage implies, serves as a kind a laboratory for practicing the "New Rhetoric."

Answers

1. Answer **C**
   Statement A: According to the first sentence of paragraph two, students are told that Americans enjoy superior freedom.
   Statement B: The passage states that students and teachers create the course together in the "liberatory classroom," which is nonhierarchical.
   Statement C: There is no mention of a social hour in connection with a nonhierarchical classroom.
   Statement D: The final sentence of paragraph one asserts that the "roadblocks to social change can be dismantled with the dialectic of New Rhetoric."

2. Answer **C**
   Statement A: According to sentence two of paragraph one, prescientific thinking places its trust in luck or good fortune.
   Statement B: Under the rubric "acceleration," the passage asserts that our fast-paced, data-saturated lifestyle prevents people from critically examining the world around them.
   Statement C: Since both A and B are correct according to the passage, C is the correct response.
   Statement D: Refer to C above.

3. Answer **B**
   Statement A: One feature of a nonhierarchical classroom as it is described in the passage is to encourage self-autonomy and by implication to deemphasize the role of authority of the teacher. There is, in any case, no mention in the passage of the teacher as role model.
   Statement B: The next-to-last sentence in paragraph two identifies this as the "primary goal" of the "liberatory classroom."
   Statement C: This is not mentioned in the passage.
   Statement D: This is not mentioned in the passage.

4. Answer **C**
   Statement A: The passage does assert that roadblocks to social change can be dismantled with the dialectic of New Rhetoric.
   Statement B: A main goal of the "New Rhetoric" as it is explained throughout the passage is to raise the students' level of social awareness, and to make them "critical builders of an improving society." Part of the process is to have them examine "these issues in writing."
   Statement C: The passage does not address the processes involved in the actual writing, which might, indeed, include the production and revision of drafts. Since this is not included in the passage, C is correct.
   Statement D: Though no formal definition of "liberatory classroom" is given, the reader must infer from the details provided in paragraph two that it is, in fact, a kind of laboratory in which principles of the "New Rhetoric" are practiced. This is clearly a logical inference.

Exercise 3

Identify the central theme or topic, details, and details about details.

DIRECTIONS: Read the sample and underline the <u>topic</u>, the <u>details about the topic</u>, and bracket (the details about the details).

Example: Just about anyone you talk to nowadays complains about the cost of his automobile insurance. It's about time that someone came to the defense of the insurance companies.
(a) The topic deals with <u>automobile</u> <u>insurance</u>.
(b) Details or key words are <u>complains</u>, <u>cost</u>, <u>defense</u>, <u>companies</u>.

DIRECTIONS: Read the sample selection and underline the <u>topic</u>, the <u>details about the topic</u>, and bracket (the details about the details). Use square brackets for [extraneous material] if desired.

Example: Just about anyone you talk to nowadays complains about the cost of his automobile insurance. It's about time that someone came to the defense of the insurance companies.

We are all familiar with the effects of inflation, but most people forget that the insurance companies are affected too. An interesting point should be noted. Even though the total costs of producing a policy have been increasing because of increased salaries, paper cost, equipment replacement, etc., the insurance companies' expense ratios have been going down.

If expenses are reduced, then why are premiums going up? Let's look at what makes up the rates that the insurance companies must charge. Automobile repair rates from labor have risen about 20 percent in the last year and a half. In addition, it has been shown that a new automobile costing $5000 would cost $20,000 if it were to be repaired with replacement parts (not including the engine). During this same period, a semiprivate hospital room has increased in cost over 22 percent and physicians' and surgeons' fees have increased 20 percent. Lawyers continue to ask for larger awards, and the courts are granting them. How can insurance companies continue to pay amounts inflated in this manner without reflecting the increase in their rates?

It is a real shame that the insurance companies don't make these facts known more widely to their customers. A widespread advertising campaign would help to explain their position and make it more tolerable when that next bill comes and has once again increased.

Method: Just about anyone you talk to nowadays <u>complains</u> about the <u>cost</u> of his <u>automobile</u> insurance. It's about time that someone came to the <u>defense</u> of the insurance <u>companies</u>.

We are all familiar with the effects of <u>inflation</u>, but most people forget that the insurance companies are affected too. An interesting point should be noted. Even though the total <u>costs</u> of producing a <u>policy</u> have been <u>increasing</u> because of (increased salaries, paper cost, equipment replacement, etc.) the insurance companies' <u>expense</u> <u>ratios</u> have been going <u>down</u>.

If expenses are reduced, then why are <u>premiums</u> going <u>up</u>? Let's look at what makes up the rates that the insurance companies must <u>charge</u>. Automobile <u>repair</u> rates for labor have <u>risen</u> about (20 percent) in the last year and a half. In addition, it has been shown that a new automobile costing ($5000) would cost ($20,000) if it were to be repaired with <u>replacement</u> <u>parts</u> (not including the engine). During this same period, a semiprivate <u>hospital</u> room has increased in cost over (22 percent) and <u>physicians'</u> and surgeons' fees have <u>increased</u> (20 percent). <u>Lawyers</u> continue to ask for large <u>awards</u>, and the <u>courts</u> are <u>granting</u> them. How can insurance companies continue to pay amounts inflated in this manner without reflecting the increase in their rates?

It is a real shame that the insurance companies don't make these facts known more widely to their customers. A widespread <u>advertising</u> <u>campaign</u> would help to explain their position and make it more <u>tolerable</u> when the <u>next</u> <u>bill</u> comes and has once again <u>increased</u>.

Method in Outline Form

(a) The topic: <u>automobile insurance</u>
(b) Details or key words:
1. complains, cost
2. defense, companies
3. inflation, policy, increasing
4. expense ratios, down
5. premiums, up
6. repair, risen, replacement parts
7. hospital, physicians, increased
8. lawyers, awards, courts, granting
9. advertising campaign, tolerable, next bill, increased

(c) Details about details:
1. (20 percent)
2. ($5000), ($20,000)
3. (22 percent), (20 percent)

Having read the passage and used the underlining technique, let us use this information to answer the type of questions used in the examination.

DIRECTIONS: Choose the best answer.

1. The main point of the passage is to

   A. come to the aid of the insurance companies.
   B. write your representatives to curb the rise of insurance rates.
   C. start a widespread advertising campaign to curtail insurance costs.
   D. imply that insurance premiums are based on many factors and are a complex issue.

2. Which of the following is contradicted by the passage?

   A. Many people complain about their insurance rates.
   B. Insurance companies' expense ratios are continuing to rise with inflation.
   C. Insurance companies are affected by the inflationary features of the economy.
   D. Salaries affect policy costs.

3. The main topic of the passage is

   A. public awareness.
   B. advertising strategy.
   C. automobile insurance rates.
   D. expense ratios.

4. Which of the following is supported by the passages?

   A. A car repaired with replacement parts would cost four (4) times as much as a new car.
   B. The public is fully aware of why their insurance premiums are increasing.
   C. Insurance premiums have risen mainly because of larger awards in lawsuits.
   D. Inflation has little effect on insurance rates.

5. Factor(s) affecting the overall pricing structure of rates could be considered as

   A. paper costs.
   B. equipment replacement.
   C. hospitalization costs.
   D. all of the above.

Answers

1. **Answer D**
   Statement A: No aid to insurance companies is advised, but it is suggested that the companies communicate to the public how rates are derived and what affects them.
   Statement B: No campaign is suggested that involves elected officials.
   Statement C: It is suggested that insurance companies explain their position on rates, but that certainly is not the main thread of the passage.
   Statement D: This is the best answer since it addresses the complex factors upon which rates are based.

2. **Answer B**
   Statement A: The passage implies that a lot of people comment on the high cost of insurance.
   Statement B: It clearly is stated in the passage that insurance companies' expense ratios have been dropping and so the statement is contradicted by the passage.
   Statement C: The key element of the passage is that insurance companies, just like the public, are affected by many economic parameters.
   Statement D: Salaries are mentioned as one factor playing a role in rate determination.

3. **Answer C**
   Statement A: The point of public awareness concerning factors affecting premiums is expressed; however, the issue is more specific.
   Statement B: Insurance companies are advised to inform the public about rate determinants, but that certainly is not the key element or topic.
   Statement C: Rates and what affects the rates and their impact on the public generally are addressed.
   Statement D: Expense ratios were commented on specifically and were made the key issue.

4. **Answer A**
   Statement A: The passage mentions that a car costing $5000 new would cost $20,000 if it were repaired with replacement parts.
   Statement B: Although public awareness is an issue, the passage neither implies nor states the level of awareness.
   Statement C: Awards due to legal procedures are clearly only one factor of this complex issue.
   Statement D: Inflation is an important factor and greatly influences the rate structure.

5. **Answer D**
   The passage clearly identifies paper costs, equipment replacement costs, and hospitalization costs as factors that affect premiums.

Exercise 4

Identify the central theme or topic, details, and details about details.

DIRECTIONS: Read the sample and underline the <u>topic</u>, the <u>details</u> <u>about</u> <u>the</u> <u>topic</u>, and bracket (the details about the details).

Example: (Anthropologists) call such <u>ceremonies</u> as weddings, funerals, and bar mitzvahs, "<u>rites</u> <u>of</u> <u>passage</u>."
(a) The topic deals with <u>ceremonies</u>, "<u>rites</u> <u>of</u> <u>passage</u>".
(b) Details of key words are <u>weddings, funerals, bar mitzvahs</u>.
(c) Details about details are (Anthropologists).

Example: Anthropologists call such ceremonies as weddings, funerals, and bar mitzvahs, "rites of passage." They are crucial to us as human beings, and in every culture they evolve to mark those crucial and critical times when our individual communal lives go through events that are both difficult and dangerous: death, life, union, separation. They are necessary features of our various traditions and cultures, crucially important in making our cultures what they are. Polish Catholic weddings and Irish Catholic funerals are famously important in defining what those two traditions truly are, and the baptisms and funerals of Protestant African Americans are just as crucial in defining those traditions. When we participate in and with those events as experienced by our neighbors and friends, we both add something and get something. We add our respect for the difference which makes our neighbor special, and we get a renewed respect for our own traditions and for what makes them unique.

Method: (Anthropologists) call such ceremonies as weddings, funerals, and bar mitzvahs, "rites of passage." They are crucial to us as human beings, and in every culture they evolve to mark those crucial and critical times when our individual communal lives go through events that are both difficult and dangerous: (death, life, union, separation). They are necessary features of our various traditions and cultures, crucially important in making our cultures what they are. (Polish Catholic weddings) and (Irish Catholic funerals) are famously important in (defining) what those two (traditions) truly are, and the (baptisms and funerals of Protestant African Americans) are just as (crucial in defining those traditions). When we participate in and with those events as experienced by our neighbors and friends, we both add something and get something. We add our respect for the difference which makes our neighbor special, and we get a renewed respect for our own traditions and for what makes them unique.

Method in Outline Form

(a) Topic: ceremonies, "rites of passage"
(b) Details or key words:
   1. weddings, funerals, bar mitzvahs
   2. crucial to human beings
   3. mark crucial and critical times
   4. necessary features of various traditions
   5. crucially important in making cultures
   6. we participate in events experienced by neighbors, friends
   7. we add respect for difference
   8. get renewed respect for own tradition, unique

(c) Details about details:
   1. (Anthropologists)
   2. (death, life, union, separation)
   3. (Polish Catholic weddings, Irish Catholic funerals, defining traditions)
   4. (Protestant African Americans, traditions)
   5. (neighbors and friends, traditions unique)

Having read and used the underlining technique let us use this information to answer the type of questions used in the examination.

DIRECTIONS: Choose the best answer.

   1. This passage implies that

      A. rituals in cultures different from our own are often so complex that we should not try to participate in them.
      B. virtually any communal ceremony, whether a wedding, funeral, or bar mitzvah, would qualify to anthropologists as a "rite of passage."

    C. rituals in the modern world have become so diluted that they rarely have the substance of the original rite.

    D. Irish Catholics would probably not welcome Polish Catholics at their wedding ceremonies.

2. Which of the following is contradicted by the information in the passage?

    A. Rites of passage in various traditions and cultures are interesting to observers because they are often colorful, but they rarely actually make the culture what it is.

    B. Union and death are two events that might qualify as events marked by communal ceremonies.

    C. Baptism in Baptist churches involves immersion, while Presbyterian baptism requires only the sprinkling of water.

    D. Food is usually a major component of communal rituals.

3. According to the passage, what is one by-product of our participating in important events of our friends and neighbors, particularly when these events originate in traditions different from our own?

    A. We come to realize that our own traditions are usually more appealing than those of diverse cultures.

    B. We learn to deal with the discomfort that often accompanies new experiences.

    C. We both add our respect for them, and we gain renewed respect for the uniqueness of our own rituals.

    D. We can often pick up bits and pieces of other languages by participating in rituals of those whose language differs from our own.

4. A Protestant christening ceremony is one of those "rites of passage" referred to in the passage which serve to mark an important event in our culture.

    A. This particular ritual, though not mentioned specifically in the passage, would qualify as one of those "rites of passage.'

    B. Protestant christening ceremonies are mentioned in the passage, but they do not qualify as "rites of passage."

    C. There is not enough information provided by the passage to allow the reader to conclude that the ceremony mentioned would qualify as a "rite of passage."

    D. The statement is contradicted by the passage.

Answers

1. Answer **B**

Statement A: Although rituals in cultures different from our own culture may seem, or actually be, more complex than rituals with which we are quite familiar, the passage does not deal with these complexities; instead it suggests that we should participate in rituals that are a part of cultures different from our own.

Statement B: The passage clearly states in the first sentence that anthropologists include the ceremonies mentioned in this response as "rites of passage."

Statement C: Though many rituals have, no doubt, become diluted in the modern world, this passage does not address this issue overtly or implicitly.

Statement D: The passage mentions Irish Catholic weddings and Polish Catholic weddings to make a point about famously defining rituals, but nowhere does it indicate who would welcome whom at a wedding ceremony.

2. Answer **A**

Statement A: The passage clearly states that rites of passage do, in fact, make the culture what it is. This response is therefore clearly contradicted by the passage.

Statement B: Union and death are referred to in sentence two as among those events that mark crucial times in communal lives.

Statement C: The difference between Baptist and Presbyterian baptismal rites is not discussed in the passage, which therefore neither confirms nor contradicts the information in this response.

Statement D: Specific components of various communal rituals are not mentioned in the passage. The presence or absence of food in rituals is neither contradicted nor confirmed.

3. Answer **C**

Perhaps the main point of the passage is to suggest that we both; give respect to a culture different from our own by participating in its rituals, and that we also gain an appreciation for what is unique in our own rituals from our participation. Responses A, B, and D are not mentioned in the passage.

4. Answer **A**

Statement A: Protestant christening ceremonies are not named specifically in the passage. However, they fit the implied definition provided in sentence one, and they fit the spirit of the definition extended through the passage for a defining cultural ritual.

Statement B: In fact Protestant christening ceremonies are not mentioned specifically in the passage in any context, and they do, in fact, fit the implied definition of a "rite of passage" developed in the passage.

Statement C: See explanation of statement A, which indicates that the passage supports the inference that a Protestant christening ceremony is a "rite of passage."

Statement D: The passage does not deal with the issue explicitly and does not contradict it by implication.

Exercise 5

Identify the central theme or topic, details, and details about details.

DIRECTIONS: Read the sample and underline the topic, the details about the topic, and bracket (the details about the details).

Example: In the first half of the 1600s, during the British Civil War, ten Puritan families, Roundheads as their critics called them, came up from Virginia to Maryland where religious diversity was more greatly tolerated and established Providence, the original settlement on the Severn River.
(a) The topic deals with the original settlement on the Severn River.
(b) Details or key words are Puritan families came to Maryland, religious diversity tolerated, established Providence.
(c) Details about details are (Roundheads from Virginia).

DIRECTIONS: Read the sample selection and underline the topic, the details about the topic, and bracket (the details about the details). Use square brackets for [extraneous material].

Example: In the first half of the 1600s, during the British Civil War, ten Puritan families, Roundheads as their critics called them, came up from Virginia to Maryland where religious diversity was more greatly tolerated and established Providence, the original settlement on the Severn River. In 1650 Providence was "erected" into a county named Annarundell after the wife of Cecil Calvert, Lord Baltimore, the Lady Anne Arundel. Annapolis, also on the Severn

River and named after Lord Baltimore's wife, was originally Anne Arundel Town, a small town but one of the new country's most important because of its extensive population of impressive lawyers, Francis Scott Key and William Pinkney to name two, and because it was the site of one of the country's earliest colleges, St. John's College, chartered in 1784 and opened in the fall of 1789. From early settlement on, the Chesapeake never went untouched by the many wars England involved herself in, but the Severn, unlike some of its sister rivers, remained mostly uninvolved, perhaps because it led to no important harbors, perhaps because its banks gave no rapid access to cities. Its role has been mostly to provide homes and spawning and nesting grounds for the rich web of plant and animal life. The river has long been a sanctuary, an estuary yawning wide into the Chesapeake where Annapolis reigns and the waters are salt.

Method: In the first half of the 1600s, during the British Civil War, ten Puritan families, (Roundheads) as their critics called them, came up (from Virginia) to Maryland where religious diversity was more greatly tolerated and established Providence, the original settlement on the Severn River. In 1650 Providence was "erected" into a county named Annarundell after the wife of Cecil Calvert, Lord Baltimore, the Lady Anne Arundel. Annapolis, also (on the Severn River) and (named after Lord Baltimore's wife), was originally Anne Arundel Town, a small town but one of the new country's most important because of its extensive population of impressive lawyers, (Francis Scott Key) and (William Pinkney) to name two, and because it was the site of one of the country's earliest colleges, (St. John's College), chartered in 1784 and opened in the fall of 1789. From early settlement on, the Chesapeake never went untouched by the many wars (England involved) herself (in), but the Severn, unlike some of its sister rivers, remained mostly uninvolved, perhaps because it led to no important harbors, perhaps because its banks gave no rapid access to cities. Its role has been mostly to provide homes and spawning and nesting grounds for the rich web of plant and animal life. The river has long been a sanctuary, an estuary yawning wide into the Chesapeake where Annapolis reigns and the waters are salt.

Method in Outline Form

(a) Topic: original settlement on the Severn River
(b) Details or key words:
 1. Puritan families came to Maryland, religious diversity tolerated, established Providence
 2. Providence "erected" into county named Annarundell after wife of Lord Baltimore, Lady Anne Arundel
 3. Annapolis originally Anne Arundel Town, small town but important because of impressive lawyers and one of country's earliest colleges
 4. Chesapeake never untouched by wars but Severn mostly uninvolved, no important harbors, no rapid access to cities
 5. role to provide homes and spawning and nesting grounds for plant and animal life
 6. river a sanctuary where Annapolis reigns and waters salt

(c) Details about details:
 1. (Roundheads) (from Virginia)
 2. (Annapolis), (on Severn River), (named after Lord Baltimore's wife)
 3. (Francis Scott Key), (William Pinkney)
 4. (St. John's College)
 5. (England involved in)

Having read the passage and used the underlining technique, let us use this information to answer the type of questions used in the examination.

DIRECTIONS: Choose the best answer.

1. Concerning the original settlement on the Severn River,

   A. one can assume that it was formed by Virginians who were attempting to escape higher taxes.
   B. it is clear that those who made it were searching for fertile land and abundant wildlife.
   C. it appears from the passage that it was formed by people in search of greater religious freedom.
   D. the passage indicates that its inhabitants shared no particular religious or political beliefs.

2. The passage suggests that Annapolis was

   A. almost from the beginning a heavily populated port.
   B. in its early years an important small town, known for its impressive lawyers and one of the country's earliest colleges.
   C. not especially important until the establishment of the Naval Academy.
   D. a summer retreat for wealthy families from Baltimore.

3. Which of the following statement(s) is/are contradicted by the passage?

   A. Puritans are also referred to as Roundheads.
   B. Settlements along the Severn River generally remained uninvolved in wars in which England was involved.
   C. St. John's College is one of the country's oldest colleges.
   D. Anne Arundel was a sister of Cecil Calvert, Lord Baltimore.

4. Which of the following is neither supported nor contradicted by the passage?

   A. Many inhabitants of settlements on the banks of the Severn traditionally earned their living from oystering and fishing.
   B. Annapolis attracted some of the country's most impressive lawyers, among them Francis Scott Key and William Pinkney.
   C. The earliest settlement on the Severn was called Providence.
   D. The Severn River provided no rapid access to cities.

5. What body of water, according to the passage, does the Severn River lead into?

   A. The Potomac River
   B. The Atlantic Ocean
   C. The Rappahannock River
   D. The Chesapeake Bay

Answers

1. Answer C
   Statement A: There is no mention of taxes either in Virginia or Maryland in the passage.
   Statement B: Though it is implied that the land on the banks of the Severn is fertile and that the wildlife is abundant, there is no suggestion in the passage that this played a role in the settlement of the land.
   Statement C: The passage does, in fact, indicate that the tolerance of religious diversity, in effect greater religious freedom, was the main reason that early settlers moved from Virginia to Maryland.
   Statement D: This is contradicted by the fact that the original ten families who first settled Providence were Puritans, and they were therefore united by their shared religious beliefs.

2. Answer **B**

   Statement A: This statement is contradicted by the passage.

   Statement B: This passage indicated in its third sentence that Annapolis was small, that it was known for its impressive lawyers, and that is was the site of one of the country's earliest colleges.

   Statement C: The Naval Academy is not mentioned in the passage.

   Statement D: There is no reference to wealthy families from Baltimore in the passage.

3. Answer **D**

   Statement A: Sentence one indicates that Puritans were known as Roundheads by their critics.

   Statement B: The passage notes specifically that the Severn, unlike some of its sister rivers, was "mostly uninvolved" in England's many wars.

   Statement C: St. John's College, chartered in 1784, is identified in the passage as one of America's oldest colleges.

   Statement D: The Lady Anne Arundel is identified in the passage as the wife of Lord Baltimore, not as his sister; the passage, therefore, contradicts this statement.

4. Answer **A**

   Statement A: There is no suggestion in the passage that people along the Severn made or make money fishing and oystering. All three of the remaining statements appear in the passage.

5. Answer **D**

   Statement A: It is not mentioned in the passage.

   Statement B: It is not mentioned in the passage.

   Statement C: It is not mentioned in the passage.

   Statement D: The Chesapeake Bay is the only body of water other than the Severn River mentioned in the passage, and the Severn is described as "yawning wide into the Chesapeake."

WRITING THE ESSAY

Since 1985, the Association of American Medical Colleges (AAMC) has been trial-testing an essay topic on the MCAT. This project was in response to a study about the professional preparation of the physician. The 1989 administrations of the MCAT included 60 minutes for the writing of two essays. In 1991 the essay became a permanent part of the MCAT.

Medical school faculties have long felt that writing skills are essential for a physician. Many have expressed the opinion that present-day students are somewhat weak in these skills. The goal of the essay topic is to see if the student has the ability and skill to write under standardized conditions. The students should be able to:

1. develop a central theme
2. synthesize material
3. separate major from minor issues
4. propose alternative solutions
5. present a theme in a flowing and logical manner
6. write in correct English, timed, at a first-draft composition level

No specific college courses to obtain essay writing skills have been advocated by anyone. The essay portion (two topics) of the examination will take 60 minutes (30 minutes/topic). It will be administered after the lunch break.

The AAMC has proposed the following guidelines for topic developments:

1. The topic should have *no* relationship to the application process or the candidate's career choice.
2. The topic should not deal with health care or religious themes.
3. Social subjects that may prejudice an evaluator due to opinions or judgmental statements made by the examinee should be avoided.
4. Questions should come from sources which would allow any candidate to respond fully despite recognized differences in social, ethnic, and geographic background.
5. Formal course content, especially in the sciences, should be avoided.

SCORING METHOD

All essays will be scored by an experienced group of readers. A minimum of four readers will rate each essay on a six-point scale. An additional reader will be used if the four original scores differ by more than one point. For reporting purposes, the scores will be averaged and converted to an alphabetical score, with the scale ranging from J to T.

An essay that *exhibits* the major characteristics of logical analysis and presentation would fall in the range from J to Q, with J representing a percentile score between 0–8 and Q representing a range of 54–65. Essays in the Q and above range clearly should display a *grasp* of the material under discussion. The T range will represent the 91–100 percentile. Papers falling into this range definitely must *demonstrate* facets essential to good writing such as purpose, goal, and conviction.

Medical schools will receive the alphabetical score, but may also obtain writing samples. Both the examinee and the schools will receive percentile data, score distribution characteristics, and confidence bands.

CHARACTERISTICS OF GOOD WRITING

E. B. White, one of America's finest writers, once observed that there is "no infallible guide to good writing." There are, however, some principles of good writing which can be learned and which, when learned, can improve virtually everyone's writing. A first requirement is that one find something of interest, preferably something original, to say about the subject at hand. Having satisfied the first requirement, the writer's second goal is to communicate his or her ideas with absolute clarity. To communicate clearly in an essay of the kind required on the MCAT one must focus on the three major components of written communication: (1) unity and coherence, (2) support of the main idea with concrete details and examples, and (3) mechanical concerns.

Unity in an essay results from having a sharply focused central idea, often referred to as a thesis. This thesis typically includes the subject about which one is writing and a predicate, which consists of the major point or points that the writer is making about the subject. The body of the essay will develop this thesis in detail, and the essay will have unity or lack of it to the degree that the writer maintains focus on the central idea. If, for example, the thesis of an essay is that justice (the subject) is blind (the predicate), the essay will be unified in direct proportion to the skill with which the writer maintains focus on this thesis—in other words, the success he or she has in avoiding excursions into subjects unrelated, or related only tangentially, to the main idea.

Closely related to unity in an essay is coherence, which refers to the integration of the various parts. When ideas in a composition flow smoothly from one idea to another and thus create the sense that each idea follows logically from the one preceding it, the essay is said to have coherence. A primary way that one achieves coherence is by using transitional words and phrases such as "moreover," "however," "therefore," "in other words," and "for example." In a good essay each sentence flows smoothly into the next, and each paragraph grows logically from the one which precedes it.

If an essay, therefore, contains those ingredients mentioned above—unity, typically resulting from a thoughtful, original thesis which runs through the essay much the way the spinal column runs through the body, and coherence, which results from the use of devices that hold sentence to sentence and paragraph to paragraph, much the way glue holds clippings on the page of a scrapbook—it will very likely be a good, strong essay. To make a good essay better and a very good one excellent requires attention to the two remaining aspects of written communication: (1) supporting, concrete details and examples, and (2) mechanics. For an essay to convey a sense of authority, general or abstract statements must be anchored in specific details. If one asserts, for example, that the American dollar is strong in the world market, he or she might observe that it is worth $1.30 in Canada. Or if one is writing about the dangers of horseback riding and jumping, he or she might cite the paralysis from the neck down of the experienced equestrian, Christopher Reeve.

The final area for concern for this discussion is mechanics, which covers such things as grammar, spelling, and punctuation. Because many mechanical errors result from carelessness, all writers should proofread as carefully as time permits. There is little disagreement among writing teachers as to the importance of revision, but in a timed essay such as that on the MCAT, there will be a minimum amount of time to devote to revision. You should, however, proofread your essay at least once and, because it will be scored as a rough draft, do not hesitate to make interlinear corrections as neatly as you can when you see that you have made a mechanical error, such as a misspelling, faulty punctuation, or a subject–verb disagreement. Neatness, while certainly a praiseworthy quality in any manuscript, is much less important on the MCAT essay than that the essay be legible.

PREPARING FOR THE MCAT ESSAY

Although the specific essay questions for the MCAT change from test to test, the general type of question remains the same. By becoming acquainted with the format of the kind of questions that have been asked in the past, you can better prepare yourself to deal with whatever specific question you get on your examination. Typically the question begins with a directive to write a *unified* essay in response to the question that follows. You are then given a statement, usually one that could be characterized as an aphorism, which is an assertion that has the ring of truth. You are then asked to explain what you think the statement means, after which you are to describe a circumstance in which the statement might not be true. Finally, in what is probably the central part of your essay, you are to discuss the conditions that must prevail in order for the statement to be considered true.

There are several underlying principles involved in this kind of question. The first is the principle of unity, referred to in the general discussion of good writing on page 339, and discussed below in the section on specific ways in which you can unify your response to the MCAT question itself. The second principle involves your ability to explain clearly what a statement means. Keep in mind that explanation involves a straightforward amplification of the statement, and it will often require that you clarify terms or stipulate definitions of words that might be open to interpretation. Explanation does not require you to analyze (to address questions of "why" the statement says what it says); that will come later in the discussion section of your essay. A third principle is a bit more subtle. You are asked to describe a situation in which the given statement may not be true. While this may appear to be an oblique way of approaching an actual discussion of the statement's truth, it is based on the principle that we often understand what something *is* by understanding, first, what it is not. In this case it is a call to consider the truth of a statement by understanding the conditions under which it is *not* true. This is actually a very useful exercise, and rather than seeing it as a hurdle to cross before you begin your discussion, take advantage of the opportunity afforded by this part to open your mind to the reality that the truth of any statement is dependent, to a certain extent, on the circumstances surrounding it.

The final part of the question, which calls on you to discuss the circumstances in which the statement *is* true, is asking you to rigorously analyze the statement by presenting conditions that appear to confirm its essential truth. The key concept here is "analysis." The question may not use the word "analyze" as a stated directive, but keep in mind the principle that when you are asked to discuss, often you are actually being asked to analyze. Analysis can use the rhetorical modes mentioned above, such as definition, description, and explanation; but analysis uses these modes finally to communicate to the reader *why* something is as it is. In what will probably be a part of your strategy in the essay, you may go a step beyond analysis into persuasion, which is the use of analysis to convince the reader that your central thesis is correct. Unless you find yourself in violent disagreement with the statement presented in the question, however, the persuasive component of your essay will be what could be referred to as "soft sell." Though there are occasions in writing when strong persuasion is called for, it is not a good idea to allow your essay for the MCAT to be dominated by an argumentative tone, if for no other reason than that the question itself begs for an objective, open-minded, and carefully reasoned response.

With the general principles discussed above in mind, examine them in the following question, which resembles the questions given before on the essay part of the MCAT:

Consider this statement:

All that is necessary for the triumph of evil is that good men do nothing.

Write a unified essay in which you perform the following tasks. Explain what you think the above statement means. Describe a specific situation in which good men were, in fact, doing something, but evil triumphed nonetheless. Discuss what you think determines when the triumph of evil is dependent on the fact that good men are doing nothing.

Clearly in order to explain what the statement in question means requires that you stipulate possible definitions for "evil" and for "good men," both of which are open to interpretation. You might, for example, equate evil with forces that bring about destruction—of life, of liberty, and of those virtues which have traditionally been held sacred in our society. Good men, in this context, would be those who believe in these virtues. The statement itself seems to rest on an unspoken acceptance among most people of these stipulated definitions. With the meaning of the key terms of this statement now understood, you could explain that the statement means that when good men—those who hold those values that promote the survival and well-being of human beings—do not actively protect those values, destructive human impulses will subvert the human race. In short, the statement is a strong warning against apathy to those who value life, liberty, and the pursuit of happiness. The strong warning comes in the form of an all-or-nothing plea: if well-meaning individuals do nothing to resist destructive forces, they will lose all; evil will triumph in spite of the good intentions of those individuals.

The second part of the question asks you to describe a situation in which good men were doing something (i.e., not doing "nothing") and yet evil triumphed nonetheless. Many illustrations of such a conceivable circumstance will come to your mind. In war-torn countries where invaders are attempting to overthrow the existing order, perhaps an order in which peaceful citizens were coexisting and enjoying life, the revolutionists may simply outnumber those who wish to uphold the status quo. These latter "good men" may, in fact, risk their lives fighting for the principles in which they believe; but "evil," in the form of the invaders, could triumph in spite of their efforts. One could also imagine a situation in which the balance between forces of good and those of evil is delicate. In such a situation, some natural disaster such as an earthquake could destabilize conditions; the evil forces could take advantage of the chaos and upset the delicate balance in favor of evil. Imagine, for example, a largely peaceful town in which order prevails. An earthquake strikes the town, and looters take over privately owned businesses and appropriate money and goods, perhaps including guns and ammunition, that belong to good people. This might enable chaos, or evil, to triumph over good. The weakness of an all-or-none statement like the one with which you are concerned is that there are exceptions to virtually every rule, and with a little imagination you are certain to discover some of these exceptions. In this case, all that you would need to do is to find a circumstance in which good men are not doing enough. They may be doing *something*, but it simply may not be sufficient. If you establish such a circumstance, you have found a flaw in the statement that *all* that is necessary for the triumph of evil is that good men do nothing.

The final part of the question asks you to discuss what you think determines when all that is necessary for the triumph of evil is that good men do nothing. Here, for the sake of unity and coherence, you should find a transition that acknowledges that in spite of the exceptions described above, the statement contains a strong element of truth. You might acknowledge that all-or-none statements like the one in question typically are employed to jar the reader into considering a worst-case scenario. You are then in a position to discuss the statement in terms of its implications or of the essential truth conveyed by the spirit of the statement. The main section of your essay, therefore, will be concerned with the consequences of apathy. What happens when people do not actively promote the values in which they believe? You could begin with the institution of the family and argue that well-meaning parents, in failing to be an active part of their children's lives, leave children vulnerable to influences that they may be unable to deal with effectively. Life and literature are full of examples that support this point, and you should cite some of these examples. Joyce Carol Oates' story, "Where Are You Going, Where Have You Been?" tells of a young girl whose parents ask their daughter superficial questions, but they fail to become involved in a meaningful way in her life. She seeks attention from causal strangers and ultimately winds up being lured from her home by the diabolical villain ironically named Arnold Friend. You could next move to examples involving social issues or conditions within our country and then within the world in which "good men" are doing little to actively promote peace or to preserve our environment. Good men and women were simply not doing enough recently in Dunblane, Scotland to prevent the senseless murder of innocent schoolchildren by a deranged sociopath. By all accounts the village is filled with good, peace-loving men and women. But there was also ample evidence that the man who opened fire on the children was known to be a potential threat. One must ask if these good people so took their peaceful lives for granted that they failed to act and, through their apathy, left open the gate, if not for the triumph of evil, then at least for its intrusion into their lives.

Remember that the question will call for a unified essay in which you are to perform several tasks. The simplest way to unify your essay is to construct an introductory paragraph in which you blueprint your essay and state your main idea or thesis. This will be helpful both for the reader and for yourself. In the time allotted you will probably be able to write an essay of approximately 500 words or less. This means that you will likely have no more than four or five well-developed paragraphs. Use transitions between paragraphs to alert the reader to the fact that you are moving on to another topic, and then be sure that you link each topic of each paragraph to the main idea in the introductory paragraph. There are, of course, many subtler ways of unifying an essay and of giving it coherence. But on this essay you will be pressed for time and will have less time to formulate elaborate rhetorical strategies. Organizing the essay around a thesis and presenting a blueprint in the introductory paragraph will help assure the essay's unity, and it will help guarantee that you do not neglect any aspect of the question. Keep in mind that the content of the essay is more important than its physical appearance. The essay will be scored as a draft. You can go back and polish it if time permits, but the most important ingredients are: (1) the quality of the essay's ideas; (2) the unity and coherence of the various parts; and (3) the appropriateness of supporting examples. The appearance of the manuscript, including mechanical details, is a distant fourth.

Two final questions often arise when students are preparing for the MCAT essay: one is that of whether or not to outline the essay before writing it; the other is whether or not there is a need for a concluding paragraph. The fact is that it is virtually always helpful to outline an essay, and it is usually hazardous not to do so. Writers compose in different ways, and they outline in different ways. Some require a comprehensive outline with details, and details about details enumerated; others need only a skeletal outline including only the main topics. Your purpose in writing this essay is to produce a final product that is organized and unified, which is precisely what an outline helps guarantee that you will do. Keep in mind the method of outlining that has worked best for you in the past, and use it for this essay. If you have not outlined your essays before writing them in the past, learn to do so now. Practice picking the main points that you would cover for the sample essay topics below, and jot them down, experimenting with various levels of detail that will be helpful for you to include.

As for the matter of a concluding paragraph for your essay, there is disagreement among experts on this subject. The traditional viewpoint is that a final paragraph which restates your main ideas and finally opens the subject for more general application can be desirable. Another viewpoint is that if you have fully and clearly explored your subject in the essay, a formal conclusion is redundant. You should be guided in your MCAT essay by two factors. The first of these is time: if you are pressed for time, the concluding paragraph is the most dispensable part of the essay. The second factor has to do with your own perception of how well you have presented your points in the rest of the essay. If, after rereading your essay, you sense that the organization has been weak, try to strengthen it with a conclusion that summarizes and restates your main points. If you decide that you do not have time for, or do not need, a concluding paragraph, at least clinch your essay with a strong sentence, one that brings it to closure. The endpoint of each unit of writing—a sentence, a paragraph, or an entire essay—is strategically the most emphatic point of that unit. You want to leave the reader of your MCAT essay with the sense that you have squarely confronted the issues raised by the question.

PRACTICE TOPICS

Use the questions below to practice your skills at outlining. After you outline the individual essays, choose at least one of the questions and, using your outline, write a full essay in response to the question. Time yourself at 30 minutes per essay.

1. Consider this statement:

Too great haste in paying off an obligation is a kind of ingratitude.

Write a unified essay in which you perform the following tasks. Explain what you think the above statement means. Describe a specific situation in which paying off an obligation quickly or hastily would not be a form of ingratitude. Discuss what you think determines when paying off an obligation with great haste is a kind of ingratitude.

2. Consider this statement:

They who are in highest places, and have the most power, have the least liberty. . . .

Write a unified essay in which you perform the following tasks. Explain what you think the above statement means. Describe a specific situation in which those who are in the highest places and have the most power, in fact, manage to have at least a fair amount of liberty. Discuss what you think determines whether those in high places who possess much power have liberty.

3. Consider this statement:

A soft answer turneth away wrath.

Write a unified essay in which you perform the following tasks. Explain what you think the above statement means. Describe a specific situation in which a soft answer might *not* turn away wrath. Discuss what you think determines the circumstance in which a soft answer does turn away wrath.

4. Consider this statement:

**Revenge is a kind of wild justice, which the more man's nature runs to,
the more ought law to weed it out.**

Write a unified essay in which you perform the following tasks. Explain what you think the above statement means. Describe a specific situation in which revenge is a kind of justice that law ought not prohibit. Discuss what you think determines the point at which law ought to weed out revenge.

ADDITIONAL TOPICS

You might find it helpful in understanding the format of the MCAT essay to take the statements below and form questions like the ones above and like those in the sample essay questions in the Model Examination sections.

1. Wise men say nothing in dangerous times.
2. Never tell your resolution beforehand.
3. They that endeavor to abolish vice, destroy also virtue; for contraries, though they destroy one another, are yet the life of one another.
4. A service beyond recompense weighs so heavy that it almost gives offense.
5. All evils are equal when they are extreme.
6. Quarrels would not last long if the fault were only on one side.

The MCAT
Model Examination A

ANSWER SHEET

DIRECTIONS: After locating the number of the question to which you are responding, fill in the circle containing the letter of the answer you have selected. Use pencil (not a ballpoint pen) to completely blacken the circle.

VERBAL REASONING

1. Ⓐ Ⓑ Ⓒ Ⓓ
2. Ⓐ Ⓑ Ⓒ Ⓓ
3. Ⓐ Ⓑ Ⓒ Ⓓ
4. Ⓐ Ⓑ Ⓒ Ⓓ
5. Ⓐ Ⓑ Ⓒ Ⓓ
6. Ⓐ Ⓑ Ⓒ Ⓓ
7. Ⓐ Ⓑ Ⓒ Ⓓ
8. Ⓐ Ⓑ Ⓒ Ⓓ
9. Ⓐ Ⓑ Ⓒ Ⓓ
10. Ⓐ Ⓑ Ⓒ Ⓓ
11. Ⓐ Ⓑ Ⓒ Ⓓ
12. Ⓐ Ⓑ Ⓒ Ⓓ
13. Ⓐ Ⓑ Ⓒ Ⓓ
14. Ⓐ Ⓑ Ⓒ Ⓓ
15. Ⓐ Ⓑ Ⓒ Ⓓ
16. Ⓐ Ⓑ Ⓒ Ⓓ
17. Ⓐ Ⓑ Ⓒ Ⓓ
18. Ⓐ Ⓑ Ⓒ Ⓓ
19. Ⓐ Ⓑ Ⓒ Ⓓ
20. Ⓐ Ⓑ Ⓒ Ⓓ
21. Ⓐ Ⓑ Ⓒ Ⓓ
22. Ⓐ Ⓑ Ⓒ Ⓓ
23. Ⓐ Ⓑ Ⓒ Ⓓ
24. Ⓐ Ⓑ Ⓒ Ⓓ
25. Ⓐ Ⓑ Ⓒ Ⓓ
26. Ⓐ Ⓑ Ⓒ Ⓓ
27. Ⓐ Ⓑ Ⓒ Ⓓ
28. Ⓐ Ⓑ Ⓒ Ⓓ
29. Ⓐ Ⓑ Ⓒ Ⓓ
30. Ⓐ Ⓑ Ⓒ Ⓓ

31. Ⓐ Ⓑ Ⓒ Ⓓ
32. Ⓐ Ⓑ Ⓒ Ⓓ
33. Ⓐ Ⓑ Ⓒ Ⓓ
34. Ⓐ Ⓑ Ⓒ Ⓓ
35. Ⓐ Ⓑ Ⓒ Ⓓ
36. Ⓐ Ⓑ Ⓒ Ⓓ
37. Ⓐ Ⓑ Ⓒ Ⓓ
38. Ⓐ Ⓑ Ⓒ Ⓓ
39. Ⓐ Ⓑ Ⓒ Ⓓ
40. Ⓐ Ⓑ Ⓒ Ⓓ
41. Ⓐ Ⓑ Ⓒ Ⓓ
42. Ⓐ Ⓑ Ⓒ Ⓓ
43. Ⓐ Ⓑ Ⓒ Ⓓ
44. Ⓐ Ⓑ Ⓒ Ⓓ
45. Ⓐ Ⓑ Ⓒ Ⓓ
46. Ⓐ Ⓑ Ⓒ Ⓓ
47. Ⓐ Ⓑ Ⓒ Ⓓ
48. Ⓐ Ⓑ Ⓒ Ⓓ
49. Ⓐ Ⓑ Ⓒ Ⓓ
50. Ⓐ Ⓑ Ⓒ Ⓓ
51. Ⓐ Ⓑ Ⓒ Ⓓ
52. Ⓐ Ⓑ Ⓒ Ⓓ
53. Ⓐ Ⓑ Ⓒ Ⓓ
54. Ⓐ Ⓑ Ⓒ Ⓓ
55. Ⓐ Ⓑ Ⓒ Ⓓ
56. Ⓐ Ⓑ Ⓒ Ⓓ
57. Ⓐ Ⓑ Ⓒ Ⓓ
58. Ⓐ Ⓑ Ⓒ Ⓓ
59. Ⓐ Ⓑ Ⓒ Ⓓ
60. Ⓐ Ⓑ Ⓒ Ⓓ

61. Ⓐ Ⓑ Ⓒ Ⓓ
62. Ⓐ Ⓑ Ⓒ Ⓓ
63. Ⓐ Ⓑ Ⓒ Ⓓ
64. Ⓐ Ⓑ Ⓒ Ⓓ
65. Ⓐ Ⓑ Ⓒ Ⓓ

PHYSICAL SCIENCES

66. Ⓐ Ⓑ Ⓒ Ⓓ
67. Ⓐ Ⓑ Ⓒ Ⓓ
68. Ⓐ Ⓑ Ⓒ Ⓓ
69. Ⓐ Ⓑ Ⓒ Ⓓ
70. Ⓐ Ⓑ Ⓒ Ⓓ
71. Ⓐ Ⓑ Ⓒ Ⓓ
72. Ⓐ Ⓑ Ⓒ Ⓓ
73. Ⓐ Ⓑ Ⓒ Ⓓ
74. Ⓐ Ⓑ Ⓒ Ⓓ
75. Ⓐ Ⓑ Ⓒ Ⓓ
76. Ⓐ Ⓑ Ⓒ Ⓓ
77. Ⓐ Ⓑ Ⓒ Ⓓ
78. Ⓐ Ⓑ Ⓒ Ⓓ
79. Ⓐ Ⓑ Ⓒ Ⓓ
80. Ⓐ Ⓑ Ⓒ Ⓓ
81. Ⓐ Ⓑ Ⓒ Ⓓ
82. Ⓐ Ⓑ Ⓒ Ⓓ
83. Ⓐ Ⓑ Ⓒ Ⓓ
84. Ⓐ Ⓑ Ⓒ Ⓓ
85. Ⓐ Ⓑ Ⓒ Ⓓ
86. Ⓐ Ⓑ Ⓒ Ⓓ
87. Ⓐ Ⓑ Ⓒ Ⓓ
88. Ⓐ Ⓑ Ⓒ Ⓓ

89. Ⓐ Ⓑ Ⓒ Ⓓ
90. Ⓐ Ⓑ Ⓒ Ⓓ
91. Ⓐ Ⓑ Ⓒ Ⓓ
92. Ⓐ Ⓑ Ⓒ Ⓓ
93. Ⓐ Ⓑ Ⓒ Ⓓ
94. Ⓐ Ⓑ Ⓒ Ⓓ
95. Ⓐ Ⓑ Ⓒ Ⓓ
96. Ⓐ Ⓑ Ⓒ Ⓓ
97. Ⓐ Ⓑ Ⓒ Ⓓ
98. Ⓐ Ⓑ Ⓒ Ⓓ
99. Ⓐ Ⓑ Ⓒ Ⓓ
100. Ⓐ Ⓑ Ⓒ Ⓓ
101. Ⓐ Ⓑ Ⓒ Ⓓ
102. Ⓐ Ⓑ Ⓒ Ⓓ
103. Ⓐ Ⓑ Ⓒ Ⓓ
104. Ⓐ Ⓑ Ⓒ Ⓓ
105. Ⓐ Ⓑ Ⓒ Ⓓ
106. Ⓐ Ⓑ Ⓒ Ⓓ
107. Ⓐ Ⓑ Ⓒ Ⓓ
108. Ⓐ Ⓑ Ⓒ Ⓓ
109. Ⓐ Ⓑ Ⓒ Ⓓ
110. Ⓐ Ⓑ Ⓒ Ⓓ
111. Ⓐ Ⓑ Ⓒ Ⓓ
112. Ⓐ Ⓑ Ⓒ Ⓓ
113. Ⓐ Ⓑ Ⓒ Ⓓ
114. Ⓐ Ⓑ Ⓒ Ⓓ
115. Ⓐ Ⓑ Ⓒ Ⓓ
116. Ⓐ Ⓑ Ⓒ Ⓓ Ⓔ
117. Ⓐ Ⓑ Ⓒ Ⓓ Ⓔ
118. Ⓐ Ⓑ Ⓒ Ⓓ Ⓔ

119. Ⓐ Ⓑ Ⓒ Ⓓ Ⓔ

BIOLOGICAL SCIENCES

120. Ⓐ Ⓑ Ⓒ Ⓓ Ⓔ
121. Ⓐ Ⓑ Ⓒ Ⓓ
122. Ⓐ Ⓑ Ⓒ Ⓓ
123. Ⓐ Ⓑ Ⓒ Ⓓ
124. Ⓐ Ⓑ Ⓒ Ⓓ
125. Ⓐ Ⓑ Ⓒ Ⓓ
126. Ⓐ Ⓑ Ⓒ Ⓓ
127. Ⓐ Ⓑ Ⓒ Ⓓ
128. Ⓐ Ⓑ Ⓒ Ⓓ
129. Ⓐ Ⓑ Ⓒ Ⓓ
130. Ⓐ Ⓑ Ⓒ Ⓓ
131. Ⓐ Ⓑ Ⓒ Ⓓ
132. Ⓐ Ⓑ Ⓒ Ⓓ
133. Ⓐ Ⓑ Ⓒ Ⓓ
134. Ⓐ Ⓑ Ⓒ Ⓓ
135. Ⓐ Ⓑ Ⓒ Ⓓ
136. Ⓐ Ⓑ Ⓒ Ⓓ
137. Ⓐ Ⓑ Ⓒ Ⓓ
138. Ⓐ Ⓑ Ⓒ Ⓓ
139. Ⓐ Ⓑ Ⓒ Ⓓ
140. Ⓐ Ⓑ Ⓒ Ⓓ
141. Ⓐ Ⓑ Ⓒ Ⓓ
142. Ⓐ Ⓑ Ⓒ Ⓓ

WRITING SAMPLE
Use separate ruled sheets of
paper.

143. Ⓐ Ⓑ Ⓒ Ⓓ
144. Ⓐ Ⓑ Ⓒ Ⓓ
145. Ⓐ Ⓑ Ⓒ Ⓓ
146. Ⓐ Ⓑ Ⓒ Ⓓ
147. Ⓐ Ⓑ Ⓒ Ⓓ
148. Ⓐ Ⓑ Ⓒ Ⓓ
149. Ⓐ Ⓑ Ⓒ Ⓓ
150. Ⓐ Ⓑ Ⓒ Ⓓ
151. Ⓐ Ⓑ Ⓒ Ⓓ
152. Ⓐ Ⓑ Ⓒ Ⓓ
153. Ⓐ Ⓑ Ⓒ Ⓓ
154. Ⓐ Ⓑ Ⓒ Ⓓ
155. Ⓐ Ⓑ Ⓒ Ⓓ
156. Ⓐ Ⓑ Ⓒ Ⓓ
157. Ⓐ Ⓑ Ⓒ Ⓓ
158. Ⓐ Ⓑ Ⓒ Ⓓ
159. Ⓐ Ⓑ Ⓒ Ⓓ
160. Ⓐ Ⓑ Ⓒ Ⓓ
161. Ⓐ Ⓑ Ⓒ Ⓓ
162. Ⓐ Ⓑ Ⓒ Ⓓ
163. Ⓐ Ⓑ Ⓒ Ⓓ
164. Ⓐ Ⓑ Ⓒ Ⓓ
165. Ⓐ Ⓑ Ⓒ Ⓓ
166. Ⓐ Ⓑ Ⓒ Ⓓ
167. Ⓐ Ⓑ Ⓒ Ⓓ

168. Ⓐ Ⓑ Ⓒ Ⓓ
169. Ⓐ Ⓑ Ⓒ Ⓓ
170. Ⓐ Ⓑ Ⓒ Ⓓ
171. Ⓐ Ⓑ Ⓒ Ⓓ
172. Ⓐ Ⓑ Ⓒ Ⓓ
173. Ⓐ Ⓑ Ⓒ Ⓓ
174. Ⓐ Ⓑ Ⓒ Ⓓ
175. Ⓐ Ⓑ Ⓒ Ⓓ
176. Ⓐ Ⓑ Ⓒ Ⓓ
177. Ⓐ Ⓑ Ⓒ Ⓓ
178. Ⓐ Ⓑ Ⓒ Ⓓ
179. Ⓐ Ⓑ Ⓒ Ⓓ
180. Ⓐ Ⓑ Ⓒ Ⓓ
181. Ⓐ Ⓑ Ⓒ Ⓓ
182. Ⓐ Ⓑ Ⓒ Ⓓ
183. Ⓐ Ⓑ Ⓒ Ⓓ
184. Ⓐ Ⓑ Ⓒ Ⓓ
185. Ⓐ Ⓑ Ⓒ Ⓓ
186. Ⓐ Ⓑ Ⓒ Ⓓ
187. Ⓐ Ⓑ Ⓒ Ⓓ
188. Ⓐ Ⓑ Ⓒ Ⓓ
189. Ⓐ Ⓑ Ⓒ Ⓓ
190. Ⓐ Ⓑ Ⓒ Ⓓ
191. Ⓐ Ⓑ Ⓒ Ⓓ
192. Ⓐ Ⓑ Ⓒ Ⓓ
193. Ⓐ Ⓑ Ⓒ Ⓓ

194. Ⓐ Ⓑ Ⓒ Ⓓ
195. Ⓐ Ⓑ Ⓒ Ⓓ
196. Ⓐ Ⓑ Ⓒ Ⓓ
197. Ⓐ Ⓑ Ⓒ Ⓓ
198. Ⓐ Ⓑ Ⓒ Ⓓ
199. Ⓐ Ⓑ Ⓒ Ⓓ
200. Ⓐ Ⓑ Ⓒ Ⓓ
201. Ⓐ Ⓑ Ⓒ Ⓓ
202. Ⓐ Ⓑ Ⓒ Ⓓ
203. Ⓐ Ⓑ Ⓒ Ⓓ
204. Ⓐ Ⓑ Ⓒ Ⓓ
205. Ⓐ Ⓑ Ⓒ Ⓓ
206. Ⓐ Ⓑ Ⓒ Ⓓ
207. Ⓐ Ⓑ Ⓒ Ⓓ
208. Ⓐ Ⓑ Ⓒ Ⓓ
209. Ⓐ Ⓑ Ⓒ Ⓓ
210. Ⓐ Ⓑ Ⓒ Ⓓ
211. Ⓐ Ⓑ Ⓒ Ⓓ
212. Ⓐ Ⓑ Ⓒ Ⓓ
213. Ⓐ Ⓑ Ⓒ Ⓓ
214. Ⓐ Ⓑ Ⓒ Ⓓ
215. Ⓐ Ⓑ Ⓒ Ⓓ
216. Ⓐ Ⓑ Ⓒ Ⓓ
217. Ⓐ Ⓑ Ⓒ Ⓓ
218. Ⓐ Ⓑ Ⓒ Ⓓ
219. Ⓐ Ⓑ Ⓒ Ⓓ

The MCAT
Model Examination A

VERBAL REASONING

9 PASSAGES
65 QUESTIONS
85 MINUTES

DIRECTIONS: The questions are based on the accompanying passages. Read each passage carefully, then answer the following questions. Consider only the material within the passage. For each question, select the *ONE BEST ANSWER* and indicate your selection by marking the corresponding letter on the Answer Form.

Passage I (Questions 1–9)

Periodic demands for educational reform, in conjunction with the corresponding efforts of the nation's public school systems to improve their instructional programs, are not an unusual phenomenon in the annals of this country's history. The most recent reform movement, however, which is viewed by many as a demand on the part of legislatures and the public for more effective schools, might be classified as unique. During the last 20 years, monumental amounts of research and discussion have been generated regarding all facets of public education.

The outcry was created in part by declining economic conditions and by the publication of such exhaustive studies of school resources and their impact as the Coleman et al., (1966) report on the *Equality of Educational Opportunity* and others (Jensen, 1969; Jenks et al. 1970; Rist, 1970; Avech, 1974), which seemed to point out the failure of the American educational system. The results of their findings caused considerable dismay in the educational community and the population at large, since they suggested that schools make little, if any, difference in the lives of the children who attend them. The socio-economic status of the individual's family (Hodgson, 1975) as well as a measure of "pure luck" (ERIC Action Brief, 1981) were credited with influencing student achievement and other educational outcomes to a much greater degree than a pupil's school experiences.

After the initial reaction of shock, neither researchers nor practitioners were content to stand by and accept the pessimistic picture that had been painted for them as a final verdict. In response, literally hundreds of studies have been conducted in schools across the country that focus on every aspect of public education.

Researchers have gone into the field in great numbers to obtain a firsthand view of the educational process in action. One early example of a now classic study that made an attempt to overcome the existing attitude of fatalism was that conducted by Weber (1971) in four Washington, D.C. schools The results indicated that by placing a consistent school-wide emphasis on the teaching of basic skills, school leaders could be influential in improving the reading achievement of disadvantaged inner-city youngsters.

Many other research efforts, both ethnographic and quantitative in nature, have produced positive results and have infused practitioners with a new hope and a renewed belief that what takes place in schools can indeed make a significant difference in both the academic lives and the personal development of the pupils that they serve.

Although the negative effects of the early findings have been lessened, they have not been wiped away. The call for further reform continues, as evidenced by the continuing wave of national, state, and public demands contained in such reports as *A Nation at Risk* (Goldberg & James, 1983) and *Making the Grade* (Graham, 1983). Consequently, the research effort has intensified and has resulted in the translation of many of its findings into positive plans of action.

1. The central thesis of the passage is:

   A. schools do not make a difference in the lives of the students who attend them.

   B. instructional programs must always be improved and updated so that educational critics will be satisfied.

Adapted from E. E. Seibel, "Principal Change Facilitator Style: Its Relationship to School Climate and Student Achievement." Doctoral Dissertation, Virginia Commonwealth University, 1986.

C. although the call for educational reform in the United States has been an ongoing process, the past 20-year period has been an extremely research-oriented time in the public education arena.

D. middle class parents should consider providing academic instruction for their children in the home setting.

2. According to this passage, what factors were partially responsible for triggering the educational reform movement that is discussed therein?

A. The fact that the majority of citizens in the United States have attended the public schools themselves and therefore knew that instructional programs needed to be changed.

B. The fact that many people wanted to teach their children at home and did not want to pay taxes to support the public school system.

C. Anger over the implication that the amount of money a family has, as well as the amount of "luck" they encounter, can make a difference in a child's education.

D. A decline in the national economy and the publication of exhaustive school resource studies.

3. The demand for educational reform and the resulting research that has been conducted over the past 20 years has been centered on:

A. public schools.
B. private schools.
C. home education.
D. correspondence courses.

4. The fourth paragraph states: "Researchers have gone into the field in great numbers to gain a firsthand view of the educational process in action." Which of the following statements would be reasonable assumptions to make as a result of that sentence?

I. Many studies have been conducted in school settings.

II. The persons conducting the research are not simply basing their results on educational theories.

III. There appears to be a great deal of interest in the educational process.

A. I only
B. II only
C. I and II only
D. I, II, and III

5. What groups might the word "practitioners," used in paragraph three, stand for?

A. doctors, dentists, lawyers
B. educators
C. superintendents, principals, teachers
D. both B and C

6. The author of this passage gives the impression that:

A. there is little hope for the successful future of public education in the United States.

B. although serious problems exist in the educational arena, progress is being made, partially, as a result of the hands-on involvement of researchers.

C. the field of education is so large that effective change cannot occur.

D. too many people are involved in doing educational research.

7. Based on the information presented in the final paragraph, it probably is reasonable to conclude that:

A. private schools provide students with a higher quality education than public schools.

B. research efforts on effective schools will continue as plans of action are implemented and evaluated.

C. the public is satisfied with the results of the effective schools movement.

D. the problem of educational reform is finite.

8. Which of the following statements is *supported by* the information presented in this passage?

A. Education reform in the United States has been ongoing.

B. Researchers clearly have shown that public education in the United States has failed.

C. Private education has taken the lead over public education.

D. Home teaching is becoming more and more popular with families who cannot afford to send their children to private schools.

9. Which of the following statements is *contradicted by* the information presented in this passage?

A. A student's family income is the major factor in determining his success in school.

B. As a result of the hundreds of studies that researchers have done in schools, they have been able to restructure public education and stop the demand for reform.

C. The negative effects of the early research (1966–1974) have been completely erased as a result of later studies, thus restoring the taxpayers' faith in public education.

D. All of the above.

Passage II (Questions 10–16)

The fairy tale of Cinderella is one of the most widely known folk stories in the world. In its various versions it captures the struggle for the young girl's passage into womanhood. It covers, in its scope, several of Karen Horney's ideas, as well as the trials, totems, and family patterns found in primitive cultures. The Cinderella story chronicles the transformation of the girl into the woman, the profane into the spiritual; ending in the heroine's resolution of her feminine powers.

The Cinderella story goes back as far as seventh-century China. It is classified among the most well-known folktales in the world, and there is a version in nearly every language. The plot is universal: Cinderella, a beautiful, kind, and loving girl, suffers within her family, and is aided by some form of magic through which she meets the man she is destined to marry. After the initial meetings with this man, she loses some article symbolic of the womb, and the man uses this article to find and betroth her.

Several of Karen Horney's theories from "The Distrust Between the Sexes" are evident in this folktale. One of the main ideas in Cinderella is the concept of the evil stepmother or foster mother. Even in instances where Cinderella's father is still living, the stepmother is allowed to abuse her. Her elder sisters are also given this privilege. This is because the mother and sisters are older and less attractive than the heroine. Cinderella's persecution is permitted because, as Horney says, ". . . it is only the sexually attractive woman of whom [man] is afraid and who . . . has to be kept in bondage." In the cultures from which the story derives, old women are not sexually threatening to men and so the stepmother is given the power (by the father) to make the heroine submissive. Horney continues: "Old women, on the other hand, are held in high esteem, even by cultures in which the young woman is dreaded and therefore suppressed." Not only is the stepmother granted more power over Cinderella due to her position, but she feels her power potentially jeopardized by the sway that Cinderella's beauty may have over men. The sisters also feel jeopardized by the heroine's sexual attractiveness, which leads to greater resentment and cruelty on their part.

Another of Horney's theories prevalent in the story is the duality of motherhood. There are two aspects of motherhood, the virgin mother who is self-sacrificing, nurturing, and selfless, and the mother goddess, warm, earthy, sensual, and fertile. Both aspects are visible in the heroine. Cinderella, as she is first seen, sleeps in the cold, empty hearth, reflective of the virgin's womb, empty until acted upon by some outside force. She is covered in ashes, dressed in rags; in general a picture of self-effacing humility. Despite the hardships put upon her by her family, she is kind to them and even tries her best to beautify her stepsisters for the ball. She is virtuous, in contrast to her stepsisters and stepmother. After marriage to the prince, in the end, the heroine does not seek any revenge on her persecutors. In some renditions, she actually invites her family to come live with her and her new husband. Further evidence of this virginal mother aspect is the part that the prince plays in her life at this point. Like the ultimate example of nurturing motherhood, Mother Mary, who waits for the male god to act upon her, Cinderella lies in wait for the prince to come and save her. He is the aid she needs to be freed of her harsh life.

The other aspect of motherhood is revealed in her when magic help arrives from the outside. She is bestowed with sensual, material things: beautiful clothes, ornaments, cosmetics; things to make her desirable to men. The heroine is also gifted with the famous shoes, reflective of the womb. This prince is usually attracted to her for her physical appearance. She is displaying her sensual, seductive, earthy side and the prince is a reward for her power to act on him with her seductive ability. This dichotomy provides some confusion to the heroine, her family, and her suitor. The journey to resolve the puzzle of her twofold womanhood is a main theme in this folklore.

The passage from a girl to a woman is only one of the several transitions that take place within our heroine. She also undergoes a spiritual transformation. In the beginning of every account, the heroine is dirty and ragged. In at least three versions, she is made to wear animal skins. These things are representative of the material, animalistic, profane world. As she is put through the trials for entering into adulthood, she is also put through trials to test her spirituality. In spite of hardships, she manages to remain pious, loving, and kind. These trials come to an end and she becomes clean and well dressed. She is described as radiant, angelic, and fairylike. The heroine is then presented to the prince. The image of the prince embracing the servant girl is heavily laden with religious meaning, especially during the period when this story became popular. This analogy was very often used by the convents of the Middle Ages to relate the relationship of the nuns to Jesus Christ. Cinderella's spiritual ascent is completed with her royal wedding.

The heroine's time of testing is not completely at an end until the two sides of her femininity merge. They have been in the process of merging since the time of her totem's arrival. Since the arrival of the totem, she has actively struggled with her two female aspects, the virginal/nurturing and the earthy/seductive. The heroine

Adapted from Heather Tuttle "If the Shoe Fits," VCU, 1990.

in each version of the tale is given a womb symbol: either a shoe or a ring. This symbol accompanies her when she meets the prince in her state of beauty and sensuality. She then loses this article with the prince, who uses it to find her. When he sees her again, she is once more virginal, modest; covered in dirt and ashes, yet she is missing this symbol of her womanhood. The prince is confused; this is not quite the girl he thought he came for. After he places the shoe on her foot (or the ring on her finger, as the case may be) he sees her as whole: sensual, earthy, yet loving and virginal. She no longer runs from him as she did in earlier encounters, when things became too intimate with the prince.

This is also a moment of recognition for Cinderella. She has discovered a unity of both female forces within her. There were clues previously as to the wholeness of her nature, but she ignored them. She managed to overlook the times when she was sensual, at the ball, and was still kind to her family, generously giving them jewelry. She failed to see her true nature when she was beautiful and yet very humble in the presence of nobility. Now she can no longer hide herself. The prince has seen her spiritual, virginal, and sensual facets and her true nature is revealed to all, including her astonished family. She has found strength in her wholeness, and the prince is both her aid in discovering herself and her reward for being discovered.

10. This passage asserts that:

    I.   only those versions of the story that are American can be used to illustrate Horney's theories.

    II.   regardless of the version of the Cinderella tale, the story tells of a young girl's passage into womanhood.

    III.   the concept of the evil stepmother or foster mother is a main ingredient in the Cinderella story.

    IV.   Cinderella's sisters typically are older than she and less attractive.

    V.   the prince finally sees only one facet of Cinderella.

    A. I, II, and III   **C.** II, III, and IV
    B. I and IV   **D.** IV only

11. According to this passage, Cinderella:

    A. contemplates revenge on her sisters and mother but doesn't carry through with it.
    B. does not seek revenge at all.
    C. gives up her need for revenge after she marries the prince.
    D. cannot bring herself to completely forgive her persecutors.

12. The author of this passage concludes the following from the fact that in at least three versions of the story, Cinderella is made to wear animal skins.

    A. She needs the warmth that these skins provide.
    B. The animal skins have nothing to do with the rites of passage that she is going through.
    C. The animal skins symbolize the profane animal world that she figuratively is leaving.
    D. She may decide to keep the animal skins.

13. Throughout the essay, but especially in the concluding paragraphs, the author suggests that Cinderella:

    A. is less complex than she had originally thought herself to be.
    B. is moving psychologically toward a condition of wholeness.
    C. intentionally exploits the prince to bring about her own growth.
    D. is weakened by her newly discovered wholeness.

14. One might draw the following conclusions from this passage:

    A. Horney probably had the Cinderella story in mind when she formulated her theories.
    B. Folktales and fairy tales such as Cinderella can be useful in illustrating aspects of psychological theories such as those of Horney.
    C. Horney's theories are valid because the plots of the various versions of the Cinderella story bear them out.
    D. Horney altered the story to make it fit her theories.

15. An appropriate title for this essay would be:

    A. "If the Shoe Fits": Horney's Theories and the Cinderella Story.
    B. The Narcissism of Cinderella.
    C. The Stepmother as Heroine.
    D. The Varieties of Magical Experience: The Shoe that Fit.

16. If one were to write an essay that used logic similar to that in this essay, that study might be called:

    A. Fairy Tales of the Western World.
    D. Jack and the Beanstalk and the Theories of Sigmund Freud.
    C. Little Red Riding Hood and Snow White.
    D. Cinematic Interpretations of Eastern and Western Folktales.

Passage III (Questions 17–24)

Probably most people enter medical school driven in large measure by their desire to help their fellow humankind. Although the prospects of achieving substantial wealth and reasonably high public esteem may be related motives, most consider that the search to live some form of the Golden Rule is an important reason for entering medical school. There is a growing perception among the general public, however, that many physicians are more interested in themselves and their families than in their patients. An understanding of the role conflicts experienced in medical school, residency training, and professional practice must begin in the earliest days of medical education.

The sociologist, Wendy Carlton, studied the development of medical students and concluded that three rather distinct perspectives, the moral, clinical, and legal, directly affect decision making by physicians. Her extensive observation suggested to her that "medical students are being socialized into using the clinical perspective to resolve clinical problems with little or no regard for the ethical aspects of their professional behavior. In particular there is a striking absence of both discussion of and concern with ethical issues, despite a growing body of literature that argues for the relevance of training in ethics for physicians in an age of technological medicine." The clinical perspective, to Carlton, meant the traditional evaluation of the patient to create a "clinical picture" and, indeed, she entitled her book *In Our Professional Opinion.*

Carlton found that medical students upon entering medical school use the moral, clinical, and legal perspectives in that order. After acquiring clinical experience they apply the ranking used by physicians: clinical, legal, and then the moral. Hospital administrators invoke the legal, the clinical, and then the moral. "Laypersons," she contended, "use the moral perspective and depend on professionals to provide the clinical and legal perspectives, though they may use information from the media in an attempt to address the clinical and legal aspects of problem solution."

There is considerable concern on the part of many that the clinical perspective described by Carlton can degenerate into a callous regard for patient interest. Shem, in 1978, presented a satirical view of the brutal world of the intern in his book, *The House of God.* Terry Mizrahi, a sociologist who observed medical house staff behavior in a large urban teaching center, felt that Dr. Shem's book "verified the overall detachment and dehumanizing resulting from the training process." Her book, *Getting Rid of Patients,* "substantiated a world of contradictions wherein the patient was oppressed while being characterized as the oppressor."

Melvin Konner, an anthropologist who entered medical school in his mid-thirties after a variety of experiences (including a two-year stint with faithhealers from the hunter-gatherers of the Kalahari desert in Africa), described his educational experiences in *Becoming A Doctor.* He characterized physicians as "tough, brilliant, knowledgable, hardworking, and hard on themselves. They are reliable and competent in situations ranging from 18-month-long management of cancer chemotherapy through 18-hour-long brain surgery to emergencies in which life may hinge on what they can do in 18 seconds. They have experienced many things that are closed to others. With very few exceptions, they are professionals."

"Perhaps they have earned the right to arrogance; they certainly feel that they have. But one wonders if they can see the self-serving aspects of their behavior." Konner goes on to emphasize the importance of "a nonphysical aspect to healing, which I am prepared to call spiritual. It relates to heart and mind, hope and will, love and courage, values and ideas, social and cultural—including religious—life. In the hospital, I learned to keep my thoughts to myself about all such matters. There, the pretense is that everyone knows about them, and it is unnecessary to talk of them. In reality, everyone 'knows' about them but practically nobody cares, except insofar as finding them the source of a good laugh. Such cynicism, which increases during the medical school years, deeply affects the young physicians' view of life—not just of illness but of the whole human experience. They have trained themselves to participate just so far and no farther with, say, a terminal cancer patient in his or her search for personal meaning; but then they cannot simply slough off this habit of diffidence when it comes to their own search for meaning, when they contemplate the course of their own lives. It is less than appealing, what this makes of them; yet I love them in some crazy way . . . I would not want my daughter or son to be one or to marry one . . . Yet of course, when I am in trouble—and notice that I do not say 'if'—I will go to them, and they will improve my chances."

The life of the medical student is challenging and at times frustrating. While intelligence and good undergraduate preparation are essential, they are not enough. Medicine is really the study of the human condition. What was once called "bedside manner" or "attitude" really means an understanding of the ingredients of human happiness. Although good health seems essential for the enjoyment of life, it is clearly not enough. And the advantages of good health frequently must be tempered by the need for reasonable diet, reasonable shelter, and love and understanding. The practice of medicine is a calling, not a business. Physician-healers must know the science of health and disease but must also know

Adapted from addresses of Dr. Stephen M. Ayres, Dean, School of Medicine, Medical College of Virginia, Virginia Commonwealth University, 1990.

what comprises the total experience that generally is called "being human." The first year of medical education, and part of the second, emphasizes the science of medicine. The patient experience towards the end of the first year of medical education, and the remaining years of education, are designed to help the student internalize the view that the practice of medicine must be based on the broadest possible understanding of the human condition. "The secret of the care of the patient is in caring for the patient."

17. The author could have chosen as a title for this passage:

A. Professional Growth of the Practicing Physician.
B. The Development of Medical Students.
C. The Life of the Medical Student.
D. The Development of the Physician.

18. The medical student of today:

A. is greatly concerned with achieving high public esteem.
B. needs only superior intelligence and good undergraduate education to succeed.
C. hopes to marry a classmate in order to have a more congenial marriage.
D. is concerned and wants to serve humanity.

19. Carlton suggests that as medical students undergo their training:

A. the ethical and moral issues predominate their decision-making process.
B. socialization elevates clinical decision making as a predominant force.
C. they are greatly influenced by hospital administrators who concentrate on legal issues.
D. they soon feel that they have earned the right to arrogance because of their thorough training.

20. In its discussion of the balance between the science of medical practice and what could be termed the art of dealing with patients, the passage implies that:

A. good health is enough for the enjoyment of life.
B. love and understanding of human emotions are not serious considerations in the overall scheme of a human being.
C. bedside manner can be learned.
D. medicine must use as its basis for practice a broad appreciation of life and humankind.

21. Which of the following statement(s) is/are *contradicted by* the passage?

A. Medical education should not consider the role conflicts experienced by students of medicine.
B. Laypersons focus quickly on the clinical and legal perspectives.
C. Physicians concentrate on their own happiness and are not hard on themselves.
D. All of the above.

22. The passage presented would be most suitable:

A. at a tenth year reunion of a class.
B. at a faculty meeting.
C. at an administrative council meeting.
D. as an introductory lecture to freshmen medical students.

23. Decision making by physicians is influenced by:

A. moral issues.
B. clinical phenomena.
C. legal opinions.
D. all of the above.

24. The passage either directly asserts or provides information that could lead to the inference that:

A. the first two years of medical school are devoted to learning the necessary science.
B. there is patient contact in the first two years.
C. there is a spiritual part to healing.
D. all of the above statements apply.

Passage IV (Questions 25–30)

Throughout the various phyla of the plant and animal kingdom, numerous species have evolved. It is apparent that sexual reproduction plays an important role in the continuation of the species and in the expression of different phenotypes within the species. This mode of reproduction is accomplished by the fusion of two gametes that will give rise to a zygote. In order for future generations to maintain the same number of chromosomes as their parents, the gametes must undergo a reduction in chromosome number. If the offspring express phenotypic traits that are different from those of their parents, there must be a rearrangement of the DNA within the chromosomes. The reduction of the number of chromosomes and mixing of the gene pool are accomplished by the process of meiosis.

The process of meiosis is characterized by a naturally occurring sequence of events that are usually artificially subdivided into ten different stages. The first five stages comprise the first or reductional division of meiosis. At the end of the reductional division, the chromosomes are reduced to one-half their original number (haploid). The last five stages comprise the second or equatorial division of meiosis. Germ cells undergoing meiosis give rise to haploid gametes that contain one representative of each type of chromosome. The chromosomes of the gametes may also demonstrate variations in genetic composition due to crossing over that takes place during the first prophase.

Replication of DNA occurs during interphase before the process of meiosis begins. The condensation and coiling of chromatin to form chromosomes marks the beginning of prophase 1, the first stage of meiosis. Homologous chromosomes pair with one another to form a structure called a bivalent. Next, each chromosome splits lengthwise to form two chromatids. The homologous pairs of chromosomes are now composed of four chromatids that are referred to as a tetrad. The chromatids of tetrads become short and thick and breaks may occur in them. The breaks are eventually repaired but segments of different chromatids may be joined together. This process, referred to as crossing over, enables segments of two different chromatids to be joined together. This enables the gametes to receive chromosomes derived from segments of both homologous chromosomes. In the second stage of meiosis or metaphase 1, the nuclear membrane disappears, a spindle apparatus forms, and the homologous pairs align along the equatorial plate of the cell. In anaphase 1, the homologous chromosomes migrate to opposite poles of the cell. Telophase 1 is characterized by the complete separation of the homologous pairs, and the spindle apparatus disappears. The nuclear membrane begins to reform and in many organisms a cytoplasmic division may occur at this stage.

After a brief interphase, prophase II begins. Prophase II is the first stage in the second or equatorial division of meiosis. It is characterized by the condensing of chromatin to form the chromosomes. During metaphase II, the spindle apparatus forms and the chromosomes line up along the equatorial plate. In anaphase II, the daughter chromosomes migrate to opposite poles of the cell. Anaphase II differs from the first anaphase in that the centromere divides and the two chromatids now become the daughter chromosomes. The daughter chromosomes separate completely and reach opposite poles of the cell in telophase II. Subsequent divisions of the cytoplasm result in the formation of two daughter cells that have a haploid number of chromosomes.

The two divisions of the germ cell during meiosis produce four gametes with one-half the original number of chromosomes.

From Hugo R. Seibel and Kenneth E. Guyer. *How to Prepare for the Medical College Admission Test*, 6th ed. Hauppauge. New York: Barron's Educational Series. Inc., 1990.

25. According to this passage, at the end of the reductional division of meiosis:

    A. four haploid sets of chromosomes are produced.
    B. the homologous pairs of chromosomes are completely separated.
    C. the chromatin duplicates and coils.
    D. the centromeres divide and daughter chromosomes move to opposite poles of the cell.

26. At which state or phase does the process known as "crossing over" occur?

    A. during the equatorial division
    B. before the tetrad separates
    C. during anaphase I
    D. during prophase II

27. The phase during which there is a duplication of the chromatin is known as:

    A. metaphase I.
    B. anaphase II.
    C. telophase I.
    D. interphase.

28. Which process from the list below makes variation in genetic composition possible?

    A. the formation of homologous pairs
    B. mitotic division of germ cells
    C. crossing over
    D. random mutations

29. Using information provided in the passage, one could reasonably conclude that:

    A. all species in both the plant and animal kingdom are capable of sexual reproduction.
    B. haploid cells are only found in animals.
    C. four functional gametes are always formed by the process of meiosis.
    D. zygote formation may produce an offspring that has the same number of chromosomes as its parents.

30. Which of the following statement(s) is/are *supported by* the passage?

    A. Meiosis is artificially subdivided into ten stages.
    B. Reproduction results in phenotypic expression.
    C. DNA duplicates before meiosis starts.
    D. All of the above.

Passage V (Questions 31–38)

Does the order of a child's birth in a family have a bearing on the type of adult he/she will grow up to be, or is the theory of ordinal position simply an interesting topic of cocktail party conversation? Although it has been the highlight of numerous debates and the subject of various studies, ordinal position remains a little-understood personality variable.

Consider the oldest child in a family of three children. Parents often claim that their firstborn has a solid head on his/her shoulders, behaves in a mature manner, and is capable of getting along with adults. This important family member often exhibits a quiet front, yet is able to take the lead, care for his/her siblings, and act like a miniature adult. Parents view the firstborn as an intelligent individual who will grow up to be a pillar of the community. A perfect illustration of the importance of being firstborn can be seen in the old custom of primogeniture that was particularly popular during the feudal period in Europe.

Primogeniture allowed the oldest member of a family, in most situations oldest male, to inherit all lands and possessions of his parents, to the exclusion of his siblings. The ordinal position of being the firstborn male therefore carried much power, as the firstborn was considered to be intelligent, level-headed, and capable of taking over as family protector and landlord once the father died. Theoretically the oldest would be unselfish and see to the care of the younger family members, but in actuality this was often not the case. Outlawed in the United States and no longer the mode of inheritance in Europe for today's population as a whole, primogeniture was in evidence as late as the 1920s and can still be seen in degree with some of Europe's royal families.

The second born child in a family of three is pictured quite differently from the oldest. This child is much more lively, less willing to take orders, does not show the same interest in adults, and often has difficulty communicating with them. He/she may even become a "problem" child in school. Teachers have been heard to complain that "B is not in the least like A was . . . ." Could it be that the second born is striking out in an attempt to find his/her own place? The problems of the second child in a family seem to intensify even more when the "baby" comes along and moves him/her into the "middle child" position. Now he/she has to contend not only with a successful older brother or sister, but also with the youngest who seems to be the favorite.

The youngest child appears not to feel the need to measure up to anyone and goes along his/her own way to develop into an often exuberant, well-rounded indi-

From Hugo R. Seibel and Kenneth E. Guyer. *How to Prepare for the Medical College Admission Test*, 6th ed. Hauppauge. New York: Barron's Educational Series. Inc., 1990.

vidual. Because he/she is the baby, the mother doesn't expect this third sibling to function like a miniature adult, and she considers "cute" a great number of the actions that were viewed as unsatisfactory in the case of the other children.

Personality traits are not the only topic of interest in the ordinal position arena. The academic ability of children in various birth positions has also received attention. One interesting study reported a comparison of mathematics grades between women who were separated into three groups: (1) firstborn, (2) at least second born but not last born, and (3) last born in a family. Women without siblings were excluded from the study. The results indicate a statistical difference in mathematics grades between groups (1) and (3) but no other significant differences. Group (1) achieved higher mathematics grades than group (3).

Theories of motivation and anxiety have been advanced to explain the difference in achievement. The motivation theory states that the oldest child receives more encouragement from the parents than is given to other children. For a time, the first child is the only child, an experience not shared by the other children. Particularly during this early period the parents may try very hard to help the child, thus striving to experience vicariously their own unfulfilled expectations. The anxiety theory adds another factor to try to explain the lower achievement of the youngest child. Not only is the youngest child not pushed, as was the case with his/her older siblings, but this lack of parental pushing may be interpreted as lack of parental interest. The youngest child may develop feelings of anxiety, and these may interfere with performance. Thus, the youngest child may suffer as a result of less parental pressure and expectations as well as suffering from self-imposed anxiety, both contributing to lower performance.

31. The central thesis of the passage is that:

A. the motivational drive (as well as the anxiety level of children) is directly linked to the order in which they are born.

B. the development of a child's personality may be affected by the ordinal position he/she holds in his/her family.

C. primogeniture, which is the custom of passing on property to the oldest male member of a family, is the vehicle used by the royal families of Europe to ensure that their fortunes will remain intact.

D. ordinal position remains a little understood personality variable despite the fact that it is a popular topic both at the research and at the debate level.

32. Based on the information given in the passage, it is reasonable to conclude that:

    A. the oldest child in a family is the child best equipped to handle stressful situations.

    B. more research needs to be conducted before any concrete judgments can be made regarding the effect that birth order has on an individual's personality.

    C. academically, the youngest child tends to be lazy because he/she has been babied by parents and siblings.

    D. married couples should become well versed in ordinal position literature so that they will have a guide to follow when they are ready to have children.

33. What is the probable reason that the author used the paragraph on primogeniture in this passage?

    A. As a means of making the passage more interesting for the reader by introducing a historical topic.

    B. In order to make the reader aware of the fact that the firstborn was expected to share his inheritance with his younger siblings.

    C. To make the reader aware of the fact that the custom was outlawed in the United States around 1920.

    D. As a means of illustrating that ordinal position, especially the place of the firstborn, has been a topic of interest for a long period of time.

34. Which of the following statements is/are *supported by* the information in the passage?

    I. Parents often claim that firstborn children behave in a more mature manner than later-born.

    II. The "baby" of the family is often a child with an outgoing personality.

    III. By the time the third child comes along, mothers no longer seem to put the same emphasis on certain aspects of behavior that they did when raising their first.

    A. I only   **C.** I and II only
    B. II only   **D.** I, II, and III

35. Which of the following statements is *contradicted by* the information given in the passage?

    A. Comparison to older siblings, by teachers and other adults, is the best method for stimulating the middle child to work harder.

    B. Second born children who later move into the "middle child" position achieve on a higher plane in school than do second born who remain in the same position.

    C. The youngest child does not feel the need to measure up to anyone.

    D. The second born child sometimes has a problem communicating with adults.

36. Information concerning the academic ability of children in various birth positions is presented in paragraphs seven and eight. This section of the passage deals primarily with:

    A. differences in mathematics achievement between males and females.

    B. differences in achievement of students between mathematics and other courses.

    C. differences in mathematics grades of females according to birth order.

    D. the effect of parental support on mathematics achievement.

37. In presenting the information in paragraph eight, the author suggests that anxiety:

    A. has no effect on mathematics achievement.
    B. decreases mathematics achievement.
    C. increases mathematics achievement.
    D. can only be imposed by others.

38. Which of the following statement(s) is/are *supported by* the passage?

    A. The example uses a family unit of five people.

    B. Being the youngest could be of advantage in becoming a well-balanced individual.

    C. Performance is related to anxiety in the youngest child.

    D. All of the above.

Passage VI (Questions 39–45)

Performance appraisals—"Who needs them? I'm doing a good job, so why does someone need to sit and put it in writing, then waste my time and theirs talking about it? If I'm doing something that they don't like, let them tell me about it when it happens." This is a typical comment heard from many employees.

The performance appraisal, if completed properly, can be one of the most useful tools a manager can use in developing and training subordinates regardless of what some employees may express. It is a compilation of the employee's strengths and weakness in one concise form. It serves to show the employee the areas in which a good job is being done and also indicates which areas need improvement. The appraisal serves as a permanent record that documents the employee's growth and progress or shows why a promotion is not offered. A performance appraisal forces a manager to discuss an employee's performance on one-to-one basis and find out more about what the employee's opinions and aspirations might be. This area is often overlooked in the busy day-in and day-out routine of business. It gives the employee a chance to see what the boss really thinks about his or her work.

An interesting and often very beneficial way of handling a performance appraisal is to give employees a blank evaluation form a few days before the appraisal interview and ask that they rate themselves. When the appraisal takes place, the manager and employee compare their evaluations and work out the areas of disagreement so that each understands the other's position. An unusual result often takes place. Not only do the manager and employee end up with a better knowledge of each other, but they often find that their evaluations are very close to being in agreement If anything, the employees usually find that they have underrated themselves. An exception to this result, which the manager must be alert to recognize, is that an unsatisfactory performer may evaluate his or her performance higher than does the manager. The appraisal interview in this situation can often be more valuable than that of the satisfactory performer. It gives the manager an opportunity to counsel an already trained employee and turn around the performance rather than having to seek out and train a replacement. The manager must evaluate the time expense, and attitude of the present employee against the time and expense of hiring and training a new employee.

Performance appraisals, properly administered, can cut down on turnover and greatly increase the morale of a department. The end result is increased productivity, which is really what we are all striving to accomplish.

Although standard procedure in industry for many years, performance appraisals have also reached higher education. In recent years college students have come to see themselves as purchasing a service, specifically that of education. They have demanded greater accountability, asking that the remuneration of faculty members be tied to teaching effectiveness. Many faculty members agree with the concept in theory but feel that measurement of teaching effectiveness is flawed.

Teaching effectiveness is often determined through evaluations by administrators, faculty colleagues, or students, or by a combination of two or more of these evaluations. Students are usually most interested in evaluations by students, believing that they are the "consumers" who are most directly affected by the quality of the "product" called teaching. Faculty members counter that evaluations by students are flawed, in that they are affected by the charisma (or lack of it) of the instructor, the level of difficulty of the subject matter, and the grades given in the course.

A more objective method has been suggested by various groups—the student performance at the end of the course. All students taking a particular course could be given a standard test; mean scores in sections taught by different instructors could then be compared and related to each instructor's teaching effectiveness. The results could be affected, of course, by the students' IQs, motivation, and prior instruction in the material covered by the course.

39. Of the positive aspects pertaining to the use of performance appraisals, which of those listed below is/are directly alluded to in the passage?

A. The performance appraisal gives the employee and the manager a time to discuss the employee's future in private.

B. Employees and managers usually can work out their differences during the appraisal interview.

C. Performance appraisals often lead to a better understanding between managers and employees and eventually can lead to increased productivity.

D. All of the above.

40. Which of the following statement(s) is/are NOT *supported nor contradicted by* the information in the passage?

A. Most large companies are now using the performance appraisal method because it has been proven a highly effective tool for dismissing unsatisfactory employees.

B. All performance appraisals are preceded by giving employees blank forms to rate themselves.

C. Managers feel that performance appraisals are a waste of time.

D. All of the above.

41. Which of the following statements is/are *contradicted by* the information in the passage?

A. A satisfactorily performing employee will rate himself or herself higher than the manager.

B. A performance appraisal only points out the weak areas of performance.

C. A performance appraisal is the most useful tool a manager uses in developing and training subordinates.

D. All of the above.

From Hugo R. Seibel and Kenneth E. Guyer. *How to Prepare for the Medical College Admission Test,* 6th ed. Hauppauge, New York: Barron's Educational Series, Inc., 1990.

42. Some faculty members, addressing concerns about the accuracy and validity of student evaluations of teaching, caution that:

    A. all suggested methods of evaluation of teaching effectiveness are quite subjective.

    B. the charisma of the instructor is a factor in evaluation of teaching effectiveness.

    C. evaluations of an instructor's teaching effectiveness are unaffected by student grades.

    D. evaluations of an instructor's teaching effectiveness are affected by the time of day when lectures are given.

43. According to the passage, greater difficulty of the course would have what effect on student ratings of teacher effectiveness?

    A. lower ratings
    B. higher ratings
    C. no effect
    D. the passage does not say

44. The author indicates that students are most interested in ratings of teaching effectiveness when determined by:

    A. evaluation by faculty colleagues.
    B. evaluation by administrators.
    C. evaluation by students.
    D. objectively determined progress of the performance of the class.

45. Regarding performance appraisals in industry and student evaluations of teaching, the passage asserts that:

    A. students view themselves as consumers.
    B. performance evaluations benefit the parties involved.
    C. performance appraisals can lead to increased productivity.
    D. all of the above are true statements.

Passage VII (Questions 46–51)

Paul Tillich, in his article "The Lost Dimension in Religion," asserts that in contemporary Western society there is an absence of spirituality; moreover, that in spite of a growing interest in religion, and because of it, the religious element as Tillich defines it has all but vanished. The popularity of "go-to-church-every-Sunday" and the televangelism of the 80s belong to the "concrete religion" of literal hermeneutics (the science of interpreting an author's words or scriptures), rituals, and institutions.

The lost dimension as Tillich describes it is the loss of each individual's asking himself or herself basic and important existential questions such as: "What is the meaning of life? Where do we come from, where do we go to? What shall we do, what should we become in the short stretch between birth and death?" This spiritual "dimension of depth" is lost to modern man, he says, and "religion as the state of being grasped by an infinite concern" is absent.

Though written 30 years ago, this observation is still insightful today, perhaps even more so. Tillich explains how spiritual depth has become lost to contemporary Man. He traces the causes to Man's relationship with Nature and with himself, a relationship in which Nature is "subjected scientifically and technically" by the whims of Man, and self-knowledge is nearly nonexistent.

But, Tillich claims that, though today's generations lack the courage to ask themselves weighty eschatological questions (dealing with final matters, such as death), previous generations had the courage to do so. On this point, Tillich is slightly evasive. Does he mean that, say, a rise in materialism and technology parallels a drop in spirituality, and that previous generations who were less materialistic and technologically oriented were more spiritual? Perhaps, but he seems to rely heavily on our technologically-oriented lives as evidence of a decline in spirituality. One might agree with him on this point but still believe that the roots go much deeper, and that our technology-based living and subsequent relationship with Nature is indeed an effect of something else as much as it is a cause of a loss of spirituality. Might not the dualistic perspective implicit in our own philosophical heritage, which seeks to divide the whole into parts, be called into question, along with the scientific method and "value-free" science? The present-day relationship between Man and Nature may well be a cause of the "loss of the dimension of depth"; but one could also argue that the seeds were sown a long time ago, so long ago that a more appropriate discussion of the loss of spiritual depth would include Man's relationship to technology as well.

The true religion, according to Tillich, moves vertically, hence "depth." It involves a personal dimension as well; personal existential questions ask for personal existential answers. And what Tillich sees in present-day religion (institutional and literalistic) is a horizontal aspect, a dimension that denies itself "basic and universal meaning" and the symbolic interpretation of sacred texts. This "horizontal" religion goes hand-in-hand with contemporary horizontal living, where technological/industrial society makes things " 'better and better,' 'bigger and bigger,' " there is "movement ahead without end," and "every moment is filled with something" whether it be television or a 40-hour-a-week job.

Adapted from Taylor Fleet. "A Critique of Paul Tillich," VCU, 1989

In the horizontal dimension, "no one can experience depth . . . [or start] becoming aware of himself." Symptomatic of this kind of life is the question of whether or not God exists, a "discussion in which both sides are wrong, because the discussion itself is wrong and possible only after the loss of the dimension of depth."

Tillich advocates a kind of personal inquiry, a soul-searching "in spite of the loss of the dimension of depth"; an asking of questions such as "What is the meaning of Life?" But Tillich, for all his discussion of spirituality, makes no reference to the intuitive side of Man's nature. Tillich seems to imply that existential questions and any answers they might find are rational in their relationship to one another, and that the latter follows logically from the former; that there is indeed an answer that can be articulated. I suspect that this perspective is still inside the cultural context that gave rise to the loss of the dimension of depth in the first place—perhaps Tillich needs to step out of that context and into a context that is intuitive and in which personal existential questions are acknowledged from a source much deeper than the rational mind. It is perhaps the intuitive/spiritual that is the true religious character that, as Tillich says, "in spite of the loss of dimension of depth, its power is present, and is most present in those who are aware of the loss . . . ."

46. The author of this passage observes that according to Tillich, contemporary society:

    A. is no longer interested in religion.
    B. suffers from a loss of spirituality.
    C. is more than willing to ask itself weighty existential questions.
    D. none of the above.

47. Which of the following, according to the passage, accurately reflects Tillich's view?

    A. True religion moves vertically.
    B. True religion is the same as present-day (institutional and literalistic) religion.
    C. Present-day society encourages individuals to ask deep questions about human existence.
    D. True religion asks questions addressing whether or not God exists.

48. Although the passage reflects general agreement with Tillich on many points, the author disagrees with Tillich on which of the following?

    A. his assertion that modern man lacks true religion
    B. his belief that people are more materialistic today than in the past

    C. his definition of spirituality
    D. his failure to take into account the intuitive side of human nature in discussing ways by which individuals can find answers to spiritual questions

49. The author finds Tillich's ideas about the lost dimension in religion as:

    A. less valid than they were when Tillich wrote them 30 years ago.
    B. at least as insightful as they were 30 years ago.
    C. interesting but too theoretical to be applied to actual human beings.
    D. illustrative of T.S. Eliot's idea that modern man lives in a spiritual wasteland.

50. An appropriate title for this essay might be:

    A. The Relevance of Tillich's Ideas Thirty Years Later.
    B. The Optimism of Paul Tillich.
    C. Tillich as Champion of Man's Intuition.
    D. The Tillich that No One Knows.

51. In contemporary "horizontal" religion, according to Tillich, there is:

    A. a de-emphasis on television in the lives of individuals.
    B. an accentuation of the small.
    C. a clear goal at the end of the individual's struggle.
    D. an emphasis on better and better and on bigger and bigger.

Passage VIII (Questions 52–58)

The temporomandibular joint is characterized as a bilateral diarthroidal articulation; that is, it is capable of both rotary (hinge) and translatory (gliding) motion. This range of motion permits movement both bodily (side) and in an anterior-posterior direction of the mandibular condyle within the glenoid fossa or cavity of this joint. The functional articulation actually occurs when each condyle contacts the articular eminence of the squamous part of the temporal bone. Both the right and left joints function as one unit, but each may move somewhat independently.

Interposed between the condyle and fossa and eminence is an articular disk or meniscus which is attached to the head of the condyle posteriorly and to the joint

From Hugo R. Seibel and Kenneth E. Guyer. *How to Prepare for the Medical College Admission Test*, 6th ed. Hauppauge. New York: Barron's Educational Series. Inc., 1990.

capsule laterally. This arrangement produces upper and lower joint compartments lined by synovium. The disk consists of dense collagenous connective tissue or may be fibrocartilaginous in nature. It fuses with the joint capsule, which is composed of dense fibroelastic connective tissue. This capsule is attached to the concave surface of the fossa, the convex surface of the eminence, and inferiorly to the neck of the concave surface of the fossa, the convex surface of the eminence; and inferiorly to the neck of the condyle. The thickened lateral part of the capsule forms the temporomandibular ligament.

The temporomandibular ligament functions to prevent excessive retraction of the mandible and thus limits border movements. Other ligaments attached to the joint include the sphenomandibular, the stylomandibular and the tiny Pinto's. The sphenomandibular ligament functions to limit closure of the jaws. It becomes taut if the vertical dimension is decreased. The stylomandibular ligament functions to limit extreme mandibular protrusion and overclosure of the jaws. The tiny ligament, attached to the capsule, disk, and sphenomandibular ligament, inserts on the malleus of the ear. Tension on it may cause some change in position of the malleus.

Each synovial compartment is lined with a vascular layer of connective tissue. In areas not exposed to pressure, the synovial membrane is thrown into numerous folds. There are two kinds of cells comprising the membrane. Type A cells are phagocytic in nature and are found among type B cells that are secretary in nature. The cavity is filled with synovial fluid, a transparent, yellowish, viscous material. The fluid is a dialysate of plasma and lymph consisting of a protein-mucopoly-saccharide complex. Debris is removed from this lubricating and nutritional fluid by the type A cells of the membrane.

52. The main topic of this passage is:

A. the unlimited movement capabilities of the temporomandibular joint.
B. the description of the functional anatomy of the joint.
C. the role of the ligaments in movements of the joint.
D. the histological characterization of various anatomic controls.

53. According to the passage, the meniscus is best described as:

A. the layer internal to the synovial compartments.
B. the connective tissue separating the lower compartment from the condyle.
C. the fibrocartilage positioned above the upper synovial cavity.
D. the attachment for the head of the condyle.

54. Unlike the articular disk, the joint capsule:

A. contains some connective tissue.
B. forms laterally into ligamentous tissue.
C. makes attachment with the joint.
D. consists of fibers and cells.

55. It can be concluded from the passage that:

A. border movements made by the mandible are restricted by ligamentous attachments.
B. overclosure of the jaws occurs frequently.
C. slack in one of the ligaments leads to tension in other ligaments.
D. protrusion involves movement of the mandible posteriorly.

56. According to the passage, the following are correct EXCEPT:

A. Phagocytes remove foreign material from the synovial fluid.
B. Only Type B cells produce the synovial fluid.
C. Pressure flattens areas of the synovial membrane.
D. Blood vessels are found among the connective tissue of synovial compartments.

57. Which of the following statement(s) is/are *supported by* the passage?

A. The temporomandibular joint is a universal joint.
B. A fair percentage of people experience discomfort in this joint during life.
C. There is no connection between this joint and the middle ear.
D. None of the above.

58. Which of the following statement(s) is/are *contradicted by* the passage?

A. The synovial fluid has similar qualities as plasma.
B. The disk has an attachment to the joint capsule.
C. Joint function is synchronized.
D. None of the above.

Passage IX (Questions 59–65)

Studies of part-time and full-time faculty members in specific states and types of institutions are numerous. A review of the literature reveals specific issues as hinges on which the implementation of policy changes may turn. Recent studies clearly show the impact of the increasing use of part-time faculty in higher education institutions. Recommendations range from converting all part-time positions to full-time ones, save those made necessary by last-minute budget increases, to moves away from the traditional tenure system to alternative systems. Recommendations revolve around: employment security; participation of part-time, temporary, and full-time "teach only" faculty in academic governance; access to academic due process (as regards appointments that clearly specify nature and conditions of appointment, rights to confer over terms and conditions, timely settlement of grievances, fair evaluation by peers to which they may have opportunity to respond); and compensation including salary and benefits.

Institutions have continued to hire part-time faculty at a rate that shows a 164 percent increase (compared to a 37 percent increase in number of full-time faculty) from 1970 to 1988. "Part-timers" have been hired because of organizationally perceived financial necessity, the desire to maintain administrative and curricular "flexibility," and the availability of academics who do not have full-time positions in their fields for various reasons. Between 40 and 45 percent of all nontenure-track positions surveyed by AAUP in 1984–85 were filled by women, whereas they held only 25 percent of the total number of full-time faculty positions covered in the survey.

What purposes are served for the institution? The writers of the 1986 "Report on Full-Time Nontenure-Track Appointments" in *Academe* say it is questionable whether any real flexibility is achieved because a substantial portion of the nontenure-eligible appointments occur in fields that are central to the institution's academic program ("core" courses, such as English Composition). Part-time adjuncts and graduate assistants perform most lower division teaching and approximately 40 percent of the undergraduate instruction taking place in American colleges and universities (Nielsen and Polishook, 1990).

The continual hiring of nontenure-eligible faculty members creates a class of insecure teachers whose status is inferior to that of both their tenure-eligible and tenured colleagues and whose role in some respects does not differ from that of teaching assistants. On the one hand, many are not required or expected to advise students, to participate in faculty personnel and budget matters, or to be involved in the development of curricula and the formulation and implementation of academic policy. They tend to receive less desirable teaching assignments, larger classes, and heavier teaching loads. Their compensation remains low, no matter how well they perform(ed). Their performance may never be reviewed.

Specifics may change with part-time and full-time "teach only" faculty appointments, yet some of the same conditions apply. They cannot develop habits of the professional academic, which includes research and revision of courses and curricula. They frequently work in unprofessional conditions (some without offices, so unable to allot "office hours" to students) and are virtually isolated from the stimulation and support of their colleagues. Because of these conditions, these instructional faculty members may lack both access to institutional resources necessary for building a research career and the incentive or pressure to become (equally) productive scholars. Many, particularly full-time "teach only" faculty members, are overworked and continually distracted by the efforts involved in looking for more secure employment conditions. Academic freedom of these teachers is also in question, as what they feel or what they may say could affect their ability to "serve the institution." To those whose appointment must be renewed at the discretion of the institution, expression of commitment to academic freedom may not be enough.

The contagion of insecurity restricts unorthodox thinking, while the rising number of those faculty reduces the cadre of those faculty, notably those with tenure, who are uninhibited in advocating changes in accepted ideas and in the policies and programs of the institutions at which they serve. (*Academe*, July/August 1986, p17a).

The presence of "temporary" faculty members who must concern themselves with their status in the institution while pursuing other employment is reflected in morale—theirs, the institution's, and that of everyone around them. The creation of this "two-tier class system" erodes sound governance practices and the fellowship of the faculty. As tenure-track faculty members perform more administrative duties, student advising, and committee work, they have less time for research and professional development. This atmosphere is generally less supportive of scholarly pursuits.

What some perceive as the increasing incidence and abuse of nontenure-track appointments when many of the best faculty recruits are choosing private sector positions instead of careers in higher education works against efforts to recruit and encourage the talented young scholars who might otherwise be more interested. These abuses may also contribute to the numbers of those who are leaving the ranks of academia. The writers who recognize this trend cite the proliferation of these temporary positions as evidence of "shortsightedness" and "unregulated growth."

59. Issues of concern regarding part-time faculty include:

    A.   job security.
    B.   academic governance.
    C.   grievance procedures.
    D.   all of the above.

Adapted from A. Nancy Avakian, Ph.D and Margaret Martin, "The Issues: Viewpoints of the Academy about Nontenure-Eligible Faculty Members," 1990.

60. The title of the passage could be:

    A. The Effect of Nontenure Track Faculty on the Educational System.

    B. Academic Freedom in Jeopardy.

    C. Viewpoints of the Academy About Non-tenure-Eligible Faculty.

    D. Reforms due to the Increase in Nontenure-Eligible Faculty.

61. Statistical data contained in the passage supports which of the following?

    A. Most part-timers are women.

    B. Part-timers have been hired at an increased rate.

    C. Flexibility has been achieved in curriculum development.

    D. Core courses are taught mainly by full-time faculty.

62. Using information provided by the author, one would be wrong to conclude that:

    A. part-time faculty is never expected to take part in curriculum development.

    B. performance review of part-time faculty is questionable.

    C. full-time "teach only" faculty has a secure base from which to function.

    D. A and C of the above.

63. Tenure-track faculty:

    A. leave most of the advising to part-timers.

    B. in the future will have more time for scholarly pursuits.

    C. are apt to initiate changes.

    D. are chosen from a large pool of the best recruits.

64. Regarding temporary faculty members, the passage either asserts directly or implies that:

    A. they have and create morale problems.

    B. they help erode the governance system in higher education.

    C. some view the hiring of this group as short-sighted.

    D. all of the above statements apply.

65. Which of the following statement(s) is/are *supported by* the passage?

    A. The theme of the discussion has been well investigated.

    B. Many reasons explain the existence of part-time faculty.

    C. Part-time faculty has had an impact on higher education.

    D. All of the above.

PHYSICAL SCIENCES

10 PROBLEM SETS OF 5–10 QUESTIONS EACH
15 PROBLEMS FOLLLOWED BY A SINGLE QUESTION
77 QUESTIONS
100 MINUTES

DIRECTIONS: The following questions or incomplete statements are in groups. Preceding each series of questions or statements is a paragraph or a short explanatory statement, a formula or set of formulas, or a definition. Read the written material and then answer the questions or complete the statements. Select the ONE BEST ANSWER for each question and indicate your selection by marking the corresponding letter of your choice on the Answer Form. Eliminate those alternatives you know to be incorrect and then select an answer from among the remaining alternatives. A periodic table is provided (see p. 583). You may consult it whenever you wish to do so.

Passage I (Questions 66–70)

An x-ray tube consists of two metal electrodes, a heated filament cathode, and an anode containing the metal target sealed under high vacuum in a glass envelope. The heated filament in the cathode emits electrons which are accelerated by a high DC voltage and collide with the positive anode target. Two different types of x-ray spectra may be seen. The continuous or "bremsstrahlung" spectrum that is always present is produced when the electron penetrates through the outer electron cloud and is abruptly accelerated by the large positive charge on the nucleus of a heavy atom. The production of x-rays increases with increasing atomic number but is typically no more than 1% efficient, the remaining energy appearing as heat in the target metal. The sharp line spectra that can be seen at higher voltages occur when the incident electrons eject an inner shell electron, such as an $n = 1$ shell electron. The spectral line is produced when an electron, say from $n = 2$, fills the vacancy in the $n = 1$ shell, emitting an x-ray photon whose energy corresponds to the energy difference between the $n = 2$ and $n = 1$ shells. The intensity of x-rays is proportional to the number of photons created. The photon energy $E = hf = hc/\lambda$ where h is Planck's constant and c is the speed of light. Figure 1 is a sketch of intensity versus wavelength for a molybdenum target with an accelerating voltage of 35,000 V.

Figure 1. X-ray intensity versus wavelength

C. the type of cathode used.
D. the type of anode material used.

67. The sharp K_α peak in Figure 1 corresponds to an electron transition from state $n = 2$ to $n = 1$, where K_β corresponds to a transition from state $n = 3$ to $n = 1$. The K_α line peak is higher than the K_β because:

A. it is due to a higher atomic number target metal.
B. K_α is the more energetic transition.
C. the K_α transition is more probable than the K_β transition, so its intensity is higher.
D. the K_α transition occurs in the valence shells instead of the inner shells.

66. Figure 1 shows that the continuous x-ray spectrum has a minimum (cut-off) wavelength. No shorter wavelengths are emitted from the tube. This minimum wavelength corresponds to:

A. the smallest number of emitted photons.
B. the highest energy photons emitted.

68. The current to the heated filament in the cathode is increased while the accelerating voltage is kept constant. This increased current increases the number of electrons striking the target increasing the overall intensity. What effect does this have on the minimum wavelength value?

    A. The minimum value will move to shorter wavelength values.
    B. It will move to longer wavelength values.
    C. There will no longer be a cutoff wavelength.
    D. The minimum wavelength will remain the same.

69. If the accelerating voltage, V_o, is increased while keeping the filament current constant, the overall intensity will also increase. What effect will this have on the wavelength position where the two peaks are observed?

    A. They will occur at the same wavelengths.
    B. The peaks occur at shorter wavelengths due to the higher energies available.
    C. They may disappear because all energies may exceed those of the $n = 3$ to $n = 1$ transition.
    D. The K_α occur at longer wavelengths but the K_β occur at shorter wavelengths.

70. Because the efficiency of x-ray production increases with increasing atomic number, Z, it would seem that lead (Z = 82) would be a better target material than tungsten (Z = 74). However, tungsten (also used in ordinary light bulb filaments) is the most common target meal, whereas lead is never used. This is because:

    A. lead has too many electrons.
    B. lead becomes radioactive.
    C. lead would melt, whereas tungsten has a very high melting point.
    D. lead will not get hot enough to produce any x-rays.

Passage II (Questions 71–76)

A safety engineering firm is producing a film for high school driver education classes. The firm uses skilled test drivers driving both small cars and larger vans. The vans weigh three times as much as the cars and have larger tires with twice the tread width. In a demonstration that tests reaction times and skid-to-stop distances and shows them on the film, three guns that fire a yellow paint onto the road are mounted on the bumpers and

fired electrically. When the driver hears the report of the first gun, he locks the brakes, and the touch of his foot on the brake pedal fires a second yellow pellet. The third pellet is fired when the car stops. The safety engineers also design several remote controlled cars and vans in order to film crash results.

71. Drivers of a car and a van brake hard and skid to a stop from 50 mph. The skid marks are measured to be the same length for both. Why are the stopping distances the same length?

    A. The mechanical work done by friction to stop both is the same.
    B. The frictional force between tires and road is three times greater for the heavier van so it slides the same distance as the car.
    C. The frictional force for the car and van are the same.
    D. The wider tires on the van require less friction force than the narrow tires on the car.

72. Two drivers in identical cars skid to a stop from speeds of 20 mph and 40 mph. How do the lengths of the skid marks compare?

    A. They are the same length.
    B. The 40 mph mark is twice as long.
    C. The 40 mph mark is four times as long.
    D. The 40 mph mark is eight times as long.

73. A remote controlled car and van are crashed head-on at the same speed. Why does the car suffer more damage in the collision?

    A. The car and van had the same momentum.
    B. The forces during collision are equal and opposite, so the smaller and weaker car suffers more damage.
    C. The van exerts a larger force on the car.
    D. The mechanical work done in stopping the car is greater.

74. The van going at a speed of 15 mph collides head-on with a car going at a speed of 45 mph. Because the van weighs three times as much, their vector momenta are equal and opposite. However, examination shows that the car suffers more damage than the van. Why?

    A. The massive van exerts a larger force on the car.
    B. The lighter car exerts a smaller force on the van.

C. The forces exerted during the collision are equal and opposite, so the weaker car suffers more damage.
D. The mechanical work required to stop the van is smaller.

75. A driver in a van skids to a stop from 20 mph and a driver in a car skids to a stop from 60 mph. How do the length of the skid marks compare?

A. The van skids three times further than the car, because it is three times heavier.
B. The car skids three times further because it is lighter and is going three times faster.
C. The car will skid nine times as far as the van.
D. They skid the same length because the speed ratio is 1:3, whereas the weight ratio is 3:1.

76. For the reaction time test, one driver is tested at 20 mph and 60 mph. It is noted that the distance between the first two paint marks is three times farther for the 60 mph test than the 20 mph test. How do his reaction times compare at 20 mph and 60 mph?

A. His reaction time at 60 mph is three times faster.
B. His reaction times remain the same.
C. His reaction time at 20 mph is three times faster.
D. His reaction time at 20 mph is one-third as long as at 60 mph.

Passage III (Questions 77–81)

An engineer is to design a small conveyor belt with attached buckets to carry fixed quantities of dog food from the first floor of the factory up to the second floor, 4.0 m above, where each sample of dog food is dumped into a sack that moves underneath the end of the conveyor belt as the bucket dumps the dog food into the sack (see the sketch on this page). The sacks then move to another part of the plant where they are sealed and packed for shipment to stores. The engineer wishes to determine the power rating of an electric motor that will drive the conveyor belt, and also needs to know what current will be drawn by the motor. Each bucket has a mass of 2 kg and can carry 8 kg of dog food. The conveyor belt should carry 30 buckets per minute to the top because that is how fast (30 sacks per minute) the sacks are moved. As a first approximation, the engineer will assume that the system is virtually frictionless. He will also assume that the mass of the buckets, themselves, can be ignored, because there are as many going down as going up at any time.

77. The engineer wants the angle of inclination to be 30°, as shown. How long should the conveyor belt be?

A. 3 m   C. 8 m
B. 6 m   D. 9 m

78. If the practical effect is to transport 30 buckets per minute from the bottom to the top of the belt, what power, in watts, is required?

A. 196 watts   C. 300 watts
B. 240 watts   D. 8,800 watts

79. If an electric motor, operated at 120 volts, drives the conveyor belt, what current will it draw, in amperes? (Neglect losses.)

A. 1.6 amperes   C. 4.2 amperes
B. 2.0 amperes   D. 8.4 amperes

80. If the engineer now assumes that he should use a motor rated 45% higher in power (to allow for friction), what should the rated power (watts) of the motor be?

A. 240 watts   C. 420 watts
B. 290 watts   D. 12,200 watts

81. If the conveyor belt runs faster so that 60 buckets per minute are raised rather than 30 buckets per minute, how should the rated power of the motor be changed?

A. It should be twice as large.
B. It should remains the same, since the mass carried in each bucket remains 10 kg.
C. It should increase by the square of 2.
D. It should increase by the square root of 2.

Passage IV (Questions 82–87)

The apparatus shown is designed for students to make measurements in mechanics. It consists of an essentially frictionless adjustable track down which different small metal blocks slide after being released from various heights, h. The blocks can collide with objects placed on the track end when the end is in the 0° (horizontal) position. The student can also allow the blocks to fly off the adjustable end section of the track at angles of 0°, 30°, and 45°. For all three angles of launch assume that the mass will land 1 meter below the track end. A photogate-timer system will allow the speed of the blocks to be measured just as they leave the track end. Some data from students is given in the table.

	Mass (grams)	Height h (meters)
Block 1	200	0.4
	200	0.77
	200	1.2
Block 2	300	0.4
	300	0.77
	300	1.2

82. Block 1 is released from a height $h = 0.77$ m and collides with (inelastically) and *sticks* to a 500-gram mass on the horizontal (0°) track end. The photogate-timer system measures their combined speed to be 1.11 m/sec. What is the speed of Block 1 *just before* impact?

A. 3.88 m/sec
B. 1.55 m/sec
C. 2.08 m/sec
D. 3.34 m/sec

83. Block 2 is now released from a height of 0.77 m and collides and sticks to the 500-gram mass. How does the combined speed of Block 2 and the mass compare with the combined speed of Block 1 and the mass from the above question?

A. It is the same.
B. It is smaller.
C. It is larger.
D. There is insufficient information to answer the question.

84. Using data from the table, show that if Block 1 and Block 2 are released at 1.2 m, their speeds at the bottom of the track are, respectively:

A. 1.85 m/sec, 2.35 m/sec.
B. 2.35 m/sec, 1.85 m/sec.
C. 3.23 m/sec, 4.88 m/sec.
D. 4.85 m/sec, 4.85 m/sec.

85. Both Block 1 and Block 2 are released from $h = 1.2$ m. Each is allowed to fly off the track end at elevation angles of 30° and 45°, so that they fly through parabolic arcs. Ignoring air friction, their speeds at the *top* of their parabolic arcs:

A. are greater for the 30° arc than for the 45° arc.
B. are smaller for the 30° arc than for the 45° arc.
C. are the same for the 30° arc and 45° arc.
D. depend on their masses.

86. Block 1 and Block 2 are again released from $h = 1.2$ m. Block 1 flies off the track end at 30° and Block 2 at 45°. Their speeds when they hit the floor 1 meter below the track end:

A. are smaller for Block 1 than Block 2.
B. are larger for Block 1 than Block 2.
C. are the same for Block 1 and Block 2.
D. depend on mass and angle, so the question cannot be answered.

87. When Block 1 and Block 2 hit the floor as in the above question, the ratio of their kinetic energies at that instant is:

A. equal.
B. 7/2.
C. 2/3.
D. 3/2.

Questions 88–95 are independent of any passage and of each other.

88. A student pushes a 20-kg box over a rough floor at a constant speed of 1 m/sec with a force of 100 N. If the student pushes with a larger force of 150 N, the box will:

   A. move at a constant speed of 1.5 m/sec.
   B. move at a constant speed of 2.25 m/sec.
   C. accelerate.
   D. decelerate.

89. Rutherford first observed nuclear transmutation when N^{14} was bombarded with alpha particles (He^4 nuclei). The reaction is written as:

$$_2He^4 + _7N^{14} \rightarrow {}_8O^{17} + ?$$

   What is the missing particle ?

   A. $_2He^4$ (alpha particle)
   B. $_1H^1$ (proton)
   C. $_0n^1$ (neutron)
   D. $_{-1}e^0$ (electron)

90. Two charged particles, A and B, are a distance r apart so that a certain force exists between them. The charge on A is tripled while the distance between the charges is also tripled. How does the force between the particles change?

   A. It does not change.
   B. It increases by a factor of 3.
   C. It decreases by a factor of 9.
   D. It decreases by a factor of 3.

91. A 3-ohm resistor and a 6-ohm resistor are connected in parallel and a 2-ohm resistor is connected in series with this combination as shown. If a current of 3 amperes is sent through the 2-ohm resistor, the currents through the 3- and 6-ohm resistors are, respectively:

   A. 3 and 2 amperes
   B. 1 and 2 amperes
   C. 2 and 1 amperes
   D. 0.5 and 2.5 amperes

92. 2 L of an ideal gas are at a pressure of 2 atm and a temperature of 20°C. If the temperature is kept constant and the pressure is increased to 3.5 atm, what is the new volume?

   A. 1.1 L C. 1.5 L
   B. 0.9 L D. 0.7 L

93. A golf ball is dropped from the top of a very tall building. (Air friction is present.) Which graph below correctly shows the velocity of the ball as a function of time?

94. A ball of mass 2 kg is thrown horizontally at a speed of 5.4 m/sec off a 10 m high roof. A second ball of mass 4 kg is thrown downward at an angle of 45° below the horizontal at the same speed. The speeds of the 2- and 4-kg balls when they hit at the bottom are, respectively:

   A. 15 m/sec, 30 m/sec.
   B. 30 m/sec, 15 m/sec.
   C. 10.8 m/sec, 21.6 m/sec.
   D. 15 m/sec, 15 m/sec.

95. A 2 cm high object is 20 cm in front of a converging lens with a focal length of +10 cm. A real image is seen. The object is now moved closer (to 15 cm in front of the lens). The new image is:

   A. larger and closer to the lens than the first image.
   B. larger and farther from the lens than the first image.
   C. smaller and closer to the lens than the first image.
   D. smaller and farther from the lens than the first image.

Passage V (Questions 96–105)

A class is to study electrical circuits. The laboratory portion is to be open-ended so that each pair of students does an experiment on their own, at their own pace. They are given resistors, batteries, voltmeters, ammeters, ohmmeters, oscilloscopes, capacitors, and inductance coils; as well as suitable general power supplies and function generators. The lecture portion covers the general theory including Ohm's law and Kirchhoff's laws for circuits, the operating properties of oscilloscopes, alternating current circuits (including RC, LC, and RLC series circuits), and the theory of induced *emf's* using Faraday's law.

96. Three 6-ohm resistors are connected in parallel and the ends of the parallel combination are connected to a 12-volt battery. What current flows through each individual resistor?

A. 6 A
B. 3 A
C. 2 A
D. 1 A

97. A set of three resistors with values of $R_1 = 1$ ohm, $R_2 = 2$ ohms, and $R_3 = 3$ ohms are given to the students. What are the highest and lowest equivalent resistances one can construct by using series and/or parallel arrangements of the resistors?

A. 6 ohms and 0.677 ohms
B. 9 ohms and 0.677 ohms
C. 6 ohms and 0.545 ohms
D. 9 ohms and 0.545 ohms

98. A small flat circular coil of 50 turns has an area of 1 cm^2 (1×10^{-4} m^2). It is placed with its circular area perpendicular to the magnetic field of a permanent magnet and is pulled out quickly in 0.1 sec. The induced voltage across the coil is found to be 0.05 volts. What is the magnetic field strength of the magnet in Tesla?

A. 2.0 T
B. 0.5 T
C. 1.2 T
D. 1.0 T

99. A 4-ohm resistor, a 3-millihenry inductor, and a 2-microfarad capacitor are connected into a series RLC circuit. An AC sinusoidal signal at the exact frequency of resonance for the above circuit is applied by a function generator (so that a maximum current results in the circuit). What is the impedance (Z) of this circuit at the resonant frequency?

A. 2.4 ohms
B. 2.6 ohms
C. 2.8 ohms
D. 4.0 ohms

100. The function generator in this circuit is set for an output of 2.0 volts at the resonant frequency. What is the AC current?

A. 0.3 A
B. 0.5 A
C. 0.8 A
D. 1.1 A

101. Two 2-ohm resistors are connected in parallel. A 4-ohm resistor is then connected in series with the parallel combination. What current is drawn from a 12-volt battery connected across the ends of this combination?

A. 2.2 A
B. 1.4 A
C. 1.8 A
D. 2.4 A

102. In the series-parallel circuit of question 101, what current flows through each individual 2-ohm resistance?

A. 2.4 A
B. 1.2 A
C. 0.8 A
D. 1.4 A

103. Resistors of 2-ohms and 4-ohms are available. How many *different* series combinations or parallel combinations of resistors can the students construct using three resistors at a time? (The sets of three resistors will be *all* in series or *all* in parallel.)

A. 8
B. 3
C. 14
D. 16

104. An uncharged capacitor is in series with a resistor. A battery is then connected across the RC combination. Which graph correctly shows the voltage across the capacitor as a function of time from the instant the battery was connected?

A.

C.

B.

D.

105. A student is given an unknown resistance and a battery of unknown voltage. She connects an ammeter in series with the resistor and connects the battery across the ammeter-resistor pair. A voltmeter is connected in parallel with the resistor. The voltmeter reading is 6 volts and the ammeter reads 0.5 A. What are the approximate values of battery voltage and resistance?

A. 3 V, 12 ohms
B. 6 V, 2 ohms
C. 6 V, 12 ohms
D. 3 V, 3 ohms

Passage VI (Questions 106–110)

Amino acids contain one or two amino functional groups and one or two carboxyl groups (depending on the particular amino aid). The first carboxyl group in a particular amino acid has a pK$_a$ of about 2.1 and the second carboxyl group (if present) has a pK$_a$ of about 4.0. The first amino group has a pK$_a$ of about 9.0 and the second amino group (if present) has a pK_a of about 10.5. (The pK_a of the amino group relates to the ionization of the protonated $R-NH_3^+$ to form $H^+ + R-NH_2$.)

Some amino acids also contain other functional groups such as phenolic-OH group, thiol group, guanidino group, imidazole group, and even aliphatic alcohol group. The ionization state of each of the functional groups in an amino acid contributes to the charge on that functional group.

For example, an un-ionized carboxyl or thiol group has a charge of zero, while either of these in the ionized state has a charge of –1. An un-ionized amino group has a charge of zero, but in its ionized state it has a charge of +1. The sum of the charges of the functional groups of amino acid gives its net charge. It is the net charge that determines whether a particular amino acid will move in an electrical field and, if so, in which direction (toward the cathode or the anode).

The ionization states of the functional groups of an amino acid may be altered by changing the pH of the solution (usually buffer solution).

An amino acid with one amino group and one carboxyl group (with no other functional groups) will have a pK_a value for each of these groups. A pH equal to the mean of the two pK_a values will cause the amino acid to have a net charge of zero. (This pH is designated pI.) At a pH below pI, the amino acid will have a net positive charge; at a pH above pI, the amino acid will have a net negative charge. When more than one amino group or more than one carboxyl group is present, the pI is the mean of the pK_a values on the two sides of the net uncharged species. Let us consider an amino acid with two carboxyl groups and one amino group, starting at a sufficiently low pH and going to higher pH.

$$A^+ \xrightleftharpoons{pK_{a1}} A^0 \xrightleftharpoons{pK_{a2}} A^- \xrightleftharpoons{pK_{a3}} A^{2-}$$

With A^0 as the uncharged species, the pI value will be the mean of pK_{a1} and pK_{a2}.

106. The isoelectric pH of an amino acid having two amino groups and one carboxyl group would be about:

A. 3.05.   C. 6.50.
B. 5.20.   D. 9.75.

107. The isoelectric point of an amino acid having two carboxyl groups and one amino group would be about:

A. 3.05.   C. 6.50.
B. 5.20.   D. 9.75.

108. At a pH of about 8, an amino acid with one carboxyl group and one amino group would:

A. move toward the anode in an electrical field.
B. move toward the cathode in an electrical field.
C. exhibit no movement in an electrical field.
D. probably move but in a direction that is not predictable.

109. Although not naturally occurring, an amino acid with two amino groups and two carboxyl groups would have an isoelectric point of about:

A. 5.20.   C. 7.80.
B. 6.50.   D. 9.75.

110. The change in net charge of amino acids from plus one or two to zero to negative one or two in response to different pH values in the medium is exploited in separation of amino acids by:

A. electrophoresis.
B. gas chromatography.
C. ultracentrifugation.
D. distillation.

Passage VII (Questions 111–115)

A balloon is filled with nitrogen gas (N_2) to a volume of 1000 mL at sea level at standard pressure. It is found that the volume of the balloon changes under a variety of conditions.

The volume occupied by any gas varies directly with the absolute temperature (^0K) and the number of moles of gas and inversely with the absolute pressure (e.g., mm mercury).

111. A decrease in volume to 900 mL would result from:

A. a 10% decrease in °C.
B. a 10% decrease in °K.
C. a 10% decrease in °F.
D. a 100% decrease in °F.

112. An increase of 10% in volume is noted in taking the balloon up a mountain; this is explained by:

A. a 10% increase in atmospheric pressure.
B. a conversion of 20% of N_2 molecules into N atoms.
C. a 10% decrease in temperature (°C).
D. a 10% decrease in atmospheric pressure.

113. Since H_2 has a molecular weight about one-fourteenth that of N_2, a similar balloon containing the same number of H_2 molecules at the same temper-

ature and pressure would have a volume _____ that of the N_2-containing balloon.

A. one-fourteenth
B. fourteen times.
C. between three and four times
D. equal to

114. If nitrogen existed in monoatomic form (i.e., N) rather than diatomic N_2 molecules, 0.05 moles of N would occupy _____ volume occupied by 0.05 moles of H_2 at the same temperature and pressure.

A. twice the
B. one-half the
C. the same
D. one-fourth the

115. If the balloon containing N_2 gas were simultaneously subjected to a 5% decrease in atmospheric pressure and a decrease in temperature from 27°C to 12°C, the volume of the balloon will:

A. increase about 5%.
B. increase about 10%.
C. not change.
D. decrease about 10%.

Passage VIII (Questions 116–121)

The colorimeter is a device for measuring the amount of light that passes through a solution. When the color (wavelength) of light is selected properly, the colorimeter is a useful tool for determining the amount of a particular light-absorbing material in solution.

A colorimeter is equipped with a meter that responds in linear fashion to the amount of light reaching it. The meter is set to zero with no light and it is found that a cuvette containing pure water gives a reading of 81 for light of a particular wavelength. When the same cuvette with an aqueous solution is placed in the light path, a reading of 72 is obtained.

116. The transmittance of the solution is:

A. 0.811.
B. 81.1.
C. 0.889.
D. 0.722.
E. 72.2.

117. The absorbance of the solution is:

A. 0.189.
B. 0.111.
C. 0.278.
D. 0.051.
E. 0.141.

118. If the light is of a particular wavelength that is specifically absorbed by the solute (or one of its functional groups), dilution of the solution with an equal volume of water will produce a new solution whose absorbance will be:

A. 0.026.
B. 0.095.
C. 0.222.
D. 0.282.
E. greater than 0.5.

119. If the path length through which light travels in the above solution is halved, the absorbance will be:

A. 0.013.
B. 0.052.
C. 0.047.
D. 0.141.
E. 0.190.

120. If the solute concentration for the first reading in this question set is doubled, the reading for this higher concentration will be:

A. 64.
B. 51.
C. 45.
D. 18.
E. 5.

121. If the wavelength of the light in this previous question is doubled, the reading will:

A. be doubled.
B. be halved.
C. show no change.
D. change by an amount that cannot be predicted.

Passage IX (Questions 122–126)

When an aqueous solution of strong base is added to an aqueous solution of strong acid, the pH remains low until most of the acid has been neutralized. Then the further addition of aqueous base results in an abrupt change of pH to a value that soon reaches a high value. Additional base has little effect on pH after the high pH has been reached.

Addition of an aqueous solution of strong base to an aqueous solution of weak acid produced different results. (These results are explained by the low degree of ionization of the weak acid.) A graph of the amount of base added and the resultant pH indicates that there is one or more areas where addition of more base produces little effect on the pH. Such pH areas are referred to as "buffering," and the inflection point of each buffering area is found to be the pK_a of the acid. There may be more than one acid function on each molecule, and thus there may be more than one inflection point (and pK_a).

As a rule, inorganic acids are usually strong acids. They would thus have no pK_a and no buffering action. They would also usually have only one acid function in the molecule. Phosphoric acid (H_3PO_4) and carbonic acid (H_2CO_3) are exceptions to both these rules.

Organic acids are often weak acids, provide buffering action, and have one or more pK_a's.

Formic acid (1 carbon) has one carboxylic acid group, oxalic acid has two carboxylic acid groups and citric acid has three.

An aqueous solution of an inorganic acid is titrated with strong base to give the following titration curve:

122. The pK_a with the lowest pH is at:

A. point 1.   **C.** point 3.
B. point 2.   **D.** point 4.

123. This acid appears to have _____ pK_a's.

A. 0   **C.** 2
B. 1   **D.** 3

124. Assuming we have covered the titration range form 0 to 14, this acid could be:

A. HF.
B. HCl.
C. H_3PO_4.
D. none of the above.

125. The greatest buffering is noted at:

A. points 1 and 2.
B. points 3 and 4.
C. points 1 and 3.
D. points 2 and 4.

126. Equal amounts of two species will be found at:

A. point 1 only.
B. point 2 only.
C. point 3 only.
D. more than one of the above.

Passage X (Questions 127–135)

A 0.01 mole of HCl is diluted to 1000 mL with water and mixed in a beaker to produce solution A. To this is added 1000 mL of water. After mixing, the resulting solution is solution B. To this is added 0.02 moles sodium propionate. After mixing, the resulting solution is solution C. To this is added 0.01 mole sodium propionate and 0.01 mole propionic acid. After mixing, the resulting solution is solution D. To this is added 1000 mL more water. After mixing, the resulting solution is solution E. To another beaker is added 0.005 mole of pyruvic acid. Water is added to a total volume of 500 mL. After mixing, the resulting solution is solution F. To solution F is added 0.005 mole of sodium pyruvate. After mixing, the resulting solution is solution G. K_a values are 1.3×10^{-5} for propionic acid, 1.4×10^{-4} for pyruvic acid, and 5.9×10^{-10} for boric acid. pK_a values are 4.89 for propionic acid, 3.85 for pyruvic acid, and 9.23 for boric acid. (For the purpose of this problem, assume no volume change occurs after the addition of small quantities of liquid or solid.)

127. The pH of solution A is:

A. 2.0.   **C.** 4.0.
B. 3.0.   **D.** 6.0.

128. The pH of solution B is:

A. less than 2.
B. between 2 and 3.
C. between 3 and 4.
D. between 4 and 7.

129. The pH of solution C is equal to the pK_a of the weak acid, propionic acid, because:

A. there are equal quantities of HCl and propionic acid.
B. the quantity of sodium propionate is twice that of propionic acid.
C. the quantity of sodium propionate equals that of propionic acid.
D. all the sodium propionate has been converted to propionic acid.

130. The pH of solution D is:

A. between 1 and 2.
B. between 3 and 4.
C. between 4 and 5.
D. greater than 5.5.

131. The pH of solution E is:

A. between 2 and 3.
B. between 4 and 5.
C. between 5 and 6.
D. greater than 6.5.

132. The pH of solution F is:

A. between 2 and 3.
B. between 4 and 5.
C. between 5 and 6.
D. greater than 6.5.

133. The pH of solution G is:

A. 1.4.   C. 4.9.
B. 3.8.   D. greater than 6.

134. The degree of ionization of pyruvic acid is:

A. 0.012.   C. 1.2.
B. 0.12.   D. greater than 2.

135. The percent of ionization of pyruvic acid is:

A. 0.12.   C. 12.
B. 1.2.   D. greater than 20.

Questions 136–142 are independent of any passage and of each other.

136. Compound A is known to have a molecular weight of 20. The molecular weight of Compound B is not known. Upon observing that gaseous Compound B will diffuse half as fast as gaseous Compound A, we can calculate the molecular weight of Compound B as:

A. 10.   C. 40.
B. 20.   D. 80.

137. In the titration of a 0.100 N solution of NaOH, it is found that 20.0 ml of a 0.200 N solution of an unknown acid will neutralize 40.0 ml of the 0.100 N NaOH. This indicates that the unknown acid is:

A. monoprotic.   C. triprotic.
B. diprotic.   D. none of the above.

138. If it is known that the pH of a solution is 4.5, we can calculate that the pOH is:

A. 4.5.   C. 9.5.
B. 7.5.   D. 12.5.

139. The pK_a of an acid HA is 4.2. The pH at which equal concentrations of A^- and HA are present in solution is:

A. 2.4.   C. 7.0.
B. 4.2.   D. 9.8.

140. A buffer is made of a weak acid ($pK_a = 5.9$) and its salt. Such a buffer functions best to suppress changes of pH on addition of acid when the pH of the solution is:

A. 3.9.   C. 7.0.
B. 5.9.   D. 8.9.

141. One liter of a gas is held at a pressure of 1 atm. If there is no change in temperature, increasing the pressure to 2 atm will result in a volume change to:

A. 2.0 liters.   C. 0.50 liters.
B. 0.95 liters. D. 0.20 liters.

142. In recovery of silver from photographic film, you have decided to dissolve the silver ion with dilute nitric acid. Addition of dilute HCl to precipitate AgCl seems to result in unacceptable losses. You might improve recovery by addition of _____ in the latter step.

A. $NaNO_3$ C. Ag_2SO_4
B. NaCl   D. sodium acetate

WRITING SAMPLE

2 ESSAYS
60 MINUTES (30 MINUTES/TOPIC)

DIRECTIONS: Your response must be a unified, organized essay; it should contain fully developed, logically constructed paragraphs. Remember quality is more important than length. Before you begin writing, make sure you have read the item carefully and understand what is being asked. Write as legibly as possible. Because your essays will be scored as first-draft compositions, you may cross out and make corrections on your response booklet as necessary. It is not necessary to recopy your essay.

Part 1

Consider this statement:

Men are dependent on circumstances, not circumstances on men.

Herodotus

Write a unified essay in which you perform the following tasks. Explain the meaning of the above statement. Describe a specific situation where circumstances might be dependent on individuals. Discuss what you think determines whether or not individuals are dependent on circumstances or vice versa.

Part 2

Consider this statement:

The voluntary death by which a man puts an end to intolerable suffering is really an act of redemption.

Ernst Heinrich Haeckel
(German biologist)

Write a unified essay in which you perform the following tasks. Explain what you think the above statement means. Describe a specific situation in which the voluntary death by which a person put an end to intolerable suffering would not be an act of redemption. Discuss what you think determines the choice of voluntary death in the face of human suffering.

BIOLOGICAL SCIENCES

10 PROBLEM SETS OF 5–10 QUESTIONS EACH
15 PROBLEMS FOLLOWED BY A SINGLE QUESTION
77 QUESTIONS
100 MINUTES

DIRECTIONS: The following questions or incomplete statements are in groups. Preceding each series of questions or statements is a paragraph or a short explanatory statement, a formula or set of formulas, or a definition. Read the written material and then answer the questions or complete the statements. Select the ONE BEST ANSWER for each question and indicate your selection by marking the corresponding letter of your choice on the Answer Form. Eliminate those alternatives you know to be incorrect and then select an answer from among the remaining alternatives.

Passage I (Questions 143–147)

The function of the thyroid gland is to produce colloidal material containing the thyroid hormones T_3 (triiodothyronine) and T_4 (thyroxin), which affect the rate of metabolism of all tissues.

The iodides consumed by the body are absorbed and carried to the iodide pool in the extracellular fluid via the circulatory system. Five basic events occur during the production of thyroid hormone: (a) trapping iodide; (b) oxidation of iodide to iodine; (c) synthesis of hormone; (d) storage of hormone in the thyroid follicle; and (e) release of hormone into the circulation. TSH (thyroid stimulating hormone) from the anterior pituitary influences the trapping mechanism. It can be stated that thyroid hormone: (a) controls the rate of metabolism; (b) controls growth, maturation, and differentiation of the organism; and (c) influences nervous system activity.

Problems associated with thyroid function are:

1. Cretinism—a congenital failure of proper development. The cretin is a dwarf physically and mentally.
2. Myxedema—an acquired thyroid deficiency in the adult. This deficiency can be due to thyroidectomy, neoplasms, or a pituitary deficiency in TSH secretion.The clinical picture is the presentation of a patient who is fairly heavy, phlegmatic, and devoid of expression; the skin is rough and dry and sensitive to cold. The patient is sluggish mentally and physically. Laboratory tests show a low basal meabolic rate, low protein-bound iodine, and a high serum cholesterol level.
3. Graves' disease—an increased activity of the thyroid gland. The patient exhibits loss of weight, nervousness, irritability, increased metabolic rate, rapid heart rate, and sweating.

A patient is brought into the emergency room and, upon examination, a thyroid goiter is discovered. You suspect that he is suffering from a thyroid disorder, and you ask the intern for a definition of *hypothyroidism*.

143. He responds that *hypothyroidism* is the general term for syndromes that reflect:

A. increased secretion of thyroid hormones.
B. decreased secretion of thyroid hormones.
C. no change in secretion of thyroid hormones.
D. increased secretion of thyroid stimulating hormone releasing factor.

144. A basal metabolism rate test is ordered that measures the rate of oxidative metabolism. In hypothyroidism, this rate is:

A. above normal.
B. normal.
C. below normal.
D. not significant in your diagnosis.

145. Because of the hypothyroidism that you suspect, you would also consider that this patient:

I. has gained weight.
II. converts less food into energy.
III. stores more food as fat.
IV. has an accelerated metabolic rate.

A. I, III, and IV only
B. II, III, and IV only
C. I, II, and III only
D. all of the above

146. The physical examination in this patient would also yield the following:

    A. The patient is mentally sluggish.
    B. The patient's skin is rough and dry.
    C. The patient's serum cholesterol level would be elevated.
    D. All of the above.

147. If hyperthyroidism were the diagnosis you would reason and find:

    A. a pituitary deficiency in TSH.
    B. a block in the oxidation of iodide to iodine.
    C. a phlegmatic patient.
    D. irritability.

Passage II (Questions 148–155)

The ABO blood grouping system is explained on the basis of a single triallelic system with genes A, B, and O operating at a single genetic locus. Phenotypic and genotypic characteristics may be expressed as follows:

Phenotype	Genotype
A	A/A; A/O
B	B/B; B/O
O	O/O
AB	A/B

The A and B genes appear to be codominant; they are dominant over O, which is recessive.

Paternity will be excluded if the child (a) has an antigen that is present in neither the mother nor the putative father, and (b) does not have an antigen that the putative father has and would have had to give to his progeny (e.g., a type O child and a type AB putative father).

Correct reassignment of infants misassigned to parents in a hospital is often achieved by looking for any of the following kinds of incompatibilities between the infants and the couples and then assigning each infant to a couple with which only compatibilities exist:

1. The child has an antigen that is present in neither spouse.
2. The child lacks one or more antigens that either spouse or both spouses would have had to give him/her.

Increased probability of exclusion of alleged paternity or of a correct parental reassignment of misassigned infants results in several kinds of blood groups, HLA, and the following kinds of genetically determined proteins are also included in the studies: hemoglobin, serum proteins, red cell enzymes, and several other enzymes.

The ABO blood group is transmitted in humans as alleles A and B that are codominant, occurring at the same autosomal locus as a recessive allele O. In some cases it may be utilized to assist in determining paternity or in reuniting a lost child with his or her biological parents.

148. A woman of blood type O claims a child of blood type AB, and alleges that the father is a man of blood type B. The most likely explanation is that:

    A. these are the biological parents.
    B. she is the mother but the man is not the father.
    C. neither is a possible parent of the child.
    D. she is not the mother but the man's blood type does not rule him out as the father.

149. If the man in question 148 is found to have previously fathered a child of blood type O, the chance that a child of the man and the woman in this question would be blood type O is:

    A. zero.   C. 33%.
    B. 25%.   D. 50%.

150. With the information from the above question, the chance that any child of the man and woman would be a girl with blood type B is

    A. zero.   C. 33%.
    B. 25%.   D. 50%.

151. The above man with a phenotype B will possess which of the following genotypes?

    A. A/O   C. O/O
    B. B/O   D. A/B

152. Phenotype may be defined as:

    A. genetic makeup of an individual.
    B. hidden traits of an individual.
    C. unrelated characteristics.
    D. visible expression of genotype.

153. Alleles are genes that:

    A. arise during the cross-over process.
    B. are linked to one chromosome only.
    C. are always sex-linked and are transmitted from mothers to their sons.
    D. occupy corresponding positions on homologous chromosomes.

154. Rh-related hemolytic anemia of the newborn (erythroblastosis foetalis) may result when the:

   A. father, mother, and fetus are all Rh negative.

   B. father and mother are Rh positive, but the fetus is Rh negative.

   C. mother is Rh negative and the fetus is Rh positive.

   D. mother is Rh positive and the fetus is Rh negative.

155. The czarina of Russia and Queen Victoria of England were normal women who produced sons suffering from hemophilia, a disease that is caused by a sex-linked recessive gene, h. The more common dominant gene, H, produces normal blood clotting. The genotype of these women must have been:

   A. HH.   **C.** hh.

   B. Hh.   **D.** none of the above.

Passage III (Questions 156–162)

Study of *W* and *F* families showing presence of syncope, electrocardiographic evidence of prolonged Q-T interval and abnormal audiogram. The propositus (Case 1) is III-10 (**arrow**). Case 2 is her cousin (III-2). Figures in parentheses indicate subject's age. Intervals (in hundredths of a second) appear directly below each subject's age. **Black** symbols indicate abnormal audiogram; hatched symbols indicate prolonged QTc interval (0.425 second) (/ / / /) or syncope (\ \ \ \); d = died. A history, physical examination and one or more electrocardiograms were obtained in all patients. An audiogram was obtained in all cases, except those marked by a star, in which hearing was only examined clinically.

Inheritance of Q-T prolongation (≥ 0.425 sec) and cardiac arrhythmias in the W. and F. families is shown in the above pedigree, which was ascertained through the proposita, III-10, who suffered cardiac arrest and had to be resuscitated 12 hours after her first delivery following an uneventful pregnancy. A major objective of the study was the determination of whether prolonged Q-T interval in these families was (1) the autosomal recessive form, Jervell, Lang-Nielsen syndrome, also characterized by high-frequency perceptive deafness, (2) Ward-Romano syndrome, an autosomal dominant form, not associated with deafness, or (3) perhaps a third type, inherited in some other fashion.*

---

*Adapted by Dr. J. I. Townsend, Virginia Commonwealth University, from "Q-T Prolongation and Ventricular Arrhythmias With and Without Deafness in the Same Family;" E.C. Mathews, A. W. Blount, and J.I. Townsend. *The American Journal of Cardiology*, (1972): 29:702.

156. Prolonged Q-T interval and cardiac arrhythmias appear to be phenotypic manifestations of the same allele, a phenomenon known as:

   A. genetic heterogeneity.

   B. genetic polymorphism.

   C. pleiotropism.

   D. phenocopies.

157. The pedigree clearly shows that the arrhythmias in the W. family are dominant because they:

   A. affect both monozygotic twins in the third generation.

   B. are sometimes associated with deafness.

   C. show unbroken lineal descent.

   D. are transmitted by both sexes.

158. Likewise, the pedigree clearly shows that deafness in the W. family is also dominant, but the arrhythmias are the result of an allele at a different locus because:

- **A.** nondisjunction occurs among the progeny of couple II- I @ 2.
- **B.** disjunction occurs among the progeny of couple II-1 @ 2.
- **C.** independent assortment occurs among the children of couple II-1 @ 2.
- **D.** meiotic drive occurs among the children of couple II-1 @ 2.

159. Careful comparative diagnostic studies of prolonged Q-T interval and cardiac arrhythmias in the W. and F. families show the syndrome to be identical in both families, yet in the F. family this dominant trait skips a generation (II-11). This skipping is a phenomenon known as:

- **A.** reduced penetrance.
- **B.** unequal crossing over.
- **C.** transversion.
- **D.** variable expressivity.

160. That prolonged Q-T interval and the arrhythmias are autosomal is shown by:

- **A.** female to male transmission in both families.
- **B.** male to male transmission in the F. family.
- **C.** lack of male to male transmission.
- **D.** male to female transmission.

161. That deafness is autosomal is shown by:

- **A.** male to male transmission.
- **B.** lack of male to male transmission.
- **C.** two affected males (II-3 and II-5) have daughters whose hearing is normal.
- **D.** an affected female (II-2) has a daughter whose hearing is normal.

162. The proposita (III-10) has by far the greatest prolonged Q-T interval (0:570 sec) in this extended pedigree. The likely explanation is that she:

- **A.** is an example of genetic anticipation.
- **B.** has a deletion of the locus on one chromosome.
- **C.** has a duplication of the locus on one chromosome.
- **D.** is homozygous for the mutant allele.

Passage IV (Questions 163–169)

Oogenesis in oviparous vertebrates (such as amphibians) is accompanied by extensive transcription. RNA is synthesized in the oocyte nucleus and subsequently processed. The resultant mRNAs, tRNAs, and ribosomes (containing rRNAs) then accumulate in the oocyte cytoplasm. Most of these RNAs (referred to as oogenetic or maternal RNAs) and ribosomes do not function in translation until after embryonic development has been initiated. Although protein synthesis is detectable in the zygote prior to the beginning of cleavage, RNA synthesis is not detected in embryonic cells until later in development (as seen in the figure below). The RNA synthesized in embryonic cells is collectively referred to as embryonic RNA.

Transcriptional inhibitors, such as the antibiotic actinomycin D, are useful tools for studying patterns of RNA synthesis in development. When cells are treated with actinomycin D, actinomycin D binds to the guanine residues of DNA and blocks the subsequent synthesis of all types of RNA, without affecting DNA synthesis and cell division. Previously synthesized and processed RNAs are not affected by such inhibitors. The relative importance of oogenetic and embryonic RNAs in protein synthesis in embryos can be determined by blocking the synthesis of postfertilization RNA synthesis with a transcriptional inhibitor. When early cleavage stage amphibian embryos are exposed to a transcriptional inhibitor, development and protein synthesis continue until the blastula stage at which point development arrests.

Relative Rate of mRNA (▲), tRNA (■) and rRNA (●) synthesis in developing embryos

163. Radiolabelled molecules are commonly used to monitor the amount and/or rate of synthetic processes in cells. A commonly employed radiolabel is tritum, H3. Which of the following tritiated molecules would be the most appropriate one for specifically monitoring RNA synthesis in amphibian embryos?

A. H3-adenine
B. H3-guanine
C. H3-thymidine
D. H3-uridine

164. Embryonic mRNA synthesis begins to be detected in amphibian embryos:

A. at the blastula stage.
B. during early cleavage.
C. at the gastrula stage.
D. during oogenesis.

165. An amphibian embryo at the gastrula stage would be actively synthesizing:

A. rRNA.
B. tRNA and rRNA.
C. mRNA and rRNA.
D. mRNA, tRNA, and rRNA.

166. Based on studies with actinomycin D, the development of amphibian embryos to the blastula stage is dependent on:

A. proteins synthesized using maternal mRNAs.
B. proteins synthesized using embryonic mRNAs.
C. the synthesis of mRNAs by embryonic cells.
D. the synthesis of tRNAs and rRNAs by embryonic cells.

167. Although actinomycin D treated embryos remain viable for a period of time and some protein synthesis can be detected in actinomycin D treated embryos, the embryos will not develop past the blastula stage. Which of the following would be the best explanation for the inability of the embryos to continue development?

A. In order to continue development the embryos need to synthesize more embryonic rRNAs and tRNAs.
B. In order to continue development the embryos need to synthesize more embryonic mRNAs and rRNAs.

C. In order to continue development the embryos need to synthesize more proteins using maternal mRNAs.
D. In order to continue development the embryos need to synthesize proteins using embryonic mRNAs.

168. Extensive stockpiling of developmentally important macromolecules (such as RNAs) prior to the initiation of development often shortens the time required for early developmental processes such as cleavage. In comparison to an organism with a similar body complexity, but which accumulated no maternal RNA in its eggs during oogenesis, the cleavage period in amphibians should be:

A. similar.
B. much longer.
C. slightly longer.
D. shorter.

169. In contrast to the situation in amphibians, only a small amount of RNA synthesis occurs during oogenesis in viviparous vertebrates (such as mammals) and the mammalian oocyte contains a minimal amount of oogenetic RNA. Synthesis of embryonic RNAs and ribosomes begins during the early cleavage stages. Therefore if mouse zygotes were exposed to a transcriptional inhibitor, development would probably arrest:

A. at the blastocyst stage.
B. at the blastula stage.
C. at the gastrula stage.
D. during the cleavage stage.

Passage V (Questions 170–176)

Blood is a fluid tissue consisting of numerous components such as red blood cells (RBCs), white blood cells, platelets, proteins and more. The cellular components comprise about 45% of whole blood, the remaining 55% is plasma.

One of the primary functions of blood is transport. Examples include nutrients, metabolic wastes, hormones, carbon dioxide, and oxygen. RBCs play a major role in transport of CO_2 and O_2. The following questions center around the RBC.

170. All of the following are characteristics of an erythrocyte, EXCEPT:

A. contains a substance composed of four proteins and a prosthetic group.
B. biconcave disc shape.
C. made in the bone marrow of adults.
D. has a nucleus and cytoplasmic organelles.

171. Sometimes called the "graveyard" of the erythrocyte, the liver and spleen contain _____, which recognize and phagocytize red blood cells at the end of their approximate 120-day life span.

A. mast cells
B. platelets
C. macrophages
D. adipocytes

172. Sometimes referred to as a microscopist's "measuring stick," an erythrocyte is abundant in most tissues and can be utilized for size comparison in a viewing field. The approximate diameter of an RBC is:

A. 7 mm.
B. 7 μm.
C. 0.7 nm.
D. 70 nm.

173. An experimenter placed some red blood cells in a hypotonic medium. What happened to the RBCs?

A. The cells swelled and burst.
B. The cells were unaffected.
C. The cells shrunk.
D. None of the above.

174. The most numerous leukocytes are the:

A. lymphocytes.
B. monocytes.
C. eosinophils.
D. neutrophils.

175. Among the defense mechanisms available to humans to ward off their destruction by the environment is (are):

I. skin.
II. white blood corpuscles.
III. antibodies.
IV. sebaceous secretions.

A. III only
B. II only
C. II and III only
D. I, II, III, and IV

176. Blood pH is influenced by respiration; experimental hyperventilation in a physiology laboratory will result in the student's blood pH being:

A. lowered.
B. raised.
C. unaffected.
D. raised to pH6.

Passage VI (Questions 177–181)

Above is a diagram of a typical capillary with a left to right blood flow as indicated. The arrows show the direction of fluid flow into and out of the capillary. On the left-hand side of the capillary, the fluid flow is from the capillary to the interstitial space. On the right side, the fluid flow is from the interstitium to the capillary. Thus, there is a constant recirculation of the interstitial fluid.

In most cases, the fluid flow from the capillary to the interstitium and back again are closely balanced. The small excess of fluid remaining in the interstitium is eventually removed by the lymphatics. The net transport of fluid (Q) in the direction of the interstitium is governed by Starling's law

$$Q = K[(P_{cap} - P_i) - (\pi_{cap} - \pi_i)]$$

where P_{cap} and P_i are the hydrostatic pressures in the capillary and the interstitium respectively. The wall of the capillary acts as a permselective membrane, therefore osmotic pressures, π_{cap} and π_I, exist on the capillary and interstitial sides respectively and contribute to the driving force for fluid movement. K is the constant of proportionality relating the driving force to fluid flow and is known as the hydraulic conductivity of the capillary.

Choose the *one best* answer.

177. A patient develops a venous blood clot in one leg which blocks return of blood. What would you predict would happen to the net fluid flow in the capillaries?

A. Fluid flow in the direction of the interstitium increases.
B. Fluid flow in the direction of the interstitium decreases.
C. Fluid flow in the direction of the interstitium is unchanged.
D. The capillary osmotic pressure will increase.

178. A patient with protein malnutrition has a lower concentration of protein in his blood. (The reflection coefficient (σ) of proteins is close to 1.) With all other things constant:

A. the hydrostatic pressure difference between the capillary and the interstitium will increase.
B. the fluid volume in the interstitium will decrease.
C. the net fluid flow will be in the direction of the interstitium.
D. the fluid volume in the interstitium stays constant.

179. An elastic bandage applied to the skin will result in:

A. a larger hydrostatic pressure difference.
B. an increased interstitial volume.
C. an increase in flow into the capillary.
D. an increased oncotic pressure difference.

180. Assuming a steady state, an infusion of urea (a nonpolar solute with a reflection coefficient of 0) results in:

A. an increase in the osmotic pressure difference.
B. an increased flow into the capillary.
C. a decrease in the interstitial volume.
D. no change in the interstitial volume.

181. The process by which a cell can move a substance from a point of lower concentration to a point of higher concentration (against the diffusion gradient) is called:

A. osmosis.   C. turgor pressure.
B. plasmolysis. D. active transport.

Passage VII (Questions 182–186)

The following relates to questions 182 and 183:

For air to flow into the lungs, alveolar gas pressure must be less than atmospheric pressure. This pressure difference can be produced in two ways. The first is by *positive pressure breathing*, as is the case when using a resuscitator. Here the pressure at the nose and mouth (the atmospheric pressure) is made greater than the alveolar gas pressure. The second method is by *negative pressure breathing*, as is the case when using the iron lung. Here alveolar gas pressure is lowered below atmospheric pressure.

Normal breathing is a form of negative pressure breathing. If intra-alveolar pressure (also called intrapulmonary pressure) is plotted while breathing, we see that during inspiration the enlarging thorax and lungs expand

the alveolar gas and its pressure transiently drops below atmospheric pressure (i.e., it becomes negative). This pressure difference causes air to flow into the lungs. Expiration involves transiently elevating the intra-alveolar pressure above atmospheric pressure. This occurs as the collapsing chest-lung system compresses the alveolar gas. Gas then flows out of the lungs.

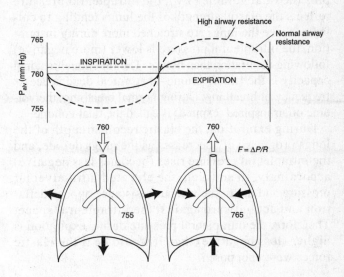

Air flow is directly proportional to the pressure difference between alveolar gas and the atmosphere, and inversely proportional to airway resistance:

$$Flow\ (F) = \frac{P_{atm} - P_{alv}}{\text{Airway Resistance (R)}}$$

Thus, the greater the airway resistance, the greater the pressure difference required to produce any given flow. High airway resistance will produce greater fluctuations in intra-alveolar pressure during inspiration and expiration.

The severity of airway resistance is reflected in the *intrapleural pressure* as well as the intra-alveolar pressure during the breathing cycle. Before inspiration begins, the intrapleural pressure reflects the elastic strength with which the lungs are tending to collapse. Of course, at this volume (the FRC) the elastic force of the lungs is balanced by the elastic strength of the chest wall tending to expand. The intrapleural pressure is slightly negative (i.e., below atmospheric pressure).

During inspiration, the elastic recoil strength of the lungs progressively increases as the lungs are stretched. This alone would lower the intrapleural pressure (i.e., make it more negative). In addition, the lowered intra-alveolar pressure (reflecting airway resistance during inspiration) and tissue viscous resistance (which opposes the inflation effort) lower the intrapleural pressure even more. Thus, during inspiration the intrapleural pressure becomes even lower (more negative) than it would if the elastic forces existed alone. Of this additional decrease in intrapleural pressure from nonelastic resistances, 80% is due to pressure needed to overcome airway resistance; tissue viscous resistance accounts for only 20% of the nonelastic resistance.

At the end of inspiration, flow stops as intra-alveolar pressure equilibrates with atmospheric pressure. At this volume (FRC + TV), functional residual capacity (FRC) plus the tidal volume (TV), the intrapleural pressure reflects the elastic strength of the lungs tending to collapse. Since the lungs are stretched more during inspiration, the intrapleural pressure is lower (more negative) following inspiration than before. The functional residual capacity is the (tidal volume–anatomical dead space) × frequency of breathing. During normal breathing, the volume of air inspired (expired) is called the tidal volume.

During expiration, the elastic recoil strength of the lungs progressively decreases as the lungs deflate, and the intrapleural pressure rises (becomes less negative) accordingly. In addition, the elevated intra-alveolar pressure and the tissue viscous resistance oppose deflation and act outward against the intrapleural space. Therefore, the intrapleural pressure during expiration is higher (less negative) than it would be if the elastic forces were unopposed.

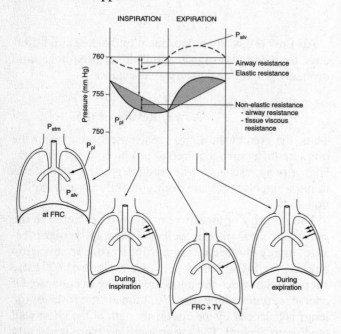

The following relates to question 184:

With a tidal volume of 500 ml, only 350 ml goes to the respiratory unit and 150 ml goes no further than the anatomic dead space. Most of the 350 ml that reaches the alveoli is involved in gas exchange, but some is a *"wasted volume"*—meaning it is a volume in excess of that needed to equilibrate with the blood passing through the capillaries of that area. A wasted volume occurs to some extent even in a healthy individual and will be produced when there is an elevated ventilation-perfusion ratio. An elevated ventilation-perfusion ratio

occurs when either the blood flow is reduced or ventilation is in excess of that needed to equilibrate the volume of blood perfusing the area. Alveolar gas in an area with a high ventilation-perfusion ratio will exhibit increased oxygen and decreased carbon dioxide concentrations because of the excess oxygen delivery and carbon dioxide removal. The wasted volume plus the anatomic dead space equals the *physiologic dead space.* Even in a healthy individual the physiologic dead space is slightly larger than the anatomic dead space.

Alveolar ventilation refers to the volume of fresh air, which reaches the respiratory unit per minute and is equal to the rate of breathing times the volume of fresh air reaching the respiratory unit per breath (i.e., the tidal volume minus the anatomic dead space). *Dead space ventilation* is the volume of fresh air, which goes no further than the anatomic dead space per minute. Alveolar ventilation plus dead space ventilation equals the respiratory minute ventilation.

Alveolar ventilation $= (TV - ADS) \times$ Frequency

$$= (500 - 150) \text{ ml} \times 12$$
breaths/min $= 4.2$ L/min

Dead space ventilation $= ADS \times$ Frequency

$$= 150 \text{ ml} \times 12 \text{ breaths/min} = 1.8$$
L/min

The following relates to question 185:

The composition of alveolar air, reflecting the oxygen uptake by blood and carbon dioxide release from blood, has a lower PO_2 (100 mm Hg) and a higher PCO_2 (40 mm Hg) than that of atmospheric or moist tracheal air. Both alveolar air and atmospheric air have the same total pressures, since these compartments are connected by open tubes of the anatomic dead space.

Alveolar air is typically represented as having a constant composition. This is justified because the fluctuations which occur in PO_2 and PCO_2 with each breathing cycle are very slight. Because the volume of fresh air entering the alveoli (350 ml) is very small compared with the "pool" of alveolar air already in the lungs (FRC = 2,200 ml), the inspired fresh air is so diluted that the PO_2 will increase and the PCO_2 will decrease by only 1 or 2 mm Hg.

Assuming a constant oxygen uptake and carbon dioxide release by the body, the content of alveolar air will reflect the ventilatory rate of the lungs. Hyperventilation makes alveolar air more like fresh air, raising alveolar PO_2 and lowering PCO_2. Hypoventilation, in contrast, produces a lower PO_2 and an elevated PCO_2 in the alveoli. Similarly, not all areas of the lung have the same PO_2 and PCO_2. While some areas are relatively hyperventilated and have a high PO_2 and low PCO_2, other areas are simultaneously hypoventilated and have a low PO_2 and high PCO_2.

The following relates to question 186:

The transportation of carbon dioxide in blood occurs by three mechanisms. It can be transported (1) in physical solution, (2) bound to amino groups of either hemoglobin or plasma proteins, or (3) converted to bicarbonate ions via its interaction with water. Carbon dioxide is transported in physical solution in both plasma and red blood cells. The amount of carbon dioxide carried as carbamino compounds in plasma is typically much less than the amount carried in red blood cells as carbamino hemoglobin. Most of the carbon dioxide is transported in the form of bicarbonate ions.

Carbon monoxide has a very high affinity (200–300 times that of O_2) for hemoglobin. It competes with oxygen for the same site on the hemoglobin molecule. With carbon monoxide bound to hemoglobin (carboxyhemoglobin) the blood's oxygen-carrying capacity is reduced, but this has no relationship to carbon dioxide transport.

182. The driving pressure (ΔP) in breathing which causes air to flow into the lungs is:

    A. atmospheric pressure (P_{atm}).
    B. the intra-alveolar (intrapulmonary) pressure (P_{alv}).
    C. atmospheric pressure minus the intra-alveolar pressure.
    D. the intrapleural pressure (P_{pl}).

183. During inspiration, intra-alveolar pressure (P_{alv}):

    A. transiently goes below atmospheric pressure (P_{atm}).
    B. transiently goes above atmospheric pressure.
    C. equals atmospheric pressure.
    D. equals intrapleural pressure.

184. The alveolar ventilation per minute refers to the amount of fresh air that reaches the alveoli of the lungs per minute. Alveolar ventilation per minute equals the:

    A. functional residual capacity × frequency of breathing.
    B. physiologic dead space × frequency of breathing.

    C. anatomic dead space × frequency of breathing.
    D. (tidal volume – anatomic dead space) × frequency of breathing.

185. Hypoventilation produces which of the following changes in alveolar gas composition?

    A. The partial pressure of oxygen increases and the partial pressure of carbon dioxide decreases.
    B. The partial pressures of both oxygen and carbon dioxide increase.
    C. The partial pressure of oxygen decreases and the partial pressure of carbon dioxide increases.
    D. The partial pressures of both oxygen and carbon dioxide decrease.

186. Carbon dioxide is transported in the blood in all of the following forms, EXCEPT:

    A. carboxyhemoglobin.
    B. dissolved carbon dioxide.
    C. bicarbonate ions.
    D. carbamino-compounds.

Passage VIII (Questions 187–191)

When a liquid is at equilibrium with the atmosphere, the contribution of its gaseous phase to the total atmospheric pressure is known as the vapor pressure for that substance. The phase transition of a liquid to a gas occurs when the kinetic energies of the molecules in the liquid phase are sufficient to overcome the attractive forces between molecules. Since the distribution of kinetic energies increases as a linear function of temperature, the rate at which gas molecules leave the gas-liquid interface also increases with temperature. The pressure exerted by escaping molecules is opposed by collision with molecules of atmospheric gases, hindering their escape if their vapor pressure is less than that of the surrounding atmosphere. In nonpolar liquids, intermolecular forces tend to increase with increasing molecular mass owing to relatively weak hydrophobic or Van der Waal's interactions. However, the intermolecular attractive forces are much greater in liquids with polar molecules, such as water and ethanol, than in relatively nonpolar liquids such as chloroform. The relatively polarity of these liquids affects their solvent capacity as well as physical properties such as melting point, boiling point, and vapor pressure. As seen in the accompanying graph, polarity is the primary determinant of vapor pressure over a range of temperatures for a series of liquids increasing in polarity while decreasing in molecular weight.

187. Compared to the vapor pressures of chloroform and water, the vapor pressure of ethyl alcohol is:

A. constant.
B. greater than either.
C. greater than that of chloroform, but less than that of water.
D. less than that of chloroform, but greater than that of water.

188. In degrees Celsius, the normal boiling point of chloroform is approximately:

A. 61.   C. 100.
B. 78.   D. 760.

189. The graph indicates that standard atmospheric pressure, in millimeters of mercury (Hg), is:

A. between 0 and 100.
B. less than 760.
C. 100.
D. 760.

190. At the top of a mountain where atmospheric pressure is less than standard atmospheric pressure, the boiling point of water is:

A. less than its normal boiling point.
B. more than its normal boiling point.
C. the same as that of chloroform and that of ethyl alcohol.
D. the same as that of chloroform.

191. At what atmospheric pressure would the boiling point of water equal the normal boiling point of ethyl alcohol?

A. 100   C. 500
B. 300   D. 700

Passage IX (Questions 192–196)

Toluene or methylbenzene is an important starting material for the synthesis of many aromatic compounds. The methyl group activates all unsubstituted carbons of the benzene ring for attack by electrophilic reagents, leading to substitution at one or more additional carbons. The *ortho, meta,* and *para* positions are substituted at different rates, depending on the capacity of the electron-donating methyl group to stabilize positively charged intermediates generated by the electrophilic attack. Unlike larger alkyl groups, the methyl group is too small to have a significant steric effect on the rate of substitution at the *ortho* position. Under appropriate conditions, the methyl group itself is often modified or derivatized, in which case, subsequent substitutions in the ring will be directed by the character of the modified group. Many different substituted products and positional isomers can be produced by manipulating reagents, reaction conditions, and the order of the various reactions. The *ortho, meta,* and *para* isomers usually differ sufficiently in properties to permit separation by standard physical methods. In any of the reactions of toluene, assume that ortho and para isomers can be separated.

192. The reaction of toluene with Br_2 in the presence of $FeBr_3$ would be expected to produce primarily:

A. benzyl bromide, $C_6H_5CH_2Br$.
B. *m*-bromotoluene.
C. *o* and *p*-bromotoluene.
D. an equimolar mixture of *m, o,* and *p*-bromotoluene.

193. The compound that undergoes electrophilic aromatic substitution more readily than toluene is:

A. chlorobenzene.   C. acetophenone.
B. nitrobenzene.   D. phenol.

194. The best sequence of reagents for conversion of toluene to *m*-nitrobenzoic acid is:

A. HNO_3-H_2SO_4, then oxidation with hot $KMnO_4$ or $K_2Cr_2O_7$.
B. Oxidation with hot $KMnO_4$ or $K_2Cr_2O_7$, followed by HNO_3-H_2SO_4.
C. Bromination of toluene with Br_2-$FeBr_3$, followed by displacement with $NaNO_2$.
D. Reaction of toluene with Br_2-$FeBr_3$, followed by oxidation with $KMnO_4$, or $K2Cr_2O_7$, and then displacement of Br by $NaNO_2$.

195. The major product of the reaction of *p*-nitro-toluene with Br_2-$FeBr_3$ is:

 A. 2-bromo-4-nitrotoluene.
 B. 3-bromo-4-nitrotoluene.
 C. *p*-nitrobenzyl bromide, *p*-$NO_2C_6H_4CH_2Br$.
 D. 2, 6-dibromo-4-nitrotoluene.

196. Which of the following resonance structures is a contributor to the intermediate formed in the nitration of toluene to form *p*-nitrotoluene?

 A. C.

 B. D.

Passage X (Questions 197–204)

The categories of necessary dietary nutrients include the essential amino acids, essential fatty acids, essential elements, and the vitamins. The nine essential amino acids for humans are found in all dietary proteins. They are called: phenylalanine, valine, threonine, tryptophan, isoleucine, methionine, histidine, leucine, and lysine. All other amino acids that are found in proteins are nonessential and can be synthesized in the body from other dietary sources. The one true essential fatty acid is linoleic. However, linoleic and arachidonic acids can help meet the nutritional requirement for this category of nutrients. Because generally all of these essential fatty acids are found in combinations of oils and fats, all three can be viewed as "essential" in a practical sense. Along with carbohydrates, we obtain both essential amino acid and fatty acids from the macronutrients (i.e., large quantities) of protein and fat respectively in our diet.

The essential elements are subcategorized as the electrolytes sodium, potassium, and chloride; the bulk essential minerals—calcium, phosphorus, and magnesium and the trace essential minerals—iron, zinc, selenium, iodine, cobalt, molybdenum, manganese, copper, chromium, and fluoride. All of these are needed, but the amount we need each day varies from micrograms to hundreds of milligrams. Vitamins are found in foods in water soluble or fat soluble forms. The former includes vitamin C, thiamine, riboflavin, niacin, vitamin B_6, folacin, vitamin B_{12}, biotin, and pantothenic acid. The fat soluble vitamins are vitamins A, D, E, and K. These are all required in the diet in trace amounts (i.e., micrograms to milligrams).

Choose the *one best* answer for each of the following:

197. Which of the following is *not* an essential nutrient?

 A. valine   C. glucose
 B. linoleic acid   D. vitamin E

198. Which of the following is *not* a vitamin?

 A. thiamine   C. niacin
 B. biotin   D. arachidonic acid

199. Which of the following is *not* a fat soluble vitamin?

 A. vitamin A   C. vitamin D
 B. vitamin B_{12} D. vitamin E

200. Which of the following is a bulk essential element?

 A. selenium   C. iron
 B. copper   D. calcium

201. A macronutrient is:

 I.   a carbohydrate.
 II. a protein.
 III a fat.
 IV. a vitamin.

 A. I only   C. I, II, and III
 B. II only   D. I, II, III, and IV

202. Regulation of the resorption of calcium from bone is controlled by the:

 A. thyroid gland.
 B. parathyroid glands.
 C. thymus.
 D. adrenal glands.

203. Undigested food is eliminated from the body by the process of:

 A. exocytosis.   C. egestion.
 B. excretion.   D. catabolism.

204. The energy released from the anaerobic respiration of a glucose molecule is less than that released from the aerobic respiration of a glucose molecule because:

 A. aerobic respiration forms many more new, strong bonds than anaerobic respiration.

B. more enzymes are required for anaerobic respiration than for aerobic respiration.

C. anaerobic respiration occurs 24 hours a day, while aerobic respiration can occur only at night.

D. anaerobic respiration requires oxygen but aerobic respiration does not require oxygen.

DIRECTIONS: Read each passage carefully, study each table, chart, or formula, then answer the question following it. Eliminate those choices that you think to be incorrect and mark the letter of your choice on the answer sheet.

Blood samples from two groups of rats were assayed for luteinizing hormone (LH) in two separate radioimmunoassays. Half the rats were intact and half were orchidectomized. Some samples in each group were collected in the morning and some were collected in the afternoon. The data are summarized in the following table:

Assay I

	Intact or Orchid X	Sampled AM or PM	LH ng/ml
1	I	AM	5.0
2	O	AM	50
3	I	PM	4.8
4	O	PM	480
5	I	AM	5.2
6	O	AM	52
7	I	PM	5.1
8	O	PM	350
9	I	AM	4.9
10	O	AM	100

Assay 2

11	I	PM	7.5
12	O	PM	75
13	I	AM	7.7
14	O	AM	770
15	I	PM	7.3
16	O	PM	250
17	I	AM	7.4
18	O	AM	100
19	I	PM	7.6
20	O	PM	640

205. Based on the above table, which of the following statements is *not supported by* the information given?

    A. Orchidectomy is followed by increased levels of LH in the blood.

    B. Blood LH levels are higher in the afternoon than in the morning.

C. The differences between LH values in these two assays are probably explained by interassay variations because the ratios between intact and orchidectomized levels are similar.

D. LH release in the orchidectomized rats may be occurring episodically.

Ovulation in the rat can be blocked by systemic administration of drugs which depress neural function. However, ovulation depends on the response of the ovaries to LH released from the pituitary gland. In the following experiment, drug X was injected subcutaneously at 13:45 hours into several groups of rats and the presence or absence of ova in the oviduct determined on the following morning. In order to pinpoint the site of action of the drug, attempts were made to restore ovulation by stimulation of the brain; injection of LRF, the hypothalamic hormone which causes pituitary LH release; and injection of LH, which induces ovulation. The results are summarized below.

Treatment	Number of Rats Treated	Number of Rats Ovulating
Drug X	10	1
Drug X + LRF	10	5
Drug X + LH	10	5
Drug X + Brain Stimulation	10	1

206. The following statements are related to the above table. Select the statement *supported by* the information given.

    A. The ovaries are responsible for the production of LH.

    B. Drug X may be blocking the release of LRF from the brain and thereby preventing the activation of pituitary LH release.

    C. Drug X may be preventing pituitary LH release in response to LRF.

    D. The effect of Drug X on the brain is greater than its effect on the ovary.

Country	Crude Birth Rate Per Thousand/Year	Crude Death Rate Per Thousand/Year
Lebanon	54	26
Egypt	50	26
India	50	25
Pakistan	49	26
USSR	43	18
East Germany	18	10

West Germany	16	16
France	35	11
Spain	19	7
Holland	45	8
Luxemburg	17	11.8
Japan	15	13

207. Which of the countries in the table shows the most rapid population growth?

A. Spain   **C.** USSR
B. Holland   **D.** Lebanon

Female albino rats weighing between 170 and 230 g were housed in pairs in wire bottom cages and received a standard diet of rat pellets and chlorinated water *ad libitum.* Unanesthetized rats were restrained and shielded with lead so that only the head and neck regions were exposed. The animals received 6400 R of X-radiation in a single dose. Following irradiation, careful check was maintained on the water and food consumption. Also, at varying intervals after exposure the animals were killed and the wet weights of their parotid salivary glands were determined. The results of these follow-ups are depicted below:

Legend:
- ●●●●● Food consumption
- – – – Water consumption
- -●-● Gland wet weight

208. Which of the following statements is true concerning the data obtained from this experiment?

A. The animals continued to consume large quantities of water up to the time of death.
B. An alteration in food consumption was already evident at 3 days after radiation.
C. Even though drinking and eating declined, the weights of the salivary glands remained unaffected until time of death.
D. Water consumption and wet weight of the glands first began to vary from control values at 8 days.

Levels of estrogens in the urine of the human female during the menstrual cycle, pregnancy, and the post-menopausal period were obtained from women during some routine work-ups during their visits to the ob-gyn clinic. The following data were obtained.

Time	Estriol μg/24 h	Estrone μg/24 h	Estradiol μg/24 h
Onset of menstruation	9	7	3
Ovulation peak	30	24	10
Luteal peak	20	18	9
Pregnancy, 150 days	10	1	.5
Pregnancy, term	35	4	2
Postmenopause	2	2	1

209. The second rise in all probability reflects an increased secretion of estrogens by the theca lutein cells of the corpus luteum.

A. This is a good assumption.
B. This is a bad assumption.
C. This is proven by the data.
D. There are no data available at all to make such an assumption.

Twenty male New Zealand albino rabbits were divided into four groups of 5 animals each and treated as follows:

Group 1: Received a subcutaneous injection of $10 \times 10^{\times 6}$ sheep red blood cells at two week intervals for a total of three injections.
Group 2: Received an intradermal injection of $10 \times 10^{\times 6}$ sheep red blood cells at two week intervals for a total of three injections.
Group 3: Received a subscapular injection of $10 \times 10^{\times 6}$ sheep red blood cells at two week intervals for a total of three injections.
Group 4: Received an intravenous injection of $10 \times 10^{\times 6}$ sheep red blood cells at two week intervals for a total of three injections.

During the six week immunization period antibody titers against sheep red blood cells were measured and the following results obtained:

Subscapular   Intravenous

210. These data show that:

  A. there is little difference in the results produced by the various routes of administration.

  B. there is little difference between subscapular and subcutaneous injection routes.

  C. the animals receiving intravenous red blood cells were immunologically incompetent.

  D. antigen clearance was most rapid in the animals receiving intradermal injections.

An experimental drug, S24953, may maintain hepatic fatty acid oxidation at a normal rate in ethanol-treated rats. The following groups were studied at 8, 16, and 32 hours after administration of ethyl alcohol and glucose. Biochemically speaking, a fatty liver is the end result of ethanol consumption.

211. Based on the above data, select the statement(s) *supported by* the information given.

  A. The experimental data point to a nearly complete prevention of ethanol-induced fatty liver by S24953.

  B. The peak of the ethanol-induced fatty liver was observed around 16 hours after consumption.

  C. Ethanol caused a 300% increase in the concentration of liver triglycerides.

  D. All of the above are supported.

A blood sample was taken from a test subject. Then a masked man came in with a gun and appeared to murder 2 persons. The test subject was visibly upset. After 30 seconds, the "victims" stood up. The subject was told of the hoax, and blood samples were taken over a period of time for counting red blood cells (RBC).

Time	RBC/mm^3 of Blood
Control (before "murder")	5.5 million
30 seconds after "murder"	5.9 million
6.5 minutes after "murder"	7.0 million
14.5 minutes after "murder"	5.6 million
18.5 minutes after "murder"	5.5 million

212. Based on the above table, select the statement *supported by* the information given.

  A. There was an increase in the RBC/mm^3 of blood of the test subject a few minutes after he thought he witnessed murder.

  B. A larger change in the RBC/mm^3 of blood would have been noted if the test subject had been placed in greater fear for his own life.

  C. Having changed from the control value, there was no return to the control value for nearly 20 minutes.

  D. Although a return of RBC/mm^3 of blood to control value was noted, a rebound would be expected within an hour after the end of the experiment.

Production of organic compounds by photosynthesis was studied in Puerto Rico. The results are given in the table below with the theoretical yield based on percentage of light captured by the plant.

	Carbohydrate Production (tons/acre)		Percentage of Sunlight
Plants	Present	Theoretical	Captured by Plant
Kelp	2.0	14	15
Cane	0.7	0.9	1.0
Plant Z	4.1	18	20

213. Within wide limits, the rate of carbohydrate production varies linearly with the incident light. If one doubled the incident light on an acre of cultivated kelp, how would the yield of kelp compare with the yield of an acre of plant Z on which the incident light was unchanged?

  A. It would surpass the carbohydrate yield per acre.

B. It would approach the carbohydrate yield per acre.

C. It would surpass the protein yield per acre.

D. It would surpass the percentage of incident light captured.

MIDDLE INCOME PEOPLE

Mean Units of Major Food Categories Consumed Per Day

Samples	Starchy Foods	Meaty Foods	Liquids
1	79	6.6	8
2	38	27	12
3	9	26	40

	Incidence of Types of Tooth Decay (percent of sample)			Type of Toothpaste Used (grams/ brushing)	
Samples	I	II	III	I	II
1	69	61	7	23	27
2	35	31	7	6	7
3	9	5	1	2	3

214. Based on the above table, select the statement *supported by* the information given.

A. Considering the group classified as starch eaters, there does not seem a noticeable difference between the types of tooth decay and the sample of population.

B. The average diet consumed results in less tooth decay.

C. Reduced toothpaste use caused a reduction in all three types of cavities.

D. Sample 3 exhibited less tooth decay.

Ten adult male guinea pigs were housed in individual cages in a room at 37°C. Five of the guinea pigs were fed an ascorbic acid deficient diet while the other five were fed standard guinea pig diet. Both groups were allowed access to water *ad libitum*. At weekly intervals the serum concentration of gamma globulin and lymphocyte reactivity were measured in both the experimental and control groups. The following graphs illustrate data collected from this experiment.

Concentration of Gamma Globulin

Lymphocyte Reactivity

215. A conclusion that can be reached from these data is:

A. there are no sex differences in the response of guinea pigs to an ascorbic acid deficient diet.

B. temperature has a marked effect on gamma globulin concentration.

C. lymphocyte reactivity in the scorbutic guinea pig is independent of gamma globulin concentration.

D. gamma globulin concentration varies inversely with lymphocyte reactivity.

216. Which hydrocarbon is a member of the series with the general formula C_nH_{2n-2}?

A. butane   **C.** benzene
B. ethene   **D.** ethyne

217. Which class of compounds has the general formula R–O–R'?

A. esters   **C.** ethers
B. alcohols   **D.** aldehydes

218. Of the functional groups listed below, which is incorrectly identified?

A. $-NH_2$ amino group

B. $-\overset{\|}{\underset{O}{C}}-CH_3$ acetyl group

C. $-\overset{\|}{\underset{O}{C}}-NH_2$ amide group

D. $-\overset{\|}{\underset{O}{C}}-OH$ hydroxyl group

219. An individual has at his disposal benzyl chloride, benzene, aluminum chloride, and sodium, and he wishes to synthesize diphenylmethane. He should react:

A. all four compounds.

B. benzyl chloride and sodium.

C. benzyl chloride, benzene, and aluminum chloride.

D. benzyl chloride, benzene, and sodium.

Model Examination A Answer Key

Verbal Reasoning

1.	C	14.	B	27.	D	40.	D	53.	A
2.	D	15.	A	28.	C	41.	D	54.	B
3.	A	16.	B	29.	D	42.	B	55.	A
4.	D	17.	D	30.	D	43.	D	56.	B
5.	D	18.	D	31.	D	44.	C	57.	D
6.	B	19.	B	32.	B	45.	D	58.	D
7.	B	20.	D	33.	D	46.	B	59.	D
8.	A	21.	D	34.	D	47.	A	60.	C
9.	D	22.	D	35.	A	48.	D	61.	B
10.	C	23.	D	36.	C	49.	B	62.	D
11.	B	24.	D	37.	B	50.	A	63.	C
12.	C	25.	B	38.	D	51.	D	64.	D
13.	B	26.	B	39.	D	52.	B	65.	D

Physical Sciences

66.	B	82.	A	98.	D	113.	D	128.	B
67.	C	83.	C	99.	D	114.	C	129.	C
68.	D	84.	D	100.	B	115.	C	130.	C
69.	A	85.	A	101.	D	116.	C	131.	B
70.	C	86.	C	102.	B	117.	D	132.	A
71.	B	87.	C	103.	A	118.	A	133.	B
72.	C	88.	C	104.	D	119.	A	134.	B
73.	B	89.	B	105.	C	120.	A	135.	C
74.	C	90.	D	106.	D	121.	D	136.	D
75.	C	91.	C	107.	A	122.	A	137.	D
76.	B	92.	A	108.	A	123.	C	138.	C
77.	C	93.	C	109.	B	124.	D	139.	B
78.	A	94.	D	110.	A	125.	C	140.	B
79.	A	95.	B	111.	B	126.	D	141.	C
80.	B	96.	C	112.	D	127.	A	142.	B
81.	A	97.	C						

Biological Sciences

143.	B	159.	A	175.	D	190.	A	205.	B
144.	C	160.	B	176.	B	191.	B	206.	B
145.	C	161.	C	177.	A	192.	C	207.	B
146.	D	162.	D	178.	C	193.	D	208.	B
147.	D	163.	D	179.	C	194.	B	209.	D
148.	D	164.	A	180.	D	195.	A	210.	B
149.	D	165.	D	181.	D	196.	B	211.	D
150.	B	166.	A	182.	C	197.	C	212.	A
151.	B	167.	D	183.	A	198.	D	213.	B
152.	D	168.	D	184.	D	199.	B	214.	D
153.	D	169.	D	185.	C	200.	D	215.	C
154.	C	170.	D	186.	A	201.	C	216.	D
155.	B	171.	C	187.	D	202.	B	217.	C
156.	C	172.	B	188.	A	203.	C	218.	D
157.	C	173.	A	189.	D	204.	A	219.	C
158.	C	174.	D						

Explanation of Answers for Model Examination A

VERBAL REASONING

1. **C.** The central theme of the passage deals with the monumental amounts of research that have been done in the field of public education over the past 20 years. Mention of the vast research effort is made in paragraphs three, four, and five, whereas paragraph six makes it clear that research will continue.

2. **D.** Paragraph two states that the outcry was created in part by declining economic conditions, as well as the publication of exhaustive studies of school resources and their impact.

3. **A.** Paragraph one makes it clear that the reform in question for this passage deals with the nation's public school systems.

4. **D.** All three statements are included in the answer. In education "the field" is considered the classroom (I). "Researchers" going into the field indicates that they are observing teachers and students in action (II). The fact that researchers have gone into the field in great numbers indicates that there is much interest in educational reform research (III).

5. **D.** The combination of **B** and **C** encompasses educators who are researchers as well as those who are practicing in the field at all levels, and names three specific sets of practitioners who are closest to school settings. The question asks, what groups, and a choice is provided to include all the combinations.

6. **B.** Paragraphs four and five discuss researchers in the field and some progress that has been made as a result of their efforts. The "tone" that the author sets in these paragraphs allows one to assume that she feels hands-on research is beneficial.

7. **B.** The paragraph states that research efforts have intensified as plans of action are *evaluated*. It is reasonable to conclude that the results of the evaluation process will lead to more specific questions that will then lead to further investigation.

8. **A.** The passage opens by telling the reader that *periodic* demands for educational reform are not unusual in this country's history. Examples of reform attempts are given throughout. The closing sentence makes it clear that researchers are continuing their efforts to find ways to improve public education.

9. **D.** Paragraph two shows that family income is a factor that influences success in school, but it is not the only factor. Although hundreds of studies have indeed been conducted, the cry for reform continues as evidenced in the last paragraph. The negative effects of the early research have been lessened as a result of recent studies, but paragraph six noted that they have not been eliminated.

10. **C.** Paragraph two traces the story back to seventh century China and goes on to state that the plot is universal. The central thesis of the passage is that all versions of the story share many ingredients, and the first paragraph asserts that one of these chronicles the transformation into womanhood. Paragraph three notes the evil stepmother as a feature common to various versions of the story.

11. **B.** A main point of the passage is that a consistent aspect of Cinderella's character is her loving and forgiving spirit.

12. **C.** No mention is made of Cinderella's need for warmth (**A** is incorrect). The skins clearly are important in a ritual sense (**B** is incorrect). Cinderella always returns to a clean, well-dressed state; and because it symbolically is essential that she give up the skins and there is no mention that she keeps them, **D** is incorrect.

13. **B.** Cinderella, as the author notes in the final paragraph, is moving toward a condition of wholeness. There is nothing to suggest that she is less complex than she had thought (**A** is incorrect), that she exploits the prince (**C** is incorrect), or that her wholeness weakens her (**D** is incorrect).

14. **B.** A central purpose of the essay is to show how various versions of this tale make concrete various aspects of Horney's theories. Nowhere is there a suggestion that Horney had in mind the Cinderella story or that Horney altered the story in any way, thus **A** and **D** are incorrect. And, though one might find that the parallel between Horney's theories and the fairy tale provide one illustration of how the theories appear to be supported by their presence in a given story like *Cinderella,* nowhere is there a suggestion that the validity of a theory could be based on a single story application such as this one. Thus **C** is incorrect.

15. **A.** Although the first part of the title is a clever play on words, it also prepares the reader for the "fit" between Horney's theories and the Cinderella tale. The three other titles are not descriptive of the pattern of argument in the essay, and in the cases of **B** and **C**, contradict information in the text.

16. **B.** In **B**, the implication is that a fairy tale will be examined in view of a set of psychological theories. **C** is incorrect in that the comparison here is between two tales, not a tale and theory. **A** and **D** suggest studies that stray from the application of psychological theory to fairy tales.

17. **D.** The best and most encompassing title would be The Development of the Physician. The passage does not deal with professional growth and the development and training of the medical student exclusively. Although it is mentioned that the first two years of the study of medicine focus on the scientific aspects and thereafter the clinical practice predominates the life of the students, it is not examined specifically.

18. **D.** The passage makes it clear that most students enter this profession because they care for their fellow man and want to serve him; in fact the passage ends on the note that "the secret of the care of the patient is in caring for the patient." Achieving public esteem is a part of becoming a physician and certainly although intelligence and a good background help, they are not enough in the making of a physician. Marriage among classmates is not discussed.

19. **B.** Moral, clinical, and legal perspectives affect decision making and are in the order used upon first entrance into school. Socialization, however, elevates the clinical perspective to resolve the myriad of clinical situations. The issue of the influence of hospital administrators is not debated in the passage. The author quotes from Konner in respect to arrogance, but no conclusion is reached in respect to the statement that their extensive training gives anyone that right.

20. **D.** Good health, although essential, is not enough for medical practice; the article stresses continuously that the overall, the broad, the human, the appreciation of life, love, and mankind must be considered and held in focus in order to serve appropriately.

21. **D.** All the statements presented in this question are definitely contradicted by the information in the passage.

22. **D.** Because this passage basically describes the development and training—philosophical, ethical, legal, and clinical—of a student, the passage would be most appropriate if it were presented during a freshman orientation lecture.

23. **D.** In paragraph two it is made clear that the studies of Carlton showed that three rather distinct perspectives, the moral, clinical, and legal, directly affect decision making by physicians.

24. **D.** It is clearly pointed out in the last paragraph that most of the first two years is devoted to the science of medicine, but that there is patient contact towards the end of year one. In paragraph six, Kenner mentions a nonphysical aspect of healing, which he calls spiritual.

25. **B.** The passage makes it clear that at the end of the reductional division the chromosomes are reduced to one-half their original number. Meiosis results in four gametes that possess one-half the chromosomal number of an adult. The production of gametes, or sex cells—egg and sperm—is known as gametogenesis. Because an individual possesses an equal amount of genetic material from both parents and the same number of chromosomes as either parent, a reduction to one-half that number must be accomplished in the development of the egg and sperm.

26. **B.** During the process of meiosis, a recombination of genetic material is possible; this is effected through crossing over, as noted in paragraph three. In crossing over, comparable portions of chromatids are exchanged; crossing over is more the rule than the exception. Replication results during the first part of meiosis in four

chromatids and two of them may exchange materials. This exchange occurs before the tetrads separate.

27. **D.** The third paragraph indicates that replication of DNA occurs during interphase before meiosis starts. Interphase is the time during which the cell grows and prepares itself for meiosis.

28. **C.** See the explanation for previous questions dealing with this passage.

29. **D.** Eggs and sperms are haploid; a fertilized egg (zygote) possesses the diploid number of the parent again. Also see explanations for previous questions.

30. **D.** The first sentence of paragraph two mentions ten stages. Paragraph one states that sexual reproduction plays an important role in the expression of different phenotypes, and paragraph three indicates that replication of DNA occurs during interphase before meiosis begins.

31. **D.** The fact that ordinal position remains a little understood personality variable is stated in the opening paragraph and sets the tone for the passage.

32. **B.** Although much research has been done on birth order, it is not possible to make *absolute* statements about any of the ordinal positions. It has not been proven, for example, that the oldest is *always* the most mature. The opening paragraph implies that more studies need to be conducted.

33. **D.** The author states that primogeniture is "a perfect illustration of the importance of being first born." Because the custom began in feudal times, it is reasonable for the reader to conclude that the paragraph was inserted to provide a sense that the subject of ordinal birth has been the subject of study for some time.

34. **D.** All statements made in the question are correct. Parents attach to their firstborn such characteristics as a solid head on his/her shoulders, a mature behavior, and the ability to associate with adults, to be able to lead, to care for siblings, and to grow up as a pillar of the community. The youngest child is freer to develop into an exuberant and free-spirited individual because mothers do not expect the youngest to function in an adultlike manner. Many actions that were frowned upon previously are now considered cute in nature.

35. **A.** Although a comparison of the middle child to the older child is made, no direct comment or evidence is presented that this helps him/her reach higher levels of achievement; in fact because of the comparison and the desire of the child to establish his own identity, he may even become a problem student. The passage makes it clear that the firstborn usually performs better, and that the youngest feels the least need to excel. It is also stated in the passage that communication with adults is typically a problem of the second born.

36. **C.** The last two paragraphs specifically deal mainly with a discussion of mathematics grades between women; three groups were analyzed: (1) firstborn; (2) second, but not last born; and (3) last born.

37. **B.** The anxiety theory tries to explain decreased achievement in mathematics of the youngest child. This child is not pushed by his parents, which could be interpreted as being due to lack of parental interest. Thus, the youngest may suffer from the lack of parental expectations as well as from a self-imposed anxiety. The combination of both factors contributes to lower performance.

38. **D.** Paragraph two cites a family with three children, and paragraph five states that the youngest child often develops into an exuberant and well-rounded individual. The last paragraph makes the point that the youngest may develop feelings of anxiety, which may interfere with performance.

39. **D.** All the statements are supported by the information in the passage.

40. **D.** The author of the passage neither supports nor contradicts the statements presented in the question.

41. **D.** All three statements are clearly contradicted by the information presented in the passage.

42. **B.** The charisma of the instructor is a factor in the evaluation of teaching effectiveness. There are objective methods available and grades do play a role in student ratings. Time of day is not discussed in the passage.

43. **D.** The difficulty of subject matter material and its effect on student ratings is not discussed in the passage.

44. **C.** Students are usually most interested in evaluations by students, believing that they are the "consumers" who are most directly affected by the quality of the "product" called teaching.

45. **D.** Paragraph five visualizes students as purchasers. Paragraph two points out that employers and employees benefit from evaluations, and paragraph four states that the end result is increased productivity.

46. **B.** In paragraph one, the author plainly asserts that Tillich believes contemporary society is characterized by an absence of spirituality, whereas, ironically, there is a growing interest in religion.

47. **A.** Tillich, according to the author, sees true religion as moving vertically, and thus being characterized by "depth." Tillich's main thesis deals with the ways in which (1) present-day religion runs counter to true religion and (2) present-day society discourages people from asking weighty eschatological questions.

48. **D.** Although the author agrees with Tillich's assertions that modern man lacks true religion and is more materialistic now than in the past, he questions in his final paragraph the strictly "rational" ways that Tillich implies are the only ways of knowing spiritual truth. Nowhere in the essay does the author quarrel with Tillich's definition of spirituality.

49. **B.** In paragraph three, the author states plainly that Tillich's ideas are perhaps even more insightful or relevant than they were 30 years ago.

50. **A.** Though the author clarifies and qualifies Tillich's positions, he asserts that Tillich is still as relevant as he was "30 years ago."

51. **D.** These are the exact words that the author quotes Tillich as using. All other answers illustrate the opposite principle.

52. **B.** The main topic of this passage is to describe how a very specialized joint participates in the movement of the mandible functions. It is a two-joint proposition, which allows for opening and closing, protrusion and retraction, and lateral deviation movements.

53. **A.** Interposed between the condyle and fossa is the articular disk or meniscus. The meniscus divides the joint into two synovial compartments; in the upper compartment a gliding motion is allowed, whereas in the lower compartment a hinge motion prevails.

54. **B.** The paragraph states that the thickened lateral part of the capsule forms the temporomandibular ligament that prevents excessive retraction of the mandible.

55. **A.** It is stated in paragraph three that the temporomandibular ligament limits border movements.

56. **B.** Although the passage indicates that type B cells are secretary in nature, it does not limit this activity to type B cells. Phagocytes do remove foreign material, blood vessels supply the joint, synovial fluid is complex, and it is indicated that where there is a lack of pressure the membrane is thrown into folds.

57. **D.** Paragraph one describes this joint to be diarthroidal, capable of hinge and gliding movements. Although it is true that many suffer from temporomandibular joint problems, the passage does not address this issue. Paragraph three mentions the malleus, which is a middle ear bone, and the fact that one of the ligaments stabilizing the joint connects to the ossicle.

58. **D.** The last paragraph likens synovial fluid to plasma and lymph. Paragraph two states that the disk fuses with the joint capsule, and paragraph one states that both the right and left joints function as one unit.

59. **D.** Recent studies clearly show an impact of the increasing use of part-time faculty; and concerns are expressed about employment security, participation in governance, access to due process, grievances, evaluations, and fair compensation.

60. **C.** This is the best answer because the article covers many aspects of the impact of nontenure-eligible faculty on the educational mission of the university.

61. **B.** Part-time faculty has been hired at a rate that shows a 164 percent increase (compared to a 37 percent increase in number of full-time faculty) from 1970–1988.

62. **D.** The statements that part-time faculty is never expected to function in curriculum matters and that full-time "teach only" faculty has a secure base are contradicted by the passage.

63. **C.** The only statement supported by the passage is that tenure-track faculty are uninhibited in advocating changes in accepted ideas and in policies and programs of the institutions.

64. **D.** All choices represent correct statements. Temporary faculty foster morale problems among themselves, the institution, and everyone else. The two-tier system has eroded sound governance practices. Some writers view the hiring of temporary faculty as shortsighted and due to unregulated growth.

65. **D.** Paragraph one points out that many have studied the issues, and paragraph two states that various reasons exist for the presence of part-time faculty. It is clear from paragraph one that evidence exists and clearly shows the impact of the increasing use of part-time faculty in higher education institutions.

PHYSICAL SCIENCES

66. **B.** The shortest wavelength corresponds to the highest photon energy, according to $E = hc/\lambda$. The maximum energy available occurs when the incident high-speed electron gives up all its energy at one time (in a bremsstrahlung process). If 80,000 volts is used to accelerate the electrons, the most energetic x-ray photon can have 80,000 eV of energy (but only a very small number of 80 keV photons will occur).

67. **C.** The K_α transitions are more probable and thus occur more often. The vertical intensity axis values are proportional to the number of photons emitted.

68. **D.** The minimum wavelength depends only on the accelerating voltage. The electrical work done in accelerating the electrons is equal to the maximum photon energy:

$$eV_0 = hc/\lambda_{min}$$

69. **A.** The peaks are characteristic of the *target* material. The photon energy emitted (say for an $n = 3$ to $n = 1$ transition) never changes. If V_0 is increased the height of the peaks (intensity) will increase. (If the voltage is decreased to a very

low value the peaks may not be seen because the incident electrons do not have enough energy to eject an inner shelf electron on the target. Thus a continuous spectrum can occur without the peaks.)

70. **C.** A high melting point metal makes a more practical target material due to the large amount of heat produced. Nearly 99% of the incoming energy is converted to heat in the target and only about 1% produces x-rays. Lead would actually be a more efficient x-ray producing target but would melt almost immediately in modern tubes.

71. **B.** The frictional work uses up all the kinetic energy. Frictional force is μmg, and frictional work is μmgs. Thus:

$$W_f = KE_i - o = KE_i \quad \text{or} \quad \mu mgs = 1/2 \, mv^2$$

thus solving for skid length, s: $s = v^2/(2 \, \mu g)$, and the skid length is proportional to the *square of the speed*. The mass drops out of the equation.

72. **C.** Because the skid length depends on speed squared, a car with twice the speed of another will slide *four* times as far.

73. **B.** The forces during the collision *are* equal and opposite according to Newton's third law of motion. Each of the other responses is incorrect for the following reasons: **A.** The more massive van has *greater* momentum at the same speed. **C.** The forces are actually *equal* and opposite. **D.** It would require *more* mechanical work to stop the van because it has larger mass. In this case, the vehicles do not stop. The large van would actually reverse the velocity of the small car and "drive" the car backwards.

74. **C.** As in the explanation for question 73, the forces during collision are equal and opposite. The other responses are incorrect because: **A.** The forces are always equal and opposite according to Newton's Third Law. **B.** Untrue, since the forces are actually equal and opposite. **D.** This is a true statement but it has nothing to do with the question asked, and does not explain why the car would suffer more damage in a head-on collision.

75. **C.** As in explanation for question 72, the skid length depends on the square of the speed.

76. **B.** In this particular experiment, the paint marks are three times farther apart when the speed (60 mph) is three times greater. Thus the

times to travel between paint marks, which is the reaction time, remain the same. (The reaction times could vary from one test to another. Here the two times happened to be identical.)

77. **C.** Elementary trigonometry states that the sine of an angle = (opposite side)/(hypotenuse). Sin 30° = 0.5, so the hypotenuse is two times as long as the opposite side.

78. **A.** The power is the work/(unit time) and the work done is equal to the total gain in gravitational potential energy. The time is 60 sec. Thus:

P(watts) = (# buckets)(10kg/bucket)(g)(4.0m)/(60s) = 196 watts.

79. **A.** Electric power, in watts, is related to voltage and current as follows:

$P = VI$. Thus $I = 196W/(120\ V)$
= 1.6 amperes.

80. **B.** The higher power motor should have a power that is 1.45 times the smaller power, i.e.:

$1.45 \times 200 = 290$ watts.

81. **A.** Because twice as much mass is raised through 4 m in one minute, the required work per minute, and thus the required power, is doubled.

82. **A.** The total momentum of the two-object "system" is conserved (constant) during this inelastic collision. The 500-gram object is at rest ($v_2 = 0$); thus $m_1v_1 + 0 = (m_1 + m_2)V$. Solving for v_1:

$$v_2 = \frac{(m_1 + m_2)V}{m_1} = 388\ \text{m/sec}$$

83. **C.** Using conservation of energy ($mgh = 1/2mv^2$), we find that the speed of Block 2 just *before* impact is the *same* as the speed of Block 1 in question 82 above (3.88 m/sec). Now the conservation of momentum principle, which we use *during the collision,* allows us to calculate the speed of the combined (stuck-together) mass after the collision. Thus $m_1v_1 = (m_1 + m_2)V$. Solving for V:

$$\frac{m_1v_1}{(m_1 + m_2)} = 1.45\ \text{m/sec}$$

(Note that v_1 is the same as in question 82 but the mass ratio is larger.)

84. **D.** Using the conservation of energy principle, $mgh = 1/2\ mv^2$, we see that when we solve for v at the bottom of the track the mass will cancel. Since h is 1.2 m for both Blocks 1 and 2, their speeds will be the same (4.85 m/sec) at the track bottom.

85. **A.** Again we use conservation of energy. However, this time the masses interchange potential energy and kinetic energy as they fly along their parabolic arcs; that is: $mgh_0 = mgh_1 + 1/2mv^2$. Since the 45° angle will cause the masses to rise higher than the 30° angle, the masses will have more potential energy and less kinetic energy at the higher angle. Conversely, the masses will have more kinetic energy and thus *greater* speeds at the top of the arc for 30°.

86. **C.** Since the speeds are the same at the track ends (see question 84) and they both fall through a vertical distance of 1 m from the track bottom, conservation of energy shows that their speeds when they strike the floor are equal also. Assume $h = 1$ m and $v = 4.85$ m/sec for both. Then:

$$1/2mv^2 + mgh = 1/2mV^2$$

(The mass will cancel, so V is the same for both blocks.)

87. **C.** Although their speeds are the same when they hit the floor, their kinetic energies are proportional to their masses. Thus, the kinetic energies ratio is:

$$\frac{1/2m_1V^2}{1/2m_1V^2} = m_1/m_2 = 2/3$$

88. **C.** When a force causes an object to move at a constant speed, the force is exactly equal to the opposing force of friction and there is no net force. (The larger 150 N force will result in a net force of 50 N that will accelerate the box, according to Newton's Second Law, $F_{net} = ma$.

89. **B.** Conservation of charge and mass requires the sum of the subscript (charge) numbers to be equal on both sides of the reaction as well as the sum of the superscript (mass) numbers to be equal. We must have then: $2 + 7 = 8 + 1$ and $4 + 14 = 17 + 1$. The missing subscript is 1, as is the missing superscript. The object is actually a proton initially, but we write the symbol for neutral hydrogen, since the proton will "grab" an electron to become hydrogen.

90. **D.** The Coulomb force between two charged particles is given by: $F = kq_1q_2/r^2$. In this case, the ratio of the new force to the old force is:

$$\frac{F_2/F_1 = k(3q_A(q_B)/(3r)^2}{kq_Aq_B/r^2} = 1/3$$

91. **C.** The current through the 2-ohm resistor must split up with the larger portion going through the smaller resistor in the parallel branch. The 3-ohm and 6-ohm resistors are in the ratio of 1 to 2, so the 3-ampere current will split into the ratio of 2 to 1—that is, 2 amperes through the 3-ohm resistor and 1 ampere through the 6-ohm resistor.

92. **A.** The Boyle's Law form of the Ideal Gas Law applies, since the temperature is constant. Thus $P_1V_1 = P_2V_2$.

$$V_2 = P_1V_1/V_2 = \frac{2 \text{ atm} \times 2L}{3.5 \text{ atm}} = 1.1 \text{ L}$$

93. **C.** Since air friction is present, the ball will reach a "terminal velocity" shown as the value of v corresponding to the horizontal dotted line.

94. **D.** The principle of conservation of mechanical energy states that the sum of the initial kinetic and potential energies equals the sum of the final kinetic and potential energies; $KE_i + PE_i = KE_f + PE_f$. Here we may take PE_f to be zero. Thus, $1/2mv_i^2 + mgh = 1/2mv_f^2$ and $v_f = 15$ m/sec, for both masses, since mass cancels and angle of launch is not involved in the calculation.

95. **B.** The thin lens formula is $1/f = 1/p + 1/q$ where f = focal length, p = object distance (from the lens), and q = image distance (from lens to image). The initial image distance is +20 cm. The magnification $m = -(q/p)$ and is initially −1. (The initial image is the same size as the object and is inverted and real.) After the object is moved to $p = 15$ cm, the new image distance is +30 cm and the magnification also increases to −1.5, so the new image is larger and farther from the lens.

96. **C.** Because the three 6-ohm resistors are in parallel, the same voltage of 12 volts is impressed across each resistor. Then by Ohm's law the current through each is given by $I = V/R = 12/6 = 2$ A. (The same method will work if all three were different resistors. Only the value of R would differ in Ohm's law.)

97. **C.** The highest resistance will result from all three in series; $R_e = R_1 + R_2 + R_3 = 6$ ohms. The smallest value will result when all three are in parallel, because the equivalent parallel resistance is always smaller than the smallest individual value.

$$1/R_e = 1/R_1 + 1/R_2 + 1/R_3 = 0.545 \text{ ohms.}$$

98. **D.** Faraday's law of electromagnetic induction gives the induced voltage (emf) as

$$E = (-) \Delta\varphi/\Delta t = NAB/\Delta t$$

Solving for B:

$$B = E\frac{\Delta t}{NA} = \frac{0.05 \times 0.1}{50 \times 1 \times 10^{-4}} = 1.0T$$

99. **D.** At resonance, where the inductive reactance, X_L and the capacitive reactance, X_C, have equal magnitudes the circuit impedance, Z, is just equal to the pure resistance R. ($Z = R = 4.0$ ohms) because:

$$Z = \sqrt{R^2 + (X_L - X_C)^2}$$

100. **B.** The AC current is found from the AC form of Ohm's law: $I = V/Z$. In this resonant circuit $Z = R$, so that $I = V/R = 2.0$ volts/4.0 ohms = 0.5 A.

101. **D.** The parallel combination has an equivalent resistance given by $1/R_p = 1/2 + 1/2$, or $R_p = 1$ ohm. When the 4-ohm resistor is connected in series, the equivalent resistance is $R_e = R_s = 4 + 1 = 5.0$ ohms. Ohm's law gives the current through the equivalent resistance:

$$I = V/R_s = 12/5 = 2.4 \text{ A.}$$

102. **B.** The full 2.4 A current drawn from the battery flows through the 4-ohm resistor but this current splits *equally* at the junction with the two 2-ohm resistors in parallel. The general method (useful when the resistances of the parallel combination are not equal) is to first find the voltage drop across the single 4-ohm resistor: $V_4 = IR = (2.4 \text{ A})(4 \text{ ohms}) = 9.6$ V. The (remaining) voltage drop across the parallel combination is: $V_p = 12$ V − 9.6 V = 2.4 V. Since the voltage is the same across parallel elements in a circuit:

$$I_2 = V_P/R = 2.4 \text{ V/2 ohm} = 1.2 \text{ A.}$$

103. **A.** Using three resistors in series the possible number of combinations is four. ($R_S = R_1 + R_2 + R_3$)(2 + 2 + 2 = 6 ohms; 2 + 4 + 2 = 8 ohms; 2 + 4 + 4 = 10 ohms; 4 + 4 + 4 = 12 ohms) In parallel there are also four possibilities; ($1/R_p = 1/R_1 + 1/R_2 + 1/R_3$) with values found from $1/R_p = 1/2 + 1/2 + 1/2$; $1/R_p = 1/2 + 1/2 + 1/4$; etc.)

104. **D.** The capacitor voltage approaches the maximum (applied) voltage, V_0 according to the expression: $V_C = V_0 (1 - e^{-t/RC})$. As t becomes very large the last term in the parentheses approaches zero and V_C approaches V_0 as a maximum limit. (The voltage across the capacitor initially rises rapidly since the battery can easily deposit charge on the capacitor plates. As more charge appears on the plates it becomes more difficult for the battery to "pump" more charge of the same sign onto a given plate.)

105. **C.** The full voltage drop occurs across the single resistance so the voltmeter reading is also the battery voltage of 6 volts. The resistance is found using Ohm's law: $R = V/I = 6/0.5 = 12$ ohms.

106. **D.** The amino groups may exist as $R\text{-}NH_3^+$ with a charge of +1 or as $R\text{-}NH_2$ with a charge of zero (0). The carboxyl group may exist as R-COOH with a charge of zero (0) or as $RCOO^-$ with a charge of –1. Thus, we might indicate the possible charged species of this amino acid at different pH's as

(+ + 0) $pK_a = 2.1$ (+ + –) $pK_a = 9.0$ (+ 0 –) $pK_a = 10.5$ (0 0 –)

$\leftarrow$ (lowest pH) ------------------ (highest pH) $\rightarrow$

We note that the third species (+ 0 –) would have a net charge of zero. The pK_a's that relate this species to those on both sides may be averaged to obtain the isoelectric point:

$$\frac{9.0 + 10.5}{2} = 9.75$$

107. **A.** The reasoning is the same as in the above question, but the species are (+ 0 0), (+ 0 –), (+ – –), and (0 – –). The pK_a's on the two sides of the electrically neutral (+ 0 –) are 2.1 and 4.0.

$$\frac{21 + 4.0}{2} = 3.05.$$

108. **A.** The isoelectric point of such amino acid would be about $\frac{2.1 + 9.0}{2} = 5.55$. It would have a net charge of zero at that pH, increasingly positive net charge as the pH decreases, and increasingly negative net charge as the pH increases. Thus, at a pH of 8, this amino acid will consist of molecules most of which exist as the species having a net charge of –1.

109. **B.** As mentioned in explanations above, the isoelectric point would be the mean of the pK_a's associated with the uncharged species. In this case:

$$\frac{4.0 + 9.0}{2} = 6.5.$$

110. **A.** Differences in the isoelectric points of various amino acids allow their separation in buffer of appropriate pH in an electrical field (electrophoresis).

111. **B.** In applying the gas laws, only the Kelvin scale may be used because of the three, it is the only one with a natural zero.

112. **D.** When going up a mountain, we could expect the possibility of either a decrease in temperature or pressure. An increase in pressure is unlikely and would result in a decrease in volume. A decrease in temperature would result in a decrease in volume. Because PV would remain constant, a 10% decrease in pressure would result in a 10% increase in volume.

113. **D.** $\frac{PV}{T} = nR$ Depending on the units of R, n can be the number of moles or the number of molecules (or atoms). Because R is a universal constant, the value of PV/T depends only on the number of molecules (or moles).

114. **C.** See explanation for question 113. Equal numbers of moles of any gas will occupy the same volume at equal temperatures and pressures.

115. **C.** $\frac{P_1V_1}{T_1} = \frac{P_2V_2}{T_2}$

$$\frac{P_1V_1}{T_1} = \frac{(0.95)P_1V_2}{(0.95)T_1}$$

$P_1V_1 = P_1V_2$ and thus $V_1 = V_2$

(Remember that T is calculated as °K (°C + 273). Thus the temperature decreased by 5%.)

116. **C.** The transmittance is defined as incident light 72/81 = 0.889.

117. **D.** The absorbance is defined as the negative logarithm of transmittance. $-\log 0.889 = 0.051$.

118. **A.** The Beer-Lambert Law states that $A = -\log T$
$= EMl$ where
A = absorbance
T = transmittance
E = a constant for the particular solute and wavelength of light
M = molarity of solution
l = path length of light
Thus absorbance varies directly with path length and with molar concentration; and decreasing the concentration by half will also halve the absorbance.

119. **A.** In the above statement of the Beer-Lambert Law it is seen that absorbance varies directly with path length. Thus, halving the path length will halve the absorbance.

120. **A.** The absorbance was 0.051. Doubling the concentration will double the absorbance to 0.102. Since absorbance = –log transmittance, and

$$\text{transmittance} = \frac{\text{reading with transmitted light}}{\text{reading with incident light}}$$

antilog (0.102) = 0.791
(0.791)(81) = 64

121. **D.** The reading, the transmittance, and the absorbance will be affected by the wavelength of light, but the direction and magnitude cannot be readily predicted.

122. **A.** Buffering is seen in two areas, indicating 2 pK_a's, at points 1 and 3.

123. **C.** See explanation for answer 122.

124. **D.** None of these would have 2 pK_a's. HF and HCl are strong acids and would not have measurable pK_a's. H_3PO_4 has 3 pK_a's.

125. **C.** Points 1 and 3, both pK_a's, show greatest buffering.

126. **D.** Points 1 and 3 are both correct, because equal amounts of two species will be found at a pK_a.

127. **A.** HCl in water is expected to be virtually 100% ionized into H^+ (or H_3O^+) and Cl^-.
pH = $-\log [H^+] = -\log (1 \times 10^{-2}) = 2$

128. **B.** Because the volume has doubled, [HCl] = 0.005 molar = 5×10^{-3}.

Because HCl is virtually completely ionized,
$$[H^+] = 5 \times 10^{-3} \text{ molar}$$
$$pH = -\log (5 \times 10^{-3})$$
$$\log 10^{-3} = -3$$
$$\log 5 = \underline{0.6990}$$
$$\text{sum} = -2.3010$$
$$-(-2.3010) = 2.3010$$

Even if you are not provided with a calculator, you should recognize that the answer must be between 2 and 3 because log (5) is a positive number between zero and one.

129. **C.** The Henderson-Hasselbalch equation states

$$pH = pK_a + \log \frac{[\text{salt}]}{[\text{acid}]}$$

The strongly ionized HCl will react with sodium propionate to yield propionic acid. Thus 0.01 moles of HCl will react with 0.01 moles of sodium propionate to yield 0.01 moles of propionic acid (HPr). An additional 0.01 moles of NaPr will remain unreacted.

$$pH = pK_a + \log \frac{[\text{salt}]}{[\text{acid}]} = 4.89 + \log \frac{(0.01)}{(0.01)} = 4.89$$

When the concentrations of weak acid and salt are equal,

$$\frac{[\text{Salt}]}{[\text{Acid}]} = 1 \text{ and } \log 1 = 0$$

At these concentrations, pH = pK_a. (The concentrations should be expressed in molarities rather than simply total moles. Reflection allows us to recognize that the end result will be the same as long as we are consistent in a single set of computations.)

130. **C.** Because the solution was at the pK_a and we added equal quantities of salt and acid, it remains at the pK_a.

131. **B.** Look again at the Henderson-Hasselbalch equation. We have diluted [salt] and [acid] equally. Thus the pH remains at the pK_a.

132. **A.** $K_a = \dfrac{[H^+][Pyr^-]}{[Hpyr]} = 1.4 \times 10^{-4}$

$$= \frac{[H^+]^2}{[HPyr]} = \frac{[H^+]^2}{0.01 \text{ molar}}$$

(Because HPyr ionized to give equal numbers of ions of H^+ and Pyr^-, their concentrations should be equal. Thus, substituting $[H^+]$ for $[Pyr^-]$ should introduce little error.)

$[H^+]^2 = (0.01) \times 1.4 \times 10^{-4} = 1.4 \times 10^{-6}$
$[H^+]$ would be approximately $+1.2 \times 10^{-3}$ by inspection.
$-\log(1.2 \times 10^{-3})$ is between 2 and 3.

133. **B.** The solution is at the pK_a value for the buffer pair because equal molar quantities of the buffer pair are present.

134. **B.** degree of ionization $= \dfrac{[H^+]}{[acid]}$

In an earlier problem in this set we calculated that when $[HPyr] = 0.01$, $[H^+] =$ about 1.2×10^{-3}

$$\dfrac{1.2 \times 10^{-3}}{0.01} = 0.12$$

135. **C.** Percent ionization = 100 (degree of ionization)
$100 \times 0.12 = 12$

136. **D.** Remember Graham's Law:

$$\dfrac{V_1}{V_2} = \sqrt{\dfrac{m_2}{m_1}}$$

$$\dfrac{1}{0.5} = \sqrt{\dfrac{m_2}{m_1}}$$

Squaring $\dfrac{1}{0.25} = \dfrac{m_2}{20} = 4$

$$m_2 = 80$$

137. **D.** $V_1 \times N_1 = V_2 \times N_2$
$(20.0)(0.200) = (40.0)(0.100) = 4$
This tells us nothing about the structure of the acid. Remember that the normality deals only with the available protons in solution rather than the molarity. The acid could be monoprotic, diprotic, or triprotic, but we have been given no information to allow us to decide.

138. **C.** $pK_w = pH + pOH = 14$
$4.5 + pOH = 14$
$pOH = 14 - 4.5 = 9.5$

139. **B.** $pH = pK_a + \log \dfrac{[salt]}{[acid]}$
When the salt (dissociated anion) and acid concentrations are equal, $\log 1 = 0$. Thus, $pH = pK_a$ or 4.2 in this case.

140. **B.** Buffering is always best at the pK_a.

141. **C.** $\dfrac{P_1 V_1}{T_1} = \dfrac{P_2 V_2}{T_2}$
Since $T_1 = T_2$, they will cancel out.

$$(1)(1) = 2V \text{ and } V = \dfrac{1}{2} \text{ or } 0.50$$

142. **B.** The step involved is a precipitation step. Increasing the Cl^- concentration will reduce the concentration of Ag^+ in solution. Remember $K_{sp} = [Ag^+][Cl^-]$ and the source of the Cl^- is irrelevant. Thus increased concentration of Cl^- must result in decreased concentration of Ag^+ in order to maintain the solubility product constant. Addition of $Ag_2 SO_4$ would probably be counterproductive, since additional Ag^+ is being added, and probably all will not be recovered.

WRITING SAMPLE

Part 1, Essay

Herodotus's viewpoint here is clearly a fatalistic one. It is easy to see the logic behind it. Because mankind does not exist separately from either the rest of existence or the past, then every time that a person acts, she is in some ways also reacting to that surrounding existence and to the history that preceded that act. It is a frustrating point of view; and, in spite of its strange truth, it is probably a viewpoint best left without too much rumination. It is the given in life and the unchangeable. A resignation to this point of view would in some ways also be a voluntary denial of one's autonomy, of one's existence.

I say "voluntary" because I believe that the opposite viewpoint is, paradoxically, just as true. If I turn my head while driving in order to check my radio dial and in doing so also slightly turn my steering wheel causing an accident with an oncoming school bus, did not my act of turning my head create a circumstance whereby that accident occurred? Of course, it did. If I had not turned my head, then I would have not turned the wheel; and if I had not turned the wheel then the bus would not have hit my car. However, from Herodotus's viewpoint, my act did not exist by itself. Had the radio not been in the car, had a different song even been on the station, then I would perhaps not have turned my head to adjust the dial. Had the bus driver waited longer at her last stop or had she not stopped for a cup of coffee on her way to work, then perhaps she would not have been at that place at that specific time. The issue is as puzzling as the issue of whether the chicken appeared first or the egg. It is the question of the identification of an original cause in a long line of causes.

What a thinking person is most likely to conclude is that individuals and their circumstances are mutually interdependent rather than mutually exclusive and that therefore a statement like that of Herodotus is, in a sense, meaningless. His is only a statement of perspective and, further, a rather negative one. But to say the opposite, that circumstances are dependent on individuals and not vice versa would be naive and ignorant. A rational person would have to accept interdependence of individuals and circumstances in order to live realistically and effectively in the world. She would then act carefully, remaining aware both that there are circumstances over which she has no control and that her act will be part of the circumstances to come.

Part 1
Explanation of First Response: 6

The paper focuses sharply on the statement and addresses each of the three writing tasks. Paragraph one explains what the statement means, paragraph two gives a specific situation in which individuals do, in fact, determine circumstances (a reversal of the assertion that "men are dependent on circumstances, not circumstances on men"), and in paragraph three reconciles the statement and the situation that illustrates that the opposite of the statement may also be true.

The paper provides an analysis of the potential dangers of all-or-none statements like the one in question. It does so by examining the logical extension of the idea that individuals are dependent on circumstances and by characterizing the implications of this assertion as "fatalistic." The logic of the paper's argument is sophisticated, on the one hand agreeing with the "strange truth" of Herodotus's point in paragraph one, but in paragraph two illustrating with a series of circumstances "dependent on individuals" that the reverse is also true. The final paragraph presents a balanced consideration of the interdependent relationship between individuals and the circumstances that they create and by which they are shaped.

The writing is clear and nicely controlled. The sentences are varied, containing simple (e.g., sentence one), compound (e.g., sentence four), and complex structures (e.g., sentence three). The first sentence of each paragraph serves as a topic sentence and gives unity to the paragraph that follows. Transitions, such as "however" in sentence five of paragraph two, provide coherence within the paragraph.

Part 2, Essay

Haeckel's quotation is an enigma because its meaning depends upon the interpretation of ambiguous words, "voluntary death," "intolerable suffering," and of course, "redemption." It is not clear whether the "voluntary death" is a suicide or a murder or any of the possibilities between these two extremes. So, even at the outset, the reader steps onto a shaky platform on which rests the remainder of Haeckel's statement. This "voluntary death" would specifically be the one that would put "an end to intolerable suffering." Because to "suffer" something is, in a sense, to

"tolerate" it, then "intolerable suffering" would be an impossibility by definition. Finally, this enigmatic but "voluntary death," voluntary perhaps only because it is caused by a human act, is "an act of redemption." Naturally, one's thoughts might turn to the religious connotations of the word. In this case, it would mean a sort of act of deliverance from evil by sacrifice. If, however, you strip the mystery of religious aura from the word, it means simply a payback. Perhaps the redemption is the cashing in of the mortal life for freedom from human suffering. Keeping all of this in mind, Haeckel's statement, though, still a puzzle of sorts, must mean that for a person to cause or to allow death in order to discontinue the suffering of pain (of one sort or another) is an exchange of the body, which is only loaned for the duration of mortality, in exchange for the freedom of the human spirit.

Now, one could argue (and people certainly have argued) endlessly about the moral right and/or wrong of this idea because it is at the core of the controversies over euthanasia, abortion, and the execution of criminals. The argument is over, the "right" or "wrong" of this "redemption." Because "'right" and "wrong" cannot really be defined but only agreed upon tentatively (as with laws), perhaps the literal meaning of the quote might be a better target for thought. The problem here is that it is not clear whose "intolerable suffering" is being referred to in the statement. For example, if I refuse to tolerate or to suffer the presence of my annoying little brother, is my killing him or allowing him to die an act of redemption? The thought is appalling, of course, but, according to Haeckel, it would, in fact, be a redemptive act (even if the sacrifice entailed is only that of my own innocence). The way that Haeckel's quotation is worded, there are no real exceptions.

Haeckel's quotation could be used to try to justify morally the act of taking a human life. But the statement does not morally justify anything; it merely defines a type of "voluntary death" as a sort of exchange. The end of a human's life is always an exchange of one state for another. So the moral question, the "choice" perhaps, is a personal one (or a legal one). Morality is not defined by absolute natural laws; it is rather defined personally (or, in a social situation, legally). What governs the choice maker or the potential actor consists of nothing more absolute and nothing less vague than his or her conscience and personal beliefs. Haeckel's quote could be used loosely to justify an act that results in death. But "used" is the key word here. Moral decision, decisions about right and wrong, are not that easy. Ultimately, the choice of a *"voluntary* death" in "the face of intolerable suffering" is determined only by the judgment and conscience of the individual, the mysterious "volunteer."

Part 2
Explanation of Second Response: 4

The paper focuses on the topic defined by the statement and addresses the three writing tasks. The first paragraph responds to the task of explaining the statement, in this case a task complicated by the need to clarify definitions of words that have multiple meanings. In the second paragraph, the paper provides what is clearly one of the most extreme examples imaginable to demonstrate that, given the phrasing of the quotation, there are no specific situations in which "voluntary death" would not be an act of redemption. Paragraph three explores the factors that determine the choice of voluntary death in the face of intolerable suffering.

There is no question that Haeckel's statement raises difficult problems, and it is clear that this essay constructs a sophisticated argument that explores the complexity of these problems. The strategy of defining ambiguous terms in paragraph one is a good one; the choice to explore the connotations of these words also is effective, though anyone who chooses to spend this much time on definition in the first paragraph should be aware of the danger of overdoing it. This essay stops just short of this. The reason that this essay received a 4 rather than a 5 or 6 is that the second task ("Describe a specific situation in which the voluntary death by which a person puts an end to intolerable suffering would not be an act of redemption") is not confronted as directly as it might be. The paper maintains that "there are no real exceptions," virtually by definition. The writer might have used his or her skill with definition clearly demonstrated in paragraph one to construct at least one hypothetical situation that would provide a conceivable exception to Haeckel's statement. In addition to the need for a specific "exceptional" situation in paragraph two, the paper could be strengthened by the use of other examples to illustrate the major points in paragraphs one and three. This paper in general, however, is tightly reasoned, and it moves logically toward the conclusion that the choice of voluntary death in the face of intolerable suffering is ultimately a moral decision, one based on conscience.

BIOLOGICAL SCIENCES

143. **B.** The thyroid hormones affect the rate of metabolism of all the tissues of the body; they control the growth, maturation, and differentiation of the organism. A goiter is any enlargement of the gland due to neoplasm or inflammatory disease. Endemic goiters are due to lack of iodine intake; this results in the increased production of TSH, compensatory hypertrophy and eventual exhaustion of the gland. Thyroxin deficiency leads to goiter; if the deficiency is not corrected cretinism in the young and myxedema in the adult may be a consequence.

144. **C.** Hypothyroidism would result in a patient who is fairly heavy, phlegmatic, is devoid of expression, and has rough and dry skin and laboratory tests would show a low basal metabolic rate, low protein bound iodine, and a high serum cholesterol level.

145. **C.** The hypothyroid patient would have shown weight gain since less food is converted into energy and more food is stored as fat.

146. **D.** See explanations for questions 143–145.

147. **D.** A hyperthyroid patient would exhibit weight loss, nervousness, irritability, increased metabolic rate, rapid heart rate, sweating, and a protrusion of the eyeballs.

148. **D.** This woman is not the mother. She can contribute only the O gene, and this child must receive an A gene from one parent and a B gene from the other parent. The man cannot be ruled out as the father with the limited information given, since he can contribute a B gene to a child.

149. **D.** If the man previously fathered a child with blood type O, then the man must have a genotype of BO. The woman can contribute only the O gene. Since the man has an equal chance of contributing the B or the O gene, there is a 50% chance of the child being type O (genotype OO) or type B (genotype BO).

150. **B.** The chance of any child of this couple being type B is 50% (see explanation for question 149). The chance that any child will be a girl is 50%. Since the blood type and the sex are independent of each other, multiply their individual chances (50% × 50% = 25%).

151. **B.** Phenotypic and genotypic characteristics may be expressed as follows:

Phenotype	Genotype
A	A/O
B	B/O
O	O/O
AB	A/B

152. **D.** Genotype refers to the genetic makeup of the organism. The genotype is expressed via phenotypic characteristics that are visible and observable under normal circumstances.

153. **D.** An allele is one of a pair of genes that occupies the same locus on homologous chromosomes.

154. **C.** Rhesus (Rh) agglutinogen is present in

humans and is represented by a dominant gene R. The agglutinogen of an Rh positive fetus passes across the placenta, enters the maternal blood stream, and elicits the production of an agglutinin (antibody) by the mother. The agglutinin passes into the circulation of the fetus and if present in sufficient concentration can produce agglutination, at times fatal to the developing fetus.

155. **B.** Hemophilia, a frequent disease of the royal houses of Europe, is a bleeding disorder transmitted through a sex-linked recessive gene. It results in abnormal coagulation; hemophilia A is the classical true hemophilia resulting from a deficiency of factor VIII. Both sexes carry a complete complement of sex-linked genes. A female, with the XX arrangement, will only exhibit a recessive gene if she has received it from both parents (a rare event with an uncommon gene), whereas in the XY male the recessive gene cannot be masked because there is no partner X and so a larger number of recessive genes are expressed. A man receives his X from his mother and passes it on to his daughters. His daughters are the carriers of sex-linked traits and their sons may be affected.

156. **C.** Pleiotropism is defined as multiple phenotypic effects of a gene (allele).

157. **C.** 1-2, who manifests prolonged Q-T interval, has 14 descendants who are also affected and six who are not. Each of the 14 affected descendants has an affected parent; both parents (II-3&10) of four are affected. The trait thus shows unbroken lineal descent and is, therefore, *dominant*.

158. **C.** *Deafness is not a pleiotropic affect of the gene producing prolonged Q-T,* for these abnormalities are observed *assorting* among the progeny of a male (II-1), who is doubly homozygous normal, and his wife (II-2), who is heterozygous for both abnormalities, that is, doubly heterozygous. Alleles segregate (Mendel's first law) from each other; non-alleles may assort. In the absence of linkage, *independent assortment* (Mendel's second law) of nonalleles occurs. Although the sample is not large enough to rule out weak linkage, it does rule out allelism.

159. **A.** Every affected descendant of the affected progenitor (I-3) of the F. family has at least one parent affected, except III-21, a son of II-11, who marks the only break in lineal descent of the trait. If the trait were recessive, the three normal mothers (I-4, II-9, and II-12) of affected children would have to be carriers. Because of the rarity of the defect and the lack of biological kinship between these women and their spouses, it is highly unlikely that they are carriers. It is probable that the trait is dominant and that the allele has slightly reduced penetrance and failed to manifest itself phenotypically in II-11.

160. **B.** If one were limited to the data on the W. family, it would be impossible to distinguish whether the defect is autosomal or X-linked. That is because we could not then rule out male-to-male transmission among the progeny of couple II-3&10, who have three arrhythmic sons. Nonetheless, prolonged Q-T and the arrhythmias are clinically indistinguishable and almost certainly determined by the same *autosomal dominant* allele as in the F. family, where male-to-male transmission shows that this dominant trait is autosomal. X-linked traits cannot be transmitted from father to son (male-to-male) because sons can receive their X chromosome (in which X-linked traits are transmitted) from only their mother, *not* from their father.

161. **C.** All of the daughters of affected males would be affected if the trait were X-linked because they received their father's X chromosome which would have contained the (dominant) mutant allele had it been X-linked. None of the daughters of the affected fathers (II-3 and II-5) are affected, thus the mutant allele is *not* in the X chromosome; the trait is autosomal.

162. **D.** Many autosomal dominant genes that produce rather mild phenotypic effects in the heterozygote produce much more extreme effects—in some cases, even lethality—in homozygotes. It is likely that *the propista* (III-10) *is homozygous* for the prolonged Q-T allele and demonstrates the more extreme phenotype frequently manifested by homozygotes for rare autosomal dominant traits.

163. **D.** Developing embryos would be actively synthesizing both RNA and DNA (the latter would be associated with chromosome duplication prior to each cell division). Radiolabelled adenine, **A**, guanine, **B**, and uridine, **D**, would be incorporated into newly synthesized RNA. Radiolabelled adenine, guanine, and thymidine, **C**, would be incorporated into newly synthesized DNA. Because uridine is incorporated into RNA but not into DNA, radiolabelled uridine should be used to monitor RNA synthesis.

164. **A.** The correct answer is chosen after studying the graph. Note that the rate of mRNA synthesis begins to increase at the blastula stage, **A,** and reaches a peak just before the gastrula stage. As is stated in the passage and also illustrated in the graph, no RNA of any type is synthesized during cleavage. Because the question specifically asks about embryonic mRNA synthesis, **D,** is inappropriate.

165. **D.** Again the correct answer is chosen after studying the graph. Embryonic RNA synthesis begins at the blastula stage. Initially mRNAs and later tRNAs begin to be synthesized. By the gastrula stage, rRNA synthesis has also begun. Therefore gastrula stage embryos would be synthesizing all types of RNA.

166. **A.** No synthesis of embryonic RNAs would occur in actinomycin D-treated embryos. Because no embryonic mRNAs would be made, the proteins that these embryonic mRNAs would code for would also not be made. The proteins made by the developing embryos would be translated from the preexisting oogenetic or maternal RNAs.

167. **D.** Again actinomycin D-treated embryos would be unable to synthesize embryonic RNAs. Because protein synthesis still occurs in these embryos, there must still be adequate rRNAs and tRNAs for translation of oogenetic or maternal mRNAs to continue. Therefore, the best explanation is that continued development requires the synthesis of proteins using embryonic mRNAs (which would not be made in actinomycin D-treated embryos).

168. **D.** Embryos with smaller stockpiles of maternal RNAs usually initiate synthesis of embryonic RNAs earlier in development and this usually results in a slower rate of cleavage. Embryos with a greater stockpile of maternal RNAs would undergo cleavage more rapidly than embryos with a smaller stockpile of maternal RNAS.

169. **D.** Because the mouse zygote contains a minimal amount of maternal RNAs and initiates synthesis of embryonic RNAs early in cleavage, one might expect actinomycin D-treated embryos to arrest very early in development.

170. **D.** is the exception. A mature red blood cell does *not* have a nucleus or cytoplasmic organelles. They are lost during erythropoiesis. Choices **A, B,** and **C** *are* characteristics of an erythrocyte.

171. **C.** Macrophages residing in the liver and spleen engulf and break down the old erythrocyte, releasing hemoglobin, which is eventually broken down into iron and bilirubin; macrophage means "Big Eater."

172. **B.** This is a fact that needs to be committed to memory.

173. **A.** A *hypotonic* medium is one that has a lower osmotic pressure than the fluid of comparison in this example; the osmotic flow is from the solution *into* the cells; causing them to swell and ultimately burst. Remember osmotic water flow goes from regions of low to high osmotic pressure. The cells would shrink if placed in a hypertonic medium, that is, the fluid (water) in the cells would flow out into the surrounding medium.

174. **D.** The percentage of white blood cells varies as listed:
Agranular cells:
1. lymphocytes — 20–25%
2. monocytes — 3–8%
Granular cells:
1. neutrophils — 65–75%
2. eosinophils — 2–5%
3. basophils — 0.5% or less

175. **D.** Humans are very well protected against the dangers of their surroundings. The external layer of skin is practically impermeable; it protects against trauma, bacteria, drying, water penetration, ultraviolet light, noxious agents, etc. White blood cells are influential in the mobilization of the immunological machinery of the body and also have the capability to engulf bacteria, etc., and destroy them. After an antigen enters the organism, the immune system counters by producing antibodies to neutralize the effect and in many cases to protect the organism against susceptibility to the same agent in the future (the basis of immunization).

176. **B.** Hyperventilation is abnormally rapid, deep breathing resulting in a loss of CO_2 and an increase in blood pH. A person would be in the state of respiratory alkalosis since a decreased blood concentration of hydrogen ion is the result of pulmonary CO_2 elimination.

177. **A.** A reduction in venous blood return to the heart will result in an elevated P_{cap}. This increase in P_{cap} results in a larger driving force for fluid flow into the interstitium. There is no reason to believe that there would be a change in the

osmotic pressures, which are largely due to proteins trapped on either side of the capillary wall. In fact, swelling of the leg secondary to the increased interstitial fluid is a common clinical finding.

178. **C.** Osmotic pressure (π) is equal to $\pi = \sigma RTC$, where R is the gas constant, T is the temperature, C is the concentration of solutes, and σ is the reflection coefficient. The reflection coefficient is an empirically determined constant that is inversely related to the permeability of a solute for the capillary wall. The lack of protein in the capillary will result in a decrease in the capillary osmotic pressure and will decrease $\Delta\pi$. This decrease will result in a net flow of fluid toward the interstitium increasing the total volume of fluid in the interstitium.

179. **C.** A constriction bandage increases P_i which results in a decreased ΔP and a net fluid flow into the capillary. P_{cap} is determined by the arterial pressures, and there is no reason for oncotic pressures to change significantly with externally applied pressure. A constriction bandage is a common form of treatment to reduce swelling (i.e., excess interstitial volume).

180. **D.** As explained in question 178, the reflection coefficient is a measure of how effectively a solute is confined by a membrane. The higher the coefficient, the greater is the solute's contribution to the osmotic pressure in that compartment. Because urea is a nonpolar solute with a reflection coefficient of 0, it is freely permeable to the capillary wall. Therefore, in the steady state, the concentration of urea will be equal on both sides of capillary. Urea will contribute nothing to the difference in osmotic pressure or the net flux of fluid.

181. **D.** Active transport requires energy and allows a cell to move material from a point of lower concentration to a point of higher concentration.

182. **C.** The driving force (ΔP) causing air to flow into or out of the lungs is the pressure difference between the atmospheric pressure (P_{atm}) and the intra-alveolar pressure (P_{alv}). The absolute atmospheric or intra-alveolar pressures do not dictate air flow, it is the pressure difference that is important. Intrapleural pressure reflects lung elastic forces as well plus any smaller pressure difference between P_{atm} and P_{alv} while breathing. Thus, the absolute value of the intrapleural pressure has no bearing on inspiration.

183. **A.** During inspiration the chest wall enlarges, expanding the lungs and the intra-alveolar air. Thus, the intra-alveolar pressure transiently drops below atmospheric pressure, pulling air into the lungs. During expiration the chest wall collapses causing the intra-alveolar pressure to transiently go above atmospheric pressure and air flows out of the lungs. When intra-alveolar pressure equals atmospheric pressure, no air will flow into or out of the lungs. The intrapleural pressure will always be lower than the intra-alveolar pressure by an amount equal to the elastic forces of the lungs. Thus, intra-alveolar pressure never goes below intrapleural pressure.

184. **D.** As defined, the alveolar ventilation equals the amount of fresh air which reaches the alveoli per minute. Thus, alveolar ventilation is the amount of fresh air reaching the alveoli per breath times the number of breaths per minute. Because part of the fresh air inspired gets no farther than the anatomic dead space (i.e. it doesn't reach the alveoli), the fresh air actually reaching the alveoli equals the tidal volume minus the volume of the anatomic dead space. The frequency of breathing times any other lung volume equals something other than the alveolar ventilation.

185. **C.** With hypoventilation, oxygen delivery to the alveolar gas is less than normal and the partial pressure of oxygen will decrease. Concurrently, the removal of carbon dioxide from the alveolar compartment is less than normal and the partial pressure of carbon dioxide will increase.

186. **A.** Most carbon dioxide is transported as bicarbonate ions. A portion is also bound to the amino groups of various proteins and transported as carbamino-compounds, mainly carbamino-hemoglobin. Some is transported in physical solution as dissolved carbon dioxide. Hemoglobin that has carbon monoxide bound to it is called carboxyhemoglobin and is unrelated to the transportation of carbon dioxide.

187. **D.** This question requires the ability to read a graph. The vapor pressure of any of the compounds at a given temperature can be found by (1) running a vertical line from that temperature on the scale of the horizontal axis (abscissa) to its intersection with the graph (curve) for that compound, (2) running a horizontal line from that point to its intersection with the vertical axis (ordinate), (3) reading or estimating the vapor pressure from the scale on the ordinate. Because the curve for ethyl alcohol lies above the curve

for water and below the curve for chloroform at every temperature on this plot, the vapor pressure of ethyl alcohol will always be read as lower than that of chloroform and higher than that of water, regardless of the temperature.

188. **A.**   This question requires (1) the ability to read a graph, (2) a precise definition of the term "boiling point" as the temperature at which the vapor pressure of a liquid just equals the atmospheric pressure, (3) knowledge that standard atmospheric pressure (i.e., one atmosphere), which approximates atmospheric pressure at sea level is by convention 760 mm (Hg). (Knowing the boiling point of water [100°C], which is one of those reference points that everyone should know, one can deduce that the vertical dotted lines define the boiling points of the respective liquids, whereas the horizontal dotted line defines the vapor pressure at the boiling temperature.) Thus, the boiling point of any compound can be found by reading from the graph the temperature (boiling point) at which a vapor pressure of 760 mm (Hg) was attained. For chloroform, this is about 61°C.

189. **D.**   This is the reverse of question 187. Knowing that the normal boiling point of water is 100°C, one can follow the perpendicular (vertical) dotted line from 100 on the abscissa to the point of intersection with the graph for water. This point coincides with the horizontal dotted line which obviously represents the vapor pressure for all of the liquids at their normal boiling points, i.e., the standard atmospheric pressure. The vapor pressure read from the ordinate is approximately 760 mm (Hg).

190. **A.**   This question also requires the definition of boiling point as the temperature at which vapor pressure of a liquid equals atmospheric pressure. Although the pressure is not stated explicitly, it is stated that the pressure is less than standard atmospheric pressure. A cursory examination of the graph for water (or either of the other two liquids) reveals that vapor pressure increases as temperature increases and vice versa. Thus, if the vapor pressure required to equal atmospheric pressure is lower, the temperature (boiling point) required to attain that pressure should also be lower.

191. **B.**   This question requires (1) determination of the normal boiling point of ethyl alcohol, (2) determination of the vapor pressure of water at that temperature, i.e., the atmospheric pressure at

which water would boil at that temperature. As in the earlier examples, the normal boiling point of ethyl alcohol (about 78°C) can be read from the intersection of the graph for ethyl alcohol with the dotted line delineating 760 mm (Hg). The dotted line passing through this temperature intersects the graph for water at a point corresponding to 200–300 mm (Hg). This is the atmospheric pressure at which water would boil at 78°C. The only answer reasonably close to this value is **B,** 300.

192. **C.**   The methyl group of toluene is an *o, p*-directing group.

193. **D.**   The hydroxyl group is a highly activating group, whereas the chloro, nitro, and acetyl groups deactivate the ring towards electrophilic aromatic substitutions.

194. **B.**   Oxidation of toluene yields benzoic acid. Nitration would yield the meta isomer because the carboxyl group is meta directing.

195. **A.**   The methyl group activates the *o, p*-positions and directs the Br to the ortho position. The nitro group is a meta directing deactivating group.

196. **B.**   The nitration of benzene involves the attack of a nitronium ion, NO^+_2, on toluene to form a cyclohexadienyl cation as the intermediate.

197. **C.**   Valine is one of the nine essential amino acids, whereas linoleic acid is the only true essential fatty acid. Vitamin E is fat soluble and found in foods. Glucose is essential, but is obtained in other forms, such as polysaccharides. Polysaccharides contain many monosaccharide units joined in long chains and among the most important are starch and cellulose. Starch is the reserve carbohydrate in plants and on complete hydrolysis it yields glucose.

198. **D.**   Linoleic, linolenic, and arachidonic acids (polyunsaturated) are listed as essential fatty acids, because they cannot be synthesized by the animal and must therefore be provided in the diet. Among the water soluble vitamins are thiamine, biotin, and niacin.

199. **B.**   The fat soluble vitamins are vitamins A, D, E, and K. The water soluble vitamins are vitamin C, thiamine, riboflavin, niacin , vitamin B_6, folacin, vitamin B_{12}, biotin, and pantothenic acid.

200. **D.** The bulk essential minerals are calcium, phosphorus, and magnesium, whereas the trace essential minerals are iron, zinc, selenium, iodine, cobalt, molybdenum, manganese, copper, chromium, and fluoride.

201. **C.** Amino acids are derived from proteins; carbohydrates that are polyhydroxy aldehydes and the simplest carbohydrate units are known as monosaccharides. The most important monosaccharide is glucose; it is obtained by the hydrolysis of starch. Fat and oil comprise one of the three main classes of food. Fats and oils are esters of glycerol with carboxylic acids.

202. **B.** Parathyroid hormone acts upon bone, eliciting changes in calcium and phosphorus. Osteoclasts are the cells stimulated by parathyroid hormone to facilitate the resorption of calcium and phosphorus from bone. Administration of parathyroid hormone to animals without parathyroids results in an increase of phosphorus excretion in the urine, a fall in serum inorgamic phosphorus levels, an increase in serum calcium, and an increase of calcium excretion in the urine.

203. **C.** Excretion concerns itself with the elimination of water (fluid) and metabolic wastes, whereas egestion is the process of eliminating undigested food materials. Catabolism is the chemical breakdown of molecules.

204. **A.** In anaerobic respiration glucose is converted to two molecules of the 3-carbon compound pyruvic acid. In aerobic respiration, glucose is converted to six molecules each of carbon dioxide and water. Anaerobic respiration is only about 3% as efficient as aerobic respiration. The anaerobic pathway is the same as the aerobic to the pyruvic acid stage.

205. **B.** LH (luteinizing hormone) is secreted by the pituitary gland. In the male, it is also called ICSH (interstitial, cell stimulating, hormone) from its effects on the testes. In our case, half of each group had its testes removed. This eliminates the feedback from testes to pituitary. Comparison of AM and PM readings for intact rats shows no significant differences in LH levels. For orchidectomized rats, levels vary widely, with no consistent AM-PM relationship.

206. **B.** Also see explanation for question 205, but note that hypothalamic areas of the brain secrete luteinizing releasing factor (LRF), which via the hypothalamo-pituitary portal system reaches the anterior pituitary to initiate luteinizing hormone production. LH then acts on the gonads to produce ova in the female. In this experiment Drug X probably blocks LRF because when LRF is administered with the drug, ovulation takes place. Statement **D** is neither supported nor contradicted by the information presented and has no impact.

207. **B.** It is obvious from the table that there is no population growth in West Germany and that the longest doubling time can be attributed to Japan; Holland has the largest excess of births over deaths, so it has the greatest rate of population growth.

208. **B.** Chemicals, X rays, cosmic rays, and so forth can exert an effect on tissues. Radiation supplemented by chemotherapy is used to treat patients with cancer, whereas ultraviolet rays may cause or facilitate the development of skin cancer. Our experiments were designed to determine if X-radiation causes an alteration in water consumption and volume of salivary glands in rats. The graph illustrates that the first parameter that was affected by 6400R was food intake; the above was evident at 3 days after irradiation. Water consumption was the least affected parameter.

209. **D.** Estrogen production by the corpus luteum diminishes drastically during pregnancy, and could stop altogether at or before parturition. There is no evidence to indicate whether the increased estrogen comes from reactivation of the corpus luteum or from some other follicle.

210. **B.** Injection routes are critical in the action of materials that stimulate immune responses. The purpose of the study was to determine the effect of different routes of administration on antibody titer. It is clear that intradermal administration produced the highest titer while there was little difference between subscapular and subcutaneous injection routes.

211. **D.** At 32 hours, liver triglycerides were little more for drug and ethanol than for glucose, so **A** is correct. **B** is correct because the ethanol graph peaks at 16 hours. **C** refers to the effects of ethanol, which produced three times as much triglycerides than glucose did.

212. **A.** The table shows that an increase in red blood cells was present at 6.5 minutes after the event. Statements **B** and **D** are neither supported nor contradicted by the data, but statement **C** is

contradicted because there was a return to control values by 18.5 minutes.

213. **B.** Photosynthesis occurs in the chloroplasts of green plants. and sugars are formed from carbon dioxide and water in the presence of light and chlorophyll. During the process, light or radiant energy is converted to chemical energy in the form of carbohydrates. The basic reaction is:

$$6 \, CO_2 + 6 \, H_2O \rightarrow C_6H_{12}O_6 + 6 \, O_2$$

In our experiment without changing the incident sunlight, the largest percentage increase that is theoretically possible is predicted for kelp; if one doubled the incident light on kelp it most likely would approach the carbohydrate yield of plant Z.

214. **D.** Even though several variables are presented, sample 3 clearly shows the occurrence of less decay. Statement **A** is neither supported nor contradicted by the information. Statement **B** is contradicted by the information. Statement **C** is consistent with the information but includes an assumption of causation that cannot be assessed using the information given.

215. **C.** The object of this experiment was to determine the effect of ascorbic acid deficiency on the immunologic system. Two conclusions can be reached from an examination of the data: the scorbutic guinea pig probably has a partial immunologic deficiency and its lymphocyte reactivity is independent of gamma globulin concentration. There was no change in GG concentration, whereas lymphocyte reactivity dropped drastically.

216. **D.** The general formula C_nH_{2n-2} applies to all members of the alkyne series. The suffix for names in this series is "yne." Ethyne is the only choice that has the correct ending.

217. **C.** Ethers have the general formula R–O–R'. The other compounds have the following general formulas:

$$\text{esters} \quad R-C \underset{\textstyle O-R'}{\overset{\textstyle O}{\vphantom{|}}}$$

esters
$$R-C\begin{smallmatrix} \parallel O \\ \diagdown \\ O-R' \end{smallmatrix}$$

aldehydes
$$R-C\begin{smallmatrix} \parallel O \\ \diagdown \\ H \end{smallmatrix}$$

alcohols   R–OH

218. **D.** This configuration:
$$-C-OH \\ \parallel \\ O$$

is characteristic of carboxyl groups. A hydroxyl group is identified by –OH.

219. **C.**
$$\varnothing CH_2Cl + \varnothing \xrightarrow{AlCl_3} \varnothing - CH_2 - \varnothing$$
Friedel-Crafts Reaction

$$\varnothing CH_2Cl + Na \longrightarrow \varnothing - CH_2CH_2 - \varnothing$$
Wurtz Reaction

The MCAT
Model Examination B

ANSWER SHEET

DIRECTIONS: After locating the number of the question to which you are responding, fill in the circle containing the letter of the answer you have selected. Use pencil (not a ballpoint pen) to completely blacken the circle.

VERBAL REASONING

1. Ⓐ Ⓑ Ⓒ Ⓓ
2. Ⓐ Ⓑ Ⓒ Ⓓ
3. Ⓐ Ⓑ Ⓒ Ⓓ
4. Ⓐ Ⓑ Ⓒ Ⓓ
5. Ⓐ Ⓑ Ⓒ Ⓓ
6. Ⓐ Ⓑ Ⓒ Ⓓ
7. Ⓐ Ⓑ Ⓒ Ⓓ
8. Ⓐ Ⓑ Ⓒ Ⓓ
9. Ⓐ Ⓑ Ⓒ Ⓓ
10. Ⓐ Ⓑ Ⓒ Ⓓ
11. Ⓐ Ⓑ Ⓒ Ⓓ
12. Ⓐ Ⓑ Ⓒ Ⓓ
13. Ⓐ Ⓑ Ⓒ Ⓓ
14. Ⓐ Ⓑ Ⓒ Ⓓ
15. Ⓐ Ⓑ Ⓒ Ⓓ
16. Ⓐ Ⓑ Ⓒ Ⓓ
17. Ⓐ Ⓑ Ⓒ Ⓓ
18. Ⓐ Ⓑ Ⓒ Ⓓ
19. Ⓐ Ⓑ Ⓒ Ⓓ
20. Ⓐ Ⓑ Ⓒ Ⓓ
21. Ⓐ Ⓑ Ⓒ Ⓓ
22. Ⓐ Ⓑ Ⓒ Ⓓ
23. Ⓐ Ⓑ Ⓒ Ⓓ
24. Ⓐ Ⓑ Ⓒ Ⓓ
25. Ⓐ Ⓑ Ⓒ Ⓓ
26. Ⓐ Ⓑ Ⓒ Ⓓ
27. Ⓐ Ⓑ Ⓒ Ⓓ
28. Ⓐ Ⓑ Ⓒ Ⓓ
29. Ⓐ Ⓑ Ⓒ Ⓓ
30. Ⓐ Ⓑ Ⓒ Ⓓ

31. Ⓐ Ⓑ Ⓒ Ⓓ
32. Ⓐ Ⓑ Ⓒ Ⓓ
33. Ⓐ Ⓑ Ⓒ Ⓓ
34. Ⓐ Ⓑ Ⓒ Ⓓ
35. Ⓐ Ⓑ Ⓒ Ⓓ
36. Ⓐ Ⓑ Ⓒ Ⓓ
37. Ⓐ Ⓑ Ⓒ Ⓓ
38. Ⓐ Ⓑ Ⓒ Ⓓ
39. Ⓐ Ⓑ Ⓒ Ⓓ
40. Ⓐ Ⓑ Ⓒ Ⓓ
41. Ⓐ Ⓑ Ⓒ Ⓓ
42. Ⓐ Ⓑ Ⓒ Ⓓ
43. Ⓐ Ⓑ Ⓒ Ⓓ
44. Ⓐ Ⓑ Ⓒ Ⓓ
45. Ⓐ Ⓑ Ⓒ Ⓓ
46. Ⓐ Ⓑ Ⓒ Ⓓ
47. Ⓐ Ⓑ Ⓒ Ⓓ
48. Ⓐ Ⓑ Ⓒ Ⓓ
49. Ⓐ Ⓑ Ⓒ Ⓓ
50. Ⓐ Ⓑ Ⓒ Ⓓ
51. Ⓐ Ⓑ Ⓒ Ⓓ
52. Ⓐ Ⓑ Ⓒ Ⓓ
53. Ⓐ Ⓑ Ⓒ Ⓓ
54. Ⓐ Ⓑ Ⓒ Ⓓ
55. Ⓐ Ⓑ Ⓒ Ⓓ
56. Ⓐ Ⓑ Ⓒ Ⓓ
57. Ⓐ Ⓑ Ⓒ Ⓓ
58. Ⓐ Ⓑ Ⓒ Ⓓ
59. Ⓐ Ⓑ Ⓒ Ⓓ
60. Ⓐ Ⓑ Ⓒ Ⓓ

61. Ⓐ Ⓑ Ⓒ Ⓓ
62. Ⓐ Ⓑ Ⓒ Ⓓ
63. Ⓐ Ⓑ Ⓒ Ⓓ
64. Ⓐ Ⓑ Ⓒ Ⓓ
65. Ⓐ Ⓑ Ⓒ Ⓓ

PHYSICAL SCIENCES

66. Ⓐ Ⓑ Ⓒ Ⓓ
67. Ⓐ Ⓑ Ⓒ Ⓓ
68. Ⓐ Ⓑ Ⓒ Ⓓ
69. Ⓐ Ⓑ Ⓒ Ⓓ
70. Ⓐ Ⓑ Ⓒ Ⓓ
71. Ⓐ Ⓑ Ⓒ Ⓓ
72. Ⓐ Ⓑ Ⓒ Ⓓ
73. Ⓐ Ⓑ Ⓒ Ⓓ
74. Ⓐ Ⓑ Ⓒ Ⓓ
75. Ⓐ Ⓑ Ⓒ Ⓓ
76. Ⓐ Ⓑ Ⓒ Ⓓ
77. Ⓐ Ⓑ Ⓒ Ⓓ
78. Ⓐ Ⓑ Ⓒ Ⓓ
79. Ⓐ Ⓑ Ⓒ Ⓓ
80. Ⓐ Ⓑ Ⓒ Ⓓ
81. Ⓐ Ⓑ Ⓒ Ⓓ
82. Ⓐ Ⓑ Ⓒ Ⓓ
83. Ⓐ Ⓑ Ⓒ Ⓓ
84. Ⓐ Ⓑ Ⓒ Ⓓ
85. Ⓐ Ⓑ Ⓒ Ⓓ
86. Ⓐ Ⓑ Ⓒ Ⓓ
87. Ⓐ Ⓑ Ⓒ Ⓓ
88. Ⓐ Ⓑ Ⓒ Ⓓ

89. Ⓐ Ⓑ Ⓒ Ⓓ
90. Ⓐ Ⓑ Ⓒ Ⓓ
91. Ⓐ Ⓑ Ⓒ Ⓓ
92. Ⓐ Ⓑ Ⓒ Ⓓ
93. Ⓐ Ⓑ Ⓒ Ⓓ
94. Ⓐ Ⓑ Ⓒ Ⓓ
95. Ⓐ Ⓑ Ⓒ Ⓓ
96. Ⓐ Ⓑ Ⓒ Ⓓ
97. Ⓐ Ⓑ Ⓒ Ⓓ
98. Ⓐ Ⓑ Ⓒ Ⓓ
99. Ⓐ Ⓑ Ⓒ Ⓓ
100. Ⓐ Ⓑ Ⓒ Ⓓ
101. Ⓐ Ⓑ Ⓒ Ⓓ
102. Ⓐ Ⓑ Ⓒ Ⓓ
103. Ⓐ Ⓑ Ⓒ Ⓓ
104. Ⓐ Ⓑ Ⓒ Ⓓ
105. Ⓐ Ⓑ Ⓒ Ⓓ
106. Ⓐ Ⓑ Ⓒ Ⓓ
107. Ⓐ Ⓑ Ⓒ Ⓓ
108. Ⓐ Ⓑ Ⓒ Ⓓ
109. Ⓐ Ⓑ Ⓒ Ⓓ
110. Ⓐ Ⓑ Ⓒ Ⓓ
111. Ⓐ Ⓑ Ⓒ Ⓓ
112. Ⓐ Ⓑ Ⓒ Ⓓ
113. Ⓐ Ⓑ Ⓒ Ⓓ
114. Ⓐ Ⓑ Ⓒ Ⓓ
115. Ⓐ Ⓑ Ⓒ Ⓓ
116. Ⓐ Ⓑ Ⓒ Ⓓ
117. Ⓐ Ⓑ Ⓒ Ⓓ
118. Ⓐ Ⓑ Ⓒ Ⓓ

119. Ⓐ Ⓑ Ⓒ Ⓓ
120. Ⓐ Ⓑ Ⓒ Ⓓ
121. Ⓐ Ⓑ Ⓒ Ⓓ
122. Ⓐ Ⓑ Ⓒ Ⓓ
123. Ⓐ Ⓑ Ⓒ Ⓓ
124. Ⓐ Ⓑ Ⓒ Ⓓ
125. Ⓐ Ⓑ Ⓒ Ⓓ
126. Ⓐ Ⓑ Ⓒ Ⓓ
127. Ⓐ Ⓑ Ⓒ Ⓓ
128. Ⓐ Ⓑ Ⓒ Ⓓ
129. Ⓐ Ⓑ Ⓒ Ⓓ
130. Ⓐ Ⓑ Ⓒ Ⓓ
131. Ⓐ Ⓑ Ⓒ Ⓓ
132. Ⓐ Ⓑ Ⓒ Ⓓ
133. Ⓐ Ⓑ Ⓒ Ⓓ
134. Ⓐ Ⓑ Ⓒ Ⓓ
135. Ⓐ Ⓑ Ⓒ Ⓓ
136. Ⓐ Ⓑ Ⓒ Ⓓ
137. Ⓐ Ⓑ Ⓒ Ⓓ
138. Ⓐ Ⓑ Ⓒ Ⓓ
139. Ⓐ Ⓑ Ⓒ Ⓓ
140. Ⓐ Ⓑ Ⓒ Ⓓ
141. Ⓐ Ⓑ Ⓒ Ⓓ
142. Ⓐ Ⓑ Ⓒ Ⓓ

WRITING SAMPLE
Use separate ruled sheets of
paper.

BIOLOGICAL SCIENCES

143. Ⓐ Ⓑ Ⓒ Ⓓ
144. Ⓐ Ⓑ Ⓒ Ⓓ
145. Ⓐ Ⓑ Ⓒ Ⓓ
146. Ⓐ Ⓑ Ⓒ Ⓓ
147. Ⓐ Ⓑ Ⓒ Ⓓ
148. Ⓐ Ⓑ Ⓒ Ⓓ
149. Ⓐ Ⓑ Ⓒ Ⓓ
150. Ⓐ Ⓑ Ⓒ Ⓓ
151. Ⓐ Ⓑ Ⓒ Ⓓ
152. Ⓐ Ⓑ Ⓒ Ⓓ
153. Ⓐ Ⓑ Ⓒ Ⓓ
154. Ⓐ Ⓑ Ⓒ Ⓓ
155. Ⓐ Ⓑ Ⓒ Ⓓ
156. Ⓐ Ⓑ Ⓒ Ⓓ
157. Ⓐ Ⓑ Ⓒ Ⓓ
158. Ⓐ Ⓑ Ⓒ Ⓓ
159. Ⓐ Ⓑ Ⓒ Ⓓ
160. Ⓐ Ⓑ Ⓒ Ⓓ
161. Ⓐ Ⓑ Ⓒ Ⓓ
162. Ⓐ Ⓑ Ⓒ Ⓓ
163. Ⓐ Ⓑ Ⓒ Ⓓ
164. Ⓐ Ⓑ Ⓒ Ⓓ
165. Ⓐ Ⓑ Ⓒ Ⓓ
166. Ⓐ Ⓑ Ⓒ Ⓓ
167. Ⓐ Ⓑ Ⓒ Ⓓ

168. Ⓐ Ⓑ Ⓒ Ⓓ
169. Ⓐ Ⓑ Ⓒ Ⓓ
170. Ⓐ Ⓑ Ⓒ Ⓓ
171. Ⓐ Ⓑ Ⓒ Ⓓ
172. Ⓐ Ⓑ Ⓒ Ⓓ
173. Ⓐ Ⓑ Ⓒ Ⓓ
174. Ⓐ Ⓑ Ⓒ Ⓓ
175. Ⓐ Ⓑ Ⓒ Ⓓ
176. Ⓐ Ⓑ Ⓒ Ⓓ
177. Ⓐ Ⓑ Ⓒ Ⓓ
178. Ⓐ Ⓑ Ⓒ Ⓓ
179. Ⓐ Ⓑ Ⓒ Ⓓ
180. Ⓐ Ⓑ Ⓒ Ⓓ
181. Ⓐ Ⓑ Ⓒ Ⓓ
182. Ⓐ Ⓑ Ⓒ Ⓓ
183. Ⓐ Ⓑ Ⓒ Ⓓ
184. Ⓐ Ⓑ Ⓒ Ⓓ
185. Ⓐ Ⓑ Ⓒ Ⓓ
186. Ⓐ Ⓑ Ⓒ Ⓓ Ⓔ
187. Ⓐ Ⓑ Ⓒ Ⓓ
188. Ⓐ Ⓑ Ⓒ Ⓓ
189. Ⓐ Ⓑ Ⓒ Ⓓ Ⓔ
190. Ⓐ Ⓑ Ⓒ Ⓓ
191. Ⓐ Ⓑ Ⓒ Ⓓ
192. Ⓐ Ⓑ Ⓒ Ⓓ
193. Ⓐ Ⓑ Ⓒ Ⓓ

194. Ⓐ Ⓑ Ⓒ Ⓓ
195. Ⓐ Ⓑ Ⓒ Ⓓ
196. Ⓐ Ⓑ Ⓒ Ⓓ
197. Ⓐ Ⓑ Ⓒ Ⓓ
198. Ⓐ Ⓑ Ⓒ Ⓓ
199. Ⓐ Ⓑ Ⓒ Ⓓ
200. Ⓐ Ⓑ Ⓒ Ⓓ
201. Ⓐ Ⓑ Ⓒ Ⓓ
202. Ⓐ Ⓑ Ⓒ Ⓓ
203. Ⓐ Ⓑ Ⓒ Ⓓ
204. Ⓐ Ⓑ Ⓒ Ⓓ
205. Ⓐ Ⓑ Ⓒ Ⓓ
206. Ⓐ Ⓑ Ⓒ Ⓓ
207. Ⓐ Ⓑ Ⓒ Ⓓ
208. Ⓐ Ⓑ Ⓒ Ⓓ
209. Ⓐ Ⓑ Ⓒ Ⓓ
210. Ⓐ Ⓑ Ⓒ Ⓓ
211. Ⓐ Ⓑ Ⓒ Ⓓ
212. Ⓐ Ⓑ Ⓒ Ⓓ
213. Ⓐ Ⓑ Ⓒ Ⓓ
214. Ⓐ Ⓑ Ⓒ Ⓓ
215. Ⓐ Ⓑ Ⓒ Ⓓ
216. Ⓐ Ⓑ Ⓒ Ⓓ
217. Ⓐ Ⓑ Ⓒ Ⓓ
218. Ⓐ Ⓑ Ⓒ Ⓓ
219. Ⓐ Ⓑ Ⓒ Ⓓ

The MCAT
Model Examination B

VERBAL REASONING

9 PASSAGES
65 QUESTIONS
85 MINUTES

DIRECTIONS: The questions are based on the accompanying passages. Read each passage carefully, then answer the following questions. Consider only the material within the passage. For each question, select the *ONE BEST ANSWER* and indicate your selection by marking the corresponding letter on the Answer Form.

Passage I (Questions 1–8)

What is the essence of graphic design? How do graphic designers solve problems, organize space, and imbue their work with those visual and symbolic qualities that enable it to convey visual and verbal information with expression and clarity? The extraordinary flowering of graphic design in our time—as a potent means of communication and a major component of our visual culture—increases the need for designers, clients, and students to comprehend its essence.

Traditionally, graphic designers looked to architecture or painting for their model. Certainly, a universal language of form is common to all visual disciplines, and in some historical periods the various design arts have shared styles. Too much dependence upon other arts—or even on the universal language of form—is unsatisfactory, however, because graphic design has unique purposes and visual properties.

Graphic design is a hybrid discipline. Diverse elements including signs, symbols, words, and pictures are collected and assembled into a total message. The dual nature of these graphic elements as both communicative sign and visual form provides endless fascination and potential for invention and combination. Although all the visual arts share properties of either two- or three-dimensional space, graphic space has a special character born from its communicative function.

Perhaps the most important thing that graphic design does is give communications resonance, a richness of tone that heightens the expressive power of the page. It transcends the dry conveyance of information, intensi-

fies the message, and enriches the audience's experience. Resonance helps the designer realize clear public goals: to instruct, to delight, and to motivate.

Most designers speak of their activities as a problem-solving process because designers seek solutions to public communications problems. Approaches to problem solving vary, based on the problem at hand and the working methods of the designer. At a time when Western nations are evolving from industrial to information cultures, a comprehensive understanding of our communicative forms and graphic design becomes increasingly critical.

The general public does not understand graphic design and art direction. Designers tell the story of a graphic designer trying to explain this job to Grandmother. The designer shows Grandmother a recent project and says, "You were asking me about what I do, Grandmother. I'm a graphic designer, and I designed this."

Pointing to the photograph in the design, the grandmother asks, "Did you draw that picture?"

"No, Grandmother, it's a photograph. I didn't draw it, but I planned it, chose the photographer, helped select the models, assisted in setting it up, art-directed the shooting session, chose which shot to use, and cropped the picture."

"Did you write what it says, then?"

"Well, no," the designer replies, "But I did brainstorm with the copywriter to develop the concept."

"Oh, I see. Then you did letter these big words?" asks the grandmother, pointing to the headline.

"Uh, no, a typesetter set the copywriter's words in type, but I specified the typefaces and sizes to be used," responds the designer.

"Well, did you draw this little picture down in the corner?"

Used with permission of Philip B. Meggs and John T. Bryan, *Type and Image*, 1989.

"No, but I selected the illustrator, told her what needed to be drawn, and decided where to put it and how big to make it."

"Oh. Well, did you draw this little, what do you call it, a trademark?"

"Uh, no. A design firm that specializes in visual identification programs designed it for the client."

The grandmother is somewhat confused about just what it is that her grandchild does and why credit is claimed for all these other people's work.

1. The object of this passage is to:

    A. convince the reader that graphic designers are artists.
    B. illustrate the fact that the general public does not comprehend what graphic designers actually do.
    C. underscore the fact that understanding graphic design is essential in an information culture.
    D. provide the reader with a glimpse of the importance of graphic design in today's culture, as well as of its diverse nature.

2. According to this passage, graphic design today:

    A. is an important communication tool, as well as a major component of our visual culture.
    B. provides employment for people such as artists, directors, photographers, and writers.
    C. depends too much on other art forms.
    D. is a traditional discipline based on architectural design.

3. The author believes that the most important function of graphic design is to:

    A. provide attractive visual displays for the public.
    B. help Western culture make the transition from a technical to a communication oriented society.
    C. give communications resonance, thus helping the designer realize clear public goals: to instruct, to delight, and to motivate.
    D. bring diversity to the art field.

4. Based on the information in the passage, what do graphic designers actually do?

    I. seek solutions to public communication problems
    II. organize space
    III. imbue their work with visual and symbolic qualities

    A. I only
    B. II only
    C. I and II only
    D. I, II, and III

5. Which of the following statements best supports the notion that graphic design is a *hybrid* discipline?

    A. The extraordinary flowering of graphic design in our time increases the need for designers who have the ability to problem solve.
    B. In graphic arts, diverse elements—including signs, symbols, words, and pictures—are collected and assembled into a total message.
    C. Graphic design transcends the dry conveyance of information.
    D. Graphic design has unique purposes and a special character.

6. The author feels that the general public does not understand the concept of graphic design. Which of the following reasons best describes why this confusion probably exists?

    A. Graphic designers confuse the general public because they have a difficult time describing what their actual role is in the production of a project.
    B. The general public is not really interested in a description of the makeup of graphic design.
    C. Confusion is caused by the fact that graphic designers do not single-handedly produce a product, such as a painting or a photograph. Their job is to *orchestrate* a variety of people and sources in order to creatively solve communication problems through visual means.
    D. The designer's end product is the only thing that the general public is concerned about.

7. Which of the following statements *least* supports the idea that graphic design is important in a communication culture?

    A. One important aspect of graphic arts is its ability to convey both verbal and visual information with clarity.
    B. Graphic arts heightens the expressive power of a page.
    C. Instruction and motivation are two goals that graphic designers have in mind when producing a piece of work.

D. Architecture and painting were considered the traditional models for graphic design.

8. According to the passage, graphic design shares the following commonality with other visual disciplines:

A. a dual nature and unique purpose.
B. the expression of verbal information.
C. heavy dependence on other art forms.
D. a universal language of form.

Passage II (Questions 9–16)

Until recently, scientific data were a convenient tool in the scientific process, with the following steps: (1) formulating a question; (2) ascertaining what is known; (3) formulating a testable hypothesis; (4) conducting observations and collecting data; (5) analyzing the data and relating them to existing information; (6) formulating a new or modified hypothesis; and (7) initiating a new round of studies until the question is answered, abandoned or restated. At various periods in the age of enlightenment, different components of the scientific method have been emphasized. Early on, propositions were formulated and debated with minimum organized observation or collection of data. The age of philosophers gave way to the age of observers, such as the astronomers who gazed at the sky and mapped the thousands of points of light, the naturalists who described and collected plants and animals, and the explorers who mapped rivers and oceans, coasts and mountains. Observers of nature gave way to the industrial age, during which inventors focused on solutions, oftentimes without well formulated questions, theory, or review of prior work. Naturalists and inventors recorded their observations in journals or log books as personalized memory aids. Inventors carried record keeping a step forward as a means of economy, to prevent repetition of failed trials. In all of these circumstances, however, the records were a convenient tool of and for the individual. Data records of concepts and observations took on a new meaning during the age of inventions. Inventors sought to profit from their creations, not only by building and selling a better "mousetrap" but also by seeking legal protection under constitutionally guaranteed rights to patent intellectual property. Records of data became a part of the documentation for priority, due diligence and breadth of a claim. Record keeping for commercialization of intellectual property now has become formalized, standardized, and required.

During the past few decades, records of data have become essential components of the documentation for regulatory agencies approving utility, efficacy, or safety of new products or appliances. Progressively, regulatory agencies have extended the scope of their oversight, specifying some aspects of experimental design, data collection, and analysis. Most recently, regulatory agencies have insisted that all data collected be retained and made available for inspection, even data from aborted or defective studies. Data keeping and storage have become ends unto themselves, initially to ensure that work paid for was actually done and subsequently to ensure that unwanted results (e.g., toxicity of a drug) were not suppressed. It is perhaps a logical extension that managers of public funds have focused upon records of data as documentation that work paid for was actually done, much as an auditor of public accounts matches purchase orders, invoices, and disbursements. The managers of public funds, lacking the technical expertise to judge the quality and value of scientific investigations, have turned to process rather than product to demonstrate their diligence in protecting the taxpayers' money. The increased reliance on process rather than output measures reflects, in part, a loss of confidence by the public in the scientific community to have the ability and the will to judge and police itself. Regrettably, there are some bases for this loss of confidence in scientific peer review, and this loss of confidence permeates the scientific community itself as well as the managers of public funds.

Regardless of the cause, an increasing emphasis is now placed on data keeping and data storage. Any discussion on scientific data presupposes that there is general agreement on the definition of *data*. Unfortunately, there is no universally accepted definition of *data*. Perhaps the best we can do is conclude that, like pornography, we know *data* when we see them, or that data are defined by some unspecified *community standard*. Are data the holographic notes entered personally and immediately by the observer? Are data the printouts from apparatus? Are data the printouts of computers that accept input from the observer or directly from apparatus? Are data the embedded pieces of tissue from a treated animal, or the stained sections made from the tissue, or the notes of the observer examining the tissue, or all of these, or none of these? What are "materials and methods" as distinguished from "data" and from interpretation? How do we meet the demand that scientists must properly keep and store data, when we do not know what data are and whether or not they can be kept and stored other than by written notes of the observer or photographs of an event? Finally, who is responsible for keeping and storing data?

9. The passage could be entitled:

A. Scientific Experimentation.
B. Scientific Method.
C. Scientific Responsibility.
D. Scientific Data.

Adapted from *Basic Science*, S. Gaylen Bradley, 1990.

10. Throughout the history of experimentation and development of new knowledge:

A. the scientific method has been painstakingly applied and followed.
B. formulating a hypothesis has been a critical element in progress.
C. emphasis within the application of the scientific method has varied.
D. scientific data has been compared, analyzed, and scrutinized.

11. Using information provided in the passage, one would NOT be justified in concluding that:

I. all scientific experimentation and observation throughout history was based on strict recording and analysis of data.
II. philosophy about matter eventually turned to the scientific approach.
III. with industrialization came a method of solving questions utilizing the scientific approach.
IV. industrialization was interested and emphasized practical solutions.

A. I, II, and III   **C.** II and IV
B. I and III   **D.** IV only

12. The passage contradicts which of the following?

I. Inventors sought constitutional protection.
II. At the present, record keeping is an essential element of society.
III. Regulatory agencies can require complete documentation of data.
IV. Failed or aborted experiments do not need to be scrutinized because they are of little benefit.

A. I, II, and III   **C.** II and IV
B. I and III   **D.** IV only

13. Which of the following statement(s) is/are *supported by* the passage?

I. The criteria for a definition of data are fairly well established.
II. Data are verified by a computer printout.
III. Data must be recorded and stored.
IV. Responsibility for data storage rests upon the investigator.

A. I, II, and III   **C.** II and IV
B. I and III   **D.** none of the above

14. Which of the conclusions listed below follow(s) from the information contained in the passage?

I. There has been an evolution in the methodology of recording data.
II. After a foiled experiment, a modified hypothesis is part of the scientific approach.
III. Data storage has been utilized as an end unto itself in order to ensure completion of a project.
IV. Managers of public funds are usually well qualified to judge scientific work.

A. I, II, and III   **C.** II and IV
B. I and III   **D.** IV only

15. The passage argues that:

A. the public's money is well protected.
B. the public has trust in the scientific community.
C. the scientific community polices itself appropriately.
D. data collection and storage are increasingly stressed.

16. The passage would support the argument that:

A. scientific data are obtained after careful experimentation.
B. computerization will enhance the accuracy of data collection and keeping it appropriately.
C. regulatory agencies, the public, and the scientific community are working together in the venture to evaluate data and use it properly.
D. none of the above statements is addressed directly by the author.

Passage III (Questions 17–24)

It has become obvious in recent years that the decision-making power in many school districts is shifting, and is becoming more liberalized as both teachers and parents realize that they are an important facet in the total school operation. They know that without their support and cooperation the system cannot continue to function smoothly.

Consequently, today's educator is no longer content to sit in the background and let decisions be made and programs formulated. New teachers want a voice, they demand a piece of the action, and they are daring enough to question the judgments of the system in their desire to achieve a better educational experience for their students as well as a more economically realistic position for themselves.

Not too many years ago, perhaps as little as a decade in some areas, the decision-making power in a school system could have been observed by quickly glancing at an organizational chart that would most probably have looked like this:

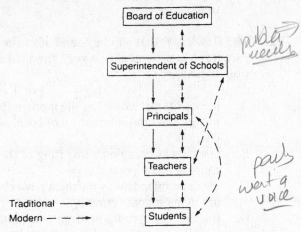

Although much simplified, the chart indicates a flow of power from the school board to the superintendent of schools down to the individual school principals and from there to the teachers and, finally, a minimal involvement of the students themselves.

The board of education was naturally found at the top, for it was assumed that this body represented the tax-paying community. Next in importance was the superintendent, whose word was considered to be law and who would, if so disposed, allow the principal some freedom to make decisions.

By the same token, those principals that prided themselves in being of a democratic nature, would then allow teachers to have a voice in selected matters and would even possibly afford students the opportunity of making minute decisions in appropriate areas.

Within the confines of the individual school, the principal was looked upon as the one person who knew more about educational matters than any other member of the staff. Therefore, he or she was spotlighted not only as the chief administrator, but as the supreme educational leader of the complex. Teachers occupied the place of facilitators, whose main job it was to take the programs that were handed down to them and see that they were carried out satisfactorily. The students were viewed as receptacles for receiving and digesting information. Their major contribution rested in being accepted to an institution of higher learning, thus making the system look good and giving the taxpayers the feeling that the money they spent was, after all, worthwhile.

The entire pattern of decision making, as presented, was based on the very real fact that the board of education controlled the purse strings of a school system.

From Hugo R. Seibel and Kenneth E. Guyer, *How to Prepare for the Medical College Admission Test*, 6th ed. Hauppauge, New York: Barron's Educational Series, Inc., 1990.

Because money has always been of supreme importance, it was considered the most logical path to follow. Few people thought to question its wisdom or bothered to seek alternatives.

The modern public has slowly come to realize that even though money is still the most crucial factor in operating an efficient school system, there are also other vital and important elements that contribute to its success.

For example, parents are demanding a voice in the operation of local schools. They favor an open door policy that affords them the opportunity to see what is going on in the classrooms and allows many of them to get involved on a parent-volunteer basis. Parents speak out in many cases by manipulating a very vital school input, over which they have strict control, namely their children. Thus we read of such things as parents keeping their offspring out of school to protest situations that they find unsuitable and intolerable. Even though these actions may not in themselves solve the problems, they do cause those in authority to sit up, take notice, and search for possible solutions at a speedy rate.

Every bit as important as the public's realization of its powers, is the teachers' realization that they too have a commodity that is of supreme importance to the system, and that is themselves. When teachers join forces and remove this vital input, school systems are forced to close and the educational machine comes to a halt. Teachers' strikes are now occurring more and more frequently in all areas of the country, and the threat of the entire profession becoming unionized is no longer a laughing matter.

Today's wise school systems have made note of these developments and are attempting to deal with them reasonably. Sharing the decision-making power by allowing more realistic and meaningful input from both parents and teachers has become a reality in many districts. Although a revised look at the power flow chart today would probably show the players in the same basic positions, it would certainly have the arrows of decision coming not only down in a direct line, but also pointing up and out, allowing for a much more liberalized flow of communication and ideas.

17. The central theme of this passage deals with:

A. the position of absolute power that is held by school boards in this country.

B. the militant attitude that is displayed by many modern teachers.

C. the shifting of decision-making power in today's school systems from that of a top down, authoritarian model to one that is more decentralized in nature.

D. increased parent interest in the public schools and the establishment of strong parent-volunteer programs.

18. The role of the teacher is presented by the author as changing from that of mere program facilitator to one of a vital voice in educational planning. This change has come about partially because:

   A. the National Education Association represents modern educators throughout the United States.
   B. teachers are more willing than ever to speak out concerning the development of new programs and policies.
   C. teachers often go on strike if their demands for new programs are not met.
   D. according to the modern side of the flow chart, teachers now discuss their ideas directly with the board of education.

19. Which one of the following statements *contradicts* the central theme of this passage?

   A. Today's students are radical and demand a share in the decision making process of local school boards.
   B. Principals are the instructional leaders in their schools.
   C. Students who get accepted to college make teachers look good.
   D. Because it has control over the purse strings, the board of education should have absolute power over all other facets of the educational machine within a school district.

20. Which of the following statements seems reasonable in light of the information presented in this passage?

   I. Parent-volunteer programs are one avenue of public involvement in local schools.
   II. Parents want to be placed above the board of education on the organizational chart.
   III. Parents are becoming a more powerful force in the operation of local schools.

   A. I and II   C. I and III
   B. II only   D. I, II, and III

21. Of the following statements, which one is NOT *supported nor contradicted by* the information presented in this passage?

   A. Parents sometimes use their children as tools for getting what they want in a school system.
   B. Teachers' strikes are taking place on a more frequent basis throughout the nation.

C. School systems of the future probably will see an equal division of power among the board of education, principals, and parents.
   D. The board of education represents the tax-paying community in any given school district.

22. The flow chart that can be found after the third paragraph is presented in a very simplified version. It pictures:

   A. the traditional as well as the modern flow of power and communication of local school districts.
   B. teachers as being on a low rung of the educational totem pole.
   C. the superintendent as the most powerful figure in the school system.
   D. the fact that students often communicate with their teachers and the principal.

23. The power that parents are beginning to exert in school systems is an important strand in this passage. What is the probable reason that parents are not represented directly on the flow chart?

   A. Parents operate as volunteers within the schools.
   B. School systems resent the influence that parents are trying to exert on them.
   C. Most organizational flow charts picture only those groups that are actual members of the organization.
   D. Parents are represented indirectly though the board of education, because that board represents the taxpaying public.

24. As a result of the information presented in this passage, the reader might conclude that in the future:

   A. the traditional decision-making power of public schools will continue to slip due to the demands made by parents and teachers.
   B. public education will become more decentralized and parents might be involved in developing school policies.
   C. it will become increasingly more difficult to determine who has the actual decision making power in a school district.
   D. all of the above.

Passage IV (Questions 25–33)

Generally, state statutes grant school administrators the legal duty to establish, maintain, and protect the school's learning environment. It is a basic tenet of school law that school authorities may exclude from school any student whose conduct interferes with or in any way disrupts the operation of the school, or who openly defies school rules, or whose conduct is willfully insubordinate, or who poses a threat of harm to himself, to other persons, or to school property.

The terms used to characterize exclusion of students from school are suspension and expulsion. Generally, suspension denotes a temporary exclusion from school with a presumption that return to school is possible. Typically, by state code provision, school authorities possess the legal prerogative to suspend students from classes and from school. Expulsion denotes a longer term of exclusion from school with a presumption of finality regarding the termination of one's status as a student. Considered the most severe student punishment available to school authorities, state statutes and local policies usually provide that only a local school board has the prerogative to expel a student.

In recent years, litigation has involved both the right of school authorities to suspend or expel, and the minimal procedural due process rights of students prior to suspension or expulsion. Following the landmark decision in *Gault,* in which the Supreme Court held that minor juvenile offenders in juvenile court were entitled to certain procedural due process protections, several lower courts began to clarify the procedural due process rights of students facing exclusion from school. The matter was ultimately treated by the United States Supreme Court in *Goss v. Lopez.*

Observing that a student possesses a property right to a public education, protected by the guarantees of the fourteenth amendment, the Supreme Court overturned an Ohio statute that allowed summary suspensions for up to ten days. In the Court's opinion, minimum procedures must be followed prior to exclusion from school. The Court held that in suspensions of ten days or less, notice of the charges and the right to be heard are required. And, if the student denies the charges, he or she must be informed of the evidence against him or her and be given the opportunity to present his or her side of the story. However, this requirement can be done informally and immediately after the incident. In *Goss,* the Supreme Court did not require that a public school system allow students to be represented by counsel, to present witnesses, or to confront and cross-examine witnesses. Nor did the Court rule on the elements of due process for suspensions of longer than ten days. The Court did observe that more procedural due process may be needed for longer suspensions.

Of major importance to the daily practice of school administrators is the Court's attitudes toward due process and school discipline, often missed by those who analyze this landmark case. First, the Court reemphasized the notion that procedural due process is a flexible legal standard, determined by the nature of the misconduct and the severity of the penalty. Second, the Court held that school officials are free to remove a student from school prior to a suspension if his or her presence is a danger to persons or property and/or is disruptive to teaching and learning.

Beyond the guidelines of the Supreme Court, a local school administrator is also bound by state statutory mandates and state court decisions, and these requirements vary. However, the following guidelines are generally accepted nationally and serve as excellent guidelines for school administrators: students must know in advance what standards of behavior are proscribed in their school and what modes of behavior are expected; they must know what specific disciplinary actions and punishments attach to violations of the rules; they must receive immediate and informed notice when they are accused of an infraction, and an opportunity to present his or her side of the story; and students must have an opportunity to appeal the decision to another administrative level within the school system. The administrator is reminded that these general elements become more formalized and technical when an expulsion is in process.

Two other student exclusion decisions from the United States Supreme Court should be briefly mentioned at this point because of their bearing on student procedural due process entitlements. The cases are *Wood v. Strickland,* and *Carey v. Piphus. Wood* involved the issue of students being allowed to sue local school board members for damages under Section 1983 for a denial of procedural due process in an expulsion hearing. In upholding the school board's actions, the Supreme Court held that individual board members could be sued if they knew or reasonably should have known that they denied students their constitutional rights or if board members acted with malicious intent.

Carey was a consolidation of two cases, both involving the suspension of a student from school. One student had violated a rule prohibiting the use of drugs at school, whereas the other student violated a rule against males wearing earrings at school. In rendering its decision in *Carey,* the Supreme Court held that students suspended from school without procedural due process are entitled to recover nominal damages of $1.00 and possibly extensive lawyers' fees. However, before any compensatory damages are awarded, a student must first submit proof of actual injury caused by the denial of due process. Punitive damages may be possible where a student can establish that school officials acted with the malicious intent to deprive him of his rights.

Adapted from H. G. Hudgins and Richard S. Vacca, *Law and Education: Contemporary Issues and Correct Decisions,* 2nd ed. Charlottesville, Virginia: The Michie Company, 1985.

25. The main topic of this passage deals with:

   A. the duty that school administrators have to establish, maintain, and protect the school's learning environment.
   B. fourteenth amendment rights.
   C. due process rights.
   D. the exclusion of students from school by means of suspension and/or expulsion.

26. According to the information presented in this passage, exclusion from school refers to:

   I. any time-out procedure directed at a student as a result of a disciplinary infraction.
   II. a temporary removal from the educational setting by means of suspension.
   III. a longer term and possibly permanent removal from the educational setting by means of expulsion.

   A. I and II   C. II and III
   B. I and III   D. all of the above

27. According to the information given in this passage, most state statutes and local policies give the prerogative of expelling a student from school to:

   A. the classroom teacher.
   B. the building administrator.
   C. the school superintendent.
   D. the school board.

28. The issue of student expulsion has produced numerous court cases. Litigation in this area generally involves:

   A. the right of school authorities to suspend or expel, as well as the student's minimal due process rights prior to suspension or expulsion.
   B. the flexible standard of the due process right as well as the length of time of the expulsion.
   C. the past disciplinary record of a student as well as the type of punitive action that was taken previously.
   D. all of the above.

29. In which of the following cases did the United States Supreme Court first treat the issue of procedural due process rights for students?

   A. *Wood v. Strickland*
   B. *Brown v. Board of Education*
   C. *Goss v. Lopez*
   D. *Carey v. Piphus*

30. Which of the following statements concerning the right to a public education is the *most* significant in *Goss v. Lopez*?

   A. Every student has the right to a public education.
   B. Public education is an inalienable right.
   C. The right to a public education is a property right.
   D. The right to a public education is protected by the fourteenth amendment.

31. Which of the following statements *contradicts* the holdings of the United States Supreme Court in *Goss v. Lopez*?

   A. Due process is a flexible standard.
   B. Due process is determined by the nature of the misconduct determined and the severity of the penalty.
   C. School authorities may not remove a student from school prior to a suspension.
   D. Minimal due process rights are required for suspensions of ten days or less, whereas more procedural due process might be needed for longer suspensions.

32. In which of the following student exclusion cases did the United States Supreme Court hold that an individual school board could be sued for knowingly denying a student his/her constitutional process rights?

   A. *Wood v. Strickland*
   B. *Brown v. Board of Education*
   C. *Goss v. Lopez*
   D. *Carey v. Piphus*

33. In which of the following student exclusion cases did the United States Supreme Court hold that suspension from school without procedural due process entitled a student to recover nominal damages and possibly extensive legal fees?

   A. *Wood v. Strickland*
   B. *Brown v. Board of Education*
   C. *Goss v. Lopez*
   D. *Carey v. Piphus*

Passage V (Questions 34–41)

Students in institutions of higher education hold diverse interests and backgrounds. There are average students as well as bright ones. Are the needs of average students different from those headed toward graduate school? Both need qualified and enthusiastic teachers.

When students evaluate teaching ability, they may or may not know a faculty member's academic qualifications or tenure status. Some nontenure-eligible faculty members have credentials comparable to tenure-track faculty members. The fact that a faculty member has a master's degree and teaches only lower level courses does not reflect on his or her teaching ability. Yet criteria used to evaluate full-time faculty members are similar to those applied to part-time faculty members. In addition, there is often an abuse of nontenure-eligible faculty members who may be requested to teach five courses a semester while receiving only 20 percent of the pay of the full-time faculty member.

Some faculty members contend that tenure is the freedom to teach, speak and write. Both tenured and nontenure-eligible faculty members, in fact, enjoy these freedoms. Academic freedom is not necessarily contingent upon tenure because the university protects the constitutional right of freedom of speech for all faculty members.

Tenure means job security, and bonds an individual to the institution. Nontenure-eligible faculty members are expected to bond with the institution; yet how can this be accomplished when they often experience employment uncertainty? The response is that tenure is not the only way to achieve bonding. Long-term contracts or "rolling contracts" are alternatives. There are some faculty members who may not want or need job security.

These are individuals in business or technical and professional fields who want to bond with a scholarly community in order to teach. They may have a primary career elsewhere or they may be pausing between career moves.

Tenure affects attitude and morale. What makes so many nontenure-eligible faculty members feel they are second-class citizens? Often they do not have offices or have not been accorded recognition for their teaching excellence. Faculty attitudes are inhibitive of change as are economic considerations. Why do nontenure-eligible faculty have to teach only lower level courses? Many nontenure-eligible faculty members may, in fact, be better equipped to teach some upper level courses. In addition, as the pool of faculty members in certain disciplines, English, for example, diminishes, the salaries needed to hire nontenure-eligible faculty members will increase. This competitive situation will encourage nontenure-eligible faculty members to voice their complaints about the lack of diverse teaching assignments or the failure to be treated as professional equals.

Pay differential between tenure track and nontenure-eligible faculty members will vary, but issues of bonding will remain on the table.

Adapted from A. Nancy Avakian. "Some Reflections on Nontenure-Eligible Faculty Members." In *Role of Nontenure-Eligible Faculty in the Academy*, 1990.

There is a need to determine the role and purpose of research in the university. Although the tripartite foundation of teaching, public service, and research is espoused, the institution's reward system leans toward research. At the same time, legislators, students, and parents cry out for excellence in teaching in order to raise the standards of quality. This conundrum must be addressed.

Nontenure-eligible research faculty experience other concerns that are not necessarily bound to tenure. They want job security during the transitional periods, i.e., from receipt of one grant to another. They lose even their second-class citizenship when job security is jeopardized. Long-term contracts are suggested in lieu of tenure.

Nontenure-eligible clinical faculty members practice usually in the medical and human services professions (dentistry, medicine, nursing, veterinary medicine, social work, clinical psychology, and counseling). In medicine and social work, much of the clinical teaching of patient care is delivered by nontenure-eligible faculty members who serve an a short-term basis. They represent the "off-site" faculty and serve as preceptors for clinical training of students. Their appointments cement the relationship between the practice and school. The clinical activities of nontenure-eligible faculty are not linked solely with the generation of income.

Tenure, for individuals in these disciplines, is usually accorded to individuals who have the M.D., Ph.D., or D.Ed. degrees. Lacking of tenure fosters the two-class system in which the vast majority of clinical care providers/teachers are, once again, made to feel they are relegated to the second class. Incentives and recognition of clinical performances are very important to clinical faculty members. Is it realistic to expect and demand excellence in all endeavors (teaching, research, public service) by the nontenure-track clinical faculty?

Usually complexity of clinical teaching and practice dictates the need for a large number of nontenure-eligible faculty members whose financial compensations vastly exceed the number of tenure positions and available resources. Does tenure have a place in clinical departments which have the potential to generate substantial income for the private practitioner?

34. Which of the following types of faculty is NOT discussed by the passage?

A. research faculty
B. clinical faculty
C. part-time faculty
D. administrative faculty

35. Addressing as it does issues related to job security of various categories of faculty, the passage supports all but which of the following conclusions?

A. Institutions should promote opportunities by which individuals may feel a bonding.

B. Multiyear contracts would be beneficial to elicit identity with the institution.

C. There is a need to clarify the roles and differences of tenure and nontenure-eligible faculty.

D. Tenure is probably the only way to achieve bonding.

36. Issues of concern regarding nontenure-eligible faculty are:

I. job security.
II. compensation.
III. evaluation.
IV. academic freedom.

A. I, II, and III   **C.** II and IV
B. I and IV   **D.** I, II, III, and IV

37. One could conclude from the information provided in the passage that:

A. responsibilities and qualifications of tenure and nontenure-eligible faculty are quite similar in many instances.

B. there is a difference between undergraduate and graduate bond students and the instructors they need.

C. tenure-track faculty are apt to initiate changes.

D. students are knowledgeable about instructor's status.

38. Which of the following statement(s) is/are NOT *supported nor contradicted by* the passage?

I. Pensions should be reviewed as separate from issues of intellectual and academic freedom.

II State legislatures must be educated or reeducated about the role of faculty.

III. Institutions should provide support for nontenure-eligible research faculty between receipt of grants.

IV. Nontenure-eligible faculty members should have access to the institution's grievance procedures.

A. I, II, and III   **C.** II and IV
B. I and III   **D.** I, II, III, and IV

39. The functions of a university are:

I. teaching
II. research
III. public service
IV. protection of the constitutional right of freedom of speech

A. I, II, and III   **C.** II and IV
B. I and III   **D.** I, II, III, and IV

40. The passage either implies or directly asserts that:

A. clinical faculty are greatly concerned with the generation of income for the institution.

B. many clinical faculty have long-term records of service.

C. nontenure-eligible faculty of both the undergraduate and professional schools feel like second-class citizens.

D. clinical faculties do not require many incentives because they serve patients.

41. Which of the following is NOT *supported by* the passage?

A. A number of nontenure-eligible faculty possess credentials comparable to tenure-track people.

B. An advanced degree does not necessarily reflect upon a faculty member's teaching.

C. Tenure does not mean bonding.

D. The reward system usually favors the researcher.

Passage VI (Questions 42–47)

Herbert Hoover's initial reputation in public life arose from his legendary success in feeding the victims of World War I. Already established as a successful consulting engineer, he had responded to overwhelming human need at the outbreak of the war and had set up the Commission for Relief in Belgium to facilitate humanitarian responses to the dislocations of German occupation. From 1914 until the American declaration of war in April 1917, Hoover administered a complex organization to raise funds, obtain food, and transport it to the needy. Along the way, he negotiated and renegotiated with the warring governments, convincing them to permit his rescue operations. At the conclusion of the war, Hoover resumed international feeding with the American Relief Administration. And, during the 1920s, when he perceived need, he responded in the same fashion—in Russia from 1921–1923, for example, and again during the Mississippi floods of 1927.

The feeding, relief, and rescue operations made him one of the most beloved and admired men in the world. But that personal prestige was of small importance to Hoover, compared with the sense of satisfaction at having "saved the lives of 1,400,000,000 human beings, mostly women and children, who otherwise would have perished."

In all of his rescue efforts, children represented Hoover's first concern. Orphaned himself by age ten, he showed a lifetime commitment to children—to making sure that all children should have the opportunity to grow up with adequately nourished bodies and minds. In public life, his efforts may be seen in the White House Conference on Child Health and Protection; in private life, he and Mrs. Hoover engaged in countless hidden charities, providing for destitute families and educating needy youngsters. Each of Hoover's relief operations also began with the concern for suffering children, and then expanded to include mothers, other women, the aged, and finally able-bodied men.

But Hoover's purpose stretched beyond mere feeding. He understood that the Four Horsemen of the Apocalypse rode together, and that Famine's grim companions could warp minds as well as bodies. Not often poetic, Hoover nevertheless printed this verse at the beginning of his great documentary study of his relief activities:

I am the stalking aftermath of all wars.
Pestilence is my companion.
Tumult and Revolution rise round my feet
We kill more than all of the guns.
I breed fears and hates that bring to man more wars.
From me comes no peace to mankind.
My legacy is to Children of Famine—
Stunted bodies and twisted minds.

The battle against starvation had critical long-term political and ideological aspects. The hungry could not long defend themselves—or defend Freedom.

The outbreak of World War II in Europe in September 1939 immediately raised the relief question again. Within less than two weeks, in conversations with representatives of the Franklin Roosevelt Administration, Hoover suggested centralizing all relief activities under a single agency, preferably the Red Cross. When invited to join the executive committee of the Red Cross, Hoover declared himself willing to accept only if the Red Cross would "take on the whole job," dealing with food, clothing, medicine, and other aspects of relief. Norman Davis, head of the Red Cross, defined its role more narrowly, arguing that there was a fundamental difference between emergency relief that had been the normal function of the Red Cross and that could be financed by private contributions, and the mass feeding and relief over an extended period that would require government financing. Hoover and Roosevelt's emissaries had reached an impasse.

42. In this passage the Red Cross:

    A. pictured itself as a broad-based, capable relief organization.

We gratefully acknowledge the help of Dr. Susan Esterbrook Kennedy, Professor of History and Geography, Virginia Commonwealth University, 1990.

    B. viewed its role as supplying emergency relief.

    C. wanted Hoover to lead the organization.

    D. depended on government to finance its operation.

43. It is quite clear from the passage that Hoover's passion was:

    A. the hungry.

    B. the homeless.

    C. the children.

    D. the indigent.

44. Hoover was trained as:

    A. a politician.

    B. a businessman.

    C. a relief specialist.

    D. an engineer.

45. Which of the following is *contradicted by* the passage?

    A. Roosevelt supported Hoover's efforts.

    B. Hoover was active in negotiating between warring governments.

    C. Hoover's efforts were broad based.

    D. Hoover helped natural disaster victims.

46. Which of the following is/are *supported by* the passage?

    I. Hoover believed that a centrally coordinated effort would serve best.

    II. Deprived people will rise to the occasion and defend their liberties.

    III. Hoover was quick to act.

    IV. Hoover did not have his family's support.

    A. I, II, and III

    B. I and III

    C. II and IV

    D. none of the above

47. Which of the following would describe/fit Herbert Hoover best?

    A. He was a socialist.

    B. He was a republican.

    C. He was a globalist.

    D. He was a humanitarian.

Passage VII (Questions 48–53)

Aristotle believed that "right reasoning" or ethical thinking could best be taught by tragedies. He particularly liked *Antigone* in this regard. He pointed out that tragedies first capture the heart of the reader by having a hero (or someone with whom we can associate) and then showing that this likable person committed an "error in judgment" *(hamartia)*. Aristotle believed in training the *heart* as well as the *mind* and that pity and fear *(pathos)* can best be aroused by a hero's downfall that is actually his fault. The "error in judgment" is all the more terrifying when we realize that it could have happened to us just as easily. Tragedies show our worst fear: good and logical people can fail!

Tragedies can test the limits of a culture to function; they can depict institutional and national failures. Tragedies can also show a particular culture to be the source of error. For instance, in the historical examples, unchecked scientific research and religious proselytizing resulting from a cultural misjudgment. Modern cultural misjudgments are the Catholic persecution in Ireland, black slavery in America, and the Jewish holocaust in Germany. Yet, in these three modern cases, it is important to realize the role of *pathos,* or empathy, in teaching wisdom. The reader must *identify with those who made the error in judgment* to be motivated toward determining that reasoning. For instance white Americans can feel guilt, humility (the "beginning of wisdom"), and uncertainty by studying slavery, whereas black Americans will feel mostly anger and resentment. Black Americans, for instance, should be introduced to the persecutions of other groups in other settings to obtain "true" or underlying wisdom about man's capacity for logical errors. Similarly, the holocaust is not a Jewish tragedy nor is the Irish persecution a Catholic tragedy in the classical sense of motivating the reader towards wanting to make good judgments. For such motivation, a person must "see" himself making the logical error, not just being a victim.

Tragedies can also show conflicts in values within one group or even within one person. Samuel Johnson criticized Shakespeare for a lack of morality in his plays; the hero often was a liar or an adulterer. What Shakespeare was actually so good at was showing the complexity of judgments in clear ways.

If tragedies are potentially effective for developing ethics and even wisdom, how can they be used in the educational arena? In his 1908 book, *Ethics,* John Dewey pointed out the "danger of either dogmatism or a sense of unreality when students are introduced abruptly to theoretical ideas." Dewey went on to propose an efficiency: ". . . he is encouraged to try them on simple problems before attempting the problems of the present." Following his lead, I propose to first introduce students to simple cases and then proceed to the more complex. Across the grades, this means beginning with picture books and one-page examples and eventually progressing to case studies in college. Of course, care must be taken to have the necessary elements of an empathetic character, moral dilemma, and mistake in judgment at all of these levels.

Sources for ethical tragedies are the Bible, classical literature, history, newspapers, books, and actual experiences. Shorter versions and profiles must be developed to make an ethical lesson in a reasonable amount of time. Uses or formats are Xerox pages, pamphlets, published articles, workbooks, and computer "what if" simulations with or without video accompaniments.

The main idea is that all these tragedies, regardless of format, must be short but not too short. For instance, John F. Kennedy wrote a book called *Profiles in Courage,* which contained about a dozen stories of U.S. senators faced with ethical dilemmas. The stories are short in length, but long enough in description to capture the heart of the reader to wish the hero well. In this way, we can take the need for such virtues as wisdom and courage "to heart."

The renewal of ethical *skills* to each generation can be helped by understanding capitalistic and market mechanisms. (Notice I did not say ethical *knowledge* because we are not trying to transmit facts but to develop right reasoning.) For instance, if teachers at a certain grade level or in a certain subject area have a case study or pamphlet "fair" where their works are displayed, the better works will become known and used increasingly. A school district, university, or state education department could encourage development, publication, and "survival of the fittest" of ethical tragedies by similar display mechanisms, sales shows, or annotated bibliographies. Eventually, a *general* curriculum could be prescribed by the state education department.

Ethical pamphlets or booklets are being proposed instead of textbooks because of the modular or "mix and match" possibilities that they allow. For instance, a high school teacher can use a pamphlet to supplement a history course at a strategic point, whereas a business teacher in college can allow students to choose among some case studies and compare one of them to a recent event. The combination of student feedback and teacher rewriting should produce better case studies for the future. In this way, we can develop a naturally self-improving mechanism or *Tao* in this important area.

Encouraging teachers in various fields to write, desktop publish, and trade ethical cases has another advantage. It not only keeps the cases current, but it encourages teachers in the present generation to put the "key ideas" together to allow wise leadership to be "unlocked" in

---

Adapted from material by Dr. James J. McGovern, Virginia Commonwealth University. Presented at the Conference on Educating the Gifted for the 21st Century (1990).

individuals in the next generation. In many ways, our teachers determine and give birth to the future.

It is primarily through education that the process of heredity, which from the beginning has caused the world to rise to higher zones of consciousness, is furthered in a reflective form and in its social dimensions. The educator, as an instrument of Creation, should derive respect and ardor for his efforts from a profound, communicative sense of the development already achieved or awaited. . . .

Pierre Teilhard de Chardin
The Future of Man

48. The material in this passage is an excerpt from a longer selection. Based on the tone of the content, which of the following statements describes the probable communication vehicle of the original piece?

A. The material comes from a methods textbook on education.
B. The material is part of a talk presented at a conference on educating gifted students.
C. The material comes from a theatrical article.
D. The material is taken from a speech given to college graduates.

49. The main theme of this passage is that:

A. studying plays or stories that have a tragic ending tends to make the reader view the lead character as a hero despite any judgment errors that he may be responsible for.
B. tragedies, such as those created by Shakespeare lack moral character because the hero generally is a liar or an adulterer.
C. the skills needed to develop ethical thinking in new generations can be fostered by studying tragedies.
D. an understanding of market mechanisms is needed to understand ethics.

50. The author's sense of the Greek word *hamartia* is:

A. unavoidable mistakes.
B. faulty logic.
C. major injustices.
D. personal grief.

51. In his book *Ethics,* John Dewey cautioned teachers to:

A. avoid dogmatism.
B. begin with theoretical overviews.
C. start with simple cases.
D. limit discussions to current situations.

52. Having teachers write their own ethical case studies:

A. allows a standard curriculum to be developed.
B. provides a free market mechanism.
C. keeps the cases current.
D. allows the writer to identify with the victim.

53. Passing on a sense of ethics from one generation to another can be accomplished by:

A. teaching a basic body of knowledge.
B. inspiring students to live good lives.
C. teachers formulating good and humane reasoning, and this skill being picked up by students.
D. reading about tragedies and other cases where evil doers suffer.

Passage VIII (Questions 54–59)

In the 1970s, Peltzman hypothesized that attempts to improve automobile safety by regulation of product design would be at least partially offset by behavioral changes induced by the mandate. In his model, more recently termed the "offsetting behavior hypothesis," the imposition of mandated safety devices reduces the probability of injury, holding driving intensity constant. Given a preference for driving intensity and an aversion to injury, one would expect drivers to increase driving intensity relative to the level chosen prior to device imposition. The increase in driving intensity thus induced tends to offset the initial gain in safety for those protected and adversely affects others. This article tests whether these expectations can be confirmed. Using the most recent insurance industry generated data, we find that models adopting air bags experience increases in relative personal injury claims and that this increase is not the result of "buyer sorting." Then, using Virginia State Police reports on all fatal crashes involving late model vehicles in the 1993 calendar year, we report a series of tests to ascertain whether driver behavior differences can be found between air-bag- and non-air-bag-equipped cars. We find that air-bag-equipped cars tend to be driven more aggressively than cars without air bags and that the additional aggressiveness appears to offset the effect of the air bag for the driver and increases the risk of death to others.

Sparked initially by Lave and Weber, and developed more completely by Peltzman, a sizable body of economic literature focused on the efficacy of government safety regulations that have developed over the last 25 years. Initially, most researchers found little or no support for the offsetting behavior hypothesis and concluded that the benefits from various proposed or mandated safety appliances exceeded their costs. By the mid-1980s, slightly more support for the offsetting behavior hypothesis in limited situations was found in a few studies. Evans, as well as Lund and O'Neill, have found some evidence that newly adopted safety devices which provide active feedback, such as studded snow tires, may influence driver behavior.

Recently, several researchers have found evidence of substantial offsetting behavior. Blomquist's work both surveyed and contributed to this literature. Subsequently, Chirinko and Harper have concluded that offsetting driver behavior is "qualitatively important to the extent that it has attenuated the effects of safety regulation on automotive fatalities." Most recently, Keeler has interpreted his inability to find that regulation significantly diminishes fatalities as support for the offset hypothesis.

The debate over the efficacy of government safety regulations has been epitomized by the discussion of air bags. No technological innovation has been so opposed initially and later so embraced by the industry as the air bag. Before the National Traffic and Motor Vehicle Safety Administration mandated the feature for front-seat occupants for the 1998 model year, the air bag had become the most controversial device since passage of the National Traffic and Motor Vehicle Safety Act in 1966. Automotive insurers and consumer advocates lobbied and litigated for their adoption, while domestic automotive manufacturers urged caution and moderation. The latter successfully persuaded the Reagan Administration in 1981 to rescind the passive restraint rule, arguing that they would not be as cost effective as the already mandated three-point belt system. Several years of additional litigation followed the rescission.

By 1990, auto manufacturers began to equip increasing numbers of models with at least one air bag in response to perceived market forces and Federal Motor Vehicle Standard 208 (49 CFR Sec. 571.208). Extensive promotion quickly redefined the state-of-the-art "safe" car as one so equipped. Because air bags are perceived to and do reduce the risk of injury to protected occupants especially in head-on collisions, the recent widespread manufacturer adoption of air bags as standard equipment provides a new data source for testing the offsetting behavior hypothesis.

Using different tests, but relying on similar data sets, Hoffer and Millner as well as Peterson and Hoffer found that relative injury and absolute collision losses for a model usually increase after the adoption of air bags as standard equipment. The authors noted that while their results are supportive of offsetting behavior, they are also consistent with buyer sorting. In the sorting model, drivers with a greater likelihood of being involved in accidents shift their purchases to air-bag-equipped models. Our task in this article is to determine which of the competing hypotheses better explains their findings. . . .

Using two independent data sets, we have found strong support for the offsetting behavior hypothesis. Our analysis of the insurance industry-based HLDI data set indicates that autos newly equipped with an air bag during the 1990-1993 model years experience significant increases in relative losses under personal injury protection coverage after controlling for upward resizings. Because these increases do not diminish over time, these results are attributed to offsetting behavior.

Second, we studied 1993 fatal accidents in Virginia. We find that risk to drivers of cars equipped with air bags in single car crashes *is not* diminished, that the percentage of occupants killed in single car air bag crashes *is* unusually high, and that drivers of air-bag-equipped cars initiate an unusually large percentage of such crashes. We conclude that drivers of air-bag-equipped-cars tend to be more aggressive than drivers of cars not so equipped, and that their added aggressiveness diminishes the protection afforded drivers of cars equipped with air bags and imposes additional risks on occupants and passengers in other vehicles.

54. Which of the following best characterizes the authors' main conclusion, drawn from their examination of statistics related to automobile accidents?

A. Drivers of automobiles equipped with air bags tend to be more aware of automobile safety and therefore drive more safely than those drivers of automobiles without air bags.

B. Although statistics suggest that drivers of automobiles equipped with air bags are involved in more accidents (percentage-wise) than those not equipped with them, this is apparently a matter of coincidence.

C. Drivers of automobiles equipped with air bags have approximately the same number of accidents (percentage-wise) as those drivers in automobiles not equipped with air bags.

D. Drivers of automobiles equipped with air bags appear to drive more aggressively than those drivers in automobiles not equipped with air bags, and this is probably attributable to their belief that they have greater protection with air bags than they would have without air bags.

Adapted from "Automobile Air Bags in the 1990's: Market Failure or Market Efficiency?" from *The Journal of Law & Economics*, 1995. Used with permission of George Hoffer.

55. In which year did automobile manufacturers, due to perceived market forces, begin to equip increasing numbers of cars with at least one air bag?

A. 1981 **C.** 1966
B. 1990 **D.** 1996

56. Which hypothesis, along with the "offsetting behavior" hypothesis has been at the center of the air-bag controversy?

A. "fatality avoidance"
B. "driver sensitizing"
C. "buyer sorting"
D. "security enhancing"

57. Which statement best characterizes the conclusions of the early or initial body of economic literature, sparked by Lave and Weber, dealing with the efficacy of government safety regulations related to automobiles?

A. The cost of safety appliances exceeded their benefits.
B. The benefits of safety appliances exceeded their costs.
C. The seatbelt is the only appliance whose value has been determined.
D. There are too many variables involved in determining the cost-benefit ratio to make more than educated guesses.

58. The authors studied fatality data from:

A. all states except Hawaii.
B. North and South Carolina.
C. Virginia.
D. randomly selected states.

59. It is fair to say that the authors of this article believe that:

A. there is little to support the "offsetting behavior" hypothesis.
B. drivers of air-bag-equipped automobiles are more aggressive than those of non-air-bag-equipped automobiles.
C. it is too early to draw conclusions about the "offsetting behavior" hypothesis.
D. drivers of air-bag-equipped automobiles are less aggressive than those of non-air-bag-equipped automobiles.

Passage IX (Questions 60–65)

As the strategic importance of an information systems component within an organization grows, so does the need for the ability to continue data processing operations in the wake of a disaster. Preparation falls into two categories: (1) backup and recovery procedures to mini-

mize risks due to storage media or other types of hardware failure, as well as loss of data due to program errors, and (2) contingency planning to provide the capability to maintain an adequate level of support, despite a prolonged lack of resources. However, experts have estimated that less than 50 percent of central data processing sites in the United States have an adequate contingency plan, largely due to its lack of immediate corporate benefit.

Cost-benefit analysis can be used to determine which disaster planning control measures an organization should consider. The framework of the analysis is based on the expected benefit of a control used for a specific threat. Obviously, the benefit must be positive (cost of control is less than expected value of control), and the cost must also be considered in conjunction with financial analysis for other unrelated corporate projects.

Determination of cost of control is done by adding the initial costs of the control measure to the present value of recurring costs over a three to five year period, based on the company's borrowing rate.

Derivation of expected value of control is less straightforward. It is the product of expected loss × control effectiveness. Expected loss is calculated by multiplying the cost of total or partial damage to a specific hardware or software component by the probability of a specific threat. This probability must be annualized by calculating the expected occurrences of the threat per year. Statistical means, consensus of experts, or use of consultants are techniques a company might use to establish this type of probability.

After all threats are determined, the ones with the greatest likelihood should receive the highest planning priority. Again, each scenario must be financially analyzed and only controls with positive payback should be weighed against competing corporate projects for possible implementation.

Various strategies for disaster recovery include: (1) no action, (2) the fortress, (3) the commercial hot site, (4) the commercial cold site, (5) the warm site, (6) reciprocal processing agreements, and (7) privately owned sites.

The fortress represents the centralized data center that has taken extreme preventive measures to ward off disaster. They do not use alternate site plans, and are therefore jeopardized in the event of a major catastrophe, such as a destructive tornado. On the other hand, they are probably very well prepared for the occurrence of disasters with higher probabilities, such as equipment failure or data loss.

The commercial hot site leases space to companies charging monthly fees for a specified number of years, including a maximum available number of weeks of usage during that time period. All computing equipment

Adapted from Ben Owen, "Systems Performance Evaluation," MCV/VCU, 1990.

necessary for critical operations is provided. The hot site offers the advantage of being able to reestablish processing operation very quickly, but drawbacks include the high cost and the possibility that another firm who also has membership at the same site may have a disaster just before you do. *def. of hot site, ad*

The commercial cold site leases building space only; no computing equipment is included. It is less expensive than a hot site lease, but may not provide proper coverage because of possible inability to lease necessary computer equipment in a widespread disaster. The shared membership arrangement could also put a firm at a disadvantage. *ad of cold site*

The warm site is a service bureau with which one contracts for specified processing time when necessary. The primary advantages of the warm site are that the equipment is already in place, and most store backups for firms in time of need, making the recovery time even faster than the hot site. The primary disadvantage of the warm site is the high cost for general services that are not well suited for specialized processing requirements. *ad of warm site*

The reciprocal agreement involves two companies who provide backup capability for one another during a disaster. This arrangement has the advantage of providing more specialized equipment, assuming that reciprocating firms have similar hardware and software processing requirements. The cost is much lower than that of commercial solutions, and the only competition comes from the host site itself. The disadvantages of this setup include the two firms possibly growing apart in terms of compatibility, and potential contract violations.

Privately owned sites are used by some large firms, and involve a private hot or cold site that is used in emergencies. The same advantages and disadvantages exist for these as do for commercial hot or cold sites, except that they are more available, and in the case of the hot site, more responsive. However, they are obviously more expensive to own.

Two of the most important management issues involved in disaster planning are who is responsible and which applications get top priority. Ideally, a disaster recovery team is formed with members representing the entire corporation, who are part-time members of this project. The leader need not necessarily be from the Information Systems area. The prioritization of application recovery can be decided by this team, or by the Disaster Planning steering committee, but should be formalized. The vehicle for this is the disaster recovery plan.

60. According to the passage:

    I.   program errors may result in data loss.

    II. the majority of data processing centers have inadequate contingency plans.

    III. corporations see no immediate benefit derived from data processing.

A. I only   C. I and II only
B. II only   D. I, II, and III

61. This passage summarizes planning considerations for computer disaster recovery. The passage deals with issues, such as:

    I.   benefits versus costs of recovery.

    II. identification of quantitative techniques employed by management.

    III. comparisons of strategies for emergency operation sites.

A. I only   C. I and II only
B. II only   D. I, II, and III

62. Among major management issues to be considered were:

    I.   responsibility for planning.

    II. prioritization of critical applications.

    III. formalization of a plan.

A. I only   C. I and II only
B. II only   D. I, II, and III

63. Which of the following statements is/are *supported by* the passage?

    I.   Statistics may be used to establish priorities in planning.

    II. Planning contingency systems must be analyzed in the total schema of a corporation's operation.

    III. Most organizations have adequate plans in case of an emergency.

A. I only   C. I and II only
B. II only   D. I, II, and III

64. Cost control must consider:

A. the initial costs of measures.
B. a time span of three to five years.
C. the borrowing rate of a company.
D. all of the above.

65. Using information provided by the passage, one could conclude that:

A. the fortress type of data storage is quite safe in most emergencies.
B. hot sites are quite costly.
C. cold sites seem to be most disadvantageous.
D. all of the above are supported.

PHYSICAL SCIENCES

10 PROBLEM SETS OF 5–10 QUESTIONS EACH
15 PROBLEMS FOLLOWED BY A SINGLE QUESTION
77 questions
100 minutes

DIRECTIONS: The following questions or incomplete statements are in groups. Preceding each series of questions or statements is a paragraph or a short explanatory statement, a formula or set of formulas, or a definition. Read the written material and then answer the questions or complete the statements. Select the ONE BEST ANSWER for each question and indicate your selection by marking the corresponding letter of your choice on the Answer Form. Eliminate those alternative you know to be incorrect and then select an answer from among the remaining alternatives. A periodic table is provided (see p. 583). You may consult it whenever you wish to do so.

Passage I (Questions 66–70)

Several labs are set up and equipped to study sound waves including audible sound as well as ultrasound (with frequencies much higher than audible frequencies). The ultrasound unit is an old A-scan type unit that can only detect the distance to a sound reflecting interface by measuring the round-trip time for a wave to travel to the interface and return. Available equipment includes function generators to produce pure sine wave tones at a fairly wide range of frequencies, several different amplifiers, microphones that can be used as the inputs into audio amplifiers and oscilloscopes, and several different speakers that can be operated from separate sources. There are also some sound deadening materials and sound baffles as well as some hard smooth surfaces to efficiently reflect sound.

66. An amplifier drives one speaker at a sound level of 82 dB. The amplifier power level is 240 watts. If the table outlet supplies 120 V rms, what current in amperes, does the amplifier draw?

   A. 2.90 A   C. 1.46 A
   B. 2.00 A   D. 9.84 A

67. A second amplifier drives a second speaker at the same power level. The two speakers are sounded at the same time. Each speaker alone would have a sound level of 82 dB. What is the decibel level of the two speakers operating together?

   A. 164 dB   C. 41 dB
   B. 85 dB   D. 123 dB

68. The ultrasound unit sends a 2.5 MHz sound wave into a 40-cm tube filled with water. The

transducer that produces the short pulse of ultrasound act as a detector of the reflected wave. The reflected and transmitted pulses are seen to be 5.4 cm apart on an oscilloscope for which the horizontal sweep time knob is set for 0.1 msec/cm. What is the velocity of sound in water?

   A. 390 m/sec   C. 3210 m/sec
   B. 455 m/sec   D. 1481 m/sec

69. A sound wave at a frequency of 3000 Hz is sent through an aluminum rod and then travels out into the air. The speed of sound in air is 340 m/sec. Find the wavelength in the air and also state whether the wavelength in aluminum is longer or shorter than in air.

   A. 0.11 m, longer in Al
   B. 6.7 m, longer in Al
   C. 0.03 m, shorter in Al
   D. 0.78 m, shorter in Al

70. The function generators can produce pure sinusoidal tones in a frequency range from 15 to 26,000 Hz. About what percentage of humans can hear this entire range of 15-26,000 Hz?

   A. 0%   C. 50%
   B. 10%   D. 100%

Passage II (Questions 71–76)

A number of apparatus are devised for the study of simple harmonic motion. Several masses can be attached to different springs and set into oscillation. The periods of these mass-spring systems are given by $T = 2\pi \sqrt{m/k}$, where k is the spring constant (N/m). A pendulum system has a bob of mass 1 kg on the end of a string 50 cm long. Bobs and strings of various masses and lengths are available. If the pendulum bob is displaced through an angle of less than about 10°, it behaves as a simple pendulum of length L with a period $T = 2\pi \sqrt{L/g}$. The speed of the pendulum bob and of the mass on the end of the spring can be measured by photogate timers.

71. The pendulum with the 1-kg bob and string length of 50 cm is starting to swing through an angle of about 9°. What is its period?

    A. 3.2 sec   **C.** 1.4 sec
    B. 6.1 sec   **D.** 5.5 sec

72. The bob is replaced with a 2-kg bob and the angle of swing is reduced to 5°. What is the period of this new pendulum?

    A. 3.2 sec   **C.** 1.4 sec
    B. 6.1 sec   **D.** 5.5 sec

73. A 500-gram mass is hung from a spring carefully so that it is at rest and the stretch of the spring is measured to be 49 cm. What is the spring constant of this spring?

    A. 100 N/m **C.** 10 N/m
    B. 40 N/m **D.** 80 N/m

74. The 500-gram mass is pulled down 5 cm from its rest position and released so that the mass executes simple harmonic motion. What is the period of this simple harmonic motion?

    A. 4.4 sec   **C.** 2.8 sec
    B. 1.4 sec   **D.** 5.6 sec

75. The 500-gram mass is replaced with a 2-kg mass which is pulled down 5 cm from its rest position and released so that the mass executes simple harmonic motion. What is the period of this simple harmonic motion?

    A. 4.4 sec   **C.** 2.8 sec
    B. 1.4 sec   **D.** 6.4 sec

76. An identical spring (with same spring constant) is attached to the 2-kg mass as shown. The mass is set into motion. What is the new period of oscillation?

    A. 1.0 sec
    B. 2.8 sec
    C. 8.8 sec
    D. 5.6 sec

Passage III (Questions 77–81)

A physics instructor devises a simple electrical circuit setup in which one can easily insert various resistors and capacitors in series and parallel combinations. One can have only resistor combinations, only capacitor combinations, or capacitor-resistor combinations. The circuit is usually used for DC (direct current) studies but can also be used for AC (alternating current) studies. The DC battery voltage is 6 volts. The AC rms voltage is 120 volts (at 60 Hz). The student inserts the resistors and/or capacitors as instructed and has available suitable ammeters and voltmeters for both the DC and AC experiments. (There are three resistors, each of 2 ohms resistance. There are also three capacitors, each of 1 microfarad capacitance.)

77. All three resistors are connected in series and the combination is connected to the 6-volt DC battery. What voltage drop occurs across each individual resistor as measured by the voltmeter?

    A. 0.33 V   **C.** 2.0 V
    B. 1.0 V   **D.** 6.0 V

78. One capacitor and one resistor are connected in parallel. The ends of this combination are then connected to the 6-V DC battery, What are the final current and voltage, respectively, across the 1 microfarad capacitor?

    A. 0 A, 6 V   **C.** 0.33 A, 6 V
    B. 0.33 A, 3 V   **D.** 6 A, 6 V

79. Two of the 2-ohm resistors are connected in parallel and the 120-V AC voltage is applied to the ends of this parallel combination. What current will the AC ammeter measure if connected so it measures only the current through one of the resistors?

    A. 1 A   **C.** 60 A
    B. 2 A   **D.** 120 A

80. Two resistors are connected in parallel and the set of parallel resistors is then connected in series with the third resistor. If this series-parallel combination is connected across the 6-volt battery, what total DC current is drawn from the battery?

    A. 0.5 A   **C.** 3 A
    B. 2 A   **D.** 6 A

81. One capacitor and one resistor are connected in series. The 120 V, 60 Hz AC voltage is then applied to this series "RC" circuit. What is the AC current through this series circuit?

A. .045 A   C. 0.72 A
B. 0.50 A   D. 40.0 A

A. 0.8 N   C. 3.2 N
B. 1.6 N   D. 4.9 N

Passage IV (Questions 82–87)

An air track with carts is used as an (almost) frictionless system to study both elastic and inelastic collisions. The purpose is to understand the principle of conservation of linear momentum as well as the conservation of energy principle. It is assumed that total kinetic energy is conserved for the collision of air track carts with spring steel bumpers. The velocities of the carts are determined by the use of photogate timers, both before and after collisions. Carts with masses of 150 and 450 g are available. Some carts have "sticky" bumpers so that they stick together after colliding (in "completely inelastic" collisions). The total kinetic energy is not conserved (constant) in these latter collisions. Two of the different mass carts have a spring that can be compressed between them. A taut string tied between the carts keeps the spring compressed. The string is burned with a match and the two carts fly apart in opposite directions.

82. When the string is burned, the 150 g cart is observed to have a velocity of 3 m/sec. What is the magnitude of the opposite velocity of the 450 g cart?

A. 0.33 m/sec   C. 3 m/sec
B. 1 m/sec   D. 9 m/sec

83. Two of the 150 g carts with the spring steel bumpers collide. Cart 2 is at rest before the collision. Cart 1 has a velocity of 2 m/sec just before they collide. What is the velocity of Cart 2 just after the collision?

A. 1 m/sec in the opposite direction
B. 1 m/see in the same direction
C. 2 m/sec in the same direction
D. 2 m/sec in the opposite direction

84. A 450 g cart passes through two photogates that are 2 m apart. It has a speed of 4.0 m/sec through the first photogate and a speed of 3.0 m/sec through the second photogate. About how much energy was lost to air friction during the passage between the gates?

A. 1.1 joules   C. 2.3 joules
B. 1.6 joules   D. 8.8 joules

85. The energy lost to air friction is also the work done "against" air friction. From the result of the preceding question, calculate the average retarding force due to air friction over the 2 m distance.

86. One end of the air track is now elevated. A 450 g cart is given a push and then passes through a photogate. It ascends the track and comes to rest at a point that is measured to be a vertical height of 0.5 m above the photogate. Ignoring air friction, what was the speed of the cart through the photogate?

A. 1.24 m/sec   C. 4.55 m/sec
B. 3.13 m/sec   D. 6.26 m/sec

87. Two of the different mass carts are tied together with the compressed spring between them. When the string is burned the 150 g cart is observed to have a velocity of 9 m/sec. What is the magnitude of the opposite velocity of the 450 g cart?

A. 3 m/sec   C. 9 m/sec
B. 1 m/sec   D. 0.33 m/sec

Questions 88–95 are independent of any passage and of each other.

88. A ray of light is incident at an angle of 30° from air onto a glass surface with an index of refraction of 1.65. The angle of refraction in the glass is found to be 17.6°. Suppose the light ray were again incident at 30° but this time the incident angle is in the glass. The refracted angle in air as the ray leaves the glass will be:

A. larger than 30°.
B. smaller than 30°.
C. between 17.6° and 30°.
D. equal to 17.6°.

89. A man fires a starter pistol and hears an echo 4 sec later from the side of a distant, very large building. He knows that the speed of sound is 344 m/sec that day. The distance to the building is:

A. 2752 m.   C. 1032 m.
B. 1376 m.   D. 688 m.

90. A 1 kg mass is revolving at an angular speed of 2 rev/sec on the end of a light rod of length 0.5 m. What are the *linear* speed and the *centripetal* force on the mass? (1 rev = 2π radians)

A. 1 m/sec and 2 newtons
B. 6.28 m/sec and 79 newtons
C. 6.28 m/sec and 34 newtons
D. 1.24 m/sec and 59 newtons

91. Radioactive Cobalt-60 decays, giving off very energetic gamma rays which have been used for many years to treat cancerous tumors. The half-life for decay is about 5.3 years. If a strong source of 5000 curies was originally furnished to the hospital, about how many curies would be left after 16 years? (The sources are actually changed more often to avoid lengthy treatment times for patients).

A. 1667 curies   C. 245 curies
B. 3333 curies   D. 625 curies

92. An object of 30-grams mass is submerged in alcohol so that its apparent mass is 20 grams. What is the approximate specific gravity of the object? (The specific gravity of the alcohol is 0.79.)

A. 1.34   C. 3.11
B. 2.37   D. 0.95

93. A diffraction grating with grating constant $d = 1.67$ microns (1.67×10^{-6} meters) is used to produce an m-th order image of a spectral line of wavelength 417 nm (1 nm = 10^{-9} meters) which is seen at a diffracted angle of 30°. What is the value of the order m?

A. 1   C. 3
B. 2   D. 4

94. You have a 1100-watt hot plate and a 1300-watt toaster oven in your kitchen apartment. If you use them at the same time on a single 120-volt circuit, what current will flow in the circuit wire?

A. 20 amperes   C. 2 amperes
B. 40 amperes   D. 5 amperes

95. Nitrogen-13 decays by positive beta decay (emission of a positron, e^+) to a different isotope as follows:

$$_7N^{13} \rightarrow {}_zX^{13} + {}_{+1}e^0 + \nu_e$$

(The neutrino, ν_e, has no mass and zero charge while the positron, the antiparticle of the electron, has such a small mass that it is treated as zero mass). What is z and also the correct chemical symbol for X?

A. 8 and O   C. 6 and C
B. 7 and N   D. 2 and He

Passage V (Questions 96–105)

Students in a medical physics class are given the assignment of planning a nuclear medicine facility. They not only design the rooms and choose the major equipment, they also will have to solve elementary problems dealing with treatment, doses, radiation protection and safety, and the general principles of the physics of typical isotopes that might be used in diagnostic nuclear medicine. They are required to be familiar with concepts of half-life, half-thickness for shielding, and the decay schemes of representative isotopes.

96. The most common isotope used in diagnostic work is Technicium. It is furnished from a generator or "cow" in which the negative beta decay of Molybdenum-99 produces the desirable metastable isotope of Technicium according to the following decay scheme:

$$_{42}Mo^{99} \rightarrow {}_zTc^A + {}_{-1}e^0.$$

What are the atomic number, Z, and mass number, A, of the Tc isotope?

A. 41, 99   C. 43, 98
B. 42, 99   D. 43, 99

97. If the Mo^{99} has a physical half-life of 67 hours, about what fraction is left after 5.5 days?

A. 0.10   C. 0.40
B. 0.25   D. 0.45

98. This isotope of Technicium has a physical half-life of 6 hours. When it is tagged onto a polyphosphate carrier used for a certain procedure, there is a biological half-life of 12 hours (for the biological excretion of the carrier). What is the "effective half-life" in this case?

A. 4.0 hours   C. 10 hours
B. 7.5 hours   D. 14 hours

99. The "cow" was milked at 8:00 AM. At 2:00 PM the activity of the milked sample is measured by a technician and found to be 200 millicuries. What was the activity of the Technicium at 8:00 AM?

A. 100 mCi   C. 300 mCi
B. 150 mCi   D. 400 mCi

100. Thallium-201 is used for myocardial perfusion studies of the heart. It decays by electron capture when the nucleus captures one of the atom's own orbital electrons (converting a proton in the nucleus into an uncharged neutron), with the emission of gamma rays used for the imaging. What are the atomic number, Z, the mass number, A, of the Mercury isotope produced in the decay of the Thallium-201?

$$_{81}Th^{201} + _{-1}e^0 \rightarrow _zHg^A + \Gamma s$$

A. 80, 201   C. 81, 201
B. 80, 202   D. 81, 203

101. The Thallium-201 half-life is 74 hours. If the sample has an activity of 80 millicuries initially, what will be the activity after 9.25 days?

A. 2.5 mCi   C. 10 mCi
B. 5 mCi   D. 20 mCi

102. One advantage of the Thallium isotope is the "low whole body absorbed dose per millicurie," which, for Tl-201 is 70 millirads/millicurie. If the recommended amount to be injected for a heart scan is 10 microcurie per Kg of body mass, what would be the whole body dose in millirads for a 70 Kg person?

A. 34 mrad   C. 72 mrad
B. 49 mrad   D. 134 mrad

103. Another feature that makes Technicium a desirable isotope for diagnostic nuclear medicine use is that it is a "pure gamma emitter." What is the meaning of the terminology "pure gamma emitter?"

A. The gamma radiation stays in the patient's tissue while the electrons are detected.
B. Particles emitted cannot escape tissue while the gamma radiation escapes.
C. The isotope decay emits only penetrating gamma radiation that can escape from tissue and be detected.
D. The isotope decay emits energetic electrons that act like gamma rays.

104. A patient is injected with Technicium and is estimated to have received a whole body dose of 400 millirads. If the "Quality Factor" is 1 for gamma radiation and 3 for low energy neutrons, what was the dose received by the patient in rem units?

A. 4 mrems   C. 1200 mrems
B. 400 mrems   D. 4000 mrems

105. The half-thickness of lead for the absorption of the gamma radiation from a particular isotope is 0.4 cm of lead. How many half-thicknesses are necessary to reduce the radiation penetration to less than 1% and how thick would the lead be?

A. 2 half-thicknesses, 1.2 cm
B. 4 half-thicknesses, 3.2 cm
C. 7 half-thicknesses, 2.8 cm
D. 11 half-thicknesses, 4.4 cm

Passage VI (Questions 106–110)

One mole each of CO_2, H_2O_2, and O_2 are in a closed container at 25°C and standard pressure.

106. The molar percentage of CO_2 is:

A. 25%.   C. 40%.
B. 33%.   D. 55%.

107. The weight percentage of CO_2 is:

A. 25%.   C. 40%.
B. 33%.   D. 55%.

108. The number of molecules of CO_2 is:

A. 1.8×10^9.   C. 9.3×10^{18}.
B. 1.0×10^{14}.   D. 6.0×10^{23}.

109. If the compounds should break down to the elements, the number of total moles of gas would be:

A. three.   C. five.
B. four.   D. six.

110. At standard temperature and pressure, the original CO_2, H_2O_2, and O_2 would occupy a volume of:

A. 1 liter.   C. 25 liters.
B. 10 liters.   D. 45 liters.

Passage VII (Questions 111–115)

Separate beakers are used for the preparation of 1 M solutions of $NaNO_3$, $BaCl_2$, NaCl, and sodium acetate.

111. The lowest pH will be:

A. $NaNO_3$.   C. NaCl.
B. $BaCl_2$.   D. sodium acetate.

112. The highest pH will be:

A. $NaNO_3$.   C. NaCl.
B. $BaCl_2$.   D. sodium acetate.

113. The closest pH's of any two of these solutions will be:

A. NaCl and $NaNO_3$.
B. NaCl and $BaCl_2$.
C. $BaCl_2$ and sodium acetate.
D. $BaCl_2$ and $NaNO_3$.

114. If the solutions of NaCl and $NaNO_3$ are mixed in one beaker and the temperature adjusted to 383°K, the contents of the beaker will most likely:

A. freeze.
B. boil.
C. exhibit precipitation of $NaNO_3$.
D. exhibit a marked color change.

115. Dilution of the $NaNO_3$ solution to 0.5 molar will bring about:

A. an increase of pH by about 2.
B. no significant change in pH.
C. a decrease of pH by about 2.
D. a decrease of pH by about 4.

Passage VIII (Questions 116–120)

The resident starts a fire in the fireplace in an apartment at 15°C. After a few minutes, he stirs his 90°C coffee with a silver spoon and quickly notes a substantial increase in the temperature of the handle of the spoon. He removes the silver spoon and stirs the coffee with a stainless steel spoon. He stands facing the fire and notes that the front of his body is becoming warm. He moves behind a screen and is much cooler. After about 45 minutes, he finds that the temperature has increased behind the screen.

116. Heat is transferred through the silver spoon by:

A. consolidation.   **C.** convection.
B. conduction.   **D.** coordination.

117. The handle of the stainless steel spoon will:

A. become as hot as quickly as is true of the silver spoon.
B. become hotter or will reach the same temperature more quickly than is true of the silver spoon.
C. not become hot as quickly as is true of the silver spoon.
D. become colder while in the coffee.

118. Heat reaching the resident while standing in front of the fire is most likely accomplished by:

A. consolidation.   **C.** convection.
B. conduction.   **D.** radiation.

119. Increase in temperature behind the screen is most likely explained by:

A. consolidation.   **C.** convection.
B. conduction.   **D.** radiation.

120. In general, the fastest transfer of heat from a heat source to another object through a gas is by:

A. coordination.   **C.** convection.
B. conduction.   **D.** radiation.

Passage IX (Questions 121–125)

The LeChatelier principle states roughly that when stress is placed upon an equilibrium system, the system will react in a direction to relieve the stress.

121. In the equilibrium reaction

$$CO(g) + Cl_2(g) \rightleftharpoons COCl_2(g),$$

the imposition of higher pressure will result in increased percentage(s) of:

A. CO.   **C.** $COCl_2$.
B. Cl_2.   **D.** A and B.

122. In the equilibrium reaction

$$2H_2S(g) \rightleftharpoons 2H_2(g) + S_2(g),$$

an increase in the applied pressure will result in (a) higher percentage(s) of:

A. H_2S **C.** S_2.
B. H_2.   **D.** B and C.

123. In the equilibrium reaction

$$H_2(g) + Cl_2(g) \rightleftharpoons 2\,HCl(g),$$

imposition of increased pressure would result in a higher percentage of:

A. H_2.   **C.** HCl.
B. Cl_2.   **D.** none of the above.

124. To an equilibrium mixture of H_2, Cl_2, and HCl in the equation in question 123, is added additional Cl_2. The result will be a (an):

A. increase in the amount of HCl.
B. decrease in the amount of H_2.
C. increase in the amount of H_2.
D. more than one of the above.

125. $X(g) + Y(g) \rightleftharpoons 2Z(g)$

If the above hypothetical reaction is at equilibrium, addition of more Z (without changing pressure or temperature) will result in:

A. presence of more X.
B. presence of less X.
C. a change in K_{eq}.
D. more than one of the above.

Passage X (Questions 126–135)

Ionization constants for weak bases may be dealt with in the same way as the ionization constants for weak acids.

$$B + H_2O \rightleftharpoons BH^+ + OH^-$$

$$K_b = \frac{[BH^+][OH^-]}{[B]} \text{ and } pK_b = -\log \frac{[BH^+][OH^-]}{[B]}$$

126. Ammonia has a K_b of 1.8×10^{-5}. Its pK_b would be:

A. between 2 and 3.
B. between 3 and 4.
C. between 4 and 5.
D. greater than 5.5.

127. A 0.01 molar solution of ammonia in water would have a pOH of:

A. between 2 and 3.
B. between 3 and 4.
C. between 4 and 5.
D. greater than 5.5.

128. The pH of the above solution would be:

A. between 3 and 5.
B. between 6 and 8.5.
C. between 10 and 11.
D. between 12 and 14.

129. Hydrazine has a K_b of 1.7×10^{-6}. Its pK_b would be:

A. between 3 and 4.   C. between 5 and 6.
B. between 4 and 5.   D. between 6 and 7.

130. A 0.001 molar solution of hydrazine in water would have a pOH:

A. between 3 and 4.
B. between 4 and 5.
C. between 5 and 6.
D. between 6 and 7.

131. The above solution would have a pH:

A. between 3 and 4.
B. between 5 and 6.
C. between 6 and 8.
D. of none of the above.

132. Assuming equal concentration (and solubility) the highest pH will be observed with an aqueous solution of a base having a pK_b of:

A. 3.5.   C. 6.2.
B. 4.8.   D. 6.8.

133. A theory of acids and bases that does NOT necessarily involve hydrogen or hydroxyl ions was developed by:

A. Arrhenius.
B. Brønsted and Lowry.
C. Gordon.
D. Lewis.

134. The base NaOH would be expected to have a pK_b of:

A. 2 ± 1.   C. 9 ± 1.
B. 5 ± 1.   D. none of the above.

135. The pH of a 0.001 molar aqueous solution of NaOH would be:

A. 3   C. 9
B. 5   D. 11

Questions 136–142 are independent of any passage and each other.

136. Which is the oxidizing agent in the reaction:

$$2Fe^{2+} + Cl_2 \rightarrow 2Fe^{3+} + Cl^-?$$

A. $2Fe^{2+}$ C. Cl^-
B. Fe^{3+} D. Cl_2

137. Which molecule is nonpolar and contains a nonpolar covalent bond?

A. F_2 C. HF
B. CCl_4 D. H_2O

138. Which compound reacts with an acid to form a salt and water?

A. CH_3Cl C. KCl
B. CH_3COOH D. KOH

139. Which bond is formed by the transfer of an electron from one atom to another?

A. ionic bond   **C.** peptide bond
B. covalent bond   **D.** hydrogen bond

140. The maximum number of electrons that a single orbital of the 3d sublevel may contain is:

A. 1   **C.** 3
B. 2   **D.** 4

141. Given the following K_{sp} values, which compound will be the least soluble in water?

A. $AgBr = 5.0 \times 10^{-13}$
B. $AgCl = 1.8 \times 10^{-10}$
C. $Ag_2CrO_4 = 1.1 \times 10^{-12}$
D. $AgI = 8.3 \times 10^{-17}$

142. Which could act either as an oxidizing agent or a reducing agent?

A. Fe^0 **C.** Fe^{3+}
B. Fe^{2+} **D.** Cu^0

WRITING SAMPLE

2 ESSAYS-TOPICS
60 MINUTES (30 MINUTES/TOPIC)

DIRECTIONS: Your response must be a unified, organized essay; it should contain fully developed, logically constructed paragraphs. Remember quality is more important than length. Before you begin writing, make sure you have read the item carefully and understand what is being asked. Write as legibly as possible. Because your essays will be scored as first-draft compositions, you may cross out and make corrections on your response booklet as necessary. It is not necessary to recopy your essay.

Part 1

Consider this statement:

It is no wise man that will quit a certainty for an uncertainty.

Samuel Johnson

Write a unified essay in which you perform the following tasks. Explain what you think the above statement means. Describe a specific situation in which a wise person would quit a certainty for an uncertainty. Discuss the circumstances that you think determine whether or not one should or should not give up certainty for uncertainty.

Part 2

Consider this statement:

Destruction is, after all, a form of creation.

Graham Greene

Write a unified essay in which you perform the following tasks. Explain what you think the above statement means. Describe a specific situation in which an act of destruction is not a form of creation. Discuss what you consider to be the circumstances that determine the relationship between destruction and creation.

BIOLOGICAL SCIENCES

10 PROBLEM SETS OF 5–10 QUESTIONS EACH
15 PROBLEMS FOLLOWED BY A SINGLE QUESTION
77 QUESTIONS
100 MINUTES

DIRECTIONS: The following questions or incomplete statements are in groups. Preceding each series of questions or statements is a paragraph or a short explanatory statement, a formula or set of formulas, or a definition. Read the written material and then answer the questions or complete the statements. Select the ONE BEST ANSWER for each question and indicate your selection by marking the corresponding letter of your choice on the Answer Form. Eliminate those alternatives you know to be incorrect and then select an answer from among the remaining alternatives.

Passage I (Questions 143–147)

The diagram below represents three generations of a human family, some of whose members have a non-lethal birth defect. Individuals 1, 3, and 4 are distantly related and come from a family in which the defect has occurred for many generations. Information on the occurrence of the defect among the ancestors of individual 2 is unavailable. The preceding four generations of the family and the siblings of individual 19 included no individuals who expressed the defect. The defect is caused by a single gene for which new mutations are very rare. The individuals with birth defects are represented by solid black symbols while the individuals who have a normal phenotype are represented by open symbols. Males are represented by squares and females are represented by circles.

143. The defect is most likely caused by:

   A. an autosomal gene for which the defective allele is recessive to the normal allele.
   B. an X-linked gene for which the defective allele is recessive to the normal allele.
   C. an autosomal gene for which the defective allele is dominant to the normal allele.
   D. an X-linked gene for which the defective allele is dominant to the normal allele.

144. The genotype of individual number 1 in the family:

   A. is most likely to contain only normal alleles.
   B. is most likely to contain only defective alleles.
   C. is most likely to contain both normal and defective alleles.
   D. cannot be determined from the pedigree.

145. The genotype of individual number 6 in the family:

   A. is most likely to contain only normal alleles.
   B. is most likely to contain only defective alleles.
   C. is most likely to contain both normal and defective alleles.
   D. cannot be determined from the pedigree.

146. The genotype of individual number 8 in the family:

   A. is most likely to contain only normal alleles.
   B. is most likely to contain only defective alleles
   C. is most likely to contain both normal and defective alleles.
   D. cannot be determined from the pedigree.

147. The genotype of individual number 9 in the family:

   A. is most likely to contain only normal alleles.
   B. is most likely to contain only defective alleles.
   C. is most likely to contain both normal and defective alleles.
   D. cannot be determined from the pedigree.

Passage II (Questions 148–157)

Many scientists think of the pituitary gland as the master gland responsible for the secretion of many different hormones. A reciprocal relationship operates between the hormones secreted by the pituitary and the hormones produced by the target organs; this delicate control of balance of production of secretory product between the pituitary and the target organs is known as "negative feedback." Among the many hormones produced by the pituitary gland are ACTH, FSH, LH, TSH, and STH. The following experiments were set up to demonstrate the actions of some of the above factors. Twenty-five, day-old immature male and female rats were subjected to the following treatment for 10 days: Group I was given a 0.5 cc saline injection; Group 2 was given a 0.5 cc FSH injection; and Group 3 was given a 0.5 cc crude pituitary extract injection. The results were recorded in table form.

MALE RATS

Group	Body Weight grams	Testes mg	Seminal Vesicles mg	Prostate mg	Thyroid mg	Adrenals mg
1	86	3750	18	71	6.0	20
2	82	5310	57	176	6.1	21
3	83	4830	24	163	7.5	27

FEMALE RATS

Group	Body Weight grams	Ovaries mg	Uterus mg	Thyroid mg	Adrenals mg
1	83	20	25	5.9	22
2	82	43	83	5.7	21
3	84	33	61	7.1	37

148. Based on the information provided, which of the following statements is/are *supported* by the data?

A. From the table it seems as if the crude pituitary extract had a lesser effect on the sex organs than did FSH.

B. Pituitary extract affected every organ under investigation.

C. Hypophysectomy probably would have resulted in a decreased weight of the organs under investigation.

D. All of the above.

149. Based on the information provided, which of the following statement(s) is/are *supported* by the data?

A. The administration of FSH alone to an immature rat will produce follicular growth, but uterine and vaginal configurations will remain infantile since LH is also needed. The experimental data indicate uterine growth, casting doubt on the purity of the FSH preparation.

B. Both FSH and LH are necessary for the production of estrogen.

C. FSH has as its target organs the organs of reproduction.

D. A and C of the above.

150. Based on the information provided, which of the following, statement(s) is/are *contradicted* by the data?

A. FSH in the male had the greatest effect on the weight of the prostate gland; the tissue is therefore most reactive to it.

B. The adrenal weight probably would drop if the animals were deprived of ACTH.

C. In these experiments, none of the hormones in the pituitary extract probably were as effective as a purified fraction of them might have been.

D. Body weights were not a significant experimental parameter.

151. Housed in the sella tursica is the:

A. pineal organ. C. olfactory bulb.
B. pituitary gland. D. optic chiasm.

152. Social stress will affect most severely the:

A. pancreas. C. adrenal.
B. pineal. D. parathyroid.

153. During the follicular phase of a normal menstrual cycle, ovarian changes occur that are due to pituitary secretions of:

A. FSH only. C. oxytocin.
B. LH only. D. FSH and LH.

154. Follicle-stimulating hormone is to estrogen as luteinizing hormone is to:

A. progesterone.
B. testosterone.
C. vasopressin.
D. luteotrophic hormone.

155. The pituitary (master) gland releases a gonadotrophic hormone that stimulates the production of testosterone by:

A. spermatogonia.
B. interstitial cells of Leydig.
C. Sertoli cells.
D. epididymis.

156. Each of the following is under control of the adenohypophysis EXCEPT the:

A. thyroid. C. testis.
B. adrenal medulla. D. adrenal cortex.

157. The sperm count of a normal 25-year-old male would be

A. one million/ml.
B. one hundred million/ml.
C. one hundred thousand/ml.
D. four million/ml.

Passage III (Questions 158–165)

The diagram illustrates a typical single neuron; the basic unit of the nervous system. Neurons connect with each other and in that manner an impulse is conducted and transmitted throughout the body. Two types of cell processes are indicated.

158. An impulse would be transmitted to another neuron by:

A. 4. C. 10a.
B. 6. D. 11.

159. Protein synthesis is carried out mainly by:

A. 2. C. 5.
B. 3. D. 7.

160. Cellular "digestive" or "suicide" packages is a common description or name for:

A. mitochondria.
B. Golgi zones or Golgi bodies.
C. lysosomes.
D. centrosomes.

161. The neurotransmitter acetylcholine is released by:

A. axon terminals.
B. dendrite terminals.
C. Golgi apparatus of neuron cell bodies.
D. Schwann cells.

162. We speak in terms of an aggregation of nerve cell bodies in the central nervous system as the site of a (an):

A. ganglion. C. cranial nerve.
B. nucleus. D. association area.

163. The neurolemma of an axon is part of the:

    A. nerve cell body.   **C.** node of Ranvier.
    B. Schwann cell.   **D.** axoplasm.

164. Which of the following germ layers gives origin to the nervous system?

    A. ectoderm
    B. mesoderm
    C. endoderm
    D. ectoderm and endoderm

165. The cell bodies of the motor neurons are located in the spinal cord in the:

    A. intermediolateral cell column.
    B. dorsal root ganglia.
    C. dorsal horn (gray matter).
    D. ventral horn (gray matter).

Passage IV (Questions 166–173)

In order for a thoracic surgeon to visualize the heart, he or she must open up the pericardium which is a sac that covers the heart. A human heart is four-chambered and is composed of right and left atria which are separated by an interatrial septum that is frequently marred by defects. In the fetus the foramen ovale is an opening in this septum and blood passes from the right atrium to the left atrium so that the pulmonary circulation may be bypassed. A patent foramen ovale may contribute to the condition known as "blue baby." Two ventricles are also present; specifically we can speak of a right ventricle that pumps deoxygenated blood to the lungs and a left ventricle that pumps oxygenated blood to the tissues of the body. Between the ventricles is located the interventricular septum.

The superior and inferior vena cava and the coronary sinus empty into the right atrium. From here blood passes into the right ventricle to be pumped into the lungs via the pulmonary arteries. Blood from the lungs is returned to the left atrium by the pulmonary veins; it then passes into the left ventricle to leave upon its contraction via the aorta to supply the arterial system of the body. The heart alternately contracts and relaxes, and this cardiac cycle is repeated about 75 times per minute; the duration of one cycle is about 0.8 second. Atrial systole (contraction) which takes about 0.1 second is followed by ventricular systole lasting about 0.3 second and absolute diastole (relaxation) follows lasting about 0.4 second.

The heart has an automatic rhythmic beat, but it is also under the influence of nerves which, however, serve only to change the force or frequency of the contractions of the muscle in accordance with the physiologic needs of the organism. The modification of the intrinsic rhythmicity is by way of the two parts of the autonomic nervous system; stimulation occurs through the sympathetic portion while homeostatic maintenance is mainly a function of the parasympathetic portion. Stimulation through the sympathetic nerves increases the rate and force of the heart beat; while slowing and reduction in force are the result of parasympathetic stimulation. Vasodilation of the coronary arteries is brought about by sympathetic stimulation while vasoconstriction is elicited by parasympathetic stimulation.

166. When a physician informs a patient that his blood pressure reading is 160/90, she refers respectively to:

    A. systolic blood pressure of the left ventricle.
    B. blood pressure in the veins of the arm.
    C. systolic and diastolic pressures of the brachial artery.
    D. systolic pressure of the aorta and diastolic pressure in the superior vena cava.

167. The vital centers for control of heart rate, respiratory rate, and blood pressure are located in the:

    A. pons.   **C.** cerebellum.
    B. medulla.   **D.** hypothalamus.

168. Blood in the pulmonary veins is rich in:

    A. oxyhemoglobin.
    B. carbaminohemoglobin.
    C. hemoglobin.
    D. uric acid.

169. Running to catch the bus to go to work has produced a rapid heart rate, an increase in the respiratory rate, and an increase in blood pressure in an individual. We can attribute these changes to:

    A. the peripheral nervous system.
    B. the central nervous system.
    C. the parasympathetic component of the autonomic nervous system.
    D. the sympathetic component of the autonomic nervous system.

170. Which of the following muscle types is NOT under the control of the autonomic (involuntary) nervous system?

    A. heart (cardiac)   **C.** skeletal (striated)
    B. smooth   **D.** arrector pili

171. The functional unit of a striated muscle is known as the sarcomere. A sarcomere on an electron micrograph is the region between:

A. two A bands. **C.** two H bands.
B. two I bands. **D.** two Z bands.

172. If we examine the three types of muscles in respect to their characteristics, which of the series below is false?

	Characteristic	Cardiac	Skeletal	Smooth
A.	No. of Nuclei	One-Several	Many	One
B.	Position of Nuclei	Central	Central	Central
C.	Striations	Present	Present	Absent
D.	Control	Autonomic	Voluntary	Autonomic

173. Heartbeat is initiated by the:

A. vagus nerve.
B. sympathetic nervous system.
C. A-V (atrio-ventricular) node.
D. S-A (sino-atrial) node.

Passage V (Questions 174–178)

Human immunodeficiency virus type-1 (HIV-1) initiates infection of a cell by binding of a viral envelope protein (gpl20) to a cell surface glycoprotein (CD4) on the cell. CD4 is found primarily on a subset of T lymphocytes. The CD4 molecules on these T lymphocytes normally function as receptors for the class II major histocompatibility complex molecules on the surfaces of antigen-presenting cells. Some cultured cell lines [including HSB(CD4+)M.23 and H9 cell lines] express CD4 and can therefore bind gp 120 protein and can be infected by HIV-1. One possible strategy for inhibition of the spread of HIV-1 infection would be treatment with small molecules that resemble the region of CD4 molecules that binds gp120 and that would therefore bind to gp120 molecules on virus particles and prevent the virus particles from binding to cells.

A series of experiments in which a class of modified dipeptides called CPFs were evaluated is shown in Figures 1 and 2. Two different CPFs (CPFDD and CPFDF) were tested. Figure 1 describes the effects of pretreatment of HSB(CD4+)M.23 cells with CPFs on the subsequent binding of fluorescent-labelled gp120. Figure 2 describes the production of HIV-1 virus (measured as viral p24 protein production by the cells) by H9 cells which were exposed to HIV-1-infected T lymphocytes in the presence of various concentrations of CPFs.

Data modified from Finberg et al, *Science* (1990): 249:289-291.

● CPFDF   ▲ CPFDD

Binding of gp120 (visualized with fluorescent antibody staining) to HSB(CD4+)M.23 cells after incubation of the gp120 with CPFDF (●) or CPFDD (▲).

● T + H9   ▲ T + H9   ■ T + H9   ▼ T alone
              + CPFDF   + CPFDD

Virus production (measured as p24 protein production) by H9 cells exposed to HIV-1 infected T cells.

174. CPFDD:

A. inhibited gp120 binding to CD4 more strongly than CPFDF.
B. inhibited gp120 binding to CD4 less strongly than CPFDF.
C. stimulated gp120 binding to CD4 more strongly than CPFDF.

D. stimulated gp120 binding to CD4 less strongly than CPFDF.

175. CPFDF:

  A. inhibited gp120 binding to CD4 more strongly than CPFDD.
  B. inhibited gp120 binding to CD4 less strongly than CPFDD.
  C. stimulated gp120 binding to CD4 more strongly than CPFDD.
  D. stimulated gp120 binding to CD4 less strongly than CPFDD.

176. According to the data presented in Figure 1, a 50 µM/L increase in the concentration CPFDD caused the largest increase in inhibition of the binding of gp120 to CD4 when the initial concentration of CPFDD was:

  A. 0.
  B. 150 µM/L CPFDD.
  C. 300 µM/L CPFDD.
  D. 800 µM/L CPFDD.

177. CPFDD:

  A. caused total (>95%) inhibition of transfer of HIV-1 from T cells to H9 cells after 6 days.
  B. caused strong (approximately 75%) inhibition of transfer of HIV-1 from T cells to H9 cells after 6 days.
  C. caused weak (approximately 25%) inhibition of transfer of HIV-1 from T cells to H9 cells after 6 days.
  D. caused no (<5%) inhibition of transfer HIV-1 from T cells to H9 cells after 6 days.

178. CPFDF:

  A. caused total (>95%) inhibition of transfer of HIV-1 from T cells to H9 cells after 6 days.
  B. caused strong (approximately 75%) inhibition of transfer of HIV-1 from T cells to H9 cells after 6 days.
  C. caused weak (approximately 25%) inhibition of transfer of HIV-1from T cells to H9 cells after 6 days.
  D. caused no (<5%) inhibition of transfer of HIV-1 from T cells to H9 cells after 6 days.

Passage VI (Questions 179–184)

The A B O blood grouping system is explained on the basis of a single triallelic system with genes A, B, and O operating at a single genetic locus. Phenotypic and genotypic characteristics may be expressed as follows:

Phenotype	Genotype
A	A/A; A/O
B	B/B; B/O
O	O/O
AB	A/B

The A and B genes appear to be codominant; they are dominant over O, which is recessive.

179. Utilizing this system, transfusions have become relatively safe. The universal recipient is considered to be type:

  A. A.   C. O.
  B. B.   D. AB.

180. Which of the following agglutinogens do these individuals carry on their red blood cells?

  A. A.   C. O.
  B. B.   D. A, B.

181. A person of blood type A can receive blood of type(s):

  A. A.   C. O.
  B. B; A.   D. A; O.

182. Two people are planning to have a family. The woman has blood type A/A and the man B/B. Their children might have the following:

  A. A and B.
  B. B only.
  C. A/B only.
  D. A and B and A/B.

183. A man with blood cell genotype B/O marries a woman with type A/B. Their offspring could have any of the following:

  A. A/B, B/B, A/O, B/O
  B. A/B and B/O only.
  C. A/O and B/B only.
  D. none of the combinations above.

184. A foreign protein, when introduced into the body is recognized and elicits an immunologic response; this substance is known as a (an):

  A. antigen.   C. complement.
  B. antibody.   D. vitamin.

Passage VII (Questions 185–189)

185. You have samples of 4 different compounds (A, B, C, and D) but they are not identified as to structure. One is 2,3-dihydroxypentane; one is 2,4-dihydroxypentane; one is 2-pentene; and one is pentane. One compound is found to react with periodate to produce aldehydes. This compound would be:

    A. 2,3-dihydroxypentane.
    B. 2,4-dihydroxypentane.
    C. 2-pentene.
    D. pentane.

186. A solution containing 2-methylpentane-1, 5-diol and 3-methylpentane-1, 5-diol is oxidized to produce dicarboxylic acids. The total number of species of dicarboxylic acids will be:

    A. 1   **D.** 4
    B. 2   **E.** 5
    C. 3

187. You have been given a sample that could be an ester, hemiacetal, or ether. If it produces two compounds on treatment with weak aqueous acid and no apparent reaction on treatment with weak aqueous base, it is

    A. the ester
    B. the hemiacetal
    C. the ether
    D. A mixture of at least two of the compounds. No single one of the indicated compounds will give these results.

188. The naturally occurring fatty acids usually have

    A. an even number of carbon atoms
    B. an odd number of carbon atoms
    C. a number of carbon atoms which will yield a whole number when divided by three
    D. carboxyl groups on both ends of a hydrocarbon chain

189. A sample of β-ketoadipic acid is reacted with lithium aluminum hydride in diethyl ether at room temperature for 24 hours. The product is

    A. butane
    B. β-hydroxyadipic acid
    C. 1,3,6-hexanetriol
    D. a mixture of 2-hexenedioic acid and 3-hexenedioic acid
    E. α-ketosuccinic acid

Passage VIII (Questions 190–194)

Many of the physiological functions of neurons are mediated by signal transduction systems. By way of intermediate messengers, transduction systems relay extracellular signals to intracellular effector elements which produce a physiologic response. Depending on their position in the relay chain, the intermediate relay elements are known as second messengers, tertiary messengers, and so on.

In the stylized neuron above, the extracellular signal (a neurotransmitter) is signified by the letter "L" (ligand). When "L" binds to its receptor, it opens the associated channel which admits extracellular calcium into the neuron. This constitutes a Receptor Operated Channel (ROC). Admission of calcium via the ROC serves to depolarize the neuron. With depolarization, the Voltage Operated Channel (VOC) can also open to admit calcium. When the cell is sufficiently depolarized, both channels close and no more calcium is admitted.

An elevation of calcium within the cell serves to activate the calcium binding protein Calmodulin (CaM). Activated CaM, in turn, activates a Calcium/ Calmodulin-dependent Kinase (CKII). A kinase is a specialized enzyme that can transfer a phosphoryl group from a high energy donor such as ATP to an appropriate substrate phosphoprotein. CKII can transfer phosphoryl groups to itself in a process known as autophosphorylation. The autophosphorylated form of CKII is active and is able to carry out multiple cellular functions including increasing neurotransmitter synthesis and release.

CKII is inactivated by dephosphorylation. The initial calcium influx also serves to activate inactive Protein Phosphatases (PP), the enzymes that remove phosphoryl groups from phosphoproteins. The activity of these phosphatases is, however, somewhat slower than the other components in the system. Thus, the complete system contains all of the elements necessary for transducing an initial extracellular signal into a physiologic response. It also contains an internal mechanism for terminating the response.

190. Increasing the activity of CKII could be best achieved by blocking step(s):

    A. 3.   **C.** 7.
    B. 5.   **D.** 3 and 7.

191. Decreasing the activity of CKII could be achieved by blocking step(s):

A. 2 only.
B. 5 only.
C. 2 or 4 or 5.
D. 7.

192. An electrode is used to depolarize the neuron to the same extent as activation of the ROC. No neurotransmitter ligand (L) is present to bind to its receptor. Calcium, present in normal extracellular concentrations, would enter the cell through:

A. the ROC.
B. the VOC.
C. ROC and the VOC.
D. none of the above.

193. The enzyme responsible for transfer of a phosphoryl group from a high energy donor to a suitable substrate is known as a:

A. phosphatase.
B. catalase.
C. transferase.
D. kinase.

194. CKII can perform its multiple cellular functions because:

A. there is more kinase than phosphatase.
B. there is more phosphatase than kinase.
C. the inactivation pathway is slower than the activation pathway.
D. the activation pathway is slower than the inactivation pathway,

Passage IX (Questions 195–199)

A student is given four unknown clear colorless liquids, each having the molecular formula $C_5H_{10}O$. Assume that the compounds shown below are in bottles labeled I-IV. The contents of these bottles are to be associated with their chemical or physical properties.

$$\begin{matrix} & O \\ & \| \\ CH_3CCHCH_3 \\ & | \\ & CH_3 \end{matrix}$$

$$\begin{matrix} CH_3CHCH_2CH=O \\ | \\ CH_3 \end{matrix}$$

I

II

$$\begin{matrix} CH_3C=CHCH_2OH \\ | \\ CH_3 \end{matrix}$$

$$\begin{matrix} & O \\ & \| \\ CH_3CH_2CCH_2CH_3 \end{matrix}$$

III

IV

195. The compound above that has the highest boiling point would be:

A. I.
B. II.
C. III.
D. IV.

196. The compound above that would react with 2,4-dinitrophenyl hydrazine to form a hydrazone and gives a positive Tollen's test with $Ag(NH_3)_2OH$ is:

A. I.
B. II.
C. III.
D. IV.

197. The compound above that on hydrogenation with H_2 in the presence of a catalyst, such as Pt or Ni, forms a chiral center, and which can be resolved into R and S enantiomers is:

A. I.
B. II.
C. III.
D. IV.

198. The reaction of acetaldehyde (ethanal) with isopropyl Grignard reagent, $CH_3CHMgBr$,
$$\quad\quad\quad\quad\quad\quad\quad\quad\quad | $$
$$\quad\quad\quad\quad\quad\quad\quad\quad\quad CH_3$$
followed by hydrolysis and then oxidation with $K_2Cr_2O_7$ would be expected to produce:

A. I.
B. II.
C. III.
D. IV.

199. The name of the compound above that would rapidly decolorize Br_2 in CH_2Cl_2 is:

A. 3-pentanone.
B. 2-methyl-2-pentanone.
C. 3-methyl-2-buten-1-ol.
D. 2-methyl-2-buten-4-ol.

Passage X (Questions 200–204)

Ten milliliters of blood were removed from a patient, and centrifugation was utilized to separate 5 ml of plasma from the blood cells. A 3-ml sample of the plasma was extracted with 100 ml of an appropriate lipid solvent. The lipid solvent was then evaporated to 10 ml, and a 0.1-ml sample was analyzed for cholesterol. The color produced in the calorimetric analysis at 560 millimicrons was exactly equal to a standard in which 0.5 mg of cholesterol was known to be present.

200. The cholesterol concentration of the patient's plasma was:

A. 200 mg cholesterol/100 ml plasma.
B. 295 mg cholesterol/100 ml plasma.

C. 867 mg cholesterol/100 ml plasma.
D. 1667 mg cholesterol/100 ml plasma.

201. In order to make the above calculations it was *not* necessary to know:

A. the volume of plasma separated from the blood.
B. the volume of plasma subjected to extraction.
C. the solvent volume after evaporation.
D. the volume of sample that was subjected to colorimetric analysis.

202. If the addition of twice the volume of standard produces more than twice the absorbance at 560 millimicrons, this is probably best explained by:

A. exceeding the linear range of the method.
B. error in pipetting.
C. error in weighing to prepare the standard solution.
D. any or all of the above.

203. Cholesterol is an intermediate in the biosynthesis of:

A. essential fatty acids.
B. steroid hormones.
C. essential amino acids.
D. prostaglandins.

204. The essential fatty acids are required in the human body in the biosynthesis of:

A. ascorbic acid.   C. estrogen.
B. bile acids.   D. prostaglandins.

DIRECTIONS: Read each passage carefully, study each table, chart, or formula, then answer the question following it. Eliminate those choices that you think to be incorrect and mark the letter of your choice on the answer sheet.

A scientist sets up the following experiment. Ten male rats are placed in each of two cages. One cage is placed in a room regulated at a constant temperature of 37°C (group A) while the other cage is placed in a similar room kept at 45°C (group B). Food and water were provided *ad libitum* to both experimental sets. Food consumption, water consumption, ACTH blood level, and heart rate were determined for a period of ten days. The following bar graphs illustrate the results.

205. The investigator after examining the four graphs can report that:

A. at a higher temperature the rats were more active.
B. the rats maintained at 37°C developed a desire for water.
C. ACTH level is not markedly affected by the experimental conditions.
D. at higher temperatures more food is required.

Animals utilized in the following experiment were golden hamsters (*Mesocricetus auratus*). Normal diet consisted of Purina laboratory chow provided *ad libitum*. Animals were divided into three groups: group A—Control; group B—Cold exposed at 5°C ± 1°C for five days; group C—Cold exposed at 5°C ± 1°C for 30 days. Body weight (BW), thyroid weight (TW), ^{131}I uptake (^{131}I), and Serum Protein Bound Iodine^{-127} (PB ^{127}I) were measured.

Groups	BW grams	TW mg/100 g BW	^{131}I Uptake 24 hours	Serum PBI μg/100 ml
A	97	5.89	5.88	4.09
B	79	5.55	15.37*	5.27*
C	110	6.25	11.06*	5.02*

*Fisher's "T" significant to .001

206. The data suggest that:

A. the morphology of the thyroid gland was not altered because no significant weight change was recorded.

B. the thyroid gland is in a physiological state of hyperactivity in cold-exposed animals.
C. hamsters in the cold are in great distress.
D. the thyroid gland is in a physiological state of hypoactivity in cold-exposed animals.

An investigation was conducted to compare early host response to transplantable tumor, as manifested by mast cell adenine release, in golden hamsters with growing tumor and in golden hamsters immunized with tumor antigen and bacteria adjuvant. The following tables summarize the results.

Comparison of adenine release in hamsters sensitized with tumor antigen and bacteria adjuvant and adjuvant controls.

TABLE 1

Groups	No. of Animals	% Release
Tumor antigen and bacteria adjuvant	40	66.51
Bacteria adjuvant	40	11.13

Comparison of adenine release in the golden hamster with growing tumor and untreated controls.

TABLE 2

Groups	No. of Animals	% Release
Tumor transplant	40	33.50
Normal controls	40	7.50

207. Based on the information given: select the statement which is *not supported by* information in the above passage.

A. While adjuvant controls had more adenine release than untreated controls, their group average was significantly below that of the animals actively sensitized to tumor.
B. Animals that received transplants released half as much adenine as those given tumor antigen and bacteria adjuvant.
C. There is a significant difference between the tumor-bearing animals and their controls indicating some degree of enhanced cellular sensitization.
D. The experiments indicate that the immunological system of the golden hamster can respond with adenine release upon challenge with antigen prepared from that tumor.

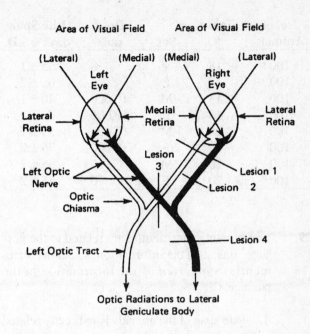

This diagram represents fiber pathways by which impulses from the retina are carried to the brain. Note components of each optic nerve and which retinal region, and corresponding visual field region, are carried by each optic nerve component.

Assume lesions 1-4 are functionally complete; that is, they result in complete sensory loss for a particular visual field region.

208. Based on location of the lesions in the previous diagram, predict what the *visual field deficit* (black region) would be for lesion #2.

The life span of poikilotherms is related to the ambient temperature. In order to investigate the process of aging in these animals one must keep meticulous records of the temperature. Various parameters, other than temperature, have been introduced into aging studies which alter the life span, and one of these, ^{60}Co gamma rays, has been widely utilized with the following results.

No. of Animals	Temp. °C	Sex	Dose rads	Life Span days ± S.D.
100	18	M	0	55 ± 1
100	18	F	0	65 ± 2
100	18	M	10,000	40 ± 1
100	18	F	10,000	65 ± 2
100	20	M	10,000	55 ± 1
100	20	F	10,000	75 ± 2
100	20	M	0	65 ± 2
100	20	F	0	75 ± 2

209. The following statement(s) are related to the passage. Based on the information, select the statement(s) *supported by* the information in the passage.

   I. Life span of the animals is indirectly related to temperature.
   II. Females generally live longer than males.
   III. Radiation affects the life span of males more than that of females.

   A. I only   **C.** I and III only
   B. III only   **D.** I, II, and III

The data below show the result of an experiment concerning cell cooperation in the immune response. The experiment attempts to determine if thymus and bone marrow cells are required for antibody to be produced against egg albumin. Various donor cells (thymus or bone marrow) are injected into recipient mice whose immune system has been rendered nonresponsive by X-irradiation. Antibody levels were then determined in the serum of the recipient animals.

Donor Cells Injected	Antibody Production
1) Thymocytes + egg albumin	0
2) Thymocytes	0
3) Bone marrow + egg albumin	0
4) Bone marrow	0
5) Thymocytes + bone marrow + egg albumin	+++
6) Spleen cells + egg albumin	+++
7) Lymph node cells + egg albumin	+++

210. Based on the information given, select the statement which is *not supported by* information in the above passage.

A. In this system, bone marrow and thymus cells are required for a mouse to make antibody to egg albumin.
B. Thymus cells or cells derived from the thymus are probably found in the spleen.
C. Thymus cells or bone marrow cells or both are capable of synthesizing antibody.
D. In the intact animal, the thymus would probably be important as a source of antibody.

Days on Drug	Strength of Drug	Factor 1	Factor 2	Factor 3	Factor 4	Factor 5	Factor 6
0	0	12.5	33.0	26.5	9.3	6.2	71
6	0.05	10.7	17.0	47.0	9.6	5.0	73
6	0.10	3.0	9.8	64.0	7.0	4.8	80
6	0.20	4.8	8.9	49.2	2.4	4.6	62
6	0.50	12.0	7.9	55.8	10.7	6.6	73
12	0.05	12.5	9.8	23.1	12.9	11.0	45
12	0.10	4.4	7.9	40.7	8.3	9.1	49
12	0.20	6.8	7.2	43.0	5.9	16.7	54
12	0.50	3.9	5.7	34.2	5.3	23.0	43

211. Based on the information given, select the statement *contradicted by* the data in the above table.

A. The 12-day treatment period consistently produced a greater effect than the 6-day period.
B. The percentage of Factor 3 increased and that of Factor 2 decreased.
C. If there was an increase in Factor 3 and a decrease in Factor 2, there was a resultant rise in the Factor 3/Factor 2 ratio.
D. The proportion of isolated Factor 4 did not show any consistent trend.

Graph 1
Drug A Administered
Average Body Weight (grams)
250 200 150 100 50
0 5 10 15 20 25 30 35 40
Days after Operation

Graph 2

212. Based on the information given, select the statement(s) *supported by* the information in graphs 1 and 2.

    A. In graph 1, the operated animals lacked a desire to eat for about one week, but then ate again to maintain their body weights at a reduced level.

    B. In graph 1, the operated group that received drug A maintained their body weight while on the drug.

    C. In graph 1, when the drug was discontinued, lack of desire to eat set in and remained until the animals' weights declined to the level of the animals that were operated on but did not receive the drug.

    D. All of the above.

The thickness of the human oral epithelium was measured in seven different areas of the oral cavity in thirty cadavers. The results are tabulated below.

Area	Average	Range
A	500μ	125–950μ
B	362μ	178–780μ
C	254μ	130–489μ
D	238μ	156–320μ
E	204μ	135–270μ
F	68μ	30–146μ
G	123μ	35–260μ

213. Based on the above table, select the statement *contradicted by* the information given.

    A. The oral epithelium has a wide range of thickness in the oral cavity.

    B. The thinnest measurement was observed in Area G.

    C. The results above are not valid because they were not attained from living subjects.

    D. The range of thickness of the oral epithelium as observed was 30–950μ.

Drug X is administered to a patient and a certain value is monitored. After 30 days of treatment the physician studies the following values:

% of Drug X Administered	Days	Mean Value of Y
0.000	0	6.51
0.025	3	6.61
0.05	3	7.39
0.10	3	7.90
0.20	3	8.00
0.025	15	9.02
0.05	15	9.07
0.10	15	9.27
0.20	15	9.53
0.025	30	10.80
0.05	30	11.80
0.10	30	12.00
0.20	30	12.51

214. Based on the previous table, select the statement *not demonstrated by* the information given.

    A. The drug has an effect.

    B. There is a dose relationship to the response.

    C. The dose administered is of critical importance as can be deduced form the values.

    D. The physician can expect values of "Y" to continue to reflect dosage.

Distribution of relative amounts of radioiodinated amino acids in thyroid homogenates after administration of graded doses of PTU for three days.

Distribution of relative amounts of radioiodinated amino acids in thyroid homogenates after administration of graded doses of PTU for six days.

215. Based on the previous graphs, select the statement(s) *supported by* the information given.

A. The percentage of labeled MIT increased and that of labeled DIT decreased; in the six-day treated group there is a rise and then a decline in the MIT detected.
B. The amount of MIT rose from 26% in the controls to 64% in the three-day experimentally treated animals.
C. A rise in the MIT/DIT ratio is observed.
D. All of the above.

216. You have at your disposal benzene, bromine, nitric acid, and sulfuric acid. If you wish to produce *m*-bromonitrobenzene, you should:

A. nitrate the benzene and then brominate.
B. brominate the benzene and then nitrate.
C. do either A or B. They work equally well.
D. forget it. You cannot obtain the desired product with these materials.

217. One mole of methyl magnesium bromide will react with one mole of substrate to give the indicated product upon hydrolysis. Which substrate and product are correct?

A. acetaldehyde → primary alcohol
B. carboxylic acid → tertiary alcohol
C. ester → ketone
D. ketone → secondary alcohol

218.
$$A + B + C \xrightarrow{\quad E(enzyme) \quad} ABCD \rightarrow D + F + E$$
$$\quad (1) \qquad (2) \qquad\qquad (3) \qquad (4)$$

In the above reaction, the enzyme-substrate complex is represented by:

A. 1.   C. 3.
B. 2.   D. 4.

219. Phenylamine is cooled to 0°C and treated with HCl and $NaNO_2$. After a few minutes of reaction time cuprous bromide is added, and the solution is heated.

What percent nitrogen is contained in the final aromatic product?

A. 20   C. 8
B. 15   D. 0

Model Examination B Answer Key

Verbal Reasoning

1.	D	14.	B	27.	D	40.	C	53.	C
2.	A	15.	D	28.	A	41.	C	54.	D
3.	C	16.	D	29.	C	42.	B	55.	B
4.	D	17.	C	30.	C	43.	C	56.	C
5.	B	18.	B	31.	C	44.	D	57.	B
6.	C	19.	D	32.	A	45.	A	58.	C
7.	D	20.	C	33.	D	46.	B	59.	B
8.	D	21.	C	34.	D	47.	D	60.	D
9.	D	22.	A	35.	D	48.	B	61.	D
10.	C	23.	C	36.	A	49.	C	62.	D
11.	B	24.	D	37.	A	50.	B	63.	C
12.	D	25.	D	38.	D	51.	C	64.	D
13.	D	26.	C	39.	D	52.	C	65.	D

Physical Sciences

66.	B	82.	B	98.	A	113.	A	128.	C
67.	B	83.	C	99.	D	114.	B	129.	C
68.	D	84.	B	100.	A	115.	B	130.	B
69.	A	85.	A	101.	C	116.	B	131.	D
70.	A	86.	B	102.	B	117.	C	132.	A
71.	C	87.	A	103.	C	118.	D	133.	D
72.	C	88.	A	104.	B	119.	C	134.	D
73.	C	89.	D	105.	C	120.	D	135.	D
74.	B	90.	B	106.	B	121.	C	136.	D
75.	C	91.	D	107.	C	122.	A	137.	A
76.	A	92.	B	108.	D	123.	D	138.	D
77.	C	93.	B	109.	B	124.	D	139.	A
78.	A	94.	A	110.	D	125.	A	140.	B
79.	C	95.	C	111.	B	126.	C	141.	D
80.	B	96.	D	112.	D	127.	B	142.	B
81.	A	97.	B						

Biological Sciences

143.	B	159.	C	175.	B	190.	C	205.	C
144.	C	160.	C	176.	A	191.	C	206.	B
145.	B	161.	A	177.	B	192.	B	207.	C
146.	A	162.	B	178.	D	193.	D	208.	B
147.	B	163.	B	179.	D	194.	C	209.	D
148.	D	164.	A	180.	D	195.	C	210.	D
149.	D	165.	D	181.	D	196.	B	211.	A
150.	A	166.	C	182.	C	197.	A	212.	D
151.	B	167.	B	183.	A	198.	A	213.	B
152.	C	168.	A	184.	A	199.	C	214.	C
153.	D	169.	D	185.	A	200.	D	215.	D
154.	A	170.	C	186.	C	201.	A	216.	A
155.	B	171.	D	187.	B	202.	B	217.	C
156.	B	172.	B	188.	A	203.	B	218.	C
157.	B	173.	D	189.	C	204.	D	219.	D
158.	D	174.	A						

Explanation of Answers for Model Examination B

VERBAL REASONING

1. **D.** At the end of the first paragraph, the author states the need for designers, clients, and students to understand the essence of graphic design. The remainder of the passage provides examples of the many objectives that this discipline accomplishes.

2. **A.** In sentence number two, the author speaks about the extraordinary flowering of this art form and describes it as a potent means of communication as well as a major component of our visual culture.

3. **C.** Paragraph four describes resonance as being the most important thing that graphic design provides. Resonance is viewed as a richness of tone that heightens the expressive power of a page.

4. **D.** Graphic design is a diverse field. The first five paragraphs include mention of each of the tasks given above. Problem solving can be found in paragraphs one and five; organization of space in paragraphs one and three; visual and symbolic qualities in paragraphs one, two, and three.

5. **B.** In paragraph three the author states that graphic design is a hybrid discipline in which, "Diverse elements, including signs, symbols, words, and pictures are collected and assembled into a total message."

6. **C.** The example of the designer explaining his job to his grandmother is used to illustrate the general public's confusion about graphic design. The answers he gives to her questions show that he has pulled together the talents of many people to produce his end result. The grandmother does not understand because she probably is used to an artist producing a work by himself rather than by coordinating the work of others.

7. **D.** Of all the statements listed, **D** has the least intense communication vocabulary in it. In a communication society, clear verbal and visual information are essential, expressive power in design conveys important messages, and instruction as well as motivation are important facets of keeping well informed.

8. **D.** In paragraph two the author says that a universal language of form is common to all visual disciplines, but that too much dependence upon other arts—such as architecture and painting—is unsatisfactory for graphic artists because their discipline has unique purposes and visual properties.

9. **D.** The passage clearly discusses all four answers to the question. The scientific method is detailed at the onset, scientific experimentation and responsibility are discussed, but definitely the author has written this text to debate and clarify the issues that surround the gathering, recording, and storing of scientific data.

10. **C.** The author makes the point that at various periods, different components of the scientific method have been emphasized. It is also emphasized that early on propositions were formulated and debated with minimum organized observation or collection of data. The above statement would eliminate the several critical elements of the strict application of the scientific method as mentioned in **A, B,** and **D** of the question.

11. **B.** The passage makes it clear that throughout history a great deal of haphazard observing, recording, and analysis have occurred. It is stated in the article that with the coming of the industrial age, inventors focused on solutions, but oftentimes they did not start with well formulated questions. The scientific method requires the above. Philosophers did give way to the age of the observers and observers gave way to the industrial age. There is no support in the passage for the claim that, as industrialization progressed, a clear scientific approach became standard for solving problems.

12. **D.** The passage does point out that inventors sought legal protection under constitutionally guaranteed rights to patent intellectual property. It is clearly stated at the end of paragraph one that record keeping now has become formalized, standardized, and required. Regulatory agencies not only can, but do require (according to the passage) that they be allowed to inspect complete records of product development. Statement IV is

contradicted in paragraphs one and two; failed experiments should be recorded to eliminate repetition, and also unwanted results (e.g., toxicity of drug) should not be suppressed because harm might result.

13. **D.** None of the statements is supported by the passage. In paragraph three, the author makes the point that there is no universally accepted definition of data. The question asked in paragraph three is "are data the printouts of computers?" But no answer is provided, and this question is raised because we don't know what data are. Can we require scientists to record and store it? The paragraph ends asking who is responsible for keeping and storing data.

14. **B.** It is quite clear from the passage that an evolutionary process has been involved in the data collection process and that data keeping and storage have become ends unto themselves in order to ensure that work paid for was actually done. No mention is made regarding the must of a modified hypothesis, and the fact that managers of public funds are clearly inadequate to judge scientific work is inescapable.

15. **D.** The passage focuses on data collection and storage and makes it quite clear that the public's money is not well protected, that the public truly has no great trust in science, and that above all, scientific peer review and policing are flawed.

16. **D.** While all three statements are viable and reasonable, they are not discussed by the author.

17. **C.** The main theme of the passage deals with the shifting of decision-making power in school districts, from one where the board of education is the most important player to one where power is shared. Paragraph one states this in the opening sentence. The remainder of the passage goes on to name the parties that are becoming more powerful, especially teachers and parents. The flow chart, which represents both traditional and modern decision-making power, graphically supports the information presented in the passage.

18. **B.** Paragraph two discusses the fact that today's teachers want to have a voice in program development as well as in determining salary scales. Later in the passage teachers are presented in an even more forceful light as their power to bring an educational system to a halt by means of strikes is noted.

19. **D.** Because the central theme of the passage discusses the fact that the board of education no longer holds absolute power in most school districts, **D** is a direct contradiction to the theme since it proposes that the power remain with the board.

20. **C.** Statement I, which talks about the emergence of parent volunteer programs in schools, and statement III, which claims that parents are becoming more powerful in schools, are both true according to the passage.

21. **C.** The *degree* of decision-making power desired by the parties described in this passage is not mentioned and therefore **C**, which calls for *equality* of power, is not supported. The statement is not contradicted because a specific degree of power is not a topic of the passage.

22. **A.** The chart presents the traditional flow of power and communication by using a solid arrow that comes from the board of education down through the students. The modern flow is represented by the broken arrows, whose direction not only goes up and down but swings out between teachers and the superintendent and students and the principal.

23. **C.** The chart presented is a simplified version of a typical organizational flow chart. Parents operate outside of the organization in the sense that they are not elected or appointed to an official position, sign no contract, and receive no salary. Although the students represented on the chart also do not sign a contract and receive no salary, the implication of a contract exists. According to law, children must attend school until age 16.

24. **D.** All three statements are conclusions that reasonably could be drawn from this passage. Paragraphs one and two talk about the present shift in decision-making power and allude to the fact that it will continue to occur. The chart shows how this has been liberalized. As parents become more involved in school affairs, the possibility of being a part of the policy-making process may become a reality. As decision making becomes more decentralized and more site based, it will become harder to point to the decision maker because the latter process will be shared.

25. **D.** Although the fourteenth amendment is the vehicle that guarantees and protects a student's

right to a public education, the main focus of this passage concerns expulsion from school, which would be a denial of that right.

26. **C.** Time-out procedures are not mentioned in this passage. Exclusion from school is the actual removal of a student from the educational setting. The difference between suspension and expulsion is described in paragraph two.

27. **D.** Expulsion from school generally is considered to be the most severe student punishment available to school administrators. In paragraph two of the passage, the author writes that state statutes and local policies usually provide that only a local school board has the prerogative to expel a student.

28. **A.** Paragraph three notes that in recent years litigation has involved both the right of school officials to exclude students as well as the rights that students have to due process prior to suspension and/or expulsions,

29. **C.** Although the matter had been treated in lower courts, *Goss v. Lopez* brought the exclusion question to the United States Supreme Court. The case is explained in paragraphs three through five.

30. **C.** Paragraph four points out that the right to a public education is a property right. Because the fourteenth amendment protects an individual's right to his/her property, the removal of a student from school would constitute an affront to his/her property.

31. **C.** Paragraph five explains that school officials *do* have the power to remove a student from the school setting, prior to suspension, if his/her presence constitutes a danger to persons or property and/or is disruptive to teaching and learning.

32. **A.** Paragraph seven discusses *Wood v. Strickland*. Although upholding the school board's actions in the case, the Court ruled that an individual member could be sued if he knew or reasonably should have known that a student's constitutional rights were denied.

33. **D.** The last paragraph discusses the fact that students have a right to nominal damages. In this case, *Carey v. Piphus,* punitive damages may also result if an official acted with malicious intent.

34. **D.** Paragraph two discussed the fact that criteria used in evaluations are similar for full-time and part-time faculty. Paragraphs seven and eight deal with research faculty, whereas the remaining paragraphs discuss clinical faculty. The issue of administrative faculty is not addressed specifically by the passage.

35. **D.** Paragraph four addresses the issues of bonding and identifying with an institution and also points out that long-term contracts would be one solution in the job security issue. The whole passage deals with the roles of several categories of faculty and the diverse issues posed and the need to find appropriate solutions. It is clearly stated in paragraph four that tenure is *not* the only way to achieve bonding.

36. **A.** Job security is discussed in paragraph four. The inequity of compensation and the evaluation criteria are addressed in paragraph two. Academic freedom is discussed in paragraph three and is a nonissue according to the author.

37. **A.** Paragraph two indicated that qualifications do not necessarily distinguish faculties and the level of the course taught does not reflect teaching ability. The argument that all students need qualified and enthusiastic instructors is made at the onset of paragraph one. Paragraph three indicates that academic freedom protects all faculty and introduction of changes is not limited. Paragraph two makes it quite clear that when students evaluate teaching, they may or may not know a faculty member's academic qualifications or tenure status.

38. **D.** None of the statements made is discussed in the passage.

39. **D.** Paragraph seven mentions the tripartite foundation of teaching, research, and public service. In paragraph three it is pointed out that the right of freedom of speech for all faculty members is guaranteed.

40. **C.** Paragraph nine makes the argument that much of clinical teaching is delivered by non-tenure-eligible faculty who serve on a short-term basis and the activities are not linked solely with the generation of income. The passage is clear on the issue of relegation of nontenure-eligible faculty to second-class citizenship. The last paragraph stresses that incentives and recognition are very important to clinical faculty members.

41. **C.** Paragraph two substantiates statements **A** and **B**. Paragraph four states that tenure means job security and bonds an individual to the institution. Paragraph nine makes it clear that the institution's reward system leans toward research.

42. **B.** Paragraph five makes it clear that the Red Cross believed that it should serve as an emergency relief organization and obtain its funds from private contributions. Hoover was invited to join the executive committee; Norman Davis was the head of the Red Cross.

43. **C.** Paragraph three points out that in all of Hoover's rescue efforts, children represented his first concern.

44. **D.** Paragraph one states that Hoover was a successful consulting engineer before he undertook his relief activities.

45. **A.** The last line of the passage leaves no doubt that Hoover's and Roosevelt's camps did not agree with each other. Paragraph one mentions that Hoover took an active part in negotiating between the warring factions and that his efforts were not limited to war victims. He helped handily the victims of the Mississippi floods of 1927.

46. **B.** Hoover (paragraph five), within less than two weeks of outbreak of hostilities, raised the relief question and suggested that one organization should provide a focal point. Paragraph four ends with the line that hungry people cannot defend themselves nor defend freedom. Paragraph three makes it clear that Mrs. Hoover supported her husband's efforts.

47. **D.** There can be no doubt in the reader's mind that Hoover was a humanitarian with an interest in helping victims.

48. **B.** This question truly should awaken the reader to the fact that the whole passage, including the references and credits, should be read. In the credit it is pointed out that the material was presented at a conference on education of the gifted for the twenty-first century.

49. **C.** Paragraph four states that tragedies are potentially effective for developing ethics and even wisdom. The last paragraph emphasizes that teachers can put key ideas together for wise leadership in individuals of the next generation. It is proposed that teachers determine and give birth

to the future. **D** tries to mislead you drastically, but careful reading of paragraph seven points out that the author distinguishes between ethical skills and ethical knowledge, which is the development of right reasoning.

50. **B.** The author in paragraph one does not speak of unavoidable mistakes major injustices, or personal grief. However, faulty logic is presented and associated with the word *hamartia*.

51. **C.** In paragraph four it is pointed out that Dewey feared a danger of either dogmatism or a sense of unreality when students are abruptly introduced to theoretical ideas. He proposes to first introduce students to simple cases and then proceed to the more complex.

52. **C.** Paragraph nine reasons that teacher preparation of material keeps the cases current, and in this way the cases help future generations.

53. **C.** Paragraphs seven through nine emphasize the combination of student feedback and teacher production of material (formulating good and humane reasoning) to be an essential skill in the passing on of a sense of ethics from one generation to another.

54. **D.** At the end of paragraph one, and again, at the end of paragraph eight, the authors state their conclusion that drivers of cars equipped with air bags tend to drive more aggressively than drivers of cars not equipped with air bags. In paragraph seven, the authors assert that the data leads to the conclusion that the increased aggressiveness is due to offsetting behavior.

55. **B.** Paragraph five asserts that 1990 was when auto manufacturers began equipping their cars with at least one air bag due to perceived market forces.

56. **C.** The authors first introduce the concept of "buyer sorting" as a competing hypothesis for "offsetting behavior" in paragraph one. Paragraph six defines and develops the "buyer sorting" concept.

57. **B.** In paragraph two, Lave and Weber's initial studies are alluded to, and the passage goes on to assert that most of the early researchers, presumably including Lave and Weber, found that the benefits of the mandated safety devices exceeded their costs.

58. **C.** In paragraph eight, the authors specifically note that they studied automobile fatality statistics for Virginia. No other state is mentioned in the passage.

59. **B.** The aggressive driving component of the authors' conclusion is perhaps the central component of all of the various conclusions presented in the passage. Paragraphs one and eight assert, as a foundation for other conclusions, that drivers of automobiles equipped with air bags drive more aggressively than those whose automobiles are not equipped with them.

60. **D.** Paragraph one makes it clear that all three statements in the question are true.

61. **D.** Paragraph two discusses the issue of cost/benefit in disaster planning measures. Paragraph three, four, and five deal with quantification, whereas, paragraph six mentions the fortress, hot, warm, cold, and privately owned sites, and the reciprocal processing agreements.

62. **D.** The last paragraph mentions that the two most important management issues involved in disaster planning are who is responsible and which applications get top priority. It is also pointed out that a formal plan should be the final outcome of the process.

63. **C.** Paragraph four points out that statistical means are a technique used by a company to establish priorities. Paragraph five emphasizes that each scenario must be financially analyzed and weighed against competing corporate projects. It is pointed out in paragraph one that less than 50 percent of central data processing sites have adequate contingency plans.

64. **D.** Paragraph three deals with the determination of cost and mentions initial costs, costs over a three- to five-year period, and a company's borrowing rate.

65. **D.** Paragraph seven stresses that the fortress system is probably very well prepared for disasters. In paragraph eight it is mentioned that hot sites are associated with high costs. Paragraph nine states that cold sites provide space only, and there is concern about proper coverage and the shared membership arrangement.

PHYSICAL SCIENCES

66. **B.** Power = voltage × current:
$I = P/V = 240$ watt/120 volts = 2.00 A.

67. **B.** 85 dB is correct. A doubling of the intensity of a sound (using 2 speakers here) corresponds to an increase of only 3 dB in apparent loudness level. The dB level is given by: $dB_1 = 10 \log_{10}(I/I_0)$. The solution is:

$$82 \text{ dB} = 10 \log_{10}(I/I_0) \text{ or } 8.2 = \log_{10}(I_1/I_0)$$

Then the dB level for two speakers (with $I_2 = 2I_1$) is:

$$dB_2 \ 10 \log_{10}(I_2/I_0) = 10 \log_{10}(2I_1/I_0)$$

Now, $\log ab = (\log a + \log b)$. Here $a = 2$ and $b = I_1/I_0$, and thus, $dB_2 = 10 \log_{10}(2) + 10 \log_{10}(I_1/I_0) = 3 + 82 \text{ dB} + 85 \text{ dB}$

68. **D.** To find the velocity we must first find the time for the sound wave to travel to the end of the water tube and return. The time is found from the pulse separation and the sweep time setting on the oscilloscope:

$$t = 5.4 \text{ cm} \times 0.1 \times 10^{-3} \text{ sec/cm} = 5.4 \times 10^{-4} \text{ sec.}$$

The velocity of sound in the water is:

$$V = 2L/t = 2(0.4 \text{ m})/(5.4 \times 10^{-4} \text{ sec}) = 1481 \text{ m/sec.}$$

69. **A.** The velocity of any wave is given by:

$$v = \text{frequency} \times \text{wavelength} = f\lambda$$

The wavelength is:

$$\lambda = 340 \text{ m/sec}/3000 \text{ Hz} = 0.11 \text{ m/sec}$$

The wavelength in aluminum is much longer because the greater "rigidity" of Al causes much higher wave velocity of about 5100 m/sec.

70. **A.** Both ends of the above frequency range are beyond the limits of human hearing. Persons with good hearing can hear frequencies from 20 to 20,000 Hz. Sounds below 20 Hz are "infrasound" and those above 20,000 Hz are "ultrasound."

71. **C.** The given formula allows calculation of the period. The string length must be in meters. $L = 0.5$ m.
$$T = 2\pi \sqrt{L/g} = 6.28 \sqrt{0.5/9.8} = 1.41 \text{ sec}$$

72. **C.** The formula for the pendulum is independent of the mass and the angle of swing (so long as the angle is *small*; 10° or less). Thus the period is unchanged, since the length of the string is still 0.5 m.

73. **C.** Hooke's Law for the elastic spring states that the stretch or elongation, x, of a spring is proportional to the stretching force, $F = kx$, where k is the "spring constant." Here, $F = mg = kx$, so that $F = 0.5$ kg $\times$ 9.8 m/sec$^2 = k \times$ 0.49 m. Thus $k = 10$ N/m.

74. **B.** We use the formula given for a mass on the end of a spring. $T = 2\pi \sqrt{m/k}$ (The 5-cm amplitude does not appear in the expression for T. It is characteristic of simple harmonic oscillators that their periods do not depend on the starting amplitudes. For the pendulum above, the amplitude was the initial angle.)

$$T = 2\pi \sqrt{m/k} = 6.28 \sqrt{0.5\text{kg}/10\text{N}/m} = 1.4 \text{ sec}$$

75. **C.** The mass is increased by a factor of 4 over the previous question. Since the mass appears under the square root sign and the root of 4 is 2, the period will double.

76. **A.** It is obvious that it will take a larger force to stretch this double-spring system a given amount. $F = k_{eff}x$, where k_{eff} is the "effective spring constant." Since the springs are identical, it will take twice as much force to stretch the spring(s) the same amount, x. Then $k_{eff} = k + k = 2k$. (If the springs were not identical, one would still add the k's together.) Using the m (0.5 kg) and k (10 N/m) from question 75:

$$T = 2\pi \sqrt{m/2k} = 1.0 \text{ sec}$$

77. **C.** The equivalent resistance for series connections of resistors is equal to the sum of the individual resistances.

$$R_s + R_1 + R_2 + R_3, \text{ and so on. Then } I = V/R_s$$
from Ohm's law; so $I = 1$ A.

The individual voltage drops are also found using Ohm's law,

$$V = 1 \text{ A} \times 2 \text{ ohm} = 2 \text{ volts.}$$

78. **A.** No DC current can flow through the capacitor. The 6 volts does appear across the capacitor (when it is fully charged).

79. **C.** For a parallel connection, the full 120 volt drop occurs across both resistors. Then $I = V/Z = V/R = 120/2 = 60$ amperes AC, is the current through each resistor. (Note that $Z = R$ for a "pure" resistance.)

80. **B.** The rules for parallel and series combinations of resistors must be used to find the equiva-

lent total resistance. ($1/R_p = 1/R_1 + 1/R_2 = 1/2 + 1/2$ and then $R_p = 1$ ohm) ($R_s = R_3 + R_p = 3$ ohms = the equivalent resistance). Using Ohm's law again,

$$I = 6 \text{ volts}/3 \text{ ohms} = 2 \text{ amperes.}$$

81. **A.** The solution to this problem requires one to calculate the impedance Z for the RC series circuit. Here $Z = \sqrt{(X_c)^2 + R^2}$ where $X_c = 1/(2\pi fC)$ where f is the 60 Hz frequency and C is 1×10^{-6} Fd. The AC form of Ohm's law then gives I = V/Z = 120/2653 = .045 amperes.

82. **B.** The energy for the motion comes from the expanding compressed spring so that energy is not "conserved" here. However, the total momentum of the two cart system is constant. Because the initial total momentum was zero, the final momentum of the system is also zero, i.e.,

$$P_i = P_f, \text{ or}$$
$$0 = m_1v_1 + m_2v_2$$
and $\quad v_2 = -m_1v_1/m_2 = -1.0 \text{ m/sec.}$

83. **C.** Because of the spring steel bumper we may assume that the total kinetic energy of the two cart system is conserved as well as the total momentum. There are two equations that apply, namely:

$$m_1v_1 + 0 = m_1V_1 + m_2V_2 \text{ and}$$
$$1/2\ m_1v_1^2 + 0 = 1/2\ m_1V_1^2 + 1/2\ m_2V_2^2.$$

All the m's are equal, so $V_1 + V_2 = 2$ m/sec and $V_1^2 + V_2^2 = 4$ m^2/sec^2. The questions are satisfied only if one of the V's is 0 and the other is 2 m/sec. The solution of these two equations shows that the first cart stops; giving up all its kinetic energy to the second cart. Hence, $V_2 = 2.0$ m/sec in the same direction as the original velocity of cart #1.

84. **B.** In this question the energy dissipated due to air friction is apparent because of the decrease in the kinetic energy of the cart.

$$E_{lost} = 1/2\ mv_i^2 - 1/2\ mv_f^2 = 1.6 \text{ joules}$$

($m = 0.45$ kg, $v_f = 3.0$ m/sec, and $v_i = 4.0$ m/sec).

85. **A.** If one equates the energy loss in explanation for question 84 to the (negative) work done by friction over the distance of $x = 2.0$ meters;

$$F_fx = 1.6 \text{ joules, then } F_f = 0.8 \text{ N}$$

86. **B.** This question deals with the interchange of energy between the forms of kinetic energy and

gravitational potential energy. The total energy is conserved but does change form.

$$KE_i = PE_f$$

$1/2\, mv^2 - 0 = mgh$. Solving this for $v = \sqrt{2gh}$ we find that $v = 3.13$ m/sec.

87. **A.** As above we use the conservation of linear momentum principle with the initial momentum of the system equal to zero. $v_2 = -10$ m/sec.

88. **A.** Snell's law of Refraction, $n_1\sin\theta_1 = n_2\sin\theta_2$, applies to this problem. Solving for $\sin\theta_2$:

$$\sin\theta_2 = (n_1/n_2)\,\sin\theta_1$$

θ_2 will be larger than θ_1 if n_1 is greater than n_2 (and vice versa). In this case, when the ray of light is incident from inside the glass $n_1 = 1.65$ is indeed larger than $n_2 = 1.0$ for air. θ_2 will be larger than 30°.

89. **D.** This is a constant velocity problem: $V = x/t$. Here we have $x = 2d$ since the sound travels the distance d to the building and returns. Thus $d = vt/2 = 688$ m.

90. **B.** The linear and angular speeds are related by the expression $v = \omega t$, where ω must be in radians/sec. In this question, $\omega = 2$ rev/sec $\times 2\pi$ rad/rev $= 4\pi$ rad/sec. The centripetal force is given by $F_c = mv^2/r$. Thus:

$$v = 0.5 \text{ m} \times 4\pi \text{ rad/sec} = 6.28 \text{ m/sec}$$
$$F_c = 1 \text{ kg} \times (6.28 \text{ m/sec})^2/0.5 \text{ m} = 79 \text{ N}$$

91. **D.** The number of half-lives is 16/5.3 or about 3 half-lives. The activity in curies is reduced by half (0.5) for each half-life, so the activity remaining is approximately 5000 curies $\times 0.5 \times 0.5 \times 0.5 = 625$ curies. The exact exponential decay formula should be used if the time is not some integer number of half-lives:

$A = A_0 e^{-0.693t/T}$
T = half-life
t = actual time
A_0 = initial activity

92. **B.** The apparent weight of an object equals the true weight minus the upward buoyant force of the surrounding fluid, $B_f = \rho gV$, where ρ is the fluid density. Since the specific gravity (SG) is equal to the density of a substance divided by the density of water ($\rho_w = 1.0$ grams/cm^3) the SG has the same value as the density in CGS units. Weight = mg; thus $W_A = W_T - \rho gV$ can be written

$m_A g = mg - SG_f gV$. (Cancel the g's.) The density of the object $\rho_0 = m/V$ so that $V = m/\rho_0 = m/SG_0$. Finally, $m_A = m - Sg_f m/SG_0$. Then $SG_0 = 2.37$.

93. **B.** The diffraction grating equation $m\lambda = d\sin\theta$ can be solved for the value of m. λ is the wavelength and θ is the angle of diffraction.

$$m = (d/\lambda)\sin\theta = 1.67 \times 10^{-6} \text{ m} \sin 30°)/$$
$$417 \times 10^{-9} \text{ m} = 1.99 = 2$$

94. **A.** Power = Voltage $\times$ Current, $P = VI$. When appliances are plugged into the same circuit, they act like resistances in parallel where the effective resistance is less than the smallest resistance. The parallel appliances will draw more current by Ohm's Law, $I = V/R_e$. This means that the power ratings will *add*: $P_e = P_1 + P_2 = 2400$ watts. The current they both draw is: $I = P_e/V = 2400/120 = 20$ amperes.

95. **C.** Nuclear reaction equations must balance *charge subscripts* and *mass superscripts* on each side of the reaction, since charge is conserved and mass-energy changes are a very small fraction of the total mass-energy. Thus: $13 = 13 + 0 + 0$ is balanced and $7 = z + 1$. So $z = 6$ and the nucleus X is carbon, C.

96. **D.** Both the total nucleon number and the total charge are constant in a nuclear reaction. The number of nucleons is the sum of all protons and all neutrons, whereas the charge number is the sum of all proton charges. Here the total charge is 42 and the total number of nucleons is 99. Thus: $42 = Z - 1$ or $Z = 43$ for Tc and $99 = A + 0$ so that $A = 99$ for Tc.

97. **B.** Given that the half-life (the time for one-half the original nuclei to decay) is 67 hours for Mo^{99}, we find that 5.5 days is very nearly two half-lives. Thus after 5.5 days only 1/4 or 0.25 remains.

98. **A.** The effective half-life is given by the expression $1/Te = 1/T_{phy} + 1/T_{bio}$ so that the effective values is always less than either T_{phy} or T_{bio}. One should be able to answer the question without knowing the exact form of the above equation by realizing that biological excretion helps rid the body of the original radioactive material at the same time it is decaying. (There is only one answer, **A**, smaller than T_{phy}.)

99. **D.** Because one half-life for Tc99m has elapsed since 8:00 the activity must have been two times

larger at 8:00 AM. (The activity in curies is the number of decays per second, 1 Ci = 3.7×10^{10} dps.)

100. **A.** As in question 96 above, the total nucleon number and total charge on each side of the decay equation are constants. Thus the number of nucleons remains 201 (201 + 0 = 201), whereas the charge on the nucleus decreases by 1 (81 − 1 = 80).

101. **C.** 9.25 days is equal to three half-lives for T1-201. The fraction remaining is then: 1/2 × 1/2 × 1/2 = 1/8. Thus 1/8 of 80 mCi remains.

102. **B.** This problem is simply a conversion problem in effect because all necessary information is given.
(70 mrad/mCi) × (10 microCi/kg) × 70 kg = ? One must convert millicuries and microcuries to the same units so that they will cancel. 10 microCi = 0.010 millicuries. The result is 49 millirads.

103. **C.** As the term implies, only gamma radiation is emitted in the decay. This is desirable because particle radiation, such as electrons and alpha particles, cannot escape the body tissue and thus cannot be detected. Such particles would expose the patient to radiation damage without any useful result.

104. **B.** Because Technicium-99m emits no particles, the whole dose is due to gamma radiation and the rem dose is the same as the rads. 400 mrads = 400 mrems.

105. **C.** The fraction penetrating must be less than 1%, i.e., less than 0.01. One can multiply 1/2 by itself until the result is less than 0.01. This requires 7 terms: 1/2 × 1/2 × 1/2 × 1/2 × 1/2 × 1/2 × 1/2 = 0.0078. Thus 7 half-thicknesses 7 × 0.4 cm = 2.8 cm of lead is required.

106. **B.** One mole of three is 33%.

107. **C.** It is necessary to recall the approximate atomic weights: C—12; 0—16; H—1. Thus the weights are 44g for CO_2, 34g for H_2O_2, and 32g for O_2. The total weight is 110g and 44/110 = 0.4 or 40%.

108. **D.** The number of molecules in a mole of any compound is 6.0×10^{23} (Avogadro's number).

109. **B.** The elements would be C, O_2, and H_2. By inspection there would be one mole of C, three moles of O_2, and one mole of H_2. The C would be a solid and there would be four moles of gas (3 + 1).

110. **D.** Under conditions of standard temperature and pressure, a mole of any gas will occupy 22.4 liters. Thus one mole each of CO_2 and O_2 will occupy a total of 2(22.4) = 44.8 liters. H_2O_2 is a liquid. One mole of H_2O_2 is only 34g and will occupy less than 0.05 liters.

111. **B.** $BaCl_2$ can reversibly hydrolyze to form 2 HCl and $Ba(OH)_2$. The HCl will be strongly ionized, providing large numbers of hydrogen ions. $Ba(OH)_2$ will be weakly ionized, providing few hydroxyl ions. There will be a net contribution of hydrogen ions. NaCl and $NaNO_3$ can each reversibly hydrolyze to form a strong base and a strong acid. There will be no net contribution of hydrogen or hydroxyl ions. Sodium acetate can reversibly hydrolyze to form a weak acid (acetic acid) and a strong base (NaOH). There will be a net contribution of hydroxyl ions.

112. **D.** See explanation for question 111. Sodium acetate can reversibly hydrolyze to form NAOH and acetic acid, producing a net contribution of hydroxyl ions.

113. **A.** NaCl and $NaNO_3$, each a salt of a strong acid and a strong base, will be essentially neutral.

114. **B.** The temperature of 383°K is equal to 110°C. Although the salts will increase the boiling point of water, it should boil at or below this temperature.

115. **B.** No significant change will be noted on dilution of this salt of a strong base and a strong acid.

116. **B.** Heat is transferred through the solid by conduction. Silver is a good conductor of heat.

117. **C.** Stainless steel is not as good a conductor of heat as is silver, and the handle of the stainless steel spoon will not become so hot so quickly.

118. **D.** Transfer of heat through a gas or vacuum is quickly accomplished in line of sight by radiation. The heat is carried at the speed of light by infrared rays.

119. **C.** The screen would block transfer of heat by radiation. Instead, the heat would be more slowly transferred as the fire heats the air, producing convection currents.

120. **D.** Transfer of heat from a heat source to another body through a gas is quickly accomplished by radiation.

121. **C.** It is noted that there are two moles of gas on the left side of the equation and one mole on the right side. Considering the fact that one mole of gas occupies a volume of 22.4 liters at standard temperature and pressure, imposition of greater pressure should favor the shift of equilibrium to the right, thus reducing the total number of moles of gas.

122. **A.** Two moles of gas are noted on the left side of the equation and three moles on the right. Thus, greater pressure should shift the equation to the left, favoring H_2S.

123. **D.** Because two moles of gas are noted on each side, a pressure change should not affect the equilibrium of the reaction.

124. **D.** A and B are both correct, Without a change in K_{eq}, the addition of either reactant on the left side will result in more of the product on the right side, which uses up some of the H_2.

125. **A.** Without a change in temperature or pressure, addition of material on side of an equilibrium equation will result in more of a product or products on the other side. This will occur without a change in K_{eq}.

126. **C.** $pK_b = -\log K_b$ = between 4 and 5 (by inspection).

127. **B.**
$$K_b = \frac{[NH_4^+][OH^-]}{[NH3]} = \frac{[OH^-]^2}{0.01}$$
$$= 1.8 \times 10^{-5}$$
$$[OH^-]^2 = (0.01)(1.8 \times 10^{-5})$$
$$= 1.8 \times 10^{-7}$$
$$[OH^-] = 4 \times 10^{-4}$$
$$pOH = -\log[OH^-] = \text{between 3 and 4}$$
$$\text{(by inspection)}.$$

128. **C.** $pH = 14 - pOH = 14 - 3.40 = 10.60$.

129. **C.** $pK_b = -\log K_b$ = between 5 and 6 (by inspection).

130. **B.**
$$K_b = \frac{[HyH^+][OH^-]}{[Hy]} = \frac{[OH^-]^2}{0.001}$$
$$= 1.7 \times 10^{-6}$$
$$[OH^-]^2 = (0.001)(1.7 \times 10^{-6})$$
$$= 1.7 \times 10^{-9}$$
$$[OH^-]^2 = \text{about } 4 \times 10^{-5}$$
pOH is between 4 and 5.

131. **D.** $pH = 14 - pOH = 14 - (\text{between 4 and 5}) = $ between 9 and 10.

132. **A.** As the smallest pK_a will give the lowest pH, the smallest pK_b will give the lowest pOH and the highest pH.

133. **D.** The Lewis theory or concept does not deal specifically with hydrogen ions or hydroxyl ions.

134. **D.** NAOH is a strong base and is assumed to be virtually completely ionized.

135. **D.** $pOH = -\log[OH^-] = -\log(1 \times 10^{-3}) = 3$
$pH = 14 - pOH = 11$.

136. **D.** The half-reactions for the given reaction are as follows:

oxidation: $2Fe^{2+} \rightarrow 2Fe^{3+} + 2e^-$
reduction: $Cl_2 + 2e^- - 2Cl^-$

An oxidizing agent is defined as the substance being reduced. In this redox equation, Cl_2 is being reduced and is the oxidizing agent.

137. **A.** Nonpolar covalent bonds are formed between atoms of the same element or atoms with the same electronegativity. The F_2 molecule has one nonpolar covalent bond only and is therefore a nonpolar molecule.

138. **D.** An acid reacts with a base to form a salt and water. KOH is a base.

139. **A.** This is a definition of an ionic bond. It results in two ions of opposite charge.

140. **B.** Although different sublevels have different maximum numbers of orbital, any one orbital can hold a maximum of two electrons.

141. **D.** The smaller the K_{sp}, the less soluble the salt. Of the four choices, AgI has the smallest K_{sp} (the largest negative exponent).

142. **B.** A substance can act as both an oxidizing agent and a reducing agent only if the oxidation state of the element can become higher and lower than it is. There are no lower oxidation states for Fe^0 and Cu^0; there are no higher oxidation states for Fe^{3+}.

WRITING SAMPLE

Part 1, Essay

A wise person, according to Johnson, is one who knows that dreams and hopes are no substitute for reality. Though it may not always be pleasant or exciting to know what the next day will bring, there is no wisdom in reaching out for something exciting or pleasant when one cannot be sure that it is there. A realist has more hope to find happiness if he takes his reality and alters it than one who casts about in the dark hoping to find a pot of gold. A person may take his last dollar and buy a lottery ticket, hoping to win a jackpot, but the wise individual will take his last dollar and use it to buy food. Though the foolish person may think that because he is desperate, good, and deserving and that God or fate will intervene on his behalf, the wise one knows that fate and God will do little to even the odds. The wise person knows he needs food more than he needs a one in seven million chance of becoming rich.

But what courage does it take to face each day that is the same as the last? Is it wise to keep one's feet firmly planted on the ground, taking no risks? To stay with what is certain out of fear of the unknown is certainly safe, but it may be unwise. Imagine a shoe retailer is approached by a partner who has developed a new last and leather that will make women's shoes more comfortable to wear, but they will appear just as stylish. The partner asks the store owner to place the new shoes in his front window, and for this favor the two will share whatever profits come from the venture in half. The shoe salesperson refuses, knowing that the shoes he has shown in his window for the last five years have brought in a steady stream of customers. Though he is not getting rich, at least he is certain that his current display works. The partner sets off to find another store owner, discovering one only three doors down from the first shop he visited. The second owner takes the risk, for he knows that nothing great is achieved without some peril. For days the first shoe salesperson sees streams of people walking by his store, and wondering where they are going, peeks outside to see them entering his competitor's shop. Word has spread, and even the first shopkeeper's regular male customers desert him for the shop down the street. Though women buy the new shoes for themselves, men pick them up for their wives; and while they are in the shop, they find it convenient to buy their own shoes there, too. The first shopkeeper goes out of business, blaming himself for not having the wisdom to have faith in a good, albeit unproved, idea.

Had the shopkeeper been wiser, perhaps what he would have seen was that this was not a matter of uncertainty. It is possible that had he been thinking, he would have recognized that it was a certainty that women would want to wear a more comfortable shoe, and that though it seemed new and risky to stock the new shoes, there was no risk involved at all. The wisdom is not in an unwillingness to make a change, it is in the unwillingness to make a change without considering the realistic possibilities of it. The chances involved in buying a lottery ticket make it such an impossible odd that the wise individual will reject the notion of spending his last dollar on it. The chances that women will prefer comfortable and stylish shoes over uncomfortable and stylish shoes, however, is not a chance at all. It is reasonable to assume that given the choice between discomfort and comfort the customer will choose comfort. A wise person knows a certainty when he sees it, and he knows that sometimes what appears to be a risk is not a risk at all. By the same token, a wise person knows when a safe offer is really a risk, and no matter how often he says, "I need this money, surely fate will let me have it. It is only fair that one who is as deserving as I should win" will not change the odds in a lottery. So the wise individual is indeed one who will not quit certainty for uncertainty, but it is the same wise individual who knows the difference.

Part 1
Explanation of First Response: 6

This essay focuses clearly on Johnson's statement and addresses each of the three writing tasks. Paragraph one explains what the statement means, paragraph two gives a specific situation in which one would not be wise to give up a certainty for an uncertainty, and paragraph three explores circumstances that determine whether it is wise or unwise to give up a certainty for an uncertainty.

The paper provides an explanation of the quotation by introducing "reality" as a qualifier for "certainty" and "dreams and hopes" for "uncertainty." This allows the author to cite concrete examples like the one that refers to the lottery to complete the explanation by referring to realistic and unrealistic acts. Through an effective example in paragraph two, the paper illustrates that safety, contrary to the implication of the quotation, may sometimes be unwise, as the first owner discovers. Finally the passage provides a balanced analysis of the things that determine whether quitting certainty for uncertainty is wise or unwise.

The writing in this essay is clear and controlled. The writer's use of concrete examples is one of the strongest features of the passage. They grow logically out of the main ideas of each paragraph and illustrate the ideas very effectively. The lottery ticket example is easy to relate to as an example of the uncertainty of taking a long shot, whereas the shoe shop example provides a clear example of a time when acting on at least mild uncertainty can be wise indeed. There is variety in the sentence structure, and the paper flows smoothly from one sentence to the next.

Part 2, Essay

Graham Greene's definition of destruction is really only an argument of semantics. Because "create" only means to bring into being, to cause to exist, then any act of change is also an act of creation. The idea is not a new one and appears in even as ancient a myth as that of the phoenix, who rises again out of the ashes of its own funeral pile. What Greene is suggesting is an alternative perspective by which one could view or interpret destruction. The connotations of "destruction" are generally negative ones. Greene is offering another option and a more optimistic one, a view of destruction as a new beginning or a sort of rebirth.

Taken only at literal face value, Greene's statement could be a dangerous one. It could be taken as an argument for anarchy, chaos, or, even more specifically, violence and murder. Of course, this would all depend on whether or not the interpreter sees "creation" as always a positive end. Further, it would depend on whether or not creation is viewed as an end or a means. For example, murder, for most people, is certainly not a positive thing. It is, however, undeniably an act of destruction. It is also undeniably an "end" of sorts, as an unalterable change. Murder is an act of destruction that separates the corporeal existence from the spiritual one. Because there is nothing really *new* that exists as a result, because it is not a means of propagating other possibilities, one could argue that murder is an act of destruction that is not, in fact, also an act of creation.

To destroy is to disintegrate or to demolish, to cause a cessation of one form of existence. What would follow would inevitably be another form of existence. For example, if I demolish my house, then I, by default, create a pile of rubble. I could even say that I have created that pile of rubble, because it did not exist before I demolished my house. To create is to bring into being. Because (granted that we are not dealing with the loss of matter) destruction is the ceasing of one thing to exist in its present state, then one is always creating a new state of being with every destruction. The taking of a life would be one possible exception because the dead body has not been cremated and there is no accounting for the spirit that has been "lost." In general, however, the relationship between destruction and creation is inevitable, as one necessitates the other.

Part 2
Explanation of Second Response: 4

This essay does a nice job with tasks one and three. Paragraph one explains the statement by giving a traditional definition of "create," commenting then on connotations of destruction, and finally suggesting how Greene offers another option for seeing acts of creation. Paragraph two expands the explanation and moves toward a general example, murder, which might not, because it is not "positive," be considered an act of creation. The final paragraph examines the circumstances that determine the relationship between creation and destruction.

The paper has many strengths. The essay is thoughtful, and it flows smoothly from sentence to sentence, paragraph to paragraph. The use of transitions, such as "however" in the final sentence, provides coherence. The paper shows sensitivity to language, particularly in its examination of the denotation and connotation of creation and destruction. The paper would have received a rating of 5 or 6 if it had dealt more directly with the second task: that of providing a specific situation in which destruction is not a form of creation. The example of murder as such remains too general. The example of the demolition of the house in the final paragraph is effective in making the paper more concrete. Other such examples in the rest of the paper would be helpful.

BIOLOGICAL SCIENCES

143. **B.** Individuals 6, 20, and 23 could be produced by dominant defective alleles (either autosomal or sex-linked) only if all three cases resulted from new mutations since the parents in all three cases have only normal phenotypes. Because mutations are specified as rare, this is unlikely. A recessive autosomal defective allele could explain all observations down through individual 18, but the presence of a defective allele in individual 19 is unlikely due to no occurrences of the defect in that individual's ancestors and the low incidence of new mutations. The sex ratio of defective individuals (all male except for one female, and she had a defective father) is highly unlikely for an autosomal recessive defective allele. The expected probability of males among defective offspring is 1/2 for a recessive autosomal allele (i.e., normal chance of male offspring), so the probability of the observed sex ratio among defective offspring is very unlikely. For these reasons, a defective autosomal recessive allele is not a likely explanation. An X-linked recessive defective allele easily explains all observations. Defective male offspring received an X chromosome containing a recessive defective allele from their mothers (most of whom are normal due to a dominant normal allele on their other X chromosome) and the recessive allele determined their phenotype since the Y chromosome contained no allele for the characteristic. Most females were normal due to a normal allele on the X chromosome received from their fathers. The defective female (9) received a defective X from both parents.

144. **C.** Female 1 must contain one normal allele (because she has a normal phenotype and she produced normal male 8) and one defective allele (because she produced defective male 6).

145. **B.** Male 6 would contain only one allele to the characteristic since he (like all normal human males) has only one X chromosome. The Y chromosome from his father lacks an allele for the characteristic. His defective phenotype must be produced by a defective allele on his X, so he contains only defective alleles.

146. **A.** Male 8 would have one allele for the characteristics (on his single X chromosome—see explanation for question 3), Because his phenotype is normal, the allele must be normal and he would contain only normal alleles.

147. **B.** Female 9 must have two X chromosomes (like all normal human females). Because her phenotype is defective, both X chromosome must contain defective alleles. Female 9 would therefore contain only defective alleles.

148. **D.** All of the statements of the question were supported by the data. Although it would have been a good assumption that crude pituitary extract would have a lesser effect than pure FSH, one must examine the data. In our case the extract did affect every organ, however, the weight increase was less than when FSH was administered. With the data available concerning the effect of pituitary extract, it is safe to assume that hypophysectomy would have resulted in decreased organ weights. Remember, FSH in the female stimulates the growth of the ovarian follicle, whereas in the male it stimulates the testes to produce sperm.

149. **D.** FSH in the female stimulates the development of the ovarian follicle and the production of estrogen; LH and prolactin are responsible for the corpus luteum, which secretes progesterone and prepares the uterus for implantation of the fertilized egg. Because uterine growth was observed in our case, it is safe to assume that FSH was not of the highest purity. Our data neither supports nor contradicts the statement that FSH and LH are necessary for estrogen secretion. Because our data shows that FSH did not affect the thyroid and adrenal glands, the statement that FSH primarily affects the reproductive organs is supported.

150. **A.** The data shows that FSH in the male had its greatest effect on the seminal vesicles and not the prostate gland. Statements (B) and (C) are not supported nor contradicted, whereas statement (D) is a truism supported by the data; body weights did not vary significantly.

151. **B.** The pituitary gland is located within the sella tursica.

152. **C.** Stress and strain will have a pronounced influence on the output of epinephrine and norepinephrine by the adrenal medulla. Activation of the sympathetic portion of the autonomic nervous system will result in increased activity by the adrenal medulla which can be considered the site of the postganglionic cell bodies of that segment of the sympathetics.

153. **D.** The reproductive cycle is under hormonal regulation; gonadotropic hormones of the pituitary (anterior lobe) stimulate the ovaries to produce a mature egg. The pituitary and ovaries have a reciprocal effect on each other. FSH (follicle stimulating hormone) from the pituitary elicits estrogen production from the developing follicle. When estrogen concentration reaches a certain blood level, it inhibits FSH production. At that time, the egg is discharged and the cells lining the follicle come under the influence of another gonadotropin LH (luteinizing hormone), which influences the development of the corpus luteum. The corpus luteum produces the hormone progesterone which influences the wall of the uterus in preparation for implantation. As the concentration of progesterone rises, LH production is checked. If fertilization has occurred, the production of FSH is curtailed throughout the period of gestation through the production of estrogen by the placenta and ovary. If fertilization does not occur, the cycle begins anew.

154. **A.** FSH stimulates morphogenesis of the follicle primarily, whereas LH is required for either estrogen or progesterone synthesis. FSH and LH are required during the follicular phase.

155. **B.** The interstitial cells are stimulated by ICSH (interstitial cell stimulating hormone, which is identical with LH in the female) a gonadotrophin of the pituitary to produce androgens. Testosterone is an androgen.

156. **B.** The pituitary secretes ACTH, FSH, LH, TSH, and STH. ACTH acts on the adrenal cortex; FSH and LH on the gonads; TSH on the thyroid, and STH on the general system. The adrenal medulla can be considered to house the post gan-

glionic neurons for part of the sympathetic portion of the autonomic nervous system and is responsible for epi- and norepinephrine production.

157. **B.** Between 3 to 4 ml of semen comprise one ejaculate which contains between 300 and 400 million sperm cells.

158. **D.** Terminal branches transmit impulses to other neurons.

159. **C.** Protein synthesis is mainly carried out by the ribosomes. Let us identify the components of the neuron numbered: (2) nucleus with nucleolus, containing the genetic material of the cell and directing the synthetic activity of the cell; (3) Golgi apparatus (zone), the packaging and concentrating area of the cell's secretory activity; (4) dendrites, the processes that pick up an impulse and carry it toward the cell body; (5) endoplasmic reticulum (rough in this case—ribosomes are attached), the synthetic machinery of the cell (proteins etc.); (6) cell membrane, semipermeable and the protector of the cell from its environment; (7) cytoplasm (specifically the area here is called the axon hillock); (8) myelin sheath (Schwann cell covered by its neurilemma, the insulator of the axon; (9) direction of conduction of art impulse; axons (10a) conduct impulses away from the cell body to the junction with the dendrites of another neuron. The junction point is known as the synaptic area; the impulse can cross the synapse only from the axon to the dendrite and no backflow is permitted; (11) terminal branches of the axon. In a lesion (cut) the process distal from the cell body would completely degenerate; retrograde degeneration would be detected in the proximal portion and the cell body, however, the proximal portion has the capacity to regenerate.

160. **C.** Lysosomes contain hydrolytic enzymes and are also known as digestive (suicide) bags.

161. **A.** The chemical mediator of cholinergic nerve impulses is acetylcholine and is released by the axon terminals.

162. **B.** The neuron is a cellular element; as a highly specialized cell, it carries out the function of neuronal transmission. A nucleus is a cluster of nerve cell bodies within the central nervous system (brain and spinal cord), whereas a ganglion is defined as a cluster of nerve cell bodies outside the central nervous system (sympathetic chain ganglia, celiac plexus, and so on).

163. **B.** The neurolemma of an axon is part of the Schwann cell (outer membrane).

164. **A.** Ectoderm is the germ layer of origin of the nervous system.

165. **D.** The gray matter of the spinal cord is divided into two (2) components: motor and receptor. The motor part is comprised of the ventral and intermediolateral columns and gives rise to the ventral roots. Ventral horn cells supply voluntary muscles; intermediolateral cells give rise to preganglionic sympathetic fibers of the thoraco-lumbar system. The receptor portion is located in the dorsal horn. The white matter of the spinal cord is composed of nerve fibers in a network of connective tissue.

166. **C.** Blood pressure is usually measured by placing the sphygmomanometer cuff around the arm compressing the brachial artery and vein. Maximum blood pressure is obtained during ventricular contraction (systole); in our case 160. Minimum blood pressure indicates ventricular rest (diastole); in our case 90.

167. **B.** The medulla is a part of the brain stem and connects to the spinal cord at the foramen magnum. The following cranial nerves are associated with the medulla: a, XII—hypoglossal nerve; b, XI—spinal accessory nerve; c, X—vagus nerve; d, IX—glossopharyngeal nerve; e, VIII—statoacoustic nerve; and f, portions of the facial nerve (VII). The vagus nerve (X) is the most important parasympathetic nerve. Stimulation of vagal fibers slows the heart rate; constricts the smooth muscles of the bronchial tree; stimulates secretion by the bronchial mucosa; and promotes peristalsis, gastric, and pancreatic secretions. Blood pressure control also involves aortic body, carotid sinus, and carotid body receptor modulation by the glossopharyngeal (IX) and vagus (X) nerves.

168. **A.** From the right ventricle blood is sent the lungs via the pulmonary arteries; this blood is rich in carbaminohemoglobin and the CO_2 will be exchanged for O_2. Blood returns from the lungs to the left auricle via the pulmonary veins; this blood has been oxygenated and is rich in oxyhemoglobin. Blood then passes to the left ventricle and then out via the aorta to supply the tissues of the body.

169. **D.** The sympathetic component of the autonomic nervous system mobilizes the body reserves in case of emergencies.

170. **C.** Skeletal (striated) muscle is under voluntary control. The autonomic nervous system innervates cardiac muscle, smooth muscle and glands. Arrector pili musculature is associated with skin and is smooth musculature.

171. **D.** A sarcomere is the region between two bands. In simple terms we are dealing with this unit: ZIAHAIZ. Contraction of the sarcomere is due to the fine filaments (actin) sliding between the thick filaments (myosin) pulling the Z bands to which they are attached. This pulls the Z bands closer together, and so the sarcomeres are shortened.

172. **B.** In skeletal muscle, the nuclei are found peripherally. To complete the chart, the speed of contraction should also be mentioned. Skeletal muscle is the fastest working, smooth muscle the slowest, and cardiac muscle occupies an intermediate position.

173. **D.** Heart beat is initiated by the S-A (sinoatrial) node, which is also known as the pacemaker.

174. **A.** Incubation of gp120 with increasing concentrations of CPFDD reduced binding of the gp120 to CD4+ cells to nearly zero (see Figure 1), so CPFDD inhibited the binding. CPFDF caused partial inhibition at low concentrations but caused much less inhibition at higher concentrations than CPFDD (see Figure 1).

175. **B.** See explanation for question 174.

176. **A.** In Figure 1, a 50 uM/L increase in CPFDD concentration caused the largest reduction in fluorescence at the beginning of the curve.

177. **B.** In Figure 2, p24 production by infected T cells + H9 cells + CPFDD was severely reduced, but was not totally prevented. After 6 days of incubation, p24 production is increasing and is greater than p24 production by infected T cells alone. Therefore the inhibition was strong but not total.

178. **D.** In Figure 2, p24 production by infected T cells + H9 cells + CPFDF was very similar to infected T cells + H9 cells. Therefore no inhibition was detectable in the experiment.

179–181. **(179-D) (180-D) (181-D).** As can be seen from the table, there are four major blood types, and the explanation as to universal donor and recipient is based on the following:

Type	Agglutinogens on Cells	Agglutinogens in Serum and Plasma
AB—can receive A, B, AB, or O (universal recipient)	A, B	none
A—can receive A, O	A	anti b
B—can receive B, O	B	anti a
O—can receive only O, but can give to all; therefore, O is the universal donor	O	anti ab

182. **C.** The ABO blood grouping system is explained on the basis of a single triallelic system with genes A, B, and O operating at a single genetic locus. Phenotypic and genotypic characteristics may be expressed as follows:

Phenotype	Genotype
A	A/A; A/O
B	B/B; B/O
O	O/O
AB	A/B

The A and B genes appear to be codominant; they are dominant over O, which is recessive.

183. **A.** See explanations for questions 179–182. One gene from each parent can produce any of the four combinations named.

184. **A.** Any substance that has the capability to elicit an immunological response, such as the production of antibody that is specific to that substance, is considered an antigen.

185. **A.** Periodate reacts with vicinal diols to produce aldehydes through chain cleavage.

186. **C.** Although there is a plane of symmetry in the resultant 3-methylglutaric acid, there is not in 2-methylglutaric acid. Thus, there are two optical isomers of the latter.

187. **B.** Ester will react with either of these reagents to give an alcohol and an acid (or its salt if treated with weak base). Hemiacetal will not react with weak base but will react with weak acid to produce an acid and an aldehyde. Ether will not react under these conditions.

188. **A.** Naturally occurring fatty acids usually have an even number of carbon atoms and have a carboxyl on one end of the hydrocarbon chain.

189. **C.** Lithium aluminum hydride reduces carboxyls, ketones, and aldehydes to alcohols.

190. **C.** Although blocking the activation of the phosphatases by blocking the effect of calcium (step 3), the CKII activation pathway would also be blocked. For this reason, (A) and (D) are incorrect. The autophosphorylation of CKII at step 5 is the final step in the activation of CKII. A block here, as suggested by **B,** would not increase but inhibit CKII activity; hence **B** is also a poor choice.

191. **C.** CKII activity could be decreased by blocking calcium influx, calmodulin activation of CKII, or autophosphorylation. There are more than the single sites suggested in (A) and (B). Blocking dephosphorylation by the phosphatase, step 7, **D,** would serve to *increase,* not decrease, CKII activity.

192. **B.** Only a Voltage Operated Channel (VOC) is opened by depolarization alone. As stated in the passage, a Receptor Operated Channel (ROC) is opened by the binding of an appropriate ligand. The question states that depolarization is produced and no neurotransmitter ligand is present, so **A** and **C** are incorrect.

193. **D.** This comes straight out of the reading: A kinase is an enzyme that transfers phosphoryl groups from a high energy donor to a suitable substrate. **A** is incorrect, because a phosphatase antagonizes the actions of a kinase by *removing phosphoryls* from phosphoproteins. Catalases and transferase, **B** and **C,** are enzymes, but their specific functions are not phosphorylating phosphorproteins. If you chose one of these answers you attempted to address more than the question asked. Stick with the simple approach and do not read anything extraneous into the question.

194. **C.** The question requires that you synthesize two pieces of given information. First, that both the CKII activation and inactivation (phosphatase) pathways are activated by calcium and, second, that the phosphatase response to calcium is slower than other components of the system. **D** suggests the reverse of this situation and is therefore wrong. It is plausible that is less phosphatase than kinase **B,** however, this is not addressed in the reading and you would have no basis for arriving at this interpretation. **A,** also not addressed in the reading, would not constitute a plausible mechanism for CKII to function. It would suggest a mechanism that would render CKII permanently nonfunctional.

195. **C.** All have the same molecular formula, and only III is capable of intermolecular hydrogen bonding.

196. **B.** II is the only aldehyde of the four. I and IV form hydrazones but do not give a positive Tollen's test.

197. **A.** On hydrogenation I is converted to:

$$
\begin{array}{c}
\text{OH} \\
| \\
\text{CH}_3\text{—C—CHCH}_3 \\
| \quad | \\
\text{H} \quad \text{CH}_3
\end{array}
$$

in which the carbon with the hydroxyl group is chiral.

198. **A.** The reaction sequence is:

$$
\text{CH}_3\text{CH=O} + \underset{\underset{\text{CH}_3}{|}}{\text{CH}_3\text{CHMgBr}} \xrightarrow[\text{H}_2\text{O}^+]{\text{then}} \underset{\underset{\text{CH}_3}{|}}{\overset{\overset{\text{OH}}{|}}{\text{CH}_3\text{CHCHCH}_3}} \xrightarrow{\text{K}_2\text{Cr}_2\text{O}_7} 1
$$

199. **C.** Compound III has a double hand to react with Br_2. The hydroxyl group is given priority in numbering.

200. **D.**
$$\frac{0.5 \text{ mg}}{0.1 \text{ ml}} = \frac{X}{10 \text{ ml}}$$

$$X = \frac{(0.5)(1)}{0.1} = 50 \text{ mg}$$

This 50 mg represents the total amount in the entire 3 ml of plasma that was extracted.

$$\frac{50 \text{ mg}}{3 \text{ ml}} = \frac{X}{100 \text{ ml}}$$

$$X = \frac{(50)(100)}{3} = 1667 \text{ mg/100 ml}$$

201. **A.** See the explanation to answer 200. The calculation is based on 100 ml plasma, not on the total amount of plasma.

202. **B.** Exceeding the linear range would ordinarily lead to a lower absorbance than expected. An error in weighing to prepare the standard solution would introduce a constant error. The remaining possibility, a pipetting error, is most likely. Pipetting errors may be positive or negative.

203. **B.** Cholesterol is an intermediate in the biosynthesis of steroid hormones, bile acids, and vitamin D. Essential fatty acids and essential amino acids must be consumed by the organism in the diet.

204. **D.** Prostaglandins are potent compounds; they are structurally unique in the respect that they contain 20 carbon atoms and are formed from essential fatty acids. They affect the nervous system, circulation, reproductive organs, and metabolism.

205. **C.** Adrenocorticotropic hormone (ACTH) is produced by the beta cells of the pituitary and stimulates the adrenal cortex to produce glucocorticoids, which increase blood sugar and liver glycogen levels. The function of the adrenal medulla is to secrete adrenalin and noradrenalin. These compounds affect the vascular system, the heart, and respiration. One must assume that being housed in an elevated temperature setting is a stressful situation and, besides an increase in water consumption due to sweating, heart rate would be elevated. ACTH levels should remain fairly steady.

206. **B.** Thyroid hormones control the rate of metabolism and the growth, maturation, and differentiation of the organism, and influence nervous system activity. Five events are associated with thyroid hormone production: (1) trapping iodine; (2) oxidation of iodide to organic iodine; (3) hormone synthesis; (4) storage of thyroglobulin; and (5) release of hormone into the circulation. Increased activity by the organ is known as hyperthyroidism. The experimenter was interested in determining the influence of cold exposure on parameters used to assess thyroid function. Cold has a significant effect on ^{131}I uptake and serum PBI and the animals were in a hyperthyroid state physiologically.

207. **C.** The statement: there is a significant difference between tumor-bearing animals and their controls indicating some degree of cellular sensitization, is not investigated and this conclusion cannot be made from the data presented; all the other statements are supported by the data.

208. **B.** The visual system is made up of the eye and complex nerve pathways for interpretation by the cerebral cortex. Seeing starts with the ganglion cells of the retina, optic nerve, optic chiasma (nasal retinal field fibers cross), optic tract, lateral geniculate body, optic radiations, and visual cortex (area 17 of occipital lobe of cerebrum). In lesion 2, the uncrossed fibers of the right optic nerve are affected and the patient would show a deficit in his/her medial optic field.

209. **D.** A careful look at the data shows that temperature could indirectly influence life span, that females tend to live longer, and that radiation has a more deleterious effect on males.

210. **D.** Bone marrow is the largest organ in the body (4.5% of total body weight); red bone marrow is hemopoietic, whereas fat is predominant in yellow bone marrow. Lymphopoiesis is a function of the thymus and occurs mostly during fetal and early postnatal life. The thymus produces circulating lymphocytes known as T cells, which migrate to lymph nodes and the spleen where they give rise to immunologically competent cells. The thymus also is thought to stimulate lymphocyte production and enhance immunological competence. Because in our experiment neither bone marrow nor thymus cells alone induced antibody production, the hypothesis of cell cooperation can be accepted. Because thymocytes did not produce a response statement, **D** is contradicted by the results.

211. **A.** Careful scrutiny of the data shows that the percentage of Factor 3 increased and that of Factor 2 decreased, with a resultant rise in Factor 3/Factor 2 ratio. No consistent trend could be seen for Factor 4. Factor 6 showed a decline in the 12-day group and that could be due to decreased amounts of Factors 2 and 3. For the various factors, the 12-day period sometimes produced more and sometimes less outcome than the 6-day period.

212. **D.** This problem can be solved easily by careful analysis as to what takes place under the three experimental conditions, comparing graph 1 to graph 2. All statements in the question are supported by the evidence.

213. **B.** Careful analysis shows that there exists a wide range of thickness in oral epithelium (30-950μ) lining the oral cavity. A quick calculation yields an average thickness of 238μ. The thinnest measurement was observed in area F and, therefore, statement **B** is contradicted by the results.

214. **C.** Examination reveals that statement C is neither supported nor contradicted by the information. That the drug has an effect and that a dose/response is present is clear, however, that the dose is of critical importance cannot be deduced from the values and, therefore, statement C is not demonstrated by the evidence.

215. **D.** The function of the thyroid is to produce the thyroid hormones T_3-triiodothyronine and T_4-tetraiodothyronine or the thyroxine. Iodine plus tyrosine yields monoiodotyrosine (MIT); the union of two units of MIT produces diiodotyrosine (DIT) and the adding of one more MIT yields triiodothyronine (T_3). If to T_3 an MIT is joined, thyroxin (T_4) is the product; if two DIT's unite, thyroxin also is formed. Scrutiny of the presented data shows that all three statements are supported by the information presented and that propylthiouracil (PTU) interferes with thyroid hormone production; PTU is an antithyroid compound used to treat patients.

216. **A.** Remember that nitro groups are deactivating, meta-directing substituents and that halogens are deactivating, ortho, para-directing substituents. If bromination precedes nitration, then very little *m*-bromonitrobenzene will result.

217. **C.** Under the stated conditions aldehyde (except formaldehyde) → secondary alcohol; carboxylic acid → methane + carboxylic acid; ester → ketone; ketone → tertiary alcohol.

218. **C.** Substrate(s) or reactants) react(s) with the enzyme to form an enzyme-substrate complex. This complex breaks down into product(s) and frees enzymes ready for formation of a new enzyme-substrate complex.

219. **D.** We have described conditions for the formation of a diazonium salt and then replacement of the diazonium salt by Br to produce monobromobenzene. (The replacement is known as the Sandmeyer reaction.) The intermediate diazonium salt is often unstable at room temperature, so a lower temperature is used.

The MCAT
Model Examination C

ANSWER SHEET

DIRECTIONS: After locating the number of the question to which you are responding, fill in the circle containing the letter of the answer you have selected. Use pencil (not a ballpoint pen) to completely blacken the circle.

VERBAL REASONING

1. Ⓐ Ⓑ Ⓒ Ⓓ
2. Ⓐ Ⓑ Ⓒ Ⓓ
3. Ⓐ Ⓑ Ⓒ Ⓓ
4. Ⓐ Ⓑ Ⓒ Ⓓ
5. Ⓐ Ⓑ Ⓒ Ⓓ
6. Ⓐ Ⓑ Ⓒ Ⓓ
7. Ⓐ Ⓑ Ⓒ Ⓓ
8. Ⓐ Ⓑ Ⓒ Ⓓ
9. Ⓐ Ⓑ Ⓒ Ⓓ
10. Ⓐ Ⓑ Ⓒ Ⓓ
11. Ⓐ Ⓑ Ⓒ Ⓓ
12. Ⓐ Ⓑ Ⓒ Ⓓ
13. Ⓐ Ⓑ Ⓒ Ⓓ
14. Ⓐ Ⓑ Ⓒ Ⓓ
15. Ⓐ Ⓑ Ⓒ Ⓓ
16. Ⓐ Ⓑ Ⓒ Ⓓ
17. Ⓐ Ⓑ Ⓒ Ⓓ
18. Ⓐ Ⓑ Ⓒ Ⓓ
19. Ⓐ Ⓑ Ⓒ Ⓓ
20. Ⓐ Ⓑ Ⓒ Ⓓ
21. Ⓐ Ⓑ Ⓒ Ⓓ
22. Ⓐ Ⓑ Ⓒ Ⓓ
23. Ⓐ Ⓑ Ⓒ Ⓓ
24. Ⓐ Ⓑ Ⓒ Ⓓ
25. Ⓐ Ⓑ Ⓒ Ⓓ
26. Ⓐ Ⓑ Ⓒ Ⓓ
27. Ⓐ Ⓑ Ⓒ Ⓓ
28. Ⓐ Ⓑ Ⓒ Ⓓ
29. Ⓐ Ⓑ Ⓒ Ⓓ
30. Ⓐ Ⓑ Ⓒ Ⓓ

31. Ⓐ Ⓑ Ⓒ Ⓓ
32. Ⓐ Ⓑ Ⓒ Ⓓ
33. Ⓐ Ⓑ Ⓒ Ⓓ
34. Ⓐ Ⓑ Ⓒ Ⓓ
35. Ⓐ Ⓑ Ⓒ Ⓓ
36. Ⓐ Ⓑ Ⓒ Ⓓ
37. Ⓐ Ⓑ Ⓒ Ⓓ
38. Ⓐ Ⓑ Ⓒ Ⓓ
39. Ⓐ Ⓑ Ⓒ Ⓓ
40. Ⓐ Ⓑ Ⓒ Ⓓ
41. Ⓐ Ⓑ Ⓒ Ⓓ
42. Ⓐ Ⓑ Ⓒ Ⓓ
43. Ⓐ Ⓑ Ⓒ Ⓓ
44. Ⓐ Ⓑ Ⓒ Ⓓ
45. Ⓐ Ⓑ Ⓒ Ⓓ
46. Ⓐ Ⓑ Ⓒ Ⓓ
47. Ⓐ Ⓑ Ⓒ Ⓓ
48. Ⓐ Ⓑ Ⓒ Ⓓ
49. Ⓐ Ⓑ Ⓒ Ⓓ
50. Ⓐ Ⓑ Ⓒ Ⓓ
51. Ⓐ Ⓑ Ⓒ Ⓓ
52. Ⓐ Ⓑ Ⓒ Ⓓ
53. Ⓐ Ⓑ Ⓒ Ⓓ
54. Ⓐ Ⓑ Ⓒ Ⓓ
55. Ⓐ Ⓑ Ⓒ Ⓓ
56. Ⓐ Ⓑ Ⓒ Ⓓ
57. Ⓐ Ⓑ Ⓒ Ⓓ
58. Ⓐ Ⓑ Ⓒ Ⓓ
59. Ⓐ Ⓑ Ⓒ Ⓓ
60. Ⓐ Ⓑ Ⓒ Ⓓ

61. Ⓐ Ⓑ Ⓒ Ⓓ
62. Ⓐ Ⓑ Ⓒ Ⓓ
63. Ⓐ Ⓑ Ⓒ Ⓓ
64. Ⓐ Ⓑ Ⓒ Ⓓ
65. Ⓐ Ⓑ Ⓒ Ⓓ

PHYSICAL SCIENCES

66. Ⓐ Ⓑ Ⓒ Ⓓ
67. Ⓐ Ⓑ Ⓒ Ⓓ
68. Ⓐ Ⓑ Ⓒ Ⓓ
69. Ⓐ Ⓑ Ⓒ Ⓓ
70. Ⓐ Ⓑ Ⓒ Ⓓ
71. Ⓐ Ⓑ Ⓒ Ⓓ
72. Ⓐ Ⓑ Ⓒ Ⓓ
73. Ⓐ Ⓑ Ⓒ Ⓓ
74. Ⓐ Ⓑ Ⓒ Ⓓ
75. Ⓐ Ⓑ Ⓒ Ⓓ
76. Ⓐ Ⓑ Ⓒ Ⓓ
77. Ⓐ Ⓑ Ⓒ Ⓓ
78. Ⓐ Ⓑ Ⓒ Ⓓ
79. Ⓐ Ⓑ Ⓒ Ⓓ
80. Ⓐ Ⓑ Ⓒ Ⓓ
81. Ⓐ Ⓑ Ⓒ Ⓓ
82. Ⓐ Ⓑ Ⓒ Ⓓ
83. Ⓐ Ⓑ Ⓒ Ⓓ
84. Ⓐ Ⓑ Ⓒ Ⓓ
85. Ⓐ Ⓑ Ⓒ Ⓓ
86. Ⓐ Ⓑ Ⓒ Ⓓ
87. Ⓐ Ⓑ Ⓒ Ⓓ
88. Ⓐ Ⓑ Ⓒ Ⓓ

89. Ⓐ Ⓑ Ⓒ Ⓓ
90. Ⓐ Ⓑ Ⓒ Ⓓ
91. Ⓐ Ⓑ Ⓒ Ⓓ
92. Ⓐ Ⓑ Ⓒ Ⓓ
93. Ⓐ Ⓑ Ⓒ Ⓓ
94. Ⓐ Ⓑ Ⓒ Ⓓ
95. Ⓐ Ⓑ Ⓒ Ⓓ
96. Ⓐ Ⓑ Ⓒ Ⓓ
97. Ⓐ Ⓑ Ⓒ Ⓓ
98. Ⓐ Ⓑ Ⓒ Ⓓ
99. Ⓐ Ⓑ Ⓒ Ⓓ
100. Ⓐ Ⓑ Ⓒ Ⓓ
101. Ⓐ Ⓑ Ⓒ Ⓓ
102. Ⓐ Ⓑ Ⓒ Ⓓ
103. Ⓐ Ⓑ Ⓒ Ⓓ
104. Ⓐ Ⓑ Ⓒ Ⓓ
105. Ⓐ Ⓑ Ⓒ Ⓓ
106. Ⓐ Ⓑ Ⓒ Ⓓ
107. Ⓐ Ⓑ Ⓒ Ⓓ
108. Ⓐ Ⓑ Ⓒ Ⓓ
109. Ⓐ Ⓑ Ⓒ Ⓓ
110. Ⓐ Ⓑ Ⓒ Ⓓ
111. Ⓐ Ⓑ Ⓒ Ⓓ
112. Ⓐ Ⓑ Ⓒ Ⓓ
113. Ⓐ Ⓑ Ⓒ Ⓓ
114. Ⓐ Ⓑ Ⓒ Ⓓ
115. Ⓐ Ⓑ Ⓒ Ⓓ
116. Ⓐ Ⓑ Ⓒ Ⓓ
117. Ⓐ Ⓑ Ⓒ Ⓓ
118. Ⓐ Ⓑ Ⓒ Ⓓ

119. Ⓐ Ⓑ Ⓒ Ⓓ
120. Ⓐ Ⓑ Ⓒ Ⓓ
121. Ⓐ Ⓑ Ⓒ Ⓓ
122. Ⓐ Ⓑ Ⓒ Ⓓ
123. Ⓐ Ⓑ Ⓒ Ⓓ
124. Ⓐ Ⓑ Ⓒ Ⓓ
125. Ⓐ Ⓑ Ⓒ Ⓓ
126. Ⓐ Ⓑ Ⓒ Ⓓ
127. Ⓐ Ⓑ Ⓒ Ⓓ
128. Ⓐ Ⓑ Ⓒ Ⓓ
129. Ⓐ Ⓑ Ⓒ Ⓓ
130. Ⓐ Ⓑ Ⓒ Ⓓ
131. Ⓐ Ⓑ Ⓒ Ⓓ
132. Ⓐ Ⓑ Ⓒ Ⓓ
133. Ⓐ Ⓑ Ⓒ Ⓓ
134. Ⓐ Ⓑ Ⓒ Ⓓ
135. Ⓐ Ⓑ Ⓒ Ⓓ
136. Ⓐ Ⓑ Ⓒ Ⓓ
137. Ⓐ Ⓑ Ⓒ Ⓓ
138. Ⓐ Ⓑ Ⓒ Ⓓ
139. Ⓐ Ⓑ Ⓒ Ⓓ
140. Ⓐ Ⓑ Ⓒ Ⓓ
141. Ⓐ Ⓑ Ⓒ Ⓓ
142. Ⓐ Ⓑ Ⓒ Ⓓ

WRITING SAMPLE
Use separate ruled sheets of
paper.

BIOLOGICAL SCIENCES

143. Ⓐ Ⓑ Ⓒ Ⓓ
144. Ⓐ Ⓑ Ⓒ Ⓓ
145. Ⓐ Ⓑ Ⓒ Ⓓ
146. Ⓐ Ⓑ Ⓒ Ⓓ
147. Ⓐ Ⓑ Ⓒ Ⓓ
148. Ⓐ Ⓑ Ⓒ Ⓓ
149. Ⓐ Ⓑ Ⓒ Ⓓ
150. Ⓐ Ⓑ Ⓒ Ⓓ
151. Ⓐ Ⓑ Ⓒ Ⓓ
152. Ⓐ Ⓑ Ⓒ Ⓓ
153. Ⓐ Ⓑ Ⓒ Ⓓ
154. Ⓐ Ⓑ Ⓒ Ⓓ
155. Ⓐ Ⓑ Ⓒ Ⓓ
156. Ⓐ Ⓑ Ⓒ Ⓓ
157. Ⓐ Ⓑ Ⓒ Ⓓ
158. Ⓐ Ⓑ Ⓒ Ⓓ
159. Ⓐ Ⓑ Ⓒ Ⓓ
160. Ⓐ Ⓑ Ⓒ Ⓓ
161. Ⓐ Ⓑ Ⓒ Ⓓ
162. Ⓐ Ⓑ Ⓒ Ⓓ
163. Ⓐ Ⓑ Ⓒ Ⓓ
164. Ⓐ Ⓑ Ⓒ Ⓓ
165. Ⓐ Ⓑ Ⓒ Ⓓ
166. Ⓐ Ⓑ Ⓒ Ⓓ
167. Ⓐ Ⓑ Ⓒ Ⓓ

168. Ⓐ Ⓑ Ⓒ Ⓓ
169. Ⓐ Ⓑ Ⓒ Ⓓ
170. Ⓐ Ⓑ Ⓒ Ⓓ
171. Ⓐ Ⓑ Ⓒ Ⓓ
172. Ⓐ Ⓑ Ⓒ Ⓓ
173. Ⓐ Ⓑ Ⓒ Ⓓ
174. Ⓐ Ⓑ Ⓒ Ⓓ
175. Ⓐ Ⓑ Ⓒ Ⓓ
176. Ⓐ Ⓑ Ⓒ Ⓓ
177. Ⓐ Ⓑ Ⓒ Ⓓ
178. Ⓐ Ⓑ Ⓒ Ⓓ
179. Ⓐ Ⓑ Ⓒ Ⓓ
180. Ⓐ Ⓑ Ⓒ Ⓓ
181. Ⓐ Ⓑ Ⓒ Ⓓ
182. Ⓐ Ⓑ Ⓒ Ⓓ
183. Ⓐ Ⓑ Ⓒ Ⓓ
184. Ⓐ Ⓑ Ⓒ Ⓓ
185. Ⓐ Ⓑ Ⓒ Ⓓ
186. Ⓐ Ⓑ Ⓒ Ⓓ
187. Ⓐ Ⓑ Ⓒ Ⓓ
188. Ⓐ Ⓑ Ⓒ Ⓓ
189. Ⓐ Ⓑ Ⓒ Ⓓ
190. Ⓐ Ⓑ Ⓒ Ⓓ
191. Ⓐ Ⓑ Ⓒ Ⓓ
192. Ⓐ Ⓑ Ⓒ Ⓓ
193. Ⓐ Ⓑ Ⓒ Ⓓ

194. Ⓐ Ⓑ Ⓒ Ⓓ
195. Ⓐ Ⓑ Ⓒ Ⓓ
196. Ⓐ Ⓑ Ⓒ Ⓓ
197. Ⓐ Ⓑ Ⓒ Ⓓ
198. Ⓐ Ⓑ Ⓒ Ⓓ
199. Ⓐ Ⓑ Ⓒ Ⓓ
200. Ⓐ Ⓑ Ⓒ Ⓓ
201. Ⓐ Ⓑ Ⓒ Ⓓ
202. Ⓐ Ⓑ Ⓒ Ⓓ
203. Ⓐ Ⓑ Ⓒ Ⓓ
204. Ⓐ Ⓑ Ⓒ Ⓓ
205. Ⓐ Ⓑ Ⓒ Ⓓ
206. Ⓐ Ⓑ Ⓒ Ⓓ
207. Ⓐ Ⓑ Ⓒ Ⓓ
208. Ⓐ Ⓑ Ⓒ Ⓓ
209. Ⓐ Ⓑ Ⓒ Ⓓ
210. Ⓐ Ⓑ Ⓒ Ⓓ
211. Ⓐ Ⓑ Ⓒ Ⓓ
212. Ⓐ Ⓑ Ⓒ Ⓓ
213. Ⓐ Ⓑ Ⓒ Ⓓ
214. Ⓐ Ⓑ Ⓒ Ⓓ
215. Ⓐ Ⓑ Ⓒ Ⓓ
216. Ⓐ Ⓑ Ⓒ Ⓓ
217. Ⓐ Ⓑ Ⓒ Ⓓ
218. Ⓐ Ⓑ Ⓒ Ⓓ
219. Ⓐ Ⓑ Ⓒ Ⓓ

The MCAT
Model Examination C

VERBAL REASONING

9 PASSAGES
65 QUESTIONS
85 MINUTES

DIRECTIONS: The questions are based on the accompanying passages. Read each passage carefully, then answer the following questions. Consider only the material within the passage. For each question, select the *ONE BEST ANSWER* and indicate your selection by marking the corresponding letter on the Answer Form.

Passage I (Questions 1–7)

In the early 1920s, dozens of F. Scott Fitzgerald's short stories such as "The Offshore Pirate," "Head and Shoulders," "Rags Martin-Jones and the Prince of Wales" as well as his first two novels, *This Side of Paradise* and *The Beautiful and Damned* contained strong, free spirited female characters; and early in his professional career he realized that he had created a type, the Fitzgerald Flapper, for which there came to be increasing public demand. "I know that the magazines want only flapper stories from me," he told his agent Harold Ober in 1922. In the years leading up to the composition of *The Great Gatsby* (1920–1924) he struggled with the difficulty of beginning his fictional work, both the popular stories for magazines like the *Saturday Evening Post*, the more serious ones for magazines like *The Smart Set* and *Scribner's Magazine*, and his novels with independent women, whose very independence fitted them in advance into the broad cultural stereotype of the American Flapper. It was inevitable, however, that Fitzgerald, who would go on to create complex female characters, among many others, like Nicole Diver in *Tender Is the Night* and Kathleen in the unfinished *The Last Tycoon*, characters who defy easy stereotyping, would have to sacrifice the flapper he had created or else *begin* over and over again with a type solidly constructed by the public whose appetite he had, for some time, satisfied. The process by which Fitzgerald created the flapper with a gallery of memorable characters, allowed her to ride the wave of popular opinion into a permanent place in the American psyche, and then laid her to rest in the service of his own artistic development is a classic study of the central dilemma of professional authorship: how one who earns his living through his writing can, at the same time, move beyond the dictates of popular culture and create enduring art.

Fitzgerald proclaimed in 1922 that "There always were flappers." And while this is, of course, true in the sense that there have always been women who openly and proudly defied the social conventions of their time, the term "flapper" as Fitzgerald is broadly using it originated in Britain in the years just before 1918, where the term characterized a young girl who had not yet been introduced into society. John O'Hara, in calling attention to the misuse of the term "flapper" in America, offers a slight variation of this usage describing "flapper" as British slang referring to "a society girl who had made her debut and hadn't found a husband." The word "flapper" came into wide currency in the postwar decade in America to describe "a girl or young woman whose conduct and dress [were] characterized by somewhat daring freedom and boldness"—particularly one who wore rouge, flapping galoshes, dresses whose hemlines were more than 9 inches above ground, and bobbed hair. The American Flapper historically is a product of what Frederick Lewis Allen in *Only Yesterday* characterizes as the revolution in manners and morals brought about by an interaction of forces related to World War I and its aftermath. Among these Allen cites the "eat-drink-and-be-merry-for-tomorrow-we-die spirit which accompanied the departure of the soldiers to the training camps and the fighting front"; the war neurosis, which led individuals to find solace in unconventional diversions like drinking, smoking, and dancing; the winning of women's suffrage in 1920; the "growing independence of the drudgeries of housekeeping," brought about by the introduction of household appliances; an increasing tendency of women to join the work force and gain a measure of financial independence. Additional forces, according to Allen, included prohibition (with its invitation to rebel against restrictions), the automobile, the confession and sex magazines, and the movies.

Adapted from "The Fitzgerald Flapper," VCU, 1995 and used with permission of Dr. Bryant Mangum.

469

The American flapper, who came into existence during the revolution of manners and morals described by Allen and who owes her name, in part, to the British flapper, came to be associated in the 1920s with the illustrations of John Held, Jr., America's leading cartoonist of the Jazz Age. In film the first flapper was Colleen Moore, who appeared in the movie *Flapperdom* in 1922, and was shortly joined by Clara Bow, the "It" girl, who came to be considered as the quintessence of the flapper. But it is Fitzgerald who is, over and over in the popular magazines of his time credited with inventing or discovering the flapper, as the following samples demonstrate. A 1921 article in *Shadowland*, entitled "Fitzgerald, Flappers and Fame," acknowledges Fitzgerald as "the recognized spokesman of the younger generation . . . since the publication of his now famous flapper tale 'This Side of Paradise.'" In a newspaper clipping from 1922 pasted in the Fitzgeralds' scrapbooks, Fitzgerald is called "The Flapper Laureate." Another from the same period is headlined, "F. Scott Fitzgerald Tells How He Discovered the Flapper." Even into the 1930s editors and reviewers continued to associate Fitzgerald with his tales of the Jazz Age and to echo the call for the flapper stories. Magazine editors continued into the mid-1930s to ask for the old Fitzgerald stories on flappers and "flask gin," but by the mid-1920s he had given up his creation for which he is now perhaps most often remembered in favor of fictional individuals that he hoped would defy stereotyping. The popular magazines of the Jazz Age, now in the bound periodicals section of most libraries, remain the most accessible shrine, though now perhaps a dusty one, to the Fitzgerald Flapper.

1. The best title for this passage would be:

   A. Social Customs of the 1920s.
   B. The Novels of F. Scott Fitzgerald.
   C. F. Scott Fitzgerald: Creator of the American Flapper.
   D. America in the Post-World War I Decade.

2. Which of the following statements best describes the origin of the term "flapper" as it is explained in the passage?

   A. It refers to a young bird, colloquially known as a "flapper."
   B. It originated in Britain and at one time referred to a young girl who had not made her entrance into society.
   C. It was originally an American term which was associated with the flapping arm movements of women who where dancing.
   D. No one is certain where the word "flapper" came from.

3. According to John O'Hara:

   A. a particular quality of the British flapper was that she had not yet found a husband.
   B. Fitzgerald did not invent the flapper.
   C. flappers had been associated in Britain with prostitution.
   D. the movies are primarily responsible for popularizing the flapper.

4. Frederick Lewis Allen attributes the development of the flapper to:

   A. the war neurosis.
   B. women's growing independence from the drudgeries of housekeeping.
   C. the postwar revolution in manners and morals.
   D. all of the above.

5. Which of the following statements is/are *supported* by the passage?

   A. Fitzgerald is the creator of the flapper in fiction.
   B. Fitzgerald was writing about flappers in the mid-1930s.
   C. Clara Bow was the first flapper in film.
   D. Fitzgerald wanted to continue writing about flappers but the public had tired of his stereotype.

6. Which of the following is/are *neither supported nor contradicted* by the passage?

   I. Fitzgerald will be remembered as a better short story writer than a novelist.
   II. Fitzgerald will be remembered for creating the flapper in fiction.
   III. John Held, Jr. was a better cartoonist than writer.
   IV. Fitzgerald gave up writing about the flapper because he wanted to create less stereotyped characters.

   A. I, II, and III   C. II and IV
   B. I and III   D. IV only

7. The passage would support:

   A. a conclusion that Fitzgerald's stories and novels written after he gave up writing about the flapper were judged by literary critics as superior to those written during his "flapper period."
   B. a conclusion that the flapper appeared both in fiction and in film.

C. a conclusion that Fitzgerald was an autobiographical writer.

D. a conclusion that the flapper was judged to be immoral by the middle-brow American reading public.

Passage II (Questions 8–15)

The dependence process begins with an initial exposure to a psychoactive drug. The drug experience allows an individual to perceive two contrasting altered states of consciousness, the normal state versus the drug-induced state. If the drug state is perceived by an individual as more pleasurable (or producing a less painful state) than the nondrug state, then such an individual may make a choice of maintaining the drug state. The word pleasurable, however, has many meanings, and may not be related to "feeling good." Thus, someone may initiate smoking tobacco, for example, not because it makes him/her feel good (most times it doesn't) but because his/her specific peer group dictates tobacco use as a means of acceptance. Belonging to the group is pleasurable, not the use of tobacco; any drug can serve such a purpose. Many examples of this drug–human interaction can be noted, and the lesson learned, is that humans take drugs for many reasons that essentially meet their own individual needs, whether it be feeling good, peer pressure, or whatever.

Therefore, drugs may not always serve primarily as reinforcers of behavior but may have important secondary reinforcing qualities as well. Regardless of the reasons for using a specific chemical agent, however, it should be understood that most drugs produce their effects via an alteration of brain neurochemistry, which can lead to other more long-term problems, especially if the drug is consumed on a chronic basis.

Once an individual takes on the responsibility of using a given chemical agent chronically, then he/she is beginning to allow other variables to take over his/her own drug taking behavior, and to some degree will lose his/her ability to control this behavior. Taking drugs repeatedly means that one swallows, injects, sniffs, or smokes a given agent at certain times, in certain places and possibly with certain people. Each time a drug is taken all these events become cumulatively conditioned with the drug forming a conditioned-stimulus (cs) complex (learned associations). If repeated enough times, the drug takes on stimulus properties initiating certain effects psychologically. Thus, if one associates smoking behavior with feeling good with friends (peer control), then one may need to smoke when those friends are not present to feel good. Conversely, the presence of friends may also act as a stimulus to smoking. What occurs is that the use of the drug can come under environmental (stimulus) control and behavior comes under drug-induced stimulus control. Over time these events can merge to a point where drug taking becomes more and more contingent upon environmental events. The example of this stimulus-complex may be too simplistic, but one may be able to significantly reduce his/her pain by going through the drug taking ritual without administering the drug. Thus, the pharmacological effects of morphine, for example, may be elicited by going through the ritual including an injection of water. Counselors feel that some heroin addicts may be addicted to the needle, and thus the term, "needle freaks." Much of these effects are difficult to detect but have been verified in controlled human experiments. We should not take these effects lightly and should suspect that similar CS complex can occur with most drugs we take.

Acute behaviorally effective doses of psychoactive drugs generally disrupt most learned behaviors. Thus, alcohol acutely disrupts the ability of any individual to drive an automobile. However, if the individual continues to drive under the influence of alcohol, then two things can occur. First, the individual will develop behavioral tolerance to the alcohol. That is, such a person will learn to adapt to the drug state and will learn how to manage his/her automobile in spite of the pharmacological effects of alcohol. As this process continues, the learning of how to drive the car and how to get to certain places (to the ABC store) can also become contingent upon the alcohol state. Thus, an individual may have difficulties finding the ABC store when sober. This phenomena is called *drug-induced state dependent learning*. Its premise is that the retention of information learned under the drug state is contingent upon the reinstitution of the drug state. There are many examples of this with most psychoactive drugs. In fact, one might consider this a form of dependence. Thus, a person may need to continue using a specific drug in order to perform specific tasks learned under the drug state.

Drugs that are abused by man appear to have very subtle but profound effects on specific neurotransmitter systems in the brain. In the normal state these chemicals, which are the means by which nerves communicate with each other, are in a very delicate balance allowing one to perceive his/her environment and make adjustments to act in accordance with his/her own needs. Psychoactive drugs tend to disrupt this balance, which in effect alters an individual's ability to respond in his/her environment.

At this point there is one theoretical model that suggests that the drug dependent person's neurochemical system is out of balance and that the individual uses a given drug to allow his/her neurochemical systems to function in a more normal fashion. This theory has been promoted as a mental health model in order to

Adapted from John A. Rosecrans, "Psychological and Neurochemical Mechanisms Involved in the Maintenance of Chemical Dependencies" *Drug Dependence Outline*, MCV/VCU, 1990.

explain the success of chemotherapy in the control of several psychotic states. However, this has yet to be substantiated in the substance abuse area.

8. This passage deals with:

   I. the acute pharmacolgical experience.
   II. the habitual drug use: the condition of drug effects as a prelude to dependency.
   III. learning aspects.
   IV. neurochemical aspects.

   A. I, II, and III   C. II and IV
   B. I and III   D. I, II, III, and IV

9. Which of the following statements is *supported by* the passage?

   A. A drink here and there really does not hurt.
   B. Your first drink starts you on your way to drug abuse.
   C. A pleasurable state is associated with euphoria.
   D. Drug use follows certain patterns.

10. Human beings partake in drugs because of:

    A. peer pressure.
    B. psychological need.
    C. depression due to marital pressure.
    D. all of the above.

11. Chemical agents consumed chronically:

    A. alter the mind.
    B. seem to act in a predictable fashion.
    C. modulate neurochemical mechanisms.
    D. have relatively short-term effects.

12. Once an individual is addicted:

    A. ritual becomes the order of the day.
    B. environmental conditions may play a dominant role.
    C. injection of a placebo replaces the chemical.
    D. the side effects decrease and use becomes less harmful.

13. According to the author:

    A. certain tasks can be better learned while under the effects of drugs.
    B. certain tasks can be better performed while under the effects of drugs.
    C. certain tasks may be difficult to perform if not under the influence of drugs.
    D. behavioral tolerance will lessen the influence of drug affliction.

14. Which of the statements is *contradicted by* the passage?

    A. Many variables play a role in the effects exhibited by drugs.
    B. Drug users lose the ability to control their own drug-taking behavior.
    C. Chemotherapy is the cure for drug use.
    D. Specific neurotransmitters are affected by drug use.

15. Drugs may often serve as:

    A. agents that make an individual feel that he/she "can take on the world."
    B. primary and/or secondary reinforcers of behavior.
    C. crutches for persons who have low self-esteem.
    D. all of the above.

Passage III (Questions 16–24)

For almost a thousand years Alexandria was the world's center of higher learning. The library eventually contained a half million scrolls, and the museum contained a zoo, botanical garden, astronomical observatory, anatomical exhibit, and treasures from around the world. Teaching was limited only to what was necessary to train researchers for the next generation. The main focus was on improving understanding so that each generation could inherit a more advanced civilization. Teaching was not an end or good in itself.

The school of Alexandria was modeled after the Lyceum of Aristotle. What Aristotle received from Plato and was passed to the school at Alexandria was a sense of optimism and dedication in seeking the truth. We know that Plato marveled at the underlying principles of mathematics, such as the Pythagorean theorem, and that he tried to find underlying principles or "truths" in other fields of study. Aristotle's improvement was to take this idea of generalization apart and show that when deduction and induction were used alternately, we had a *method* of finding underlying principles.

The first librarian was Herodotus of Ephesus, who with these new methods of logic dared to edit Homer's *Iliad* and *Odyssey*. The second librarian was Eratosthenes of Cyrene who, to mention one specific item, measured the size of the earth. First, he measured the angle of the sun (six degrees) at midday on midsummer's day at Alexandria because he knew from previous trips to Cyrene (near today's Aswan Dam) that the sun shone to the bottom of its wells (zero degrees) on that very day and time each year. Then, he only had to measure the distance between these two places to calculate the circumference of the earth ($60/360 = $ distance/circumference).

The third librarian, Aristophanes of Byzantium, commissioned 70 scholars to translate the Bible into Greek; and this translation, used by Jesus Christ, became known as the *Septuagint*. (There is other evidence to suggest that the "flight into Egypt" took place in Alexandria.) The fourth librarian was Aristarchus of Samosthrace who developed the eight parts of speech and wrote commentaries on the works of Homer, Pindar, and Aristophanes of Athens.

Returning to the faculty, we should not fail to aknowledge what we owe to Euclid beyond geometry. Euclid, who was commissioned to start a school of mathematics around 300 B.C., established a mode of accumulating understanding by starting with a few axioms and theories, stacking conclusions into workable structures of knowledge. Examples today would be the Periodic Chart of Elements, the Myers-Briggs Personality Types, and the concept of management schools, to name a few structures or inferential models in different disciplines.

Apollonius and Archimedes were in the next generation of scholars. Whereas Apollonius gave us the conic sections, Archimedes gave us number systems (myriads) capable of counting the sands of the earth. That same generation included Aristarchus of Samos who taught that the earth moved around the sun and whose name appeared in the margin of a book used by Copernicus while studying at Bologna in the seventeenth century.

During the following century, Hipparchus of Nicea calculated the length of the year to within minutes and the length of the month to a few seconds. Around 150 A.D. Claudius Ptolemy wrote 13 books on astronomy, called the *Almagest*. This set also explained that finding a descriptive model for understanding was more important than accounting for every fact or observation. In his books on astrology, he summarized the beliefs of the Greeks, Egyptians, and Persians and gave us the horoscopes and Zodiac signs used today. Also around 150 A.D. Galen came to Alexandria to study. He was the authority on medicine for more than a thousand years; when physicians found parts of the body to differ from his descriptions, they concluded that the person was abnormal.

During the early days of Alexandria, prisoners were dissected alive. However, evil was not limited to "pagans" but discrimination and killing occurred between Jews and Greeks, Christians and Egyptians, and so on. Around 400 A.D., a Christian mob under Cyril ripped the flesh off the mathematician Hypatia because her beliefs were not like theirs.

Whereas understanding could be accumulated in libraries and transmitted by books from generation to

generation, wisdom (seeing the importance of doing good for others, i.e., human truths) has to be reinspired again and again by individuals in each generation.

Through the centuries, religion and classical humanism have contended to underwrite the meaning of wisdom. Sometimes, religion (morality) provided the rationale for justice, at other times, humanism (ethics). Whatever, the lesson from Alexandria's past is that whenever a true sense of the underlying principles of morality *or* ethics was not present, minorities and individuals suffered. Thus, during periods of ebbing or pluralistic religious beliefs (like today), ethics becomes necessary to form a behavorial consensus, to "hold these truths." Accordingly, the university's first mission is not to acquire new understandings nor to teach many students, but to reinspire wisdom at an effective level in each new generation.

16. Which statement best summarizes the attitude at the ancient library-museum at Alexandria?

   A. It was bascially a teacher-training school.
   B. It was an academy of philosophers.
   C. It was a natural history museum.
   D. It was mostly a scholarly research institute.

17. Plato's sense of "truth" was:

   A. what was revealed by God.
   B. limited to mathematical proofs.
   C. underlying principles in any field.
   D. what was agreed to by consensus.

18. Eratosthenes was able to measure the angle of the sun at two distant places on the earth's surface *simultaneously* by:

   A. measuring at one place at midday on midsummer's day a year after measuring at the other place at the same time and date.
   B. having two teams measure angles at the same time and date.
   C. calculating the transit of the sun between measurements.
   D. calculating the movement (turning) of the earth between measurements.

19. One argument given that the "flight into Egypt" of Jesus Christ took place in Alexandria was:

   A. Jesus Christ spoke Greek.
   B. Jesus Christ knew the Greek version of the Bible.
   C. Jesus Christ used the accentuation and punctuation of Alexandria.
   D. Jesus Christ was against plagiarism.

Adapted from Dr. James McGovern, "Alexandria: The First Research University," MCV/VCU, 1990.

20. What statement best fits Claudius Ptolemy?

    A. He was an ancient astronomer.
    B. He was an ancient astrologer.
    C. He was both an astronomer and astrologer.
    D. He was a historian.

21. A key difference between understanding and wisdom is:

    A. wisdom is ancient; understanding is modern.
    B. understanding can be accumulated across the generations; wisdom must be renewed in each generation.
    C. understanding deals with things, whereas wisdom deals with people.
    D. wisdom is subjective; understanding is objective.

22. The author's main point seems to be:

    A. that the study of ethical truths is needed in today's religiously pluralistic world.
    B. that we should all have the wisdom to adopt one religion or another.
    C. that religious beliefs and ethical reasoning will always be at odds.
    D. that people need both morality and ethics today.

23. From a historical point of view, this passage provides the reader with:

    A. the names of important figures who lived in Alexandria.
    B. a running commentary of the 1000 years during which Alexandria was the world's center of learning.
    C. statements made by the great philosophers Aristotle and Plato regarding the teaching of wisdom to new generations.
    D. documentation regarding the destruction of the library of Alexandria by Omar I in 642 A.D.

24. One of the great schools in Alexandria was in the disciplines of mathematics. It was founded by:

    A. Euclid.   **C.** Aristotle.
    B. Omar I.   **D.** Eratosthenes.

Passage IV (Questions 25–30)

Charles James Correll (February 2, 1890–September 26, 1972), radio comedian and co-creator with Freeman Gosden of *Amos 'n Andy* was the son of Joseph Boland Correll and (though there are some inconsistencies about his mother's first name) Julia A. Fiss Correll. He was born in Peoria, Illinois, where he grew up in a stable, working class family. While still in school, he worked as an usher in a local vaudeville house and developed an interest in show business. After graduating from Peoria's public high school, he began to follow his father's trade as a bricklayer. In his spare time, however, he played piano in Peoria's silent movie houses and sang, danced, and took small parts in local shows.

In 1918, after being noticed by the director of a local show, Correll was offered a job with the Joe Bren Company of Chicago. Bren specialized in producing minstrel shows as fundraisers for charitable groups in small cities. For the next 6 years Correll traveled the country, directing productions for Bren. In 1919, doing a show in Durham, North Carolina, he first met Freeman Gosden, who had just been hired by Bren and was to be trained by Correll. The two became friends, often sharing an apartment during summers when both men were in Chicago, preparing for the next season. In 1924 both men were brought to Bren's Chicago home office, Gosden to manage Bren's new circus division, Correll to manage the shows division.

Sharing an apartment, Correll and Gosden began to write musical reviews together, and they worked up a "song and chatter" act. In March, 1925, they began an 8-month series of weekly appearances on Chicago's radio station WEGH. Soon they were doing occasional appearances in shows and on radio programs in St. Louis, in Columbus, Ohio, and other places in the midwest. During the summer of 1925 they both resigned from the Bren Company and began concentrating on a career in vaudeville. However, the Chicago *Tribune's* radio station offered them $200 a week, and in November 1925, they began a series of nightly broadcasts on WGN.

At the suggestion of the station's management, Correll and Gosden used their experiences with minstrel shows to work up a "radio comic strip" about two African American boys, and on January 12, 1926, *Sam 'n Henry* began a series of nightly 10-minute broadcasts on WGN. The show was an immediate hit. In 1928, however, a rival Chicago newspaper lured Correll and Gosden away from WGN, though the *Tribune* retained all rights to *Sam 'n Henry* and continued broadcasting the show with two new men.

At the Chicago *Daily News's* radio station WMAQ, on March 19, 1928, Correll and Gosden began broadcasting six nights a week with a 15-minute show about two African American men living in Harlem. *Amos 'n Andy* focused on the misadventures of Amos Jones, played by Freeman Gosden as energetic, enterprising, and honest, and Andrew H. Brown, played by Correll as indolent but good-hearted. Gradually, the team added characters, but until the 1940s all the writing and voices were done by Correll and Gosden.

The show was a huge success, and with the help of the *Tribune's* publicity staff, in 1929 Correll and Gosden even put out a book (*All About Amos 'n Andy and Their Creators Correll and Gosden*) to satisfy Chicago listeners' curiosity. Within a short time NBC was offering Correll and Gosden $100,000 a year, and on August 19, 1929, Pepsodent toothpaste began sponsoring *Amos 'n Andy* on NBC's Red network.

Amos 'n Andy became network radio's first huge success. Within a few years, Correll and Gosden had moved to California where they appeared in movies, published books of *Amos 'n Andy* dialogue, and lived the life of Hollywood stars. Despite protests about the racial stereotyping of *Amos 'n Andy*, especially from the African American Press, Correll and Gosden's show remained popular throughout the Great Depression and into the 1940s. Short, stocky, and dark haired (later gray), Correll became the relaxed, gregarious half of the partnership, balancing Freeman Gosden's more temperamental, difficult, and creative personality.

Correll enjoyed his success. He bought a large, lavish home in Beverly Hills; he indulged in expensively stylish clothes, and became an enthusiastic golfer. After a divorce from his first wife, Marie Janes (whom he married in 1927), he married the dancer, Alyce Mercedes McLaughlin in 1937. They eventually had four children.

With World War II, listenership began to drop. In February, 1943, after changing networks and sponsors several times, *Amos 'n Andy* left the air. In October it returned as a half-hour weekly variety program featuring guest stars, an orchestra, outside writers, and a studio audience. This show continued with NBC until 1948 when Correll and Gosden, along with Jack Benny and other stars, left NBC. For $2.5 million Correll and Gosden sold CBS the rights to *Amos 'n Andy* for the next 20 years, and they also received star salaries to play the chief parts.

Within a few years, television ended the success of their variety show, but from 1954 into the 1960s, Correll and Gosden stayed on CBS radio with a new show, The Amos and Andy Music Hall, mixing skits with popular records. On November 25, 1960 they left the air permanently.

In the mid-1950s, CBS developed a situation comedy based on *Amos 'n Andy* characters. Correll and Gosden were creative consultants, but the cast was entirely African American. The show had modest success with audiences, but it was embroiled in constant racial controversy. The NAACP protested the show vehemently, and the cast had frequent problems with the scripts. Neither Correll nor Gosden was prepared for the kind of bitterness that the TV show had engendered, and both men, especially Gosden, felt deeply wounded by some accusations.

Adapted from "Charles James Correll," VCU, 1995 and used with permission of Dr. Nicholas Sharp.

After the TV series ended and their last radio show was over, Correll and Gosden remained friends, living near each other in quiet retirement in their Beverly Hills homes. Correll continued throughout his life to maintain warm and friendly connections with his midwestern roots, and returning to Chicago, he died there at the age of 82.

25. Which of the following is supported by the passage?

    A. Correll's interest in vaudeville came through his mother and father, both of whom were performers.
    B. Correll was independently wealthy and took up vaudeville because he could find nothing else that interested him.
    C. Correll's interest in vaudeville began when he was an usher in a vaudeville house.
    D. Correll preferred his father's profession of bricklaying to show business, but he was better at entertainment than at bricklaying.

26. According to the passage, which quality more characterizes Gosden than it does Correll?

    A. He was more even-tempered.
    B. He was more temperamental.
    C. He was a better pianist.
    D. He was the funniest.

27. What event marked the beginning of the first decline of popularity of the *Amos 'n Andy Show*?

    A. The Great Depression
    B. The arrival of Correll's first child.
    C. Gosden's hospitalization.
    D. World War II.

28. What does the passage indicate happened to the *Sam 'n Henry Show* after Correll and Gosden left radio station WGN?

    A. They carried their show with them to rival station, WMAQ.
    B. WGN retained rights to the show and continued it without Correll and Gosden.
    C. Correll and Gosden retained rights to the show but changed its name to the *Amos 'n Andy Show.*
    D. The show was cancelled.

29. From the Great Depression onward, the *Amos 'n Andy Show* was criticized for its racial stereotyping. According to the passage, which of the

words below best describes Correll's response to this criticism?

A. Angry   C. Wounded
B. Vindictive   D. Indifferent

30. In retirement, both Correll and Gosden were financially secure. What was the state of their friendship in the later years of their lives?

    A. Their friendship was weakened by the turmoil and controversy caused by the show, and they drifted apart.
    B. They remained friends and lived near each other in Beverly Hills.
    C. They quarreled bitterly over money and parted enemies.
    D. They occupied adjoining suites in the Beverly Hilton until Correll returned to Peoria.

Passage V (Questions 31–37)

The process involved in the recovery from either chronic alcohol or substance abuse is a long one, mainly a lifetime pursuit. AA teaches that an alcoholic can never drink again, and it is generally held that relapse occurs more often when someone stops going to "meetings." Although empirical observations such as these have caused a considerable amount of doubt in the past, a measure of light is now being shed on the situation.

For example, some of the answers to the puzzle of the recovery process are suggested in two articles published in the first issue of the *Informer* by O'Brien and Rosecrans. They focus primarily on the environmental contingencies that cause drug dependent individuals problems when trying to stop using a specific chemical. Thus, the drug-dependent individual is faced with many problems outside of his or her own internal need to feel good. For example, drug effects such as their self-administration, and the withdrawal syndrome following chronic use, can be elicited by external stimuli previously associated with previous drug use. A heroin-dependent individual in recovery may experience severe withdrawal symptoms if he or she enters a bar or restaurant previously associated with heroin withdrawal. Furthermore, an alcoholic when not under the influence of alcohol may have difficulty finding his or her car when parked during an alcoholic bout, but can remember where it is when drinking is resumed. This latter phenomena is better known as drug-induced state dependent learning, a pharmacological effect well documented in the human literature.

Thus, when one considers what a drug can do to an individual internally, and in conjunction with his or her

environment, one wonders how anyone could become drug-free under the burden of such effects. However, it does happen many times over regardless of the odds. Thus, is recovery a magical phenomena, or is it scientifically based? The answer is not simple. One experiment conducted in rats may help us appreciate what might be going on during the recovery process. In this study, Esposito *et al.* (*Science 224: 306–309 (1984)* at the National Institute of Mental Health were evaluating how electrical stimulation (like ECS) affects energy metabolism in rat brains. Two groups of rats were studied; one group was allowed to stimulate itself by pressing a lever (self-stimulation); the other group was stimulated within the same parameters, but the stimulation was elicited by the experimenter. The second group, thus, had no part in the electrostimulation of their brains. Interestingly, even though both groups of rats received the same level of stimulation, the brain area distribution pattern of increases in energy metabolism were quite different and contingent upon whether rat or experimenter turned on the stimulator.

This experiment is important, not because it provided a specific set of data, but because it demonstrated that a specific change in brain energy metabolism was controlled by each individual rat. The effect on energy metabolism was quite different when elicited by the experimenter. This simple experiment suggests that each individual, to recover from drug dependency, must operate on him or herself. This concept may have importance for two other reasons. First, treatment works only when the individual decides to take on recovery. Although this may appear to be a logical statement, many good professionals, including some in the areas of medical and mental health, do not appear to appreciate the difference between treatment and recovery. Secondly, during the recovery process, the individual is basically altering his or her behavioral conditioning and neurochemistry, which will allow the process to go forward. This can be done by extinguishing or altering the stimulus properties of the drugs that the individual is dependent on. "Don't drink and go to meetings." In scientific terms, the reinforcing effects of drugs are extinguished by not using them, and the stimulus properties are altered by joining forces with people who have also changed their environments. In addition, the social reinforcement and support in AA is also important to recovery because one is substituting alcohol or drugs with people, a much finer euphoriant. Therefore, success in recovery may not

Adapted from John A. Rosecrans, *Drug Dependence Outline*, MCV/VCU, 1990.

be as magical as was once thought, and may have a very precise and orderly basis. The awareness and knowledge of this scientific base can be helpful to both client and therapist.

31. An appropriate title for this passage could be:

   A. Withdrawal Syndrome.
   B. Behavioral Conditioning and Withdrawal.
   C. The Recovery Process.
   D. Environmental Contingencies and Drug Use.

32. Recovery from drug addiction:

   A. involves a lifelong process.
   B. is modulated by environmental factors.
   C. can be associated with withdrawal symptoms.
   D. includes all of the above.

33. According to the author:

   A. certain tasks can be better learned while under the influence of psychoactive drugs.
   B. certain tasks are easily performed while under the influence of drugs.
   C. certain tasks may be difficult if not under the influence.
   D. learning and performing of tasks are not drastically affected by drug use.

34. Which statement(s) is/are *supported by* the passage?

   A. Neurochemical mechanisms play a role in drug addiction and recovery.
   B. Environmental conditions may have drastic effects on an individual.
   C. The individual is a key determinator.
   D. All of the above.

35. According to the passage:

   A. the addiction process is well understood.
   B. the recovery process is well understood.
   C. recovery is the reverse of addiction and depends solely on substitution of compounds.
   D. none of the above statements is supported.

36. Most health professionals:

   A. agree on the treatment plans of withdrawal and recovery.
   B. appreciate that treatment and recovery are at times different.
   C. are comfortable with the fact that neurochemical mechanisms are determining factors.
   D. feel that AA does the best job in curing alcoholics.

37. The passage implies that the solutions to the drug addiction and recovery are found:

   A. in the individual.
   B. in experimental models.
   C. in organizations.
   D. in environmental factors.

Passage VI (Questions 38–44)

Physicians like Hippocrates, Thomas Browne, and John Gregory emphasized that physicians must do the "right thing" for their patients, and most physicians take this to mean curing illness and preventing death. Gregory refreshingly reminds us that physicians are not always perfect. "I may reckon among the moral duties incumbent on a physician, that candor, which makes him open to conviction, and ready to acknowledge and rectify his mistakes. An obstinate adherence to an unsuccessful method of treating a disease, is based on a high degree of self-conceit, and a belief of the infallibility of a system." Erik Erikson takes the Golden Rule as his "baseline . . . for wise and proper conduct" and points out that even though systematic ethicists may believe the concept too simple, the rule has "marked a mysterious meeting ground between ancient peoples surrounded by oceans and eras and is a theme hidden in the most memorable sayings of many thinkers." The Talmudic version of the Golden Rule, "What is hateful to yourself, do not to your fellow man" is similar to the Christian "Love thy neighbor as thyself." The Golden Rule is not a sufficient ethical principle, however, because it conceptualizes the idea that what is good for the physician is good for the patient. It expresses *beneficence,* which means that the physician, because of specialized knowledge and motivation, knows what is best for each patient.

The principle of beneficence, however, must be tempered by the countervailing idea of *autonomy.* The idea of human rights is a relatively recent development in social evolution. When physicians and priests were one and the same, the principle of beneficence was taken for granted. Patients were expected to do what they were told and "doctors orders" became an everyday expression. The ethical principle of autonomy echoes Rousseau, Washington, and Jefferson in emphasizing the patient's primacy in making moral judgments about himself. The courts have generally held that constitutional rights permit an individual to determine what happens to himself and his property; many of these rights have been codified in what has been called a "Patient's Bill of Rights."

Rousseau pointed out that a social contract was necessary because of the inherent inequality among human beings. Some are wise, whereas others are dull, some are strong, whereas others are weak. This inequality is particularly striking in the patient-physician relationship. Physicians have wide knowledge and experience, whereas the patient may understand his own needs and value but has little information about his clinical state. Only detailed conversations with patients and their families can narrow this gap in such a way that people can make truly autonomous judgments about their own care.

Physicians frequently appear to ignore the required balance between the principles of beneficence and autonomy. A physician recommends radical mastectomy for breast cancer. No options are provided because the physician believes he knows best. The patient asks for a second opinion and the physician refuses saying "I cannot take care of you unless I can make all important decisions." Here is presumed beneficence gone amok. A moment later the patient refuses all surgery and the physician says kindly, "It's your life and you are free to do anything you like." Here the physician is ignoring the obvious worried statement of the patient and threatening abandonment if the patient does not obey.

Aside from the physician's obvious arrogance and insensitivity, the key question must be: Is the patient completely autonomous when she refuses all treatment and walks out of the doctor's office? She has been told that she has cancer and must have what she believes to be a destructive surgical procedure. Fear of disfigurement and death have produced uncontrollable anxiety that causes her to attempt escape from the situation. True beneficence in this situation demands that the physician seek out the patient, and her family, and make certain that repeated efforts are made to present the true gravity of the situation. Beneficence does not mean the quick delivery of a series of commands, but implies shared responsibility, patient education, and understanding, and gentle persuasion where necessary. *Indeed, correctly interpreting the proper balance between these two moral principles in any given situation could be considered one of the key responsibilities of the practice of medicine.*

The beneficence/autonomy concept must be related to the burden/benefit relationship of any proposed action. The balance between the risks or burden of continued treatment relative to any anticipated benefits must be carefully considered. Sometimes life itself, or the treatment proposed to sustain life, is so burdensome that the patient claims the right to allow the dying process to proceed. Granting seriously ill patients, or their families, the right to refuse life-lengthening treatment is an important human issue that is central to professional practice. In many respects, the judicial system is ahead of most physicians in understanding the issues under discussion. Artificial feeding, for example, a technique that many would consider to be part of the basic humane care required for all patients may also become burdensome in certain situations where any benefits from such intervention is minimal.

Obviously, the accuracy of a group of physicians to predict that meaningful life is no longer possible for the individual is central to any such decision. Such a need raises the issue of who can determine what is "meaningful life" and how can physicians best learn how to decide when the burden outweighs the benefit of any course of action.

38. Which of the following statement(s) is/are *supported by* the passage?

　A. The Golden Rule is not a sufficient ethical statement.
　B. Most physicians emphasize curing illness and preventing death.
　C. The Golden Rule views the physician as knowing what is best for the patient.
　D. All of the above.

39. Which of the following would probably have been chosen by the author as a title for this passage?

　A. The Development of the Medical Decision Making Process
　B. Physician Reasoning and Autonomy
　C. The Practice of the Golden Rule
　D. Moral Reasoning and Medical Decision Making

40. Regarding human rights, which statement(s) is/are NOT *supported by* the passage?

　A. Hippocrates lived before that principle was established.
　B. Physicians must attempt to defeat the disease first and then explain their protocol.
　C. The courts generally have backed the physician as to knowing what is best for the patient.
　D. All of the above.

Adapted from Dr. Stephen M. Ayres, "Moral Reasoning and Medical Decision Making," MCV/VCU, 1990.

41. From information provided in the passage, one would be justified in concluding that:

   I. patients are perfectly capable of making autonomous judgments.

   II. beneficence implies understanding.

   III. Rousseau believed that people are quite similar.

   IV. beneficence and autonomy go hand in hand to achieve good medical practice.

   A. I, II, and III   **C.** II and IV only

   B. I and III   **D.** IV only

42. Hippocrates is cited as one of several who believed that physicians should do the "right thing" for their patients. Which other specific beliefs, thoughts, or perceptions are directly attributed to Hippocrates in the passage?

   I. He perceived medicine as a tripartite relationship between patient, disease, and doctor.

   II. He believed that disease was determined to a great extent by the patient's environment and way of life.

   III. He believed that there was nothing sacred about sickness and that each malady followed a distinct pattern (three stages).

   IV. He thought of the physician as nature's helper who should reinforce the body's own defenses.

   A. I, II, and III   **C.** II and IV

   B. I and III   **D.** I, II, III, and IV

43. According to the passage, which of the following is/are correct?

   I. Life itself at times can be burdensome.

   II. Patient education is an essential element in true beneficence.

   III. The courts have a better grasp of the right to die concept than the physician.

   IV. Basic humane treatment must always be provided no matter what the benefit is.

   A. I, II, and III   **C.** II and IV

   B. I and III   **D.** I, II, III, and IV

44. The author of the passages argues for:

   I. education.

   II. balance.

   III. consultation.

   IV. patient rights.

   A. I, II, and III   **C.** II and IV

   B. I and III   **D.** I, II, III, and IV

Passage VII (Questions 45–51)

Another kind of editorial begins in the April 1942 issue. It was the first to acknowledge America's entry into World War II. This informed youth how they could contribute to the war effort and attempted to inspire them to make such contributions. In an editorial "Little Things Can Help Win the War," the points were simple—stay healthy so you can work hard; assume minor responsibilities so adults can take major roles; save your pennies and dimes to buy Defense Stamps; and "most important of all," be confident. Confidence would provide "vision to see beyond today and its efforts and worries to the glorious day when we can all say, 'We, too, have fought a good fight and, all pulling together for the right cause, . . . we have won!' "

War effort editorials emphasized the need for collecting scrap metal and rubber, for maintaining fitness, and for growing "victory gardens."

To stress the need for staying fit, Hecht published the first guest editorial in *True Comics*. Colonel Theodore P. Bank, chief of the Athletic and Recreation Branch, Special Services Division of the War Department, wrote "The Importance of Physical Fitness Today." Bank mentioned time and effort being wasted because army recruits were unfit and work days were being lost in factories "because of sickness or injuries which are traceable directly to (young people's) lack of physical fitness."

On youth's involvement in food production, Hecht invited another guest writer, Wayne H. Darrow, director, U.S. Agricultural Labor Administration. His piece "You Can Help the Farmer Win the War," was carried on the first page of the August 1943 issue rather than on the inside front cover. Darrow wrote:

When the harvest is in this fall, everyone who has toughened his hands at farm work will be able to say that he has helped to win the war. Out on our farms this year there is a man's and a woman's job waiting for many thousand boys and girls. Our soldiers, sailors, and marines are counting on the farmers. Can the farmers count on you?

It could be thought that Hecht used editorials merely to sell magazines and to advance patriotism. He was indeed a skillful promoter, and he wanted the United States to win the war, but these aspects were less important than his major goal—a world of democracy, unity, and concord. He was an avid internationalist, a globalist.

In February 1943, in the midst of his war effort editorials, he wrote "It's Your World." The arguments were unusual, perhaps even risky for his own well-being,

From Dr. William E. Blake, Jr., "True Comics," VCU, 1990.

made as they were when the battle was at last shifting in favor of the Allies. This would not seem an appropriate moment to hint to children that the United States must bear some responsibility for the war. However, he attacked the retreat of the United States into isolationism following World War I. "So we celebrated our victory, crawled into our national shell and left the young democracies set up by the Versailles peace treaty to get along the best they could," he wrote. He continued the argument, "We hope and believe that never again will we be guilty of such failure to stand by. For one thing, we know now that withdrawing from our responsibilities after the last war was in a great measure responsible for World War II." He urged young people "to make this battle-scarred planet a safe and sane place to live in."

A similar article in January 1944 pointed out the rapid development of transportation and communication making the world smaller. "Learn to write, read, and speak another langauge—or two or three, if you can," he wrote. According to Hecht, advantages would be easier travel and more friendships in foreign countries. But also the linguist would be able to explain the principles of democracy.

In the following issue Hecht wrote another daring piece, which aroused hostility among some Americans. There was nothing subtle in the title, "An International Police Force." He maintained nations should not be free to act as they pleased. Nations should take their grievances to an international court and let judges decide. He advocated an international police force to enforce court decisions. "We can't have it both ways," he concluded. "We can't have lasting peace and at the same time insist upon all those national 'rights' which make the waging of wars inevitable."

March 1944 was the last issue of *True Comics* to carry an editorial. Paper had become scarce, and all comic magazines were forced to cut the number of pages. Features had to be discontinued and editorials seemed the most dispensable item.

Circulation figures for *True Comics* are available for each year of its publication, but it is impossible to know how widely young people were reading the editorials or what sort of impact they made.

The idea of a comic book with true stories was unique. Other publishers responded, turning our similar products, but *True Comics* stood alone in carrying editorials. These essays were clear witness to the broad, humanistic, and internationalist values and goals held by George J. Hecht; his determination to spread those ideals; and his confidence in the ability and willingness of American youth to read, to learn, and to do.

45. Which statement(s) is/are *supported by* the passage?

    I.   The passage essentially is a history lesson.
    II.   America's war effort is described.
    III. Youth and fitness are the main themes.
    IV.   The fate of a comic book is described.

    A. I, II, and III   C. II and IV
    B. I and III   D. IV only

46. The publication was unique because it incorporated:

    A. true stories.
    B. color photographs.
    C. editorials.
    D. war stories.

47. The editorials stressed:

    A. recycling.
    B. patriotism.
    C. fitness.
    D. all of the above.

48. The publisher of this series could be considered a(an):

    A. communist.
    B. idealist.
    C. internationalist.
    D. socialist.

49. In providing information related to the editorials contained in *True Comics* during the World War II period, the author of this passage asserts that:

    A. the publisher was the first to portray America's entry into World War II in comic form.
    B. the publisher hoped to reach the young.
    C. the publisher himself wrote the editorial on fitness.
    D. isolationism was proposed.

50. The feature of this publication was abandoned because:

    A. the editor changed.
    B. of competition.
    C. a paper shortage occurred.
    D. the war ended.

51. Which of the following is *contradicted by* the passage?

    A. The editor believed that America's youth were willing to be responsible.
    B. A linguist would serve democracy well.
    C. The editor was somewhat of a free spirit.
    D. A United Nations would prevent all future wars.

Passage VIII (Questions 52–58)

Herbert Hoover, engineer, self-made man, and great humanitarian hero of the First World War, went on to serve as food czar of the United States during its active war years, and returned to the international rescue business with the cessation of hostilities. As secretary of commerce during the prosperous 1920s, Hoover continued his commendable record of public service.

The 1930s, however, were less kind to his reputation. Elected president in 1928, he enjoyed a scant eight months in office before the collapse of the stock market created a catalyst for the onslaught of the Great Depression. The appearance of failure in combatting that economic and human tragedy, made worse by the Democrats' smear campaign, blighted his name. Despite his assertions that the depression had been beaten by the Summer of 1932, the voting public repudiated him in the presidential election of that year.

Out of office, he remained silent for a time and then took the offensive, first criticizing the New Deal and eventually even attacking President Franklin D. Roosevelt. An unsuccessful seeker of the Republican nomination in 1936 and 1940, Hoover struggled to make his voice heard as a critic of what he called unliberal policies. When war broke out in Europe in 1939, he assumed the dual role of passionate opponent of active United States involvement in the conflict and advocate of humanitarian relief to those caught behind enemy lines.

Poland, Finland, Belgium, Holland, and Norway solicited Hoover's assistance almost immediately. He quickly established organizations to aid each of them with money, food, and other forms of nonmilitary support. But even in 1939, his efforts encountered obstacles, both real and propagandistic—in particular a nasty set of rumors about competition with the Red Cross. In 1940, the Hoover relief machine ran up against even more formidable opponents when Winston Churchill and Franklin Roosevelt assumed the posture that relief to these nations would lighten the burden that ought to fall upon their Nazi conquerors. Besides, said Churchill, the Germans would only steal whatever relief supplies were sent to those suffering under occupation.

For the first half of 1940, Hoover combined these relief efforts with a quiet campaign to get the Republican presidential nomination. Although he and his partisans would deny it in 1940 and later, Hoover engaged in a vigorous and carefully orchestrated program, directed toward bringing him a draft. But he would see himself as the victim of deliberate sabotage at the convention when the coveted nomination went to Wendell Willkie. Virtually ignored during the campaign, Hoover returned passionately to the cause of relief, offering the "Hoover

We gratefully acknowledge the help of Dr. Susan Esterbrook Kennedy, Professor of History and Geography, Virginia Commonwealth University, 1990.

Plan" for experimental feeding, which could be stopped instantly in the event of Nazi interference. But the official United States position remained negative. By the end of 1940, Hoover formed the National Committee on Food for the Small Democracies as a propaganda and lobbying organization to press for relief via the Hoover Plan.

Meanwhile, Hoover became increasingly alarmed at the growing danger that the United States might be drawn into an active role in the fighting. He continued to believe, as he had from the outbreak of hostilities, that Britain could not be defeated, that Germany could not win, and that a negotiated peace was possible. He concluded, therefore, that there was no need for American entry. But he distrusted Roosevelt's policies. Although Hoover's active opposition to war was nowhere near so vehement as it would become in 1941, that theme interweaves with his desire for office and his commitment to relief to present a highly complex scenario of his activities and motivations in 1940, and with it, a commentary on the state of the nation from the viewpoint of a still-influential citizen.

52. An appropriate title for this passage could be:

A. Herbert Hoover the statesman.
B. Dirty Politics.
C. Herbert Hoover the Humanitarian.
D. Herbert Hoover—Relief, Politics, and War.

53. Which of the following statements is NOT *supported nor contradicted by* the passage?

A. Hoover was a genius as an organizer.
B. Hoover was a humanitarian.
C. The Democrats ran an honest campaign in 1932.
D. Hoover felt that once being president was enough.

54. The passage pictures Roosevelt as:

A. a clean politician.
B. a humanitarian.
C. a self-made man.
D. not sympathetic to Hoover's efforts.

55. Which statement is *contradicted by* the passage?

A. Despite the ups and downs of his career, Hoover's name remained unblemished.
B. Hoover was part of the political scene for a long time.
C. Hoover did not have party support in his quest for reelection.
D. Other nations sought Hoover's help.

56. Which of the following items is/are not addressed in the passage?

    A. The Hoover Plan was more appropriate.
    B. The Marshall Plan was more appropriate.
    C. The Berlin Airlift solved a severe problem.
    D. All of the above.

57. The passage offers support for all but which of the following observations?

    A. Hoover competed with the Red Cross.
    B. Churchill opposed Hoover's efforts.
    C. Hoover opposed propaganda.
    D. Hoover acted quickly when it came to relief.

58. Which statement applies to the passage as a whole?

    A. Hoover is pictured as a committed individual.
    B. The author is sympathetic and fair.
    C. It is a quick overview of a long record of humanitarian service.
    D. All of the above.

Passage IX (Questions 59–65)

Two ash samples received September 1989 and two ash samples received November 1989 were ignited to determine carbon content and then analyzed for mineral content. Data from the ash mineral analysis were used as input to the Bickelhaupt resistivity prediction model developed for the U.S.E.P.A. An additional computer run was performed to predict the resistivity of an ash that would result from burning 30% waste fuel containing 0.5% magnesium oxide along with the coal normally burned. The resistivity of the ash is an important factor in the performance of the air pollution control equipment used to control particulate emission from the combustion process.

The samples taken in September 1989 were taken from the hoppers of Units 15 and 16. The samples were taken while Unit 16 was having opacity problems to determine if resistivity problems related to ash chemistry were responsible for the performance problems. The analysis showed the ash mineral composition of the samples was virtually identical. The primary difference between the two ash samples was the loss on ignition, which was 23.33% for Unit 16 and 30.80% for Unit 15. The loss on ignition is presumed to be from unburned carbon.

With all of the carbon removed, the two samples are predicted to have approximately a 10^{11} ohm-cm resistivity at 450°F. This resistivity would lead to high sparking, and possible back corona in both units. Optimum resistivity for these units at their 450°F gas temperature is estimated to be about 7×10^9 ohm-cm. This resistivity is lower than the 2×10^{10} ohm-cm, which is normally quoted as optimum for precipitators running at lower temperatures. The lower resistivity is required due to the lower dielectric strength of the flue gases at 450°. The lower dielectric strengths will promote back corona in ash layers sooner than units running in the 200° to 250°F range.

The high resistivity predicted for the carbon free ash will change dramatically with the carbon levels indicated by the loss on ignition tests. Laboratory tests and field data from other ashes have shown large reductions in resistivity from similar carbon levels. The reductions are typically one to three orders of magnitude if the carbon is finely divided and well mixed with the ash. The benefits of the carbon are usually observed at higher gas temperatures, such as the 450°F$^+$ temperatures at which Units 15 and 16 are normally run. The higher unburned carbon levels on Unit 15 are believed to be responsible in part for the better performance of Unit 15 in September. A faulty spark sensing circuit on the automatic voltage controllers for the outlet field of Unit 16 also was later found to have contributed to poor performance of the unit.

Ash samples from November 1989 were also analyzed. The higher sodium and iron content of the November ash samples resulted in an ash with a resistivity that was about five to six times less resistive than the September samples. ESP performance during this period of lower predicted resistivities was reported to be good.

Increases in ash magnesium oxide were estimated based on the following:

Fuel: 70% coal, 30% residue
Ash: 5.3%   0.5%

$$(5.3 \times 70) + (0.5 \times .30) \ = \text{total ash}$$
$$3.71 \ \ + \ \ \ 0.15 \ = 3.86\% \text{ total ash.}$$

On a percentage basis, the coal contributes 3.71/3.86 or 96.1% of the total ash, and the residue contributes 0.15/3.86 or 3.9% of the total ash. The 3.9 ash from residue was assumed to be mostly magnesium oxide. This was added to the sample with the highest magnesium oxide content to create the analysis for hypothetical Sample #5. The increase in magnesium oxide caused the

Adapted from a report by W. J. Borowy, VCU, 1990.

predicted resistivity to increase about four times. The increase of resistivity will probably not cause operational problems with the favorable ash produced when the November samples were taken. However, low power levels and high opacity may be a problem if ash quality is similar to that encountered in September. If high resistivity problems occur when burning the high magnesium residue, injection of sodium sulfite (Na_2S) to increase the sodium oxide levels in the ash to 1.5% will lower resistivities to an acceptable level.

59. Data from the ash analysis was input into a computer model developed by:

A. U.S.D.A.   C. U.S.D.O.T.
B. U.S.D.O.E.   D. none of the above.

60. The primary difference between ash samples was:

A. one was from waste fuel and one was from coal.
B. the samples were collected at two different temperatures.
C. the loss on ignition.
D. none of the above.

61. What is the percent basis contribution of the coal to the total amount of ash produced?

A. 3.9%   C. 96.1%
B. 3.71%   D. 69.1%

62. A hypothetical sample #5 was created that increased the resistivity of the sample. What oxide was increased to create this sample?

A. sodium oxide   C. calcium oxide
B. iron oxide   D. magnesium oxide

63. What was the date of the first ash samples received?

A. September 1989   C. November 1989
B. November 1987   D. none of the above

64. Which of the following statement(s) is/are *supported by* the information in the passage?

I. Carbon content of the ash affects the electrical resistivity of the ash.
II. Magnesium oxide lowers the electrical resistivity of the ash.
III. Sodium oxide raises the electrical resistivity of the ash.

A. I only   C. I and II only
B. II and III only   D. I, II, and III

65. What is the probable reason this passage was written?

A. to discuss hazardous components of coal ash
B. to predict water treatment characteristics of a waste stream
C. to determine the impact of future fuel composition changes on electrical characteristics of fly ash
D. to calculate the composition of feed stock necessary in the production of resistors used in the electronics industry

PHYSICAL SCIENCES

10 PROBLEM SETS OF 5–10 QUESTIONS EACH
15 PROBLEMS FOLLOWED BY A SINGLE QUESTION
77 QUESTIONS
100 MINUTES

DIRECTIONS: The following questions or incomplete statements are in groups. Preceding each series of questions or statements is a paragraph or a short explanatory statement, a formula or set of formulas, or a definition. Read the written material and then answer the questions or complete the statements. Select the ONE BEST ANSWER for each question and indicate your selection by marking the corresponding letter of your choice on the Answer Form. Eliminate those alternatives you know to be incorrect and then select an answer from among the remaining alternatives. A periodic table is provided (see p. 583). You may consult it whenever you wish to do so.

Passage I (Questions 66–71)

A human centrifuge is used to test and train pilots and astronauts to withstand the large "g-forces" experienced during flight. The centrifuge arm length is such that the subject moves in a large circle of radius 9 m. The maximum angular velocity is 4 radians/sec. The subject normally faces inward toward the center of the circular path. ("eyeballs in").

During a test, the subject's respiratory and metabolic rate rise. The energy released per liter of oxygen consumed in human metabolism averages about 20,000 J/L.

66. What is the maximum linear (tangential) speed of the subject along the circular path at the maximum angular velocity of 4 radians/s?

    A. 18 m/sec   C. 36 m/sec
    B. 25 m/sec   D. 226 m/sec

67. A pilot of mass 82 kg (180 lbs) experiences 8 "g's" during one test for a period of 2 minutes. What is centripetal force, in newtons, acting on the pilot?

    A. 16 N   C. 960 N
    B. 660 N   D. 6400 N

68. In the earth frame of reference, what centrifugal force acts *on the pilot* during the test?

    A. The centrifugal force *on the pilot* is equal and opposite the centripetal force on the pilot.
    B. The centrifugal force *on the pilot* is 1 "g" larger than the centripetal force on the pilot.
    C. The centripetal force *on the pilot* is 1 "g" smaller than the centripetal force on the pilot.
    D. There is *no* centrifugal force *on the pilot*.

69. The pilot's metabolic rate rises to 450 W and remains at that level during the 2 minute test period. What is the approximate number of liters of oxygen consumed by the pilot during the test period?

    A. 3 L   C. 6 L
    B. 4 L   D. 10 L

70. What force acts on the back of the pilot's seat?

    A. 0 N   C. 960 N
    B. 88 N   D. 6400 N

71. The pilot now faces outward ("eyeballs out"). What effect does this have on the centripetal force acting on the pilot?

    A. The centripetal force now points outward.
    B. The seat back now exerts an outward force.
    C. The centripetal force is replaced by the centrifugal force (now supplied by the pilot's seat harness).
    D. The centripetal force is unchanged (now supplied by the pilot's seat harness).

Passage II (Questions 72–77)

A periscope viewing system is to be used to observe the behavior of primates in a large environmentally controlled room on the upper floor of a large research facility. The periscope, like those used on submarines, is essentially a large, folded-path, low power telescope (using prisms to fold the light path). A sketch of the preliminary design appears below. Like all Newtonian telescopes, it uses a relatively long focal length objective lens to form a real image in front of the eyepiece lens (of shorter focal length). The observer looks through the eyepiece lens to see the final image, in the same manner that one would use a magnifying glass. The distance between the lenses is approximately equal to the sum of their focal lengths. The eyepiece, in this design, can be moved forward or back in order to focus on the primates as they move closer to or further away from the objective lens.

72. The total tube length of the three sections is to be 4 m. The objective lens available has a focal length of 3 m. What should the focal length of the eyepiece lens be?

   A. 0.75 m   **C.** 1.33 m
   B. 1 m   **D.** 7 m

73. A visitor seeing the sketch points out an important flaw that will require a design change. What is the flaw?

   A. The focal length of the eyepiece lens is too short.
   B. The images of the primates will be inverted.
   C. The objective lens should be a diverging lens.
   D. The prisms cannot be used in this way.

74. What will be the approximate magnification of this periscope?

   A. 0.67 ×   **C.** 3 ×
   B. 1 ×   **D.** 300 ×

75. The prisms (45-45-90° prisms) turn the light path through 90° by "total internal reflection" from the inside hypotenuse faces of the prisms when the incident angle is 45° as in the sketch. Can one use crown glass with an index of refraction of 1.52 for the prism?

   A. Yes, because the critical angle for crown glass is 47°.
   B. Yes, because the critical angle for crown glass is 41°.
   C. No, because the critical angle for crown glass is exactly 47°.
   D. No, because the critical angle for crown glass is 41°.

76. Describe the properties of the image that one sees with this preliminary design.

   A. real, inverted, magnified
   B. real, upright, magnified
   C. virtual, upright, same size as object
   D. virtual, inverted, magnified

77. The telescope is focused on a primate rather far away on the far side of the large habitat. As the primate moves rather closer to the telescope, what must the observer do to see the primate clearly?

   A. No change, the image remains clear.
   B. Move the eyepiece away from the objective.
   C. Move the eyepiece closer to the objective.
   D. Use an inverting eyepiece because the image flips.

Passage III (Questions 78–82)

A large vertical cylindrical tank of water about 75 m tall is used by the U.S. Navy to train submariners in techniques used to safely escape sunken submarines in shallow waters. The tanks are used for physiological experiments also. Until very recently all submariners had to undergo a yearly physical test to show that they could escape from a depth of several feet of water (without the use of any artificial breathing apparatus). The sailors enter an air lock and wait while the air pressure is increased until it equals the water pressure at the bottom of the tank. The bottom four feet of the air lock is filled with water. The door to the tank is then opened and the sailors take a final breath (of the high pressure air), swim out the door, and rise slowly to the surface. The trip to the surface takes several minutes. (During this time the swimmer exhales continuously.) The density of the water is 1000 kg/m^3.

78. If the water is incompressible, what pressure does the water exert at the bottom of the 75 m tall tank?

   A. 3.6×10^5 N/m^2 **C.** 72×10^5 N/m^2
   B. 7.35×10^5 N/m^2 **D.** 75×10^5 N/m^2

79. One atmosphere of pressure (atm) = 1.01×10^5 N/m^2. Approximately how many atmospheres are exerted by the pressure at the bottom of the tank?

   A. 72.0 atm   **C.** 7.3 atm
   B. 8.36 atm   **D.** 0.836 atm

80. A glass viewport of are 65 cm^2 is located near the bottom of the tank at 70 meters below the surface. What is the force on the viewport in newtons?

A. 4110 N   C. 4460 N
B. 450 N   D. 5660 N

81. If the sailor's total lung capacity is 6.3 liters and he takes in this volume of air at the pressure in the air lock, to what approximate volume, in liters, will the air expand as he rises to the surface (where the absolute pressure is 1 atmosphere)?

A. 52 liters   C. 540 liters
B. 67 liters   D. 670 liters

82. Because air contains 21% oxygen by volume, what is the partial pressure of oxygen in the lungs at the bottom of the 75 m escape tank?

A. 2.12×10^4 N/m^2 C. 1.76×10^5 N/m^2
B. 1.57×10^5 N/m^2 D. 1.01×10^6 N/m^2

Passage IV (Questions 83–87)

A brewery builds a cylindrical tank with 12 large electrical resistance heaters for the purpose of boiling city water to obtain distilled water. Each heater has a resistance of 15 ohms and normally draws a 20 A current. The tank radius is 1.1 m and the normal depth of water will be 2.0 m. An access hatch of 30 cm radius is designed to withstand a maximum gauge pressure of 31,000 N/m^2. When the tank is full the water pressure on the tank bottom is normally 19,500 N/m^2 when the tank is open to the air at 1 atm (1 atm = 1.01 3 105 N/m^2). The tank can be pressurized so that the water will boil at a higher temperature than 100°C.

83. The tank is filled to the normal 2 m depth and then pressurized so that the maximum gauge pressure of 31,000 N/m^2 is exerted on the tank bottom. Of this maximum pressure, how much is due to pressurization?

A. 126,300 N/m^2 C. zero
B. 8200 N/m^2 D. 11,400 N/m^2

84. What total electrical power, in watts, is supplied to all 12 resistance heaters at a current of 20 A?

A. 40,000 W   C. 49,000 W
B. 72,000 W   D. 52,000 W

85. What is the normal water volume in the cylindrical tank?

A. 7.6 m^3 C. 6.5 m^3
B. 4.2 m^3 D. 14.1 m^3

86. The water enters the tank at 50°C and boils at 105°C due to pressurization. If the current is increased until the 12 heaters are supplying 110,000 watts, how long will it take 5 m^3 (mass = 5,000 kg) of water to heat through the 55°C rise? The heat needed to change the temperature of 1 kg of water by 1°C is its "specific heat" (c = 4190 joules/kg · °C).

A. 1.5 hours   C. 2.9 hours
B. 3.4 hours   D. 6.2 hours

87. The tank can be filled to the normal 2 m depth (and volume) in 13 minutes by a pipe through which the fill water flows at a speed of 1.0 m/sec. What is the cross-sectional *area* of the cylindrical fill pipe?

A. 1.1 m^2 C. 0.05 m^2
B. 0.01 m^2 D. 0.9 m^2

Questions 88–95 are independent of any passage and of each other.

88. Two children of masses 35 kg and 20 kg are on a seesaw board 2 m long with the pivot at the center. How far from the pivot must the 35 kg child sit on one side if the smaller child is sitting on the other end of the board?

A. 0.81 m   C. 0.72 m
B. 0.35 m   D. 0.57 m

89. A centrifuge starts from rest and reaches a final angular speed of 57,300 rev/min in 2 minutes. (Recall that 1 rev = 2π radians.) What is the angular acceleration of the centrifuge?

A. 50 rad/sec^2 C. 3000 rad/sec^2
B. 32 rad/sec^2 D. 12 rad/sec^2

90. A 4 kg block is initially moving at 5 m/sec when the applied force is removed, and the block slides to rest on a rough floor with a coefficient of friction of 0.4. How much work is done by the friction force in stopping the block?

A. 400 joules   C. 100 joules
B. 50 joules   D. 220 joules

91. A small insect is 4.8 cm from a +6.0 cm focal length lens. Find the position of the image relative to the lens.

A. 24 cm on the same side as the insect
B. 32 cm on the opposite side
C. 12 cm on the same side as the insect
D. 18 cm on the opposite side

92. Forces of 2 newtons act for 4 seconds on masses of 3 kg and 6 kg, which are initially at rest on frictionless surfaces. What are the respective momenta of the 3 kg and 6 kg masses at the end of the 4 sec periods.

A. 6 and 12 kg-m/sec
B. 8 and 8 kg-m/sec
C. 12 and 6 kg-m/sec
D. 12 and 24 kg-m/sec

93. The isotope $_{29}Cu^{64}$ is unusual in that it can decay by γ, β^-, and β^+ emission. (The β^+ is a positron or positive electron, while the β^- is the usual electron.) What is the resulting nuclide for each case? $(\gamma, \beta^-, \beta^+)$

A. Ni^{63}, Co^{64}, Fe^{63} C. Cu^{64}, Zn^{64}, Ni^{64}
B. Ni^{64}, Zn^{63}, Co^{64} D. Ni^{64}, Cu^{64}, Zn^{64}

94. The index of refraction of water is $n_w = 1.33$. The speed of light in a certain substance is 83% of its value in water. What is the index of refraction, n_u, of this substance?

A. 1.6   C. 1.1
B. 1.8   D. 2.1

95. Two light bulbs with ratings of 60 watts and 100 watts are operated on a 120-volt circuit. What are the respective resistances of the 60-watt and 100-watt bulbs?

A. 120 and 220 ohms
B. 240 and 144 ohms
C. 120 and 440 ohms
D. 144 and 440 ohms

Passage V (Questions 96–105)

A set of laboratory experiments designed to physically involve the students is planned for a high school physics course. They are to verify Newton's laws of motion and the conservation laws for linear and angular momentum. A pair of low carts on which the student sits are fitted with two complete skateboard wheel sets each. A laser beam and photogate can measure the velocities of such large objects using a commercial computer timing system. The forces required are measured with calibrated spring scales. The experiments are performed in the gymnasium to make use of its large smooth floor area. The instructor has devised a pulley and falling mass system to provide the constant forces to accelerate the cart student systems, but most of the time she has the student provide the accelerating forces by walking backward while keeping the force reading constant on a spring scale. The experience of providing a constant force while accelerating gives the pulling student a "feel" for the real meaning of acceleration.

96. A student practices until he can pull a classmate at constant speed to just overcome friction. This requires a force of 9 N when the mass of cart-student is 90 kg. The student then accelerates the cart-student by pulling with a constant force of 18 N. What is the measured acceleration?

A. 0.1 m/sec^2 C. 1.2 m/sec^2
B. 0.8 m/sec^2 D. 4.2 m/sec^2

97. Two students of different masses sit on carts close together. They push off from one another and their velocities are measured just after they separate. The 60 kg student-cart has a speed of 1.2 m/sec. The other student-cart has an opposite speed of 0.8 m/sec. What is the mass of the second student-cart?

A. 40 kg   C. 110 kg
B. 90 kg   D. 120 kg

98. A student-cart of mass 80 kg has an initial speed through a photogate of 2 m/sec. The frictional forces bring the cart to rest after it travels 8 m. What is the average total friction force that acted over the 8 m distance?

A. 10 N   C. 40 N
B. 20 N   D. 60 N

99. A student stands on a rotating frictionless stand with two large weights in his hands. While holding his arms in close to his sides, another student starts him spinning with a rotational angular velocity of 0.3 rev/sec. He then sticks his arms out straight at shoulder height and his angular velocity slows to 0.2 rev/sec. What is the ratio of his moment of inertia about his vertical spin axis when his arms are extended to his moment of inertia when his arms are at his sides?

A. 0.6   C. 1.5
B. 0.8   D. 2.5

100. A student-cart has a mass of 80 kg and an initial speed of 2 m/sec. Another student then drops a 20 kg bag of sand onto the lap of the student on the cart. What is the new velocity of the student-cart-bag?

A. 0.9 m/sec   **C.** 1.2 m/sec
B. 1.0 m/sec   **D.** 1.6 m/sec

101. Two students whose cart-student masses are 120 kg and 80 kg sit on the essentially frictionless carts. They hold the ends of a light rope and pull until the carts bump together. They meet at their common center-of-mass. If they start 2 m apart, how far from the starting point of the heavier 120 kg mass is the meeting point?

A. 0.4 m   **C.** 1.2 m
B. 0.8 m   **D.** 1.4 m

102. One student-cart of mass 80 kg has an initial speed of 4 m/sec and collides with another 80 kg student-cart which is at rest. The two carts lock together (due to a coupling mechanism) and move off together. What is their common velocity?

A. 0.5 m/sec   **C.** 2 m/sec
B. 1 m/sec   **D.** 2.5 m/sec

103. A student-cart of mass 100 kg is accelerated at 0.8 m/sec^2 by the falling mass system that supplies a horizontal force of 90 N to a cord attached to the front of the cart. What is the friction force opposing the motion?

A. 3 N   **C.** 60 N
B. 10 N   **D.** 90 N

104. The 90 N force that accelerates the cart at 0.8 m/sec^2 in the above problem is supplied by the tension in a cord passing over a frictionless pulley system to a weight that falls vertically. What is the mass of the falling weight?

A. 5 kg   **C.** 40 kg
B. 10 kg   **D.** 100 kg

105. In another trial, an 80 kg student-cart is to be accelerated from rest over a 10 m distance. The students calculate that the net force (including the tension in the cord and the opposing friction

force) accelerating the cart is 100 N. What is the speed of the 80 kg student-cart at the end of the 10 m distance?

A. 2 m/sec   **C.** 5 m/sec
B. 4.5 m/sec   **D.** 10 m/sec

Passage VI (Questions 106–110)

Water is a weakly ionized compound having a $K_a = 1.0 \times 10^{-14}$. In the absence of added H^+ or OH^- ions, the $[H^+] = [OH^-]$. (It is recognized, of course, that H^+ actually is present for the most part in hydrated form as H_3O^+.) The K_a of benzoic acid is 6.6×10^{-5}.

106. The pH of pure water is:

A. 3.0   **C.** 7.0
B. 5.0   **D.** 9.0

107. Addition of 0.0001 moles of benzoic acid to a beaker containing 1 liter of water will result in benzoic acid solution of pH:

A. between 3 and 4.
B. between 4 and 5.
C. between 5 and 6.
D. between 6 and 7.

108. The pOH in question 107 would be:

A. between 4 and 5.
B. between 5 and 6.
C. between 6 and 7.
D. greater than 7.

109. If 1×10^{-12} moles of benzoic acid are dissolved in one liter of water, the pH will be about:

A. 6.   **C.** 8.
B. 7.   **D.** 9.

110. If 5×10^{-13} moles of sodium hydroxide are dissolved in the above one liter aqueous solution of 1×10^{-12} moles of benzoic acid, the pH will be:

A. between 4 and 5.
B. between 5 and 6.
C. between 6 and 7.
D. between 7 and 8.

Passage VII (Questions 111–115)

A solution of $AgNO_3$ (1×10^{-6} molar) is prepared. To this is added K_2CrO_4 until precipitation of Ag_2CrO_4 begins. The K_{sp} of Ag_2CrO_4 is 9×10^{-12}.

111. The precipitate begins at a K_2CrO_4 concentration of about:

A. 1×10^{-6}. C. 1×10^{-1}.
B. 1×10^{-3}. D. 1×10^{1}.

112. Addition of NaCl will bring about:

A. additional precipitation of Ag_2CrO_4.
B. a reaction that will dissolve the Ag_2CrO_4 precipitate.
C. precipitation of AgCl only if its K_{sp} is exceeded.
D. A and C.

113. Increasing the temperature will usually:

A. bring about more complete precipitation.
B. change the K_{sp}.
C. change the formula of the precipitate.
D. not be easily accomplished until ongoing precipitation is complete.

114. If the K_{sp}'s of AgBr, AgCl, and AgI are respectively 7.7×10^{-13}, 1.56×10^{-10}, and 1.5×10^{-16}, the addition of the sodium salt of which of these halides would first bring about precipitation of an insoluble salt?

A. NaBr
B. NaCl
C. NaI
D. all about the same (within a factor of 10)

115. If the sodium salts of the 3 halides in question 114 were added to a concentration that is one-half of that needed to bring about precipitation of that particular silver salt, the result would be:

A. precipitation of only the least soluble silver halide.
B. percipitation of part of each of the three silver halides.
C. precipitation of a portion of the two least soluble silver halides.
D. no precipitation.

Passage VIII (Questions 116–120)

Many metals react with oxygen to form oxides. Some of these oxides, such as Na_2O, CaO, and SrO, react with water to form basic solutions. (These oxides are called basic oxides or basic anhydrides.)

Many nonmetals can react with oxygen to form oxides as well. These nonmetal oxides, however, react with water to form acidic solutions. Thus, they are called acid anhydrides.

116. Phosphorus would be expected to react with oxygen to form an oxide that will:

A. react with water to form an acidic solution.
B. react with water to form a basic solution.
C. react with water to form a neutral solution.
D. not react with water.

117. Nitrogen will react with oxygen to form an oxide (N_2O_5) that will:

A. react with water to form an acidic solution.
B. react with water to form a basic solution.
C. react with water to form a neutral solution.
D. not react with water.

118. One mole of Ca will react with oxygen to form an oxide that will react with water to form:

A. one mole of acid in solution.
B. one mole of base in solution.
C. two moles of acid in solution.
D. two moles of base in solution.

119. The solution in the question would require _____ for neutralization.

A. one mole of HCl
B. one mole of NaOH
C. two moles of HCl
D. two moles of NaOH

120. Burning of coal (without use of sufficient scrubbers) in the production of electricity is believed by many to be a major cause of "acid rain." If so, this is most likely because of the production of:

A. oxides of sulfur.
B. carbon dioxide.
C. carbon monoxide.
D. sodium oxide.

Passage IX (Questions 121–125)

Colligative properties of solutions are those properties that depend on the concentration of molecules or ions in solution rather than on their identities.

121. The freezing point of 1000g of water would be lowered most by the addition of one mole of:

   A. ethylene glycol.   C. Na_2SO_4.
   B. sodium chloride.   D. ethyl alcohol.

122. Calculations of freezing point depression resulting from solutes are based on:

   A. molarity.   C. mole fraction.
   B. molality.   D. A and B.

123. Colligative properties include:

   A. boiling point elevation.
   B. freezing point depression.
   C. osmotic pressure.
   D. more than one of the above.

124. It is noted that the addition of 46g of a solute to 1000g of water will lower the freezing point of water to $-2°C$. It could be predicted that the addition of 92g of the same solute to an identical 1000g of water in another container will:

   A. lower the freezing point to $-4°C$.
   B. lower the freezing point to $-8°C$.
   C. produce a freezing point of $0°C$.
   D. produce a freezing point of $+2°C$.

125. Several beakers are prepared, containing 1000g of the same solvent in each. Five grams of non-ionizing solutes are added, one solute to each beaker. The greatest effect on boiling point will be noticed with the solute with the:

   A. highest molecular weight.
   B. highest melting point.
   C. lowest molecular weight.
   D. lowest melting point.

Passage X (Questions 126–135)

In a neutral atom, the number of orbital electrons is equal to the number of protons in the nucleus (atomic number). Orbital electron configurations may be shown in shorthand form and may be used to predict reactivity and valence. Krypton, for example, may be shown as $1s^22s^22p^63s^23p^63d^{10}4s^24p^6$. Neon is $1s^22s^22p^6$.

126. A neutral atom of the element $1s^22s^22p^63s^1$ would be expected to:

   A. readily lose an electron to become an ion with a charge of +1.
   B. readily lose two electrons to become an ion with a charge of +2.
   C. readily gain three electrons to become an ion with a charge of -3.
   D. be an unreactive (noble) element.

127. The above element has an atomic number of:

   A. 8.   C. 18.
   B. 11.   D. 19.

128. A neutral atom of the element $1s^22s^22p^63s^23p^63d^{10}4s^24p^5$ would be expected to react by:

   A. losing one electron.
   B. losing two electrons.
   C. gaining one electron.
   D. gaining three electrons.

129. An atom of atomic number 9, having an electron configuration of $1s^22s^22p^6$, would be:

   A. a neutral atom.
   B. an ion with a charge of +1.
   C. a noble element.
   D. an ion with a charge of -1.

130. An atom of atomic number 11, having an electronic configuration of $1s^22s^22p^63p^1$, would be:

   A. a neutral atom at ground state.
   B. an ion with a charge of +1.
   C. a neutral atom at an excited state.
   D. an ion with a charge of -1.

131. Noble elements include all of the following EXCEPT:

   A. helium.   C. neon.
   B. argon.   D. scandium.

132. The number of quantum numbers possessed by each orbital electron is:

   A. one.   C. three.
   B. two.   D. four.

133. The possible number of values of magnetic quantum number is:

A. one. C. three
B. two. D. four.

134. The possible number of values of spin quantum numbers is:

A. one. C. three
B. two. D. four.

135. In a particular atom, the number of electrons that possess all four quantum numbers identical to those of another electron is:

A. zero. C. two.
B. one. D. three.

Questions 136–142 are independent of any passage and of each other.

136. If one wished to remove substantially all of the chloride ions from an aqueous solution, this could be done by the addition of an aqueous solution of:

A. KNO_3. C. $AgNO_3$.
B. Na_2SO_4. D. starch.

137. If it is known that H_2S is a weak acid that ionizes to form $2H^+$ and S^{2-}, lowering the pH of a solution of H_2S by adding HCl should:

A. raise the S^{2-} concentration.
B. lower the S^{2-} concentration.
C. have no effect on S^{2-} concentration.
D. not be possible.

138. Which of the following aqueous solutions will have the lowest freezing point?

A. 1 M NaCl. C. 1.5 M glucose.
B. 0.3 M Na_2SO_4. D. H_2O.

139. Consider this reaction: $Fe^{2+} \rightleftarrows Fe^{3+} + e^-$. Which of the following is correct?

A. The reaction toward the right is an oxidation.
B. The reaction toward the right is a reduction.
C. The reaction toward the left is a reduction.
D. A and C are correct.

140. The hydronium ion is:

A. a protonated water molecule.
B. formed by removal of H^- from a water molecule.
C. an ion with the formula of H_2O^+.
D. an uranium byproduct.

141. How many milliliters of 0.5N NaOH are required to neutralize 50 ml of 0.25N HCl?

A. 25 C. 0.25
B. 50 D. 2.5

142. A zwitterion is a molecule containing:

A. both cationic and anionic functions.
B. more than one cationic or anionic function.
C. polar and nonpolar groups.
D. a Z^+ charge.

WRITING SAMPLE

2 ESSAYS—TOPICS
60 MINUTES (30 MINUTES/TOPIC)

DIRECTIONS: Your response must be a unified, organized essay; it should contain fully developed, logically constructed paragraphs. Remember quality is more important than length. Before you begin writing, make sure you have read the item carefully and understand what is being asked. Write as legibly as possible. Because your essays will be scored as first-draft compositions, you may cross out and make corrections on your response booklet as necessary. It is not necessary to recopy your essay.

Part 1

Consider this statement:

Probably all laws are useless; for good men do not want laws at all, and bad men are made no better by them.

Demonax

Write a unified essay in which you perform these tasks. Explain the meaning of the above quote. Give specific examples of a time when good people would want laws and when bad ones would be made better by them. Discuss the purpose of a set of imposed laws, what makes them useful or useless in serving this purpose.

Part 2

Consider this statement:

And thus your freedom when it loses its fetters becomes itself the fetter of a greater freedom.

Kahlil Gibran

Write a unified essay in which you complete the following tasks. Explain what you think the above statement means. Describe a specific situation in which freedom that has lost its fetter does not become the fetter of a greater freedom. Discuss the manner in which one type of freedom might put a restraint or a confinement on another type of freedom.

BIOLOGICAL SCIENCES

10 PROBLEM SETS OF 5–10 QUESTIONS EACH
15 PROBLEMS FOLLOWED BY A SINGLE QUESTION
77 QUESTIONS
100 MINUTES

DIRECTIONS: The following questions or incomplete statements are in groups. Preceding each series of questions or statements is a paragraph or a short explanatory statement, a formula or set of formulas, or a definition. Read the written material and then answer the questions or complete the statements. Select the ONE BEST ANSWER for each question and indicate your selection by marking the corresponding letter of your choice on the Answer Form. Eliminate those alternatives you know to be incorrect and then select an answer from among the remaining alternatives.

Passage I (Questions 143–151)

The pituitary gland is responsible for the secretion of thyroid stimulating hormone (TSH), which elicits an increased production of thyroid hormone from the gland; this thyroid hormone then may inhibit the pituitary via a negative feedback. Under hyperthyroid conditions, the following tests would give elevated values:
1. Basal metabolic rate (BMR)
2. Protein bound iodine (PBI)
3. Radioactive iodine uptake (RAI)

143. When TSH secretion falls, the secretion by the thyroid of thyroid hormone:

    A. stays the same.
    B. increases.

    C. decreases.
    D. will feed back upon the pituitary.

144. According to the schema given, if a normal individual is given an injection of TSH, his/her thyroid hormone production will first

    A. show no noticeable change.
    B. increase.
    C. decrease.
    D. lead to a decrease in pituitary TSH output.

Use the information in the flow chart and paragraph above, and in the following charts, to answer questions 145–147.

145. In which of the graphs is there evidence of thyroid malfunction?

    A. I   **C.** I and III
    B. I and II   **D.** III

146. Which graph(s) probably represent(s) the case of a typical hyperthyroid person?

    A. II   **C.** I and III
    B. I   **D.** II and III

147. Which of the graphs lead(s) you to believe that there is a breakdown in the normal thyroid-pituitary functional relationship?

A. I and III   **C.** II
B. III   **D.** II and III

148. A lack of iodine in the diet usually is associated with which disorder?

A. acromegaly   **C.** rickets
B. goiter   **D.** skin rash

149. Thyroid stimulating hormone (TSH) is produced by which of the following?

A. acidophils (alpha cells)
B. basophils (beta cells)
C. delta cells
D. chromophobes

150. Which of the following statements concerning the thyroid are correct?

A. The gland is derived from the pharynx (foramen cecum of the tongue).
B. Colloid is located extracellularly.
C. T_3-triiodothyronine and T_4 thyroxine are the active principles.
D. All of the above.

151. Hypersecretion of which hormone will result in acromegaly (giantism)?

A. TSH—thyroid stimulating hormone
B. STH—somatotropin (growth hormone)
C. ACTH—adrenocorticotrophic hormone
D. thyroxin

Passage II (Questions 152–156)

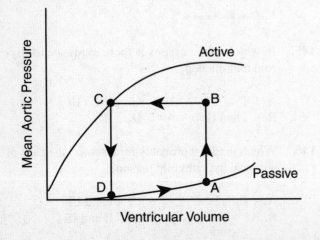

As the left ventricle of the heart contracts, it generates a pressure, which when more than that in the aorta causes the ejection of a volume of blood. The action of the ventricle can be represented as the relationship between the volume of blood in the ventricle and the intraventricular pressure. The relationship between ventricular pressure and volume is known as the Frank-Starling law of the heart and is shown at left.

The lower curve represents the pressure volume relationship when the heart is being passively filled with blood during diastole (i.e., at rest). The upper curve represents the pressure-volume relationship as a result of contraction (i.e., systole). The volume at Point A is known as the end diastolic volume, which is the volume of blood in the ventricle immediately preceding contraction. During systole, the ventricle contracts, but no blood is ejected until the pressure in the ventricle exceeds the pressure in the aorta. This phase of the cardiac cycle is known as isovolumetric contraction and is represented by line segment AB. When the aortic valve opens (Point C), blood is ejected without further increase in the ventricular pressure (line segment BC). Therefore, this phase of contraction is isotonic and results in the ejection of a volume of blood known as the stroke volume.

When the pressure that the ventricle can generate exactly equals the aortic pressure, the ejection of blood ceases, and the ventricle undergoes isovolumetric relaxation as represented by the line segment CD. The blood from the atrium then fills the ventricle, and the pressure increase is the result of passive resistance of the ventricle (curve DA).

152. Assuming a constant mean aortic pressure, patients with renal failure may have an increased blood volume which results in an increased end diastolic volume in the ventricle. What effect does this increase have on cardiac function?

    I. ventricular work remains constant
    II. stroke volume increases
    III. end systolic volume increases
    IV. ventricular work increases

A. I, II, and III only   **C.** II and IV only
B. I and III only   **D.** IV only

153. Patients with hypertension have a higher mean aortic pressure. If end diastolic volume stays contant:

    I. stroke volume increases.
    II. ventricular work increases.
    III. end systolic volume decreases.
    IV. ventricular work may or may not increase.

A. I, II, and III only   **C.** II and IV only
B. I and III only   **D.** IV only

154. Patients with heart failure have an active pressure curve (i.e., upper curve) which is shifted downward and to the right as compared with that of normal. Assuming the end diastolic volume and the mean aortic pressure remain constant and the ventricle is capable of ejecting blood:

    I. stroke volume decreases.
    II. end systolic volume increases.
    III. ventricular work decreases.
    IV. end systolic volume decreases.

    A. I, II, and III only   **C.** II and IV only
    B. I and III only   **D.** IV only

155. With time, the blood volume of patients with heart failure tends to increase resulting in an increased end diastolic volume with a continued downward shift in the active pressure curve (i.e., upper curve). The increase in the end diastolic volume, as compared with the case of a failing ventricle without compensation referred to in the preceding question, will result in:

    I. a stroke volume which may or may not increase.
    II. an increase in cardiac work.
    III. a decrease in end systolic volume.
    IV. an increase in stroke volume.

    A. I, II, and III only   **C.** II and IV only
    B. I and III only   **D.** IV only

156. With a constant mean aortic pressure and as compared to normal, a compensated failure will show:

    I. an increase in stroke volume.
    II. a stroke volume which may or may not decrease.
    III. a decrease in cardiac work.
    IV. an increase in end systolic volume.

    A. I, II, and III only   **C.** II and IV only
    B. I and III only   **D.** IV only

Passage III (Questions 157–163)

In a laboratory experiment, red blood cells were placed into 0.5 M solutions and the appearance of the solutions was observed two hours later with the naked eye.

Solution	Cells
0.5 M glucose	no change
0.5 M sucrose	no change
0.5 M urea	hemolysis of RBCs
0.5 M glycerol	hemolysis of RBCs

157. How can the solutions of urea and glycerol be described with respect to the red blood cells?

    A. isotonic   **C.** hypertonic
    B. hypotonic   **D.** none of the above.

158. The reason for these results is that:

    I. the number of particles in the urea and glycerol solutions is greater than that in the glucose and sucrose solutions.
    II. glucose and sucrose form coatings around the red blood cells, which prevent their breaking.
    III. glucose and sucrose enter the cells but are immediately metabolized, therefore water does not enter the cells.
    IV. urea and glycerol can enter the cell, water follows them into the cell because it is then in greater concentration outside.

    A. I and II only   **C.** III and IV only
    B. I and III only   **D.** IV only

159. The property of the cell membrane that allows for this phenomenon to be demonstrated is called:

    A. diffusion.   **C.** impermeability.
    B. osmosis.   **D.** semipermeability.

160. The process by which a cell can move a substance from a point of lower concentration to a point of higher concentration (against the diffusion gradient) is called:

    A. osmosis.   **C.** turgor pressure.
    B. plasmolysis.   **D.** active transport.

161. Which of the following structures are NOT considered modifications of the cell membrane?

    A. basement membrane
    B. terminal bars
    C. desmosomes
    D. intercalated discs

162. The plasma membrane of animal cells:

    A. is usually rigid.

    B. has selective channels made of proteins.

    C. it too thin to be seen by the use of any microscope.

    D. is composed only of proteins and carbohydrates.

163. Dialysis (as is used for the treatment of chronic kidney ailments) differs from the process of osmosis in the respect that:

    A. both solvent and solute pass through the membrane.

    B. solute selectively passes through the membrane only.

    C. solvent selectively passes through the membrane only.

    D. gases are the only substances that pass the membrane and blood is cleansed.

Passage IV (Questions 164–168)

The diagram below represents three generations of a human family, some of whose members have a non-lethal birth defect. The defect is caused by a single gene for which new mutations are very rare. The individuals with birth defects are represented by solid black symbols, whereas the individuals who have a normal phenotype are represented by open symbols. Males are represented by squares and females are represented by circles.

164. The defect is most likely caused by:

    A. an autosomal gene for which the defective allele is recessive to the normal allele.

    B. an X-linked gene for which the defective allele is recessive to the normal allele.

    C. an autosomal gene for which the defective allele is dominant to the normal allele.

    D. an X-linked gene for which the defective allele is dominant to the normal allele.

165. The genotype of individual number 1 in the family:

    A. is most likely to contain only normal alleles.

    B. is most likely to contain only defective alleles.

    C. is most likely to contain both normal and defective alleles.

    D. cannot be determined from the pedigree.

166. The genotype of individual number 4 in the family:

    A. is most likely to contain only normal alleles.

    B. is most likely to contain only defective alleles.

    C. is most likely to contain both normal and defective alleles.

    D. cannot be determined from the pedigree.

167. The genotype of individual number 7 in the family:

    A. is most likely to contain only normal alleles.

    B. is most likely to contain only defective alleles.

    C. is most likely to contain both normal and defective alleles.

    D. cannot be determined from the pedigree.

168. The genotype of individual number 8 in the family:

    A. is most likely to contain only normal alleles.

    B. is most likely to contain only defective alleles.

    C. is most likely to contain both normal and defective alleles.

    D. cannot be determined from the pedigree.

Passage V (Questions 169–178)

Blood is the fluid that circulates around in blood vessels to provide for gas exchange, waste removal, and nutrient procurement by the cells of the body. Blood is composed of various types of cells and cell fragments (referred to as formed elements) and a fluid called plasma. The formed elements include erythrocytes or RBCs (red blood corpuscles), various types of leucocytes or WBCs (white blood cells), and thrombocytes or platelets.

In a clinical setting a number of tests are conducted on blood. One of these is to determine the packed cells volume or *hematocrit* (which is defined as the volume of formed elements relative to the total volume of blood). In order to determine an individual's hematocrit, 10 milliliters of blood are collected and placed in a heparinized centrifuge tube. Heparin is used to prevent clotting. The tube is spun for 15–20 minutes at 2500 rpm to sediment all the formed elements. The tube is then examined to determine the volume (in milliliters) of the packed formed elements. On the average, blood consists of approximately 45% formed elements and approximately 55% plasma; in other words, each 10 ml of blood will contain 4.5 ml of formed elements. The average "normal" packed cell volume or hematocrit is therefore 45% (i.e., 4.5 ml is 45% of 10 ml). Most of the sedimented formed elements are RBCs. A small region of WBCs and platelets will be located at the top of the region of formed elements; this layer is often referred to as the "buffy" coat.

A patient was seen by a physician who ordered a hematocrit as part of the patient's lab workup. Ten millimeters of blood were collected and treated as previously described. The diagram below shows the hematocrit tube at the end of centrifugation.

169. Region A consists of:

    A. fibrin clot material.
    B. plasma.
    C. serum.
    D. WBCs.

170. Region B consists predominantly of:

    A. fibrin clot material.
    B. plasma.
    C. RBCs.
    D. WBCs.

171. The lower 5.5 ml consists predominantly of:

    A. fibrin clot material.
    B. platelets.
    C. RBCs.
    D. WBCs.

172. The hematocrit of this patient is:

    A. 45%.   **C.** 4.5 ml.
    B. 55%.   **D.** 5.5 ml.

173. The hematocrit of this patient is:

    A. normal.
    B. above normal.
    C. lower than normal.
    D. cannot be determined from the information given.

174. The components of the blood responsible for binding and carrying oxygen would be located in:

    A. region A.   **C.** region C.
    B. region B.   **D.** regions A and C.

175. The cellular components of the blood responsible for fighting infections would be located in:

    A. region A.   **C.** region C.
    B. region B.   **D.** regions B and C.

176. The components of the blood responsible for initiating blood clotting would be located in:

    A. region A.   **C.** region C.
    B. region B.   **D.** regions B and C.

177. The major component found in region A would be:

    A. water.   **C.** sodium chloride.
    B. hemoglobin.   **D.** glucose.

178. The hematocrit of the patient, as compared to the normal value, suggests that the patient:

    A. lives at a high altitude.
    B. has sickle cell anemia.
    C. has pernicious anemia.
    D. has recently undergone excessive X ray treatment.

Passage VI (Questions 179–183)

A muscle fiber is a single muscle cell. Each fiber is composed of numerous cylindrical fibrils running the entire length of the fiber. The fibril exhibits light and dark bands—I and A bands respectively. The I band is bisected by the M line. There is a somewhat lighter band within the A band that is called the H band. These striations are produced by the arrangement within the fibril of myofilaments; myosin is the thick myofilament, whereas actin is considered the thin myofilament.

179. A sarcomere is the area between:

A. two A bands.   C. two I bands.
B. two H bands.   D. two Z bands.

180. During contraction the lengths of the thick and thin myofilaments:

A. increase.
B. decrease.
C. remain the same.
D. first increase, then decrease.

181. If we could imagine observing a muscle contraction under a light microscope, we would see the narrowing of the:

A. H and I bands.   C. Z bands.
B. A bands.   D. H bands only.

182. If the muscle were deprived of ATP, which of the following would NOT be affected?

A. the sodium pump of the muscle membrane
B. the calcium pump of the sarcoplasmic reticulum
C. the length of the myosin filaments
D. the velocity of shortening

183. What is the internal activator substance that is released during excitation—contraction coupling?

A. ATP   C. Ca^{2+}
B. Mg^{2+} D. H^+

Passage VII (Questions 184–189)

During the inflammatory reaction, immune and paraimmune system cells circulating in microvessels adhere to the endothelium of these vessels in areas of tissue injury. The adherent cells then migrate across the endothelium into the injured tissue. The adherence of the cells to the endothelium is stimulated by cytokines such as tumor necrosis factor, TNF. The immune and paraimmune system cells may adhere to endothelial cells through binding of CD-18 molecules on the surfaces of the immune and paraimmune system cells to GMP-140 glycoproteins on the surfaces of endothelial cells. A series of experiments to evaluate these hypotheses is shown in figures 1–3. Figure 1 reports the binding of neutrophils, monocytes, and lympho-

cytes to plastic dishes coated with varying amounts of GMP-140. Figure 2 shows neutrophil adhesion to plastic dishes under varying conditions. Figure 3 shows neutrophil adhesion to cultured layers of vascular endothelial cells in the presence of varying concentrations of GMP-140 in the test solution.

Figure 1

Adherence of neutrophils (▲), monocytes (●), and lymphocytes (■) to plastic dishes that had been coated with varying amounts of GMP-140.

Figure 2

Effects of pretreatment of plastic dishes or neutrophils on the attachment of neutrophils to plastic dishes.
1—neither cells nor dish were pretreated
2—dish coated with GMP-140; no treatment of cells
3—dish coated with GMP-140 then treated with rabbit antibodies which bind to GMP-140
4—dish coated with GMP-140 then treated with rabbit antibodies which do not bind to GMP-140
5—dish coated with GMP-140; cells treated with antibodies which bind to CD-18
6—dish coated with GMP-140; cells treated with antibodies which do not bind to CD-18

Figure 3

Effect of GMP-140 pretreatment on the binding of neutrophils to cultured endothelial cells.

Prior to the assay, aliquots of either neutrophils or endothelial cells were incubated with GMP-140 and subsequently washed by centrifugation. For the assay, pretreated neutrophils were mixed with untreated endothelial cells (●) or untreated neutrophils were mixed with treated endothelial cells (■).

184. As the concentration of GMP-140 used to coat plastic dishes was increased:

- A. the number of neutrophils attaching to the plastic tended to increase.
- B. the number of neutrophils attaching to the plastic tended to decrease.
- C. the tightness of binding of neutrophils to the plastic tended to increase.
- D. the tightness of binding of neutrophils to the plastic tended to decrease.

185. Plastic dishes that were not coated with GMP-140:

- A. did not bind monocytes.
- B. allowed attachment of about $1/4$ of the monocytes.
- C. allowed attachment of about $1/2$ of the monocytes.
- D. allowed attachment of most of the monocytes.

186. Coating of plastic dishes with GMP-140:

- A. caused the largest increase in binding of neutrophils.
- B. caused the largest increase in the binding of lymphocytes.

- C. caused the largest increase in the binding of monocytes.
- D. caused approximately equal increases in binding of all cells.

187. The data presented:

- A. strongly support the hypothesis that neutrophils bind to GMP-140 on the surface of endothelial cells.
- B. strongly support the hypothesis that neutrophils use GMP-140 on the neutrophil surface to attach to endothelial cells.
- C. strongly refute the hypothesis that neutrophils bind to GMP-140 on the surface of endothelial cells.
- D. strongly refute the hypothesis that neutrophils use GMP-140 on the neutrophil surface to attach to endothelial cells.

188. The data presented:

- A. strongly support the hypothesis that neutrophils bind to CD-18 on the surface of endothelial cells.
- B. strongly support the hypothesis that neutrophils use CD-18 on the neutrophil surface to attach to endothelial cells.
- C. strongly refute the hypothesis that neutrophils bind to CD-18 on the surface of endothelial cells.
- D. strongly refute the hypothesis that neutrophils use CD-18 on the neutrophil surface to attach to endothelial cells.

189. Based on the data and information presented, a human patient who had a genetic defect that prevented synthesis of GMP-140 would probably be most severely impaired in:

- A. phagocytosis of bacteria.
- B. killing of virus-infected cells by natural killer cells.
- C. cell-mediated immune responses to most targets.
- D. humoral immune responses to most targets.

Passage VIII (Questions 190–194)

Enzymes have often been referred to as biological catalysts. They have many properties in common with other catalysts.

190. Enzymes are generally:

- A. carbohydrates.
- B. proteins.
- C. lipids.
- D. nucleic acids.

191. Enzymes function in reactions by:

    A. increasing the net energy yield.
    B. raising the energy level of the products.
    C. decreasing the energy of activation.
    D. changing the thermodynamic nature of a reaction, thus making a reaction thermodynamically favorable when it would not otherwise be so.

192. The nature of enzymes requires that the enzyme is:

    A. used up in quantities greater than those of substrate that is converted to product.
    B. used up in quantities approximately equal to those of substrate that is converted to product.
    C. used up in quantities significantly less than those of the substrate that is converted to product.
    D. essentially not used up and must be replaced only in small quantities.

193. Activity of enzymes is often regulated by covalent modification. This is most often accomplished by:

    A. phosphorylation/dephosphorylation.
    B. sulfation/desulfation.
    C. substitution of one cation for another.
    D. substitution of one anion for another.

194. The response of most enzymes to being boiled in an aqueous solution is:

    A. substantially increased activity.
    B. substantially decreased activity.
    C. an increase of about 1 unit in isoelectric point.
    D. no noticeable change is detected.

Passage IX (Questions 195–199)

All of the possible ketopentose sugar isomers have been synthesized in a research project. The ketopentose isomers have been reduced with sodium borohydride, converting the ketone function to an alcohol.

195. The total number of 2-ketopentose isomers is:

    A. two.   C. six.
    B. four.   D. eight.

196. The total number of isomers of the sugar alcohols produced by sodium borohydride reaction is:

    A. two.   C. four.
    B. three.   D. five.

197. If all the sugar alcohols in the previous question were selectively oxidized so that the number 3 hydroxyl was converted to a ketone, there would be _____ chiral center(s) in each molecule.

    A. one   C. three
    B. two   D. four

198. The pentose(s) found in RNA usually consists of:

    A. deoxyribose.   C. various pentoses.
    B. ribose.   D. glucose.

199. If the sugar alcohols in question 196 were oxidized to convert carbon numbers 1 and 5 to carboxyls, the number of chiral centers would be:

    A. none.   C. two.
    B. one.   D. three.

Passage X (Questions 200–204)

The synthesis of proteins and nucleic acids is seen as being directed by a series of coded messages. The messages must be sent, received, and decoded.

200. The primary source or repository of information concerning synthesis of nucleic acids and proteins is considered to be:

    A. protein.   C. RNA.
    B. DNA.   D. peptides.

201. In the polymer that directs protein biosynthesis, there is a requirement of _____ unit(s) (or monomers) to code for each amino acid.

    A. one   C. three
    B. two   D. four

202. In a chromosome of higher animals there is (are) _____ strand(s) of DNA.

    A. one   C. three
    B. two   D. four

203. If 100 somatic cells of higher animals are allowed to divide once in ^2H_2O (water containing only deuterium), _____ of the cells will have only DNA containing deuterium.

A. none   **C.** one half
B. one fourth   **D.** all

204. Ultimately, sythesis of protein requires:

A. DNA.   **C.** protein.
B. RNA.   **D.** all of the above.

DIRECTIONS: Read each passage carefully, study each table, chart, or formula, then answer the question following it. Eliminate those choices that you think to be incorrect and mark the letter of your choice on the answer sheet.

Maloney sarcoma tumors were implanted in Brown Norway (BN), Lewis (Le), and Lewis-Brown Norway (LBN) rats. Studies were then done to determine the types and amounts of host serum antibodies produced against the protein components of the virus contained in the tumor cells. The following data are from one such experiment.

**ANTIPROTEIN 30 ACTIVITY IN SERA
OF TUMOR BEARING BN, Le, and LBN RATS**

Host	AgB Phenotype	Mg Equivalent Anti-p30 Antibody	
		Day 25 Post Implant	Day 31 Post Implant
BN	3/3	3.5 ± 0.8	5.3 ± 1.7
LBN	1/3	2.4 ± 0.4	4.5 ± 1.4
Le	1/1	0.4 ± 0.1	0.4 ± 0.2

205. The following statements are related to the information presented. Select the statement *supported by* the information given.

A. Brown Norway rats produced more anti-p30 antibody at both 25 and 31 days than the other two hosts.
B. On the basis of this information, Brown Norway rats are more resistant to cancer than either LBN or Le rats.
C. All three hosts produced more anti-p30 antibody at 31 days than they did at 25 days.
D. An AgB phenotype containing threes seems to be related to lower anti-p30 production

The graphs represent experimental results obtained when the pituitary gland was removed (A), the ovaries were removed (B), and lesions were placed in the hypo-

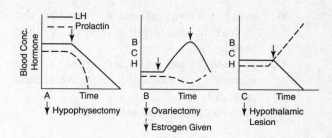

thalamus (C), that part of the brain most closely related to the pituitary gland. The hormones LH and prolactin were measured in blood by radioimmunoassay.

206. It can be concluded from these results that:

A. prolactin is produced by the ovaries.
B. LH release stimulates prolactin release.
C. ovarian hormones inhibit LH release, but not prolactin release.
D. presence of the ovaries inhibits removal of LH from the blood.

The urophysis of teleosts secretes a neurohormone directly into the blood circulatory system. This secretory apparatus is believed functional in osmoregulation in fishes from marine and freshwater habitats. Fifteen blueback herring (*Pseudoharengus aestivalis*) were maintained in a marine aquarium at temperatures of 40°–45°C. The fish were subjected to increasing salt concentration to a final concentration equal to twice that of seawater. At each concentration four of twelve urophyses were dissected and extracted, and electrophoresis on polyacrylamide gels were performed. Two specific bands of protein were identified as being specific to the urophysis. The amount of protein was determined by microdensitometry. The results are shown in the graph.

207. The experiment indicates that:

A. the protein material was unaltered in the urophysis of fish subjected to varying concentrations of seawater.

B. protein 1 was affected more by the increasing concentration of seawater than protein 2.

C. protein 2 was affected more by the increasing concentration of seawater than protein 1.

D. the data could not be analyzed.

An investigator had been studying the interrelationship (cooperation) of various cell types in tissue culture in the immune response to an antigen. The experiments conducted attempted to determine if spleen and mast cells were required for the production of antibody against a pollen. Various donor cells (spleen and mast cells) were injected into recipient rabbits whose immune system had been rendered nonresponsive by whole body X-irradiation. Antibody levels were determined in the serum of the recipients.

Experimental Groups	Antibody Level
A. Spleen and pollen	0
B. Spleen	0
C. Mast cells and pollen	0
D. Mast cells	0
E. Spleen and mast cells and pollen	++
F. Bone marrow and pollen	++
G. Thymocytes and pollen	++

208. The following statements are related to the information presented above. Select the statement *not supported by* the information given.

A. In the system under investigation, spleen and mast cells together are required for antibody production.

B. Spleen cells are probably found in the thymus.

C. Spleen cells or mast cells are essential to the antibody production against pollen.

D. In the intact animal, the mast cells would probably be important as a source of antibody.

Four groups of rats were maintained under identical conditions. Three of the groups received drugs in their drinking water over a period of five weeks. The day before autopsy each rat received one microcurie of ^{131}I. At autopsy the thyroid glands from each group were pooled and weighed. Iodinated intermediates were isolated and their radioactivity determined. Remember iodide is trapped, oxidized, proteinated, and stored as part of the thyroid hormone.

^{131}I CONTENT
(counts/min./100 mg Thyroid Tissue)

Groups	Drug	Iodine Ion	Monoiodo-tryosine	Trilodo-thyronine	Thyroxine	Av. Throid Wt. mg/100 g body wt.
1	None	6,120	10,140	7,520	35,990	14
2	A	55	46	13	62	76
3	B	40,976	10	9	14	88
4	C	1,592	2,025	1,970	8,985	4

209. Which group was treated with thryoxine, an inhibitor of the production of thyroid stimulating hormone by the pituitary gland?

A. Group 2   **C.** Group 4

B. Group 3   **D.** none of the above

After growing turkey red wheat for two years on a dry land farm, John Calendar had accumulated enough capital to move his family to a more fertile area. The first crops he planted on the new 1,000-acre farm did well. The following bar graphs indicate his production of wheat and corn over the last five years. Bushels are plotted on the abscissa, and the numbers of acres planted in both crops are shown in parentheses.

210. What was the average yearly proportion of wheat production to corn production?

A. 3/2   **C.** 10/9

B. 7/8   **D.** 5/7

Three greenhouses were constructed to examine different light cycles and their effects on the growth of several plants.

211. Plant X requires 15 hours of light per day for at least three weeks to exhibit a red coloration in its leaves. It may exhibit this highly desired feature in:

    A. greenhouse 1.
    B. greenhouse 1 and 2.
    C. greenhouse 2 and 3.
    D. all of the above.

One hundred ml of blood was drawn from a healthy male donor. Following centrifugation (4°C) and removal of the "buffy coat" by aspiration, hemoglobin was extracted from the pelleted red blood cells. The extracted hemoglobin was then divided into equal aliquots and these were treated as follows:

Aliquot 1: Analyzed on the day of extraction by polyacrylamide gel electrophoresis, followed by densitometer scanning of the stained gel

Aliquot 2: Stored for 30 days at room temperature

Aliquot 3: Stored for 30 days at 4°C

Aliquot 4: Stored for 30 days as a 50% solution (V/V) in glycerol at −20°C

At the end of the 30-day storage period, each of the aliquots was analyzed in the same way as aliquot 1. The following densitometer tracings were obtained:

Freshly Extracted Hemoglobin   Room Temperature 30 Days   4°C 30 Days   Glycerol −20°C 30 Days

212. From these data it is clear that:

    A. none of the storage conditions were able to maintain hemoglobin in an absolutely unchanged state.
    B. hemoglobin peptides are strongly affected by heating.
    C. hemoglobin contains peroxidase activity.
    D. hemoglobin coupled with oxygen has a longer self life than hemoglobin coupled with CO_2.

Blood samples from 10 female rats were withdrawn at 5 PM on the day of proestrus, when LH levels in the blood should be high if ovulation were to occur that night. The blood was assayed by double-antibody radioimmunoassay for LH. An antibody specific for LH is allowed to bind with the LH in the sample, then is partially displaced by radiolabeled LH whose binding to the limited amount of anti-LH is inversely proportional to the amount of unlabeled LH present (see standard curve). The antigen-antibody complex is precipitated with an antibody to the anti-LH, and the number of counts per minute bound in the precipitate is determined after the supernatant containing the unbound labeled LH has been poured off. The blood samples from 5 untreated rats (which ovulated) had cpm of 4000, 3000, 5000, 4000, and 3000, whereas those from 5 drug-treated animals had 5000, 13,000, 15,000, 3000, and 13,000.

213. It can be concluded from this study that:

    A. the untreated rats had very little LH in their blood compared to the treated group.
    B. the drug does not block ovulation.
    C. the dose of the drug used in this study inhibits LH release in most of the animals.
    D. ovulation occurred in three out of five of the treated rats.

Selective protein transport from the maternal circulation to the rat fetus is thought to occur via the visceral yolk sac. The maternal proteins are transferred to the yolk sac cavity and then must pass through the visceral endoderm, the visceral basement membrane (VBM), and the vitelline capillary endothelium to reach the fetal blood. Proteins X, Y, and Z were injected into a pregnant rat on day 12 of gestation and then were localized in the layers of the visceral yolk sac at 2 minutes, 6 hours, and 12 hours following injection. The results below demonstrate where each protein was localized at the three postinjection intervals.

Protein	Visceral Endoderm	VBM	Vitelline Endothelium	Fetal Blood
X	2 min.	6 hrs.	12 hrs.	—
Y	2 min., 6 hrs., & 12 hrs.	—	—	—
Z	2 min.	6 hrs.	12 hrs.	12 hrs.

214. Based on the information given, select the statement *not supported by* the information given above.

   A. All three proteins were absorbed at the same rate by the visceral endoderm.
   B. The transport of protein X is blocked by the visceral basement membrane.
   C. The visceral endoderm appears to block the transport of protein Y.
   D. Protein X appears to be transported through the visceral endoderm.

The following graph represents an experiment designed to measure the rate of collagen synthesis in developing chondrocytes. Chondrocytes were isolated from developing sterna of chick embryos and incubated in culture media containing proline–^{3}H, a precursor of collagen. Specimens were fixed after various time intervals and prepared for autoradiography. The graph represents number of silver grains counted (µm/square of organelle).

215. The following statements are related to the information presented. Select the statement *supported by* the information given.

   A. The radioactive label found in the rough endoplasmic reticulum is transferred directly into the extracellular collagen without passing through the Golgi complex.
   B. Radioactive isotope is incorporated into the extracellular collagen within 2 hours.
   C. Collagen is a highly stable molecule and is not degraded.
   D. The amount of rough endoplasmic reticulum in the cell increases during collagen synthesis.

216. Amino acids found in higher animals are usually:

   A. optically inactive.
   B. of the L-series.
   C. of the D-series.
   D. a racemic mixture.

217. Carbohydrates found in higher animals (such as glucose, fructose, and galactose) are usually:

   A. optically inactive.
   B. of the L-series.
   C. of the D-series.
   D. a racemic mixture.

218. D-glucose and L-galactose, both aldohexoses, could be said to be:

   A. epimers.   C. enantiomers.
   B. diastereomers. D. A and B.

219. Foods with the highest number of kcal/g are the:

   A. carbohydrates. C. fats.
   B. proteins.   D. nucleic acids.

Model Examination C Answer Key

Verbal Reasoning

1.	C	14.	C	27.	D	40.	D	53.	A
2.	B	15.	B	28.	B	41.	C	54.	D
3.	A	16.	D	29.	C	42.	D	55.	A
4.	D	17.	C	30.	B	43.	A	56.	D
5.	A	18.	A	31.	C	44.	D	57.	A
6.	B	19.	B	32.	D	45.	D	58.	D
7.	B	20.	C	33.	C	46.	C	59.	D
8.	D	21.	B	34.	D	47.	D	60.	C
9.	B	22.	A	35.	D	48.	C	61.	C
10.	D	23.	B	36.	C	49.	B	62.	D
11.	C	24.	A	37.	D	50.	C	63.	A
12.	B	25.	C	38.	D	51.	D	64.	A
13.	C	26.	B	39.	D	52.	D	65.	C

Physical Sciences

66.	C	82.	C	98.	B	113.	B	128.	C
67.	D	83.	D	99.	C	114.	C	129.	D
68.	D	84.	B	100.	D	115.	D	130.	C
69.	A	85.	A	101.	B	116.	A	131.	D
70.	D	86.	C	102.	C	117.	A	132.	D
71.	D	87.	B	103.	B	118.	B	133.	C
72.	B	88.	D	104.	B	119.	C	134.	B
73.	B	89.	A	105.	C	120.	A	135.	A
74.	C	90.	B	106.	C	121.	C	136.	C
75.	B	91.	A	107.	B	122.	B	137.	B
76.	D	92.	B	108.	D	123.	D	138.	A
77.	B	93.	C	109.	B	124.	A	139.	D
78.	B	94.	A	110.	A	125.	C	140.	A
79.	C	95.	B	111.	D	126.	A	141.	A
80.	C	96.	A	112.	C	127.	B	142.	A
81.	A	97.	B						

Biological Sciences

143.	C	159.	D	175.	B	190.	B	205.	A
144.	B	160.	D	176.	B	191.	C	206.	C
145.	C	161.	A	177.	A	192.	D	207.	C
146.	B	162.	B	178.	A	193.	A	208.	D
147.	A	163.	A	179.	D	194.	B	209.	C
148.	B	164.	A	180.	C	195.	B	210.	B
149.	B	165.	C	181.	A	196.	B	211.	C
150.	D	166.	B	182.	C	197.	B	212.	A
151.	B	167.	C	183.	C	198.	B	213.	C
152.	C	168.	C	184.	A	199.	C	214.	B
153.	D	169.	B	185.	B	200.	B	215.	B
154.	A	170.	D	186.	C	201.	C	216.	B
155.	C	171.	C	187.	A	202.	B	217.	C
156.	C	172.	B	188.	D	203.	A	218.	B
157.	B	173.	B	189.	A	204.	D	219.	C
158.	D	174.	C						

Explanation of Answers for Model Examination C

VERBAL REASONING

1. **C.** The entire passage presents the thesis that Fitzgerald created the American flapper through his short stories and novels. It is true that the flapper is a part of the social history of America in the post-World War I decade and thus a vehicle of social customs in America during the time; but this is not a major point of the passage. The author mainly attempts to establish the claim that Fitzgerald, not John Held, Jr. and not various flappers in film, invented or created this character type. Though there are allusions to Fitzgerald's novels, the passage mentions them only in passing, and thus **B** would be incorrect.

2. **B.** Paragraph two of the passage chronicles the origin and evolution of the term "flapper," clearly locating one of its early associations with women in Britain who had not yet been introduced into society, the answer supplied by **B**. It is actually also true, according to the *Oxford English Dictionary,* that the word may have originally come from the term that designated a young bird (**A**), a "flapper," but this information is not supplied by the passage and, therefore, would not be a correct answer for this question. Some have also suggested that the flapping arm movements of dancing flappers prompted the name. Again, however, the passage does not include this bit of information, and **C**, therefore, would be an incorrect response.

3. **A.** John O'Hara notes that the term "flapper" had been misused and that it had designated a girl who had not yet found a husband. His comment suggesting this variation is found in paragraph two.

4. **D.** The social historian, Frederick Lewis Allen, cited numerous conditions, summarized in paragraph two, which contributed to the development of the flapper. All of those cited, as well as others, are included in paragraph two.

5. **A.** As outlined in the explanation to question one (above), the central thesis of the passage is that Fitzgerald was the creator, through his fiction, of the type known as the American Flapper.

6. **B.** The passage does not deal with comparative studies of the worth of Fitzgerald's novels as opposed to his short stories, nor does it address the relative merits of John Held, Jr.'s cartoons versus his writing. Therefore, I and III are neither supported nor contradicted by the passage, which does, however, deal in detail with Fitzgerald's role in developing the flapper and with his ultimate decision to discontinue the stereotype because it limited him in the creation of complex characters. This information is presented in paragraph one.

7. **B.** While it is a fact that literary critics were harsh in their evaluation of Fitzgerald's flapper stories (**A**), that Fitzgerald was an autobiographical writer (**C**) and that certain segments of the middle-brow reading public thought that the flapper was immoral (**D**), the passage addresses none of these issues. Paragraph three does, on the other hand, address the fact that there were well-known flappers in film. Thus the correct response is **B**.

8. **D.** Paragraphs one and two could be entitled acute pharmacological experience, whereas paragraph three deals with drug effects as a prelude to dependency. Paragraph four discussed learning aspects, and paragraphs five and six deal with neurochemical aspects.

9. **B.** Paragraph one makes it perfectly clear that the dependence process starts with the initial exposure. It is also emphasized that after taking a drug an individual may feel pleasure (or less pain), but that the word pleasurable has many meanings and may not be related to "feeling good."

10. **D.** Paragraph one emphasizes that people take psychoactive drugs for many reasons that essentially meet their own individual needs, whether it be feeling good, peer pressure, or whatever.

11. **C.** Paragraphs two and five make the statement that most drugs produce their effects via an alteration of brain neurochemistry, which can lead to other more long-term problems. Alteration of the mind is not specific, and drugs do not act in a very predictable way.

12. **B.** Paragraph three discusses the phenomenon of conditioned stimulus and points out that the use of a drug can come under environmental control. Although the role of ritual is mentioned, it certainly is not the order of the day. Placebo does not routinely replace the chemical substance. No mention is made anywhere in the passage as to side effects.

13. **C.** Paragraph four deals with learned behaviors. There is no implication that learning or performing of tasks is enhanced by the consumption of psychoactive drugs. The point is made that there is the development of behavioral tolerance and that persons learn to adapt to the drug state to a degree. The example is given of an individual having difficulty finding the liquor store when sober. No credence is given in the passage to the statement that behavioral tolerance lessens the effects of drug affliction.

14. **C.** Paragraph two emphasizes that chronic drug use will introduce variables that may take over drug taking behavior, and that individuals will lose ability to control this behavior. The last paragraph mentions that chemotherapy is a modality in use, but no cure is implied. The passage as a whole focuses on the neurochemical imbalance elicited by drug use; paragraph five states that drugs have profound effects on specific neurotransmitter systems.

15. **B.** Although the reader may reach similar conclusions as those presented in statements **A** and **C**, the only statement that is specifically made by the author is statement **B.** Paragraph two states that drugs do not always serve as primary reinforcers of behavior, but have important secondary reinforcing qualities.

16. **D.** Paragraph one indicates that at Alexandria teaching was limited to only what was necessary to train researchers for the next generation. The focus was on improving understanding so that each generation could inherit a more advanced civilization.

17. **C.** Paragraph two makes it clear that Plato marveled at the underlying principles of mathematics and tried to find underlying principles or "truths" in other fields of study.

18. **A.** Paragraph three deals with the second librarian Eratosthenes who measured the size of the earth; he measured the angle of the sun (six degrees) at midday on mid-summer's day at Alexandria because he knew from previous trips to Cyrene (near today's Aswan Dam) that the sun shone to the bottom of its wells (zero degrees) on that very day and time each year. He only had to measure the distance between these two places to calculate the circumference of the earth.

19. **B.** Paragraph four indicates that Aristophanes, the third librarian, commissioned 70 scholars to translate the Bible into Greek and that this translation, which became known as the *Septuagint*, was used by Jesus Christ. The point is also made that evidence suggests that the "flight into Egypt" took place in Alexandria.

20. **C.** Paragraph seven tells us that Ptolemy wrote 13 books on astronomy, and that in his books on astrology he summarized the beliefs of the Greeks, Egyptians, and Persians and gave us the horoscope and Zodiac signs used today.

21. **B.** Paragraph nine makes the argument that wheras understanding could be accumulated in libraries and transmitted by books from generation to generation, wisdom has to be reinspired again and again by individuals in each generation.

22. **A.** The last paragraph indicates that during periods of ebbing or pluralistic religious beliefs (like today), ethics become necessary to form a behavioral consensus, to "hold these truths."

23. **B.** Paragraph one describes the great library and museum of Alexandria. The remaining paragraphs discuss the great figures who played a role in making Alexandria the center of higher learning for almost a thousand years.

24. **A.** The school of mathematics was founded by Euclid around 300 B.C.

25. **C.** Paragraph one tells of his boyhood in Peoria, and of his early job as usher in a vaudeville house through which he first became interested in show business. His father was a bricklayer, and there is no evidence in the passage that either his mother or father ever worked in show business.

26. **B.** In paragraph seven we are told that Correll's relaxed, gregarious half of the partnership balanced Gosden's more temperamental and creative temperament.

27. **D.** The first sentence in paragraph nine informs the reader that listenership began to drop following the beginning of World War II.

28. **B.** Though the passage provides few details regarding the possible evolution of the *Sam 'n Henry Show* into the *Amos 'n Andy Show,* the author of the passage states explicitly in paragraph four that the *Tribune* retained the rights to *Sam 'n Henry* and ran it with two other men.

29. **C.** Both Correll and Gosden were surprised by the controversy surrounding the show, and the passage indicates in the last sentence of paragraph 11 that Gosden, especially, was wounded by it.

30. **B.** We learn in the final paragraph that Correll and Gosden maintained a close friendship into their later years, living close to each other in Beverly Hills until Correll returned to Illinois and, at the age of 82, died.

31. **C.** A thorough reading of the passage will leave the reader with only one major theme. The writer has clearly focused on the recovery process and its many facets.

32. **D.** Paragraph one indicates that a long-term proposition is encountered in the recovery from addiction. It is a lifetime pursuit and, as AA points out, relapse frequently occurs when people stop attending meetings. Drug use and recovery depend on many factors, and the environment plays a major role in both. As is common with many compounds taken for a long period (psychoactive drugs or steroids administered under supervision), stoppage usually results in withdrawal symptoms.

33. **C.** Under no circumstances is the point made that drug use enhances learning or the performing of tasks. Psychoactive drugs are definitely detrimental to all aspects of an individual's functioning. The point is made that there is a drug-induced state dependent learning and the example is that a person sober might have a problem finding the car, but when under the influence the person "may" remember where it is.

34. **D.** Every statement is substantiated by the passage. Drugs or electrical stimulation produce their effects via an alteration of the brain's neurochemistry. The environment, it is pointed out in paragraph two, plays a key role in the addiction and recovery process. Paragraph four emphasizes that the individual determines to a great extent his/her own fate.

35. **D.** Neither addiction nor recovery are simple or well understood processes. Recovery, as paragraph four indicates, involves commitment on the part of the user to stop using the drug and to reinforce his actions by changing and utilizing environmental and social phenomena to help him in the lifelong process.

36. **C.** The passage does not address treatment of drug addiction. Paragraph four does point out that many good professionals do not appear to appreciate the difference between treatment and recovery. No indication is given that AA is the appropriate avenue to cure alcoholics. Paragraphs three and four should leave no doubt in the reader's mind that neurochemical aspects are determining factors in addiction, treatment, and eventual recovery.

37. **D.** Individual variations and commitment are emphasized. Animal experiments are essential. Organizations like AA, as is pointed out in paragraph four, help in the substitution of the drug with people and provide social reinforcement. Throughout the passage environmental aspects are highlighted.

38. **D.** The passage in paragraph one emphasizes that the Golden Rule is not a sufficient ethical principle because it fosters the idea that what is good for the physician is good for the patient. Paragraph one also emphasizes that physicians must do the "right thing" and indicates that most feel that this means curing illness and postponing death. Gregory does point out that physicians are not perfect and should acknowledge and rectify their mistakes.

39. **D.** Although the passage touches upon medical decision making, reasoning and autonomy of the patient, the application and interpretation of the Golden Rule, the central theme is philosophical and the best and most encompassing title would be "Moral Reasoning and Medical Decision Making."

40. **D.** None of the statements posed are supported by the passage. The passage points out that Hippocrates preached the Golden Rule and that certainly is part of the principle of human rights. A very strong argument is made in paragraphs four and five in favor of the physician explaining in an appropriate, understanding, sensitive, compassionate, and thorough manner the disease process to the patient and reaching a mutual consensus in order to deliniate an appropriate course of action suitable for the individual, the family, and accepted medical practice. Paragraph two makes it quite clear that the courts generally have held that the constitutional rights permit an

individual to decide what happens to himself, and these rights have been called the "Patient's Bill of Rights."

41. **C.** Throughout the passage it is stressed that a give and take attitude must exist in the decision making process, and paragraph three points out that Rousseau advocated a social contract because human beings are different. Paragraph four leaves no doubt that beneficence and autonomy must be weighed and applied to reach a decision.

42. **D.** Although every statement is correct and was espoused by Hippocrates, the passage does, however, not deal with them and so it neither contradicts nor supports the information presented in the question.

43. **A.** Paragraph six emphasizes that burden/ benefit aspects of treatment must be weighed. Sometimes life itself, or the treatment proposed to sustain life, is so problematical that patients opt for the right to die. It was previously pointed out that education of the patient is essential for proper medical practice. Paragraph six makes the point that the courts understand the concept of the right to die better than most physicians. The paragraph gives the example of artificial feeding, which may become so problematical in the respect that any benefit from the intervention is minimal.

44. **D.** There should be no doubt in the reader's mind that the passage argues strongly for education, a balance in the decision making process, consultation between physician and patient, and among physicians, and above all that patients' rights should never be negated.

45. **D.** The last paragraph makes it perfectly clear that the history of a comic book (*True Comics*) is detailed.

46. **C.** The last paragraph points out that the idea of a comic book with true stories was unique, but *True Comics* stood alone in the respect that it carried editorials.

47. **D.** A thorough reading leads the reader to conclude that besides selling magazines, the publisher preached recycling, patriotism, and fitness.

48. **C.** Paragraph three ends with the statement that the publisher was an avid internationalist, a globalist.

49. **B.** Paragraph one clearly indicates that it was an editorial in the comic book that was the first acknowledgement of America's entry into World War II. The editor was interested in reaching the young and making them aware of how they could contribute to the national effort.

50. **C.** Paragraph eight mentions that paper had become scarce and all comic books were forced to cut the number of pages, and editorials seemed dispensable.

51. **D.** The last paragraph makes it perfectly clear that Mr. Hecht had confidence in the ability and willingness of American youth. It is pointed out in paragraph six that a linguist would be able to explain the principles of democracy. The whole passage deals with the ideas and ideals of a strong willed and daring individual; the first sentence of paragraph seven should be convincing. Although the editor talks about international courts and forces, he does not propose the notion that such cooperation would prevent all future wars.

52. **D.** Of the four titles listed "Herbert Hoover— Relief, Politics, and War" is the most appropriate one. Herbert Hoover was the food czar of the United States during World War I and thereafter helped with international relief efforts. He became president in 1928 and after his loss to Roosevelt in 1932 continued a role in the political arena. He was afraid that the United States would enter World War II and hoped for a negotiated peace.

53. **A.** Although it is true that Hoover had many contacts and was a brilliant organizer, our passage really does not focus on this issue at all. Paragraph one pictures Hoover as a humanitarian and paragraph two mentions that the Democrats ran a smear campaign. Hoover as is mentioned in many places in the passage actively sought the presidency continuously.

54. **D.** Roosevelt ran a smear campaign against Hoover (paragraph two). No mention of humanitarianism and of being self-made is made in the passage. It is, however, clear from paragraph four that Roosevelt opposed the relief efforts.

55. **A.** Paragraph two mentions that Hoover's name was blighted by the 1932 campaign. Hoover was influential from World War I until his death. Paragraphs three and five detail the convention defeats, and four indicates that Poland, Finland, Holland, Belgium, and Norway solicited his help.

56. **D.** All three statements made are not addressed by the passage.

57. **A.** Paragraph four mentions that a nasty set of rumors hinted that Hoover's relief efforts competed with the Red Cross; in this paragraph both Roosevelt's and Churchill's oppositions are mentioned. The National Committee on Food for the Small Democracies was a propaganda organization. Paragraph four points out that Hoover acted quickly to aid with money, food, and other such supplies.

58. **D.** There can be no doubt in the reader's mind that Hoover was service oriented, had a long record, and was committed. No sides were taken by the author, and in that respect a fair and sympathetic job was done.

59. **D.** The opening paragraph states the computer model was developed by the U.S.E.P.A.

60. **C.** Paragraph two states that the primary difference was the loss on ignition.

61. **C.** Paragraph six states that the coal contributed 3.71/3.86 or 96.1% of the total ash.

62. **D.** Magnesium oxide was added in the hypothetical sample to increase resistivity as indicated in paragraph six.

63. **A.** Paragraph one states that two ash samples were received September 1989 and two ash samples were received November 1989.

64. **A.** Paragraph six indicates that magnesium oxide increased resistivity, whereas sodium oxide lowers resistivity.

65. **C.** The laboratory work and the computer modeling work was done to predict the effects of a change in chemical composition of a waste fuel on the electrical resistance of the ash produced.

PHYSICAL SCIENCES

66. **C.** The tangential (linear) velocity of an object moving around a circular path (velocity tangent to the circle) is proportional to the angular velocity.

    $v = r w$, where r is the radius (9 m in this case) and w is the angular velocity (which must be in radians/sec for use in this formula).

67. **D.** A "g" force is equal to the actual weight, mg, of a person or object, so:
    8 "g's" = $8(82 \text{ kg})(9.8 \text{ m/sec}^2)$ = 6429 N.

68. **D.** The centrifugal force is the "equal and opposite force" of Newton's third law and thus does NOT act *on* the *pilot*. It is the force that the pilot exerts *on* the *back of his seat*.

69. **A.** Power in watts is the rate of energy use, thus the energy, $E = P \times t$ or $E = 450 \text{ watts} \times 120 \text{ sec}$ = 54,000 joules and liters of O_2 consumed = 54,000 J/(20,000 J/L) = 2.7 L.

70. **D.** According to Newton's third law, the pilot exerts a force of 8 "g's" on his seat back. Notice that this *is* the centrifugal force and it *is* a real outward force on the seat back. (The pilot, in his rotating "frame of reference," feels as if a large outward force is pushing him into the seat back. This force is a "fictitous" force because the only real force acting on him is the inward centripetal force.)

71. **D.** The necessary inward-pointing centripetal force is unchanged. Nothing has changed except the device that supplies the centripetal force.

72. **B.** It is given in the passage that the telescope length is approximately equal to the sum of the focal lengths. If the total length is 4 m, then the value of f_e is 4 m − f_o = 1 m.

73. **B.** The objective lens forms a real, inverted image. The eyepiece acts in the same way that a magnifying glass does. The observer looks through the eyepiece and sees a final, virtual image that has the same orientation as the first image (that is, the final image is still inverted). This can be corrected by inserting a third lens, known as an erecting lens, between the objective and eyepiece.

74. **C.** The magnification of a simple Newtonian telescope is the ratio of the objective focal length to the eyepiece focal length:

    $$M = f_o/f_e = 3/1 = 3 \times.$$

75. **B.** This question requires an understanding of total internal reflection. The critical angle is the incident angle for which Snell's law of refraction predicts a refracted angle of 90°, for light rays traveling from a medium of larger index of refraction toward a medium of lower index of refraction. Here the light ray is incident inside the glass prism toward air of index, n_{air} = 1. Using Snell's law:

    $n_{glass} \sin \emptyset_c = n_{air} \sin 90°$, and because n_{glass} = 1.52; $\sin \emptyset_c = 1/1.52$ and $\emptyset_c = 41°$.

76. **D.** The objective lens is a projection lens, producing an inverted real image. The first image lies within the focal length of the eyepiece, which

therefore acts as a magnifying flass, forming a virtual, enlarged image. The eyepiece does not invert the image.

77. **B.** As the object (primate) moves closer to the objective, the real image formed by the objective is further away from the objective, i.e., closer to the original position of the eyepiece. To see the image clearly, the eyepiece must be moved "back" away from the objective in order to focus the second (virtual) image clearly. (It is the eyepiece that is adjustable in telescopes and binoculars.) This is similar to holding this printed page too close to your eyes to see clearly. If you hold the page still and move your head away you will be able to see the print clearly.

78. **B.** The pressure is due to the weight of a column of fluid 75 m tall. $P = dgy$; where $d =$ density of the liquid, and y is the depth below the surface; g is the acceleration of gravity, 9.8 m/sec^2.

79. **C.** This is a simple conversion problem:

$$7.35 \times 10 \text{ N/m}^2 \times \frac{1 \text{ atm}}{1.01 \times 10^5 \text{ n/m}^2} = 7.3 \text{ atm}$$

80. **C.** Pressure is force divided by area, or $P = F/A$; so $F = PA$. It is necessary to convert the area from cm^2 to m^2 (by multiplying by 10^{-4}m^2/cm^2). Thus $F = 6.86 \times 10^5$ N/m$^2 \times$ 65 cm$^2 \times 1 \times 10^{-4}m^2/cm^2 = 4460$ N.

81. **A.** Treating the air as an ideal gas, we see that $P_1V_1 = P_2V_2$, or $V_2 = P_1V_1/P_2$. Notice that we must use the absolute pressures in this expression. Then $P_1 = 8.36 \times 10^5$ N/m^2 and $P^2 = 1.01 \times 10^5$ N/m^2.

82. **C.** The partial pressure is the same fraction (0.21) of the total absolute pressure of 8.36×10^5 N/m^2 as the fraction of oxygen by volume in ordinary air.

83. **D.** The added pressure, above atmospheric, on the top surface of the water appears at all points in the fluid (Pascal's principle). The total pressure, above atmospheric, on the bottom is 31,000 N/m^2 and is the sum of the added pressure and the pressure due to the weight of the water. The added pressure is thus:

$P_{added} = P_{total} - P_{water}$

$= 31,000 \text{ N/m}^2 - 19,600 \text{ N/m}^2$

$= 11,400 \text{ N/m}^2$.

84. **B.** The electrical power per heater is:

$P = I^2R = (20 \text{ A})^2(15 \text{ ohms}) = 6000$ watts.

The 12 heaters supply 72,000 watts.

85. **A.** The volume of a cylinder is equal to the product of the area of the base times the height:

$V = Ah = \pi(r^2)h$
$= \pi(1.1 \text{ m})^2 (2\text{m})$
$= 7.6 \text{ m}^2$.

86. **C.** Power is the electrical work/sec. The work increases the temperature of the water according to $W = mc\Delta t = Pt$.

Then

$t = mc\Delta t/P$

$= (5,000 \text{ kg})(4,190 \text{ J/kg} \cdot °\text{C})(55°)/(110,000 \text{ J/sec})$

$= 10,475 \text{ sec} = 2.9 \text{ hr}.$

87. **B.** The volume flow rate (in cubic meters/sec) is the product of the cross-sectional area of the pipe times the flow velocity:

$V/t = Av,$ $v = 1.0$ m/sec,
$V = 7.6 \text{ m}^3,$
$t = 13 \text{ min} = 780 \text{ sec},$
$A = V/vt = 7.6 \text{ m}^3/(1 \text{ m/sec})(780 \text{ sec})$
$= 0.01 \text{ m}^2.$

88. **D.** This is a mechanical equilibrium problem involving a torque calculation. The board is supported at its center of mass and would be balanced without the children. We need consider only the torques about an axis through the pivot caused by the weights of the children. We asssume that the "counterclockwise" torque due to the heavy child is positive and the "clockwise" torque due to the light child is negative. We then sum them to zero. Measured from the pivot to the line of the force, the lever arm or "moment arm" for the 35 kg child is x, and the lever arm for the 20 kg child is 1 m.

Summing the torques, 35 kg $\times$ g $\times$ x − 20 kg $\times$ g $\times$ 1 m = 0. Thus $x = 0.57$ m.

89. **A.** The angular acceleration is the change in angular velocity divided by the time taken, or $\alpha = (\varpi_f - \varpi_i)/t$. Converting ϖ to rad/sec:

$\varpi_f = 57{,}300$ rev/min $\times 2\pi$ rad/rev $\times$ 1 min/60sec = 6000 rad/sec

$\alpha = (6000$ rad/sec $- 0)/120$ sec $= 50$ rad/sec^2

90. B. Under the conservation of energy principle, the initial kinetic energy will be entirely converted into work done by friction in stopping the block. (The energy is dissipated as frictional heat.)

$\frac{1}{2}mv^2 = \frac{1}{2} \times 4$ kg $\times (5$ m/sec$)^2 = 50$ joules

91. A. We can find the image using the thin lens formula $1/f = 1/p + 1/q$, where f = focal length, p = object distance (object to lens), and q = image distance (lens to image). Then $1/q = 1/6 - 1/4.8$, so $q = -24$ cm. Since q is negative, the image is virtual and on the same side of the lens as the insect.

92. B. The product of force and time, Ft, is the *impulse* and equals the *change in momentum* of an object, $p_f - p_i$. The initial momentum of both masses is zero. Since F and t are the same for both masses, their final momenta must be the same, so 2 N $\times$ 4 sec = 8 kg-m/sec. (Note that the 3 kg mass is moving faster but has the same momentum as the 6 kg mass.

93. C. Gamma (γ) emission is the emission of a photon from an excited nucleus and will change neither the charge nor mass number. The resulting nuclide is the (unexcited) Cu^{64}. Emission of a negative electron, β^-, from the nucleus leaves it with one additional unit of positive charge so that the atomic number, z, increases by 1. The result is $_{30}Zn^{64}$. Emission of a positron, β^+, leaves the nucleus with one less positive charge and z decreases by 1. The result is $_{28}Ni^{64}$. Note that the mass changes are so small for beta decays that the superscript mass number (64) remains the same in all three cases.

94. A. The index of refraction is $n = c/v$, where c is the speed of light in a vacuum (3×10^8 m/sec) and v is the speed of light in the material. Here, $v_s = 0.83\, v_w$. Or $v_s = 0.83\, c/n_w = c/n_s$. Cancel c and solve for $n_s = 1.6$.

95. B. Electrical power is the product of voltage and current: $P = VI$. Since $I = V/R$, by Ohm's Law we can write $P = V^2/R$. For the 60-watt bulb, $R = V^2/P = (120V)^2/60$ W = 240 ohms. For the 100-watt bulb, $R = V^2/P = (120V)^2/100$ W = 144 ohms.

96. A. Newton's second law states that the net force equals the product of mass and acceleration: $F_{net} = ma$. In this case the net force is the difference between the applied force (18 N) and the force of friction (9 N): $F_{net} = F_a - F_f = 18 - 9 = (90)a$.

97. B. The total momentum of the two-cart system is zero before the students push off, and remains zero after they separate. Then: $0 = m_1v_1 + m_2v_2$. Thus, $v_2 = 60$ kg(1.2 m/sec)/(0.8 m/sec).

98. B. The initial kinetic energy is used up in doing work against the frictional force as the student-cart is brought to rest. Using the conservation of energy principle: $F_f x = 1/2\ mv^2$, where $x = 8$ m. Then : $F_f = 20$ N.

99. C. We know that the total angular momentum of the student is conserved (constant). Because he is capable of changing his moment of inertia about the vertical axis of spin by extending his arms or pulling them in, we can find the ratio of the moments of inertia by using the conservation law in the form: $I_1 \Omega_1 = I_2 \Omega_2$. Then $I_2/I_1 = \Omega_1/\Omega_2 = 1.5$.

100. D. Linear momentum is conserved in this problem. The addition of mass causes a decrease in the velocity as given by: $m_1v_1 = (m_1 + m_{sand})V_2$. $V_2 = 1.6$ m/sec.

101. B. The center-of-mass will not move because the forces exerted by pulling on the rope are internal forces to the two-cart system. It is nearer the larger mass, and is found by using the formula for the cm: $X_{cm} = (m_1x_1 + m_2x_2)/(m_1 + m_2)$. We are allowed to place the origin of the coordinate system anywhere we choose. Placing the origin at the original position of the larger mass, $x_1 = 0$ and $x_2 = 2$ m. $X_{cm} = (0 + (80)(2))/(200$ kg$) = 0.8$ m.

102. C. Conservation of momentum applies to this completely inelastic collision as follows: $m_1v_1 = (m_1 + m_2)V$. Then $V = (80$ kg$)(4$ m/sec$)(80 + 80) = 2$ m/sec.

103. B. The net force accelerates the 100 kg mass according to Newton's Third Law. The net force here is the difference between the applied 90 N force and the opposing friction force. $F_{net} = 90 - f = ma = 100$ kg $\times 0.8$ m/sec^2. Solving for f we find that $f = 10$ N.

104. B. The falling weight can be isolated so that we can apply Newton's third law to it alone. The weight force due to the mass acts downward and the 90 N tension upward. The third law then shows that: $mg - 90 = ma$, which we solve for the unknown mass, m. $m(g - a) = 90$ N. $m(9.8 - 0.8) = 90$. Then $m = 10$ kg.

105. **C.** The work done in accelerating the cart is equal to the gain in kinetic energy: $F_{net}x = 1/2\ mv^2$, or $(100$ N$)(10$ m$) = (1/2)\ 80v^2$ and then $v = 5$ m/sec.

106. **C.** Both $[H^+]$ and $[OH^-] = 1.0 \times 10^{-7}$. The pH = 7.0.

107. **B.** $K_a = \dfrac{[H^+][B^-]}{[HB]} = 6.6 \times 10^{-5} = \dfrac{[H^+]^2}{0.0001}$

$[H^+]^2 = 6.6 \times 10^{-9} = 66 \times 10^{-10}$

Because the square root of 66 is about 8, $[H^+] = 8 \times 10^{-5}$ or between 1×10^{-4} and 1×10^{-5} pH = $-\log [H^+]$ and is between 4 and 5. Although water itself contributes $[H^+] = 1 \times 10^{-7}$, this is negligibly small in comparison to the H^+ from benzoic acid. Thus, in this example, the H^+ from water may be neglected.

108. **D.** pH + pOH = 14
Although in pure water pH = pOH, that is not the case here. Because pH is between 4 and 5, however, this pOH will be between 9 and 10.

109. **B.** $K_a = \dfrac{[H^+]^2}{1 \times 10^{-12}} = 6.6 \times 10^{-5}$

$[H^+]^2 = 6.6 \times 10^{-17} = 66 \times 10^{-18}$
$[H^+]$ = about 8×10^{-9} or 0.08×10^{-7}.

This is very small compared to the $[H^+]$ of 1.0×10^{-7} supplied by ionization of water. Thus the pH approximates 7.

110. **A.** Henderson-Hasselbalch formula

$$pH = pK_a + \log \frac{[salt]}{[acid]}$$

When the concentrations of salt and acid are equal, pH = pK_a. By inspection of $K_a = 6.6 \times 10^{-5}$, its negative log would be between 4 and 5. Thus the pK_a and the resulting pH are between 4 and 5.

111. **D.** $K_{sp} = 9 \times 10^{-12} = [Ag^+]^2\ [CrO_4^=]$
$= (1 \times 10^{-6})^2\ [CrO_4^=] = 9 \times 10^{-12}$
$[CrO_4^=] = 9$ or approximately 1×10^1

112. **C.** Addition of Cl^- ions will bring about precipitation of AgCl when its K_{sp} is exceeded.

113. **B.** The K_{sp} is given for a particular temperature and will change with temperature. It may speed

the reaction but will not likely bring about more complete precipitation.

114. **C.** The K_{sp} with the smallest number represents the one with the lowest solubility.

115. **D.** The K_{sp}'s are independent of each other. If the K_{sp} of one is not reached, no precipitation will occur.

116. **A.** Phosphorus, a nonmetal, will react with oxygen to form an oxide. This oxide will react with water to form an acidic solution.

117. **A.** Nitrogen, a nonmetal, will react with oxygen to form an oxide. This oxide will react with water to form an acidic solution.

118. **B.** One mole of Ca will form one mole of CaO by oxidation. This will form one mole of $Ca(OH)_2$ by reaction with water.

119. **C.** One mole of $Ca(OH)_2$ will require two moles of HCl for neutralization.

120. **A.** Oxides of sulfur are produced during burning of coal. These acid anhydrides react with water to form acids. Carbon dioxide can react with water to form the weak acid, carbonic acid. There is already a substantial amount of carbon dioxide in the atmosphere. Although carbon dioxide above the earth may contribute to other problems, it has not been suggested to contribute to acid rain.

121. **C.** One mole of each would exert the same effect, but only if they are ionized. NaCl produces 2 ions per molecule, and Na_2SO_4 produces 3 ions per molecule. Colligative properties depend on the number of particles.

122. **B.** Molality (moles of solute per 1000 g of solvent) is used in calculations of colligative properties. Further calculations are required if there is ionization.

123. **D.** All of these are colligative properties.

124. **A.** Without knowing the identity of the solute, we know that twice the amount will lower the freezing point twice as much.

125. **C.** If the weight is the same, the nonionizing solute with the lowest molecular weight will have the largest number of dissolved molecules.

126. **A.** Loss of a single electron in the 3s orbital leaves the stable electronic configuration of the noble gas, neon.

127. **B.** In a neutral atom, the number of electrons in orbitals equals the number of protons in the nucleus. The latter defines the atomic number.

128. **C.** Gain of an additional electron would give the stable electronic configuration of the noble element, krypton.

129. **D.** Note that the number of electrons exceeds the atomic number (and the number of protons) by one. Thus, this would be an ion with a charge of −1.

130. **C.** The fact that the number of electrons is equal to the atomic number indicates that this is a neutral atom. The fact that the outermost electron is in the 3p orbital rather than the expected 3s orbital indicates that the atom is in an excited state.

131. **D.** Noble elements include helium, neon, argon, krypton, xenon, and radon.

132. **D.** Each orbital electron possesses four quantum numbers—principal, angular momentum, magnetic, and spin.

133. **C.** Possible values of magnetic quantum number are −1, 0, and +1.

134. **B.** Possible values of spin quantum number are $+\frac{1}{2}$ and $-\frac{1}{2}$.

135. **A.** No two electrons in an atom possess all four identical quantum numbers.

136. **C.** Silver ions will react with chloride ions and precipitate as $AgCl$.

137. **B.** $H_2S \rightleftarrows 2H^+ + S^{2-}$. By the common ion effect, lowering the pH (increasing the H^+ concentration) will lower the S^{2-} concentration by displacing the reaction to the left.

$$K_i = \frac{[H^+]^2[S^{2-}]}{[H_2S]}.$$

If $[H^+]$ increases, $[S^{2-}]$ must decrease.

138. **A.** Freezing point depression in water depends only on the number of solute particles per unit volume

1 *M* NaCl = 2 × 1 × 6.02×10^{23} particles per liter

0.3 *M* Na_2SO_4 = 3 × .3 × 6.02×10^{23} particles per liter
1.5 *M* glucose = 1 × 1.5 × 6.02×10^{23} particles per liter
0.5 *M* $BaSO_4$ = 2 × 0.5 × 6.02×10^{23} particles per liter
Dividing by 6.02×10^{23} we can see that the comparative figures are NaCl, 2; Na_2SO_4, 0.9; glucose, 1.5; and $BaSO_4$, 1.0. Thus, the NaCl solution has the greatest number of particles per unit volume (considering the ionization of NaCl, Na_2SO_4, and $BaSO_4$), and it will have the lowest freezing point.

139. **D.** A reaction in which electrons (e^-) are removed is termed an oxidation reaction; the adding of electrons to an atom or molecule is termed a reduction reaction.

140. **A.** The hydronium ion, H_3O^+, is a protonated water molecule. $2H_2O \rightleftarrows H_3O^+ + OH^-$

141. **A.** As long as the volume units are the same, $N_1V_1 = N_2V_2$

$$V_2 = \frac{N_1V_1}{N_2} = \frac{(50)(0.25)}{0.50} = 25 \text{ ml}$$

142. **A.** This is a definition of the zwitterion; an example is the amino acid, glycine.

WRITING SAMPLE
Part 1, Essay

One must point out that Demonax begins his assertion with "probably." The statement then takes on a more questioning or probing tone, as if he is asking for a contradiction. This tone colors an attitude that is already filled with a sort of shrugging resignation or apathy. Demonax clearly believes that laws do not serve their intended purpose. It seems that, to him, that purpose would be to change the nature of people who are not "good." He says, in effect, that good individuals do not need laws in order to be good and that bad ones will remain bad with or without laws.

This is probably true. However, it is not clear that Demonax explored the possibility that laws might serve another purpose. Among some probable other things, laws serve as guidelines by which individuals can operate in social groups. Even a very good person might want to know on which side of the street she should drive. Laws might also be a deterrent to bad behaviors as well. A bad person who might steal the purse of an elderly blind woman might be deterred by the knowledge that the law calls for a prison sentence for so doing. The individual is made no better by the law, but the life of the blind woman might be.

Laws are useful as a set of guidelines, rules, or agreements, accepted by a group of people who wish to live interdependently. They save time for people who otherwise would have to continuously be deciding upon the methods to use in everyday social interactions. More controversial, but also inevitable, is the fact that they also uphold a moral code that is agreed upon hopefully by the majority. Without any laws, we would, in fact, be less free to move about in more important endeavors because we would be constantly battling each other for time and space. Imagine an interstate highway with no traffic regulations, for example. Or imagine trying to maintain possession of one's home if there were no laws to say that it was your home between the time when you left for work and the time when you returned from work. As an effort to change the nature of a human being, laws are, indeed, probably useless. But, as an effort to change the nature of our social lives, they are clearly invaluable and mean the difference between living in civilization and living in chaos.

Part 1
Explanation of First Response: 5

The paper focuses on the statement and addresses each of the three writing tasks. In the first paragraph the writer begins the explanation of the statement by noting that it is qualified with the word "probably," an explanation that is completed with a paraphrase of the quotation. The second paragraph presents specific situations in which laws do, in fact, serve good purposes. The final paragraph balances the extremes, exploring those things about laws that make them useful for people living together in social situations, which is a pragmatic position, but arguing that laws probably do not change human beings.

This is a tightly reasoned essay that makes good use of concrete examples. The writing is clear, and the sentences are nicely paced. Paragraph two is potentially a strong one, with its example of the elderly woman's purse; but it would benefit from a bringing together of ideas at the end, a sentence to clinch the paragraph. With fuller development of this paragraph and a brief expansion of the idea in paragraph one that, to Demonax, laws do not serve their intended purpose, the essay would receive a 6 rather than a 5.

Part 2, Essay

With the thought of the concept of freedom comes naturally the question, from what? Freedom does not exist without the possibility, really the latent presence of restraint. What Gibran says is that an increase in one freedom would necessarily imply a restraint on another. This is because an increase in a person's freedom always means also an increase in his domain of respon-sibility. For example, as an infant, a person could be seen as either totally free or totally without freedom. An infant is totally free from responsibility and obligation, yet totally dependent on and restrained by his caretakers. What Gibran understands is that, the greater one's realm of existence and the broader one's scope of knowledge, the greater also is one's realm and scope of responsibility. As you commit an act, the act becomes a part of you, a fetter perhaps, and certainly a history or past to which you are then forever confined and from which you never will be free.

From this point of view, there are certainly no possible examples of a freedom that implies no restraints, for existence itself implies a certain restraint. Even a freedom to die would imply a restraint from the opportunity to live. The point is that one thing or act at a point in the realm of time and space forbids the existence of another at that point. With every act and thought then, we redefine our own existence; with definition comes restraint, and with restraint comes the inhibition of some freedom.

What Gibran is apparently trying to do is to point beyond an immediate goal of freedom to the new existence beyond it. For example, once a person is free of the yoke of his parents and family, that freedom puts a new and greater yoke, that of responsibility on his shoulders throughout the remainder of his life. Gibran is not arguing against freedom, however, but is suggesting a more mature, wiser view of freedom than that of freedom as an end in itself. As one's vision expands, one will have greater and greater freedoms. But with that vision will also come knowledge and with knowledge will come responsibility. And so, as we seek to broaden our scope of existence, we also seek to make our burden a bit heavier. And this becomes a good thing.

Part 2
Explanation of Second Response: 4

The paper addresses all three objectives, and it does an especially nice job with one and three. Paragraph one focuses sharply on the explanation of the quotation. This is perhaps the most difficult of the tasks for this quotation because of its seeming paradox. The paragraph also provides the example of the infant, who could be considered either totally free or totally without freedom. Paragraph two does not confront the second task as directly as does paragraph one. Though there is a clear attempt here to explore the possibility of a freedom that would not imply a burden or an obstacle to a greater freedom, the paragraph stops short of providing a specific situation that illustrates the point. If there were a more direct confrontation of the second task, this essay would receive a higher rating. Paragraph three reconciles the extremes and examines the implications of the state-ment.

The writing in this paper is clear and well controlled. Each of the paragraphs is organized around a topic that gives unity to the paper. Its sentences are varied and flow nicely from one to the next. The weakest aspect of the paper is that it lacks concrete details to illustrate its points from the beginning of paragraph two to the end. With the addition of such details and with a direct confrontation of the task in paragraph two, its rating would move to 5 or 6.

BIOLOGICAL SCIENCES

143. **C.** Thyroid stimulating hormone (TSH) produced by the pituitary gland stimulates the thyroid gland to produce its hormones T_3 (triiodothyronine) and T_4 (tetraiodothyronine or thyroxine). TSH modulates the iodide trapping mechanisms; hypersecretion results in goiter and exophthalmos, whereas hyposecretion leads to diminished thyroid function and lethargy.

144. **B.** See explanation for question 143.

145. **C.** When thyroxin is administered, one would expect that the iodide uptake would decrease; in graph I it stayed level, whereas in graph III an increase of uptake is exhibited. Both experimental conditions indicate some evidence of thyroid malfunction.

146. **B.** A hyperthyroid individual would not be expected to show additional uptake because the gland already is working at an elevated level. When thyroid hormone was administered as in our experiments, normally the uptake should have decreased; it stayed the same however.

147. **A.** When thyroxin is administered, TSH production diminishes and RAI uptake should drop. This did not occur in graph I while graph II demonstrates the expected normal. Graph III shows an increase in uptake indicating that the pituitary is not responding to the negative inhibitory feedback that thyroxin elicits; TSH production should decrease at the time of thyroxine administration.

148. **B.** Acromegaly is a result of pituitary oversecretion of growth hormone. Lack of iodine will result in goiter development of the thyroid gland. Rickets is due to vitamin D deficiency. A skin rash is not a specific lesion that can be associated with only one specific cause as the others listed.

149. **B.** Acidophils produce somatotropic hormone (STH) and luteotropic hormone (LTH) or prolactin. Beta cells produce thyroid stimulating hormone (TSH), adrenocorticotropic hormone (ACTH), and melanocyte stimulating hormone (MSH). Delta cells produce luteinizing hormone (LH) (called interstitial cell stimulating hormone in the male), and follicle stimulating hormone (FSH). Chromophobes are considered resting cells.

150. **D.** All statements are correct. The thyroid originates from the foramen cecum region of the tongue. Its structural unit is the follicle, a unit of epithelial cells that surround a colloid space. Colloid is located extracellularly and contains thyroglobulin. T_3 and T_4 are the active thyroid principles and are released into the bloodstream and carried on proteins to the tissues.

151. **B.** Acromegaly and (or) giantism is due to overactivity of the alpha cells of the pituitary, which secrete growth hormone. If a person is affected before puberty, he or she will develop into a fairly well-proportioned giant. After maturity, an increase in the size of the hands and feet and massive development of the bones comprising the face are consequences. In the adult, strictly speaking, the term acromegaly must be applied to this condition.

152. **C.**

If aortic pressure is unchanged and end diastolic volume increases, the stroke volume or the difference between end diastolic volume and end systolic volume is larger. Ventricular work is equal to:

Work = Pressure • Stroke Volume = Force/Area • Volume = Force • Length

or the area under the curve. The kinetic energy of the ejected blood can be ignored because it represents ≈5% of the total energy and stays constant under most conditions. The area subtended by the pressure-volume loop increases as does the work in this case. Because the contractility of the heart represented by the upper curve remains constant, the end systolic volume also remains constant.

153. **D.**

Whereas the pressure to eject blood must increase, the volume of blood the ventricle ejects is less. Therefore, the ventricular work depends on the exact nature of the two curves. Because the ventricle cannot maintain the required pressure at low volumes, the total volume of blood ejected is less and the end systolic volume is increased.

154. **A.**

In this case, the ventricle is incapable of generating the same pressure at low volumes. Therefore, the volume of blood ejected is less (i.e., the stroke volume is smaller), and the end systolic volume is correspondingly larger. Note that this question is a play on words. If the stroke volume decreases with a constant end diastolic volume, the volume left in the ventricle after contraction will be more. The ventricular work is reduced because the pressure remains constant while the volume of blood ejected falls so that the product of the two decreases.

155. **C.**

The key to this question is to remember which two cases are being compared. The increase in end diastolic volume allows the failing ventricle to increase the stroke volume as compared to the uncompensated case. With a constant pressure, an increase in stroke volume causes an increase in the work (i.e., pressure • stroke volume). Because the aortic pressure is constant and the active pressure curve is unchanged in the two cases, the volume remaining in the ventricle at the point at which the ventricle stops ejecting blood will remain constant.

156. **C.**

The key to this question, as in question 155, is that one must remember what conditions are being compared. Increasing the end diastolic volume sufficiently could theoretically allow a failing ventricle to eject a larger stroke volume than is the case in normals. However, the compensation for a failing ventricle usually is not sufficient for this to occur under physiological conditions. Because the stroke volume is indeterminate relative to the normal condition, the ventricular work is also indeterminate given a constant mean aortic pressure. Because by definition a failing ventricle cannot maintain the same pressure at low volumes, the end systolic volume must increase in comparison to that of normal.

157. **B.** The definitions of isotonic, hypotonic, and hypertonic need to be recalled. Remember that the structure placed in a medium is surrounded by a semipermeable membrane; the structure is permeable to small particles (e.g., certain inorganic ions and water), but not to large particles (fat and protein molecules). An isotonic environment exerts the same osmotic pull as the medium does on the other side of a semipermeable membrane. It consequently has to possess the same concentration of particles and, therefore, the net gain or loss of water during osmosis is zero. If the red blood cells were placed in a hypotonic solution, hemolysis would occur because a hypotonic solution would exert a lesser osmotic pull than the medium

on the other side of a semipermeable membrane (the inside of the RBC); the medium would possess a smaller concentration of particles and consequently would lose water during osmosis. In our case, the red blood cells were hypertonic in relation to the medium and exerted a larger osmotic pull than the medium on the other side of the semipermeable membrane because it possessed a greater concentration of particles and consequently accumulated water during osmosis.

158.   **D.**   In this experiment, urea and glycerol did enter the red blood cell and water consequently followed because it was in greater quantity outside and tried to establish an equilibrium.

159.   **D.**   Cell membranes are described as semipermeable because they allow some materials to pass while they block others. All materials that pass membranes must be either a liquid or dissolved in a liquid. Molecules also must be fairly simple, but molecular size is not the limiting factor because amino acids pass less readily than do many smaller molecules. Osmosis is the passage of liquids through a membrane; usually water through the semipermeable membrane. Diffusion is the passage of molecules from a more concentrated environment to a less concentrated region; equalization is usually the end result.

160.   **D.**   Active transport involves the diffusion of molecules against a gradient; this is an energy consuming phenomenon. The process of moving substances from an area of lower concentration to where they are in a higher concentration is selective, and requires respiration. Osmosis and diffusion are described in the explanation for question 159. Turgor pressure involves the passage of water into a cell at a faster rate than it can leave; the cell becomes plump and filled (turgid). At times the force results in bursting the structures. Plasmolysis is defined as a shrinking of protoplasm due to the loss of water from a cell.

161.   **A.**   Layers of material (probably mucopolysaccharide) secreted by the cell are found on the surface of the cell. The most prominent layer is the basement membrane, or basal lamina. These structures are boundaries and must be traversed by material entering and leaving the cell. Cells must be held together; adjacent cell membranes interdigitate and intercellular cement is utilized. A desmosome is a specialized area of connection between adjacent cellular membranes (macula adherens). A terminal bar is a dense area surrounding the apical cellular surface. It includes the tight junction (zona occludens) and the loose junction (zona adherens). In cardiac muscle, several cardiac muscle cells join end to end at a specialized junctional zone known as an intercalated disc.

162.   **B.**   Some of the proteins embedded in the lipid layers of membranes are shaped to form channels with "gates," which open only to certain materials or under certain conditions.

163.   **A.**   Osmosis is a process in which solvent passes from an area of lower solute concentration to an area of higher solute concentration. In dialysis solvent and solute both pass through the membrane.

164.   **A.**   The defect cannot be dominant because individual 5 was produced by two normal parents who would have no defective alleles if the defect is dominant (either autosomal or X-linked). The defect is unlikely to be X-linked recessive because unless a new mutation occurred, individual 5 should have received a normal allele for the gene on her X from her father (individual 2) and therefore could not express a recessive X-linked defect. Therefore the most likely possibility (using the assumptions of a single controlling gene and very rare mutations) would be an autosomal gene for which the defective allele is recessive to the normal allele.

165.   **C.**   Unless a new mutation occurred, individual 1 would have to have one normal allele (which produced the normal phenotype) and one defective allele (which was contributed to individual 5 along with a defective allele from individual 2) to produce individual 5's defective phenotype.

166.   **B.**   Individual 4 would have to contain two defective alleles to produce the defective phenotype.

167.   **C.**   Individual 7 would have to contain at least one normal allele to produce her normal phenotype. Her other allele cannot be determined with certainty from the data given. Because her parents are probably both heterozygotes (see above), she has a $1/3$ probability of having two normal alleles and a $2/3$ probability of having one normal and one abnormal allele.

i.e., $Nn \times Nn$

$1/4\, NN$: $2/4\, Nn$: $1/4\, nn$

defective phenotype
$2/3$ of normal phenotype
$1/3$ of normal phenotype

Therefore she is most likely to contain one normal and one defective allele.

168. **C.**   Individual 8 would have to contain one normal allele (to produce his normal phenotype) and one abnormal allele (because he contributed one of the two defective alleles in each of offspring 14 and 18).

169. **B.**   The upper region consists of the fluid portion of the blood, the plasma.

170. **D.**   The thin "buffy" layer is the white blood cells and platelets.

171. **C.**   After centrifugation, the packed volume of formed elements was 5.5 ml. As stated previously, most of the formed elements are RBCs.

172. **B.**   After centrifugation, the volume of packed formed elements of the patient was 5.5 ml. Because hematocrit is defined as the relative volume of formed elements, the hematocrit of this patient is 55% (i.e., 5.5 ml out of 10 ml, or 55% of the total blood volume, was occupied by formed elements).

173. **B.**   The hematocrit of this patient, 55%, is higher than the normal average value of 45%.

174. **C.**   Region C consists of RBCs. These cells contain hemoglobin, which binds and carried oxygen.

175. **B.**   Region B, the "buffy" coat, consists of WBCs and platelets. The WBCs consist of a number of cell types, some of which are responsible for fighting infections.

176. **B.**   Region B, the "buffy" coat, consists of WBC and platelets. The platelets are responsible for triggering the cascade of events that results in the formation of blood clots.

177. **A.**   The major component of blood plasma is water.

178. **A.**   Because the patient's hematocrit is higher than the normal value, the patient has more formed elements, largely RBCs, than a normal individual. Because RBCs are responsible for binding and carrying oxygen, a higher hematocrit might suggest that the individual has a higher physiological demand for oxygen. Such a condition is seen in individuals living at high altitudes where the oxygen concentration of the air is lower (compared to the oxygen concentration of air at sea level).

179. **D.**   A sarcomere, the area between two Z bands, is the functional unit of muscle; it is the region between two Z lines and consists of an A band and half of two abutting I bands.

180. **C.**   According to the sliding filament theory (Huxley) the sarcomere response to excitation involves the sliding of thin and thick myofilaments past one another making and breaking chemical bonds with each other as they go. Neither the thick nor thin myofilaments change in length.

181. **A.**   If we observed this contraction under the light microscope, we would see the narrowing of the H and I bands during contraction while the width of the A band would remain constant.

182. **C.**   The immediate energy source for contraction is ATP which can be hydrolyzed by actomyosin to give ADP, P_1, and the energy which is in some way associated with cross-bridge motion. The ultimate source of the ATP is the ATP produced by the intermediary metabolisms of carbohydrates and lipids. As mentioned in previous answers the lengths of the myosin filaments would NOT be affected by ATP.

183. **C.**   Calcium ions released following an action potential in the fiber membrane and T-tubules bind with troponin. Calcium-troponin binding removes the inhibition of actomyosin formation. The sarcoplasmic reticulum concentrates calcium ions (Ca^{2+}) within its lumen, but depolarization of the T-tubule membrane induces the nearly terminal cisternae of the sarcoplasmic reticulum to release this Ca^{2+} into the sarcoplasm among the myofilaments. The Ca^{2+} becomes associated with the troponin of the thin myofilament, bringing about contraction.

184. **A.**   As shown in Figure 1, the percent of neutrophils bound increased from about 20% to about 50% as GMP-140 concentration increased. Tightness of binding, (C) and (D), was not measured, although it could contribute to the increased number of attached cells.

185. **B.**   Figure 1 indicates that about $1/4$ of monocytes attached at a GMP-140 concentration of zero.

186. **C.**   According to Figure 1, coating with GMP-140 caused little change in lymphocyte attachment, increased neutrophil attachment from about 20% up to about 50%, and increased monocyte attachment from 25% to about 75%.

187. **A.** Because GMP-140 coating of dishes increased neutrophil attachment (Figure 1), the neutrophils clearly attach to GMP-140. Pretreatment of neutrophils with GMP-140 (Figure 3) decreased attachment of the neutrophils to cultured endothelial cells, indicating that the GMP-140 binding sites on neutrophils are involved in endothelial attachment.

188. **D.** Treatment of neutrophils with antibody against CD-18 had no effect on attachment of neutrophils to GMP-140-coated dishes, so CD-18 on neutrophils is apparently not involved.

189. **A.** Neutrophils and macrophages (derived from monocytes) are most important in phagocytosis and if these cells could not easily leave vessels in inflammation sites, phagocytosis of bacteria should be impaired. Lymphocytes would not be affected because they do not appear to depend on GMP-140, so natural killer activity (due to large granular lymphocytes), cell-mediated responses (using helper T lymphocytes and cytotoxic T lymphocytes), and humoral responses (using helper T lymphocytes and B lymphocytes) should not be heavily affected. Some reduction in cell-mediated and humoral responses could occur due to reduction in macrophages available to serve as antigen-presenting cells and/or cytokine sources.

190. **B.** Enzymes are generally protein in nature, thus largely polymers of amino acids. Some other material may be present as well. The recent recognition of a small number of nucleic acids (ribozymes) that act as enzymes does not invalidate the question.

191. **C.** Enzymes function in reactions by decreasing the energy of activation. The net energy yield (positive or negative) is not affected, and a thermodynamically unfavorable reaction will not proceed simply by addition of an enzyme.

192. **D.** Enzymes are considered not to be used up in reaction. Incidental loss or destruction of enzyme does not require replacement however.

193. **A.** Covalent modification would not include changes of ions. Phosphorylation/dephosphorylation is often used as a means of regulation of activity of various enzymes. Sulfation/desulfation is seldom if ever employed.

194. **B.** The response of most enzymes to being boiled in aqueous solution is substantially decreased activity as a result of enzyme denaturation. (Remember that enzymes are proteins in general.) More moderate increase in temperature increases the activity of an enzyme.

195. **B.** The number of possible isomers is four. Note that positions 3 and 4 are chiral and thus may have the hydroxyl group on either side. Thus $2 \times 2 = 4$.

196. **B.** Although there appear at first glance to be three chiral centers, this is not so; the number 3 carbon is *not* attached to four nonidentical groups. Thus only four isomers appear to be possible, but it can be seen that two of these are identical and thus there are two optically active isomers and one optically inactive isomer.

197. **B.** There are two chiral centers.

198. **B.** Ribose is found in RNA, contributing to the name, ribonucleic acid. Deoxyribose is found in DNA.

199. **C.** As seen in the explanation for question 196, there are only two chiral centers (carbons 2 and 4).

200. **B.** DNA is the primary source of information. It is usually considered that DNA directs the synthesis of RNA and that RNA directs the synthesis of protein. DNA also directs its own replication. In some cases (for example the retroviruses), RNA can direct the synthesis of DNA.

201. **C.** RNA directs the synthesis of protein (see above) and three nucleotide bases are required to code for each amino acid.

202. **B.** Paired strands of DNA are found in the chromosomes of higher animals.

203. **A.** None of the cells will have only DNA containing deuterium. Each cell will have two strands of DNA for each chromosome, and one strand of each pair will contain deuterium.

204. **D.** As stated above, DNA is required to code for RNA and RNA is required to code for protein. The enzymes that actually carry out the biosynthesis are protein. (It might be argued that DNA is not required, but *ultimately* DNA is required for RNA synthesis.)

205. **A.** This study investigated the response of antibody produced by a host against the protein of the virus inducing tumor. Statements **C** and **D** are contradicted by the evidence. There is no information

to either confirm or deny statement **B**, however, it is clear that Brown Norway rats produced antibody at both time periods and, therefore, statement **A** is supported by the data presented.

206. **C.** From the experimental data, one can conclude that prolactin and LH are both produced by the pituitary, and that the hypothalamus stimulates LH release, but inhibits prolactin release, and that ovarian hormones inhibit LH release, but not prolactin release. Lactogenic hormone or luteotrophic hormone (LTH) or prolactin is secreted by the acidophils (alpha cells) of the pituitary. This hormone: (1) promotes growth of the breast, which has been stimulated already by estrogen and progesterone; (2) promotes and maintains lactation; (3) helps in maintenance of the corpus luteum; and (4) promotes maternal instinct.

207. **C.** The experiment was performed to determine the effect of salinity concentrations on the secretory proteins of the urophysis. The data shows that protein 2 was affected more (twice) by the increasing concentration of seawater than protein 1.

208. **D.** Careful analysis of the data shows that in the system under investigation, spleen cells and mast cells together are required for antibody production, that spleen cells are probably found in the thymus and that X-irradiation is an important tool in immunological work. Statement **C**, implying that spleen cells or mast cells are essential to the antibody production against pollen is contradicted by the data because bone marrow and pollen and thymocytes and pollen show a response. Statement **D** is not supported or contradicted by the experiment, even though mast cells are known to produce histamine and their activity is controlled by certain nasal sprays limiting their effects after exposure to certain substances.

209. **C.** Beta cells of the pituitary produce thyroid stimulating hormone, which stimulates the thyroid to produce its hormones T_3 (triiodothyronine) and T_4 (tetraiodothyronine or thyroxin). Iodides consumed in food and water are absorbed and carried to the iodide pool in the extracellular fluid via the circulatory system. Five events are involved in hormone production: (1) trapping iodide; (2) oxidation of iodide to organic iodine; (3) synthesis of hormone; (4) storage as the thyroglobulin moiety; and (5) release of the active principle into the circulation. TSH greatly influences the trapping mechanism; thiocyanates block trapping, whereas thiouracil blocks the oxidation and synthetic steps. The data show that Group 4

received thyroxine, which inhibited TSH production, whereas Group 2 was treated with thicoyanate, which affected the iodine pump. Group 3 received propylthiouracil, an inhibitor of iodine oxidation; in Group 2 iodine is not taken up and no radioactivty can be measured.

210. **B.** The five-year total of wheat was 49; for corn it was 56. The ratio is thus $7/8$.

211. **C.** Scanning of the graphs comparing the number of daylight hours clearly shows that only in greenhouses 2 and 3 are there provided 15 hours of light per day for several weeks, which is necessary for Plant X. If the question would have been that Plant Y will only bear fruit when the period of darkenss is 8 hours or less, it could not have born fruit in greenhouse 1. However, if Plant Z will only form flowers and seeds when exposed to days of no more than 15 hours in length, it certainly could not have been native in areas simulated by greenhouses 2 and 3.

212. **A.** Blood is composed of cells and plasma. Plasma constitutes about 55% of blood volume, and cellular elements about 45%. The normal red blood cell hematocrit is about 36–45%. Hemoglobin, a complex molecule of iron and protein, is a key element of the RBC; the RBC carries oxygen from the lungs to the tissues and transports carbon dioxide from the tissues to the lungs. In the breakdown of hemoglobin, bilirubin is excreted and iron is retained. The purpose of the experiment was to test the effect of different storage conditions on hemoglobin composition as revealed by gel electrophoresis. Although none of the storage conditions were able to maintain hemoglobin in an absoutely unchanged state, storage at –20°C in glycerol allowed the least change from the fresh configuration.

213. **C.** The suppressed plasma levels of FSH and LH during the follicular phase of the menstrual cycle are due to the negative inhibitory effects of estrogen being secreted from developing follicles. The small, abrupt rise in plasma estrogen is believed to trigger the ovulatory LH surge (by suspension of negative or positive feedback). During the luteal phase, estrogen and progesterone again establish the negative-feedback suppression and luteal failure occurs on day 26. The higher levels of bound LH in the treated animals indicate that these animals had lower LH levels; the drug seems to inhibit LH release.

214. **B.** Examination of the data shows that all three proteins were absorbed at the same rate (2 minutes) by the visceral endoderm; the visceral endoderm appeared to block the transport of protein Y, whereas protein X appeared to be transported through it. The statement that the visceral basement membrane blocked the transport of protein X is not supported by the data because it is found at the next level, namely, the vitelline endothelium. The vitelline endothelium does, however, block protein X from entering the fetal blood.

215. **B.** The fiber components of connective tissue add strength and support. They are collagenous, elastic, and reticular in nature; collagen fibers are the most numerous fiber type. The graphs show that labeled proline starts to appear in the collagen in under 2 hours, so **B** was supported by the evidence. Statements **A** and **C** were contradicted by the information given, and **D** is neither supported nor contradicted.

216. **B.** Glycine has no chiral center, but other amino acids in higher animals are ordinarily of the L-series.

217. **C.** Carbohydrate monosaccharides found in higher animals are generally of the D-series.

218. **B.** Epimers differ in configuration at only one carbon. Enantiomers are nonsuperimposable mirror images. Diastereomers are nonsuperimposable nonmirror images.

219. **C.** The number of kcal/g for the classes of food material are: carbohydrates, 4; proteins, 4; and fats, 9. The nucleic acids are not considered as a class of food.

The MCAT
Model Examination D

ANSWER SHEET

DIRECTIONS: After locating the number of the question to which you are responding, fill in the circle containing the letter of the answer you have selected. Use pencil (not a ballpoint pen) to completely blacken the circle.

VERBAL REASONING

1. Ⓐ Ⓑ Ⓒ Ⓓ
2. Ⓐ Ⓑ Ⓒ Ⓓ
3. Ⓐ Ⓑ Ⓒ Ⓓ
4. Ⓐ Ⓑ Ⓒ Ⓓ
5. Ⓐ Ⓑ Ⓒ Ⓓ
6. Ⓐ Ⓑ Ⓒ Ⓓ
7. Ⓐ Ⓑ Ⓒ Ⓓ
8. Ⓐ Ⓑ Ⓒ Ⓓ
9. Ⓐ Ⓑ Ⓒ Ⓓ
10. Ⓐ Ⓑ Ⓒ Ⓓ
11. Ⓐ Ⓑ Ⓒ Ⓓ
12. Ⓐ Ⓑ Ⓒ Ⓓ
13. Ⓐ Ⓑ Ⓒ Ⓓ
14. Ⓐ Ⓑ Ⓒ Ⓓ
15. Ⓐ Ⓑ Ⓒ Ⓓ
16. Ⓐ Ⓑ Ⓒ Ⓓ
17. Ⓐ Ⓑ Ⓒ Ⓓ
18. Ⓐ Ⓑ Ⓒ Ⓓ
19. Ⓐ Ⓑ Ⓒ Ⓓ
20. Ⓐ Ⓑ Ⓒ Ⓓ
21. Ⓐ Ⓑ Ⓒ Ⓓ
22. Ⓐ Ⓑ Ⓒ Ⓓ
23. Ⓐ Ⓑ Ⓒ Ⓓ
24. Ⓐ Ⓑ Ⓒ Ⓓ
25. Ⓐ Ⓑ Ⓒ Ⓓ
26. Ⓐ Ⓑ Ⓒ Ⓓ
27. Ⓐ Ⓑ Ⓒ Ⓓ
28. Ⓐ Ⓑ Ⓒ Ⓓ
29. Ⓐ Ⓑ Ⓒ Ⓓ
30. Ⓐ Ⓑ Ⓒ Ⓓ

31. Ⓐ Ⓑ Ⓒ Ⓓ
32. Ⓐ Ⓑ Ⓒ Ⓓ
33. Ⓐ Ⓑ Ⓒ Ⓓ
34. Ⓐ Ⓑ Ⓒ Ⓓ
35. Ⓐ Ⓑ Ⓒ Ⓓ
36. Ⓐ Ⓑ Ⓒ Ⓓ
37. Ⓐ Ⓑ Ⓒ Ⓓ
38. Ⓐ Ⓑ Ⓒ Ⓓ
39. Ⓐ Ⓑ Ⓒ Ⓓ
40. Ⓐ Ⓑ Ⓒ Ⓓ
41. Ⓐ Ⓑ Ⓒ Ⓓ
42. Ⓐ Ⓑ Ⓒ Ⓓ
43. Ⓐ Ⓑ Ⓒ Ⓓ
44. Ⓐ Ⓑ Ⓒ Ⓓ
45. Ⓐ Ⓑ Ⓒ Ⓓ
46. Ⓐ Ⓑ Ⓒ Ⓓ
47. Ⓐ Ⓑ Ⓒ Ⓓ
48. Ⓐ Ⓑ Ⓒ Ⓓ
49. Ⓐ Ⓑ Ⓒ Ⓓ
50. Ⓐ Ⓑ Ⓒ Ⓓ
51. Ⓐ Ⓑ Ⓒ Ⓓ
52. Ⓐ Ⓑ Ⓒ Ⓓ
53. Ⓐ Ⓑ Ⓒ Ⓓ
54. Ⓐ Ⓑ Ⓒ Ⓓ
55. Ⓐ Ⓑ Ⓒ Ⓓ
56. Ⓐ Ⓑ Ⓒ Ⓓ
57. Ⓐ Ⓑ Ⓒ Ⓓ
58. Ⓐ Ⓑ Ⓒ Ⓓ
59. Ⓐ Ⓑ Ⓒ Ⓓ
60. Ⓐ Ⓑ Ⓒ Ⓓ

61. Ⓐ Ⓑ Ⓒ Ⓓ
62. Ⓐ Ⓑ Ⓒ Ⓓ
63. Ⓐ Ⓑ Ⓒ Ⓓ
64. Ⓐ Ⓑ Ⓒ Ⓓ
65. Ⓐ Ⓑ Ⓒ Ⓓ

PHYSICAL SCIENCES

66. Ⓐ Ⓑ Ⓒ Ⓓ
67. Ⓐ Ⓑ Ⓒ Ⓓ
68. Ⓐ Ⓑ Ⓒ Ⓓ
69. Ⓐ Ⓑ Ⓒ Ⓓ
70. Ⓐ Ⓑ Ⓒ Ⓓ
71. Ⓐ Ⓑ Ⓒ Ⓓ
72. Ⓐ Ⓑ Ⓒ Ⓓ
73. Ⓐ Ⓑ Ⓒ Ⓓ
74. Ⓐ Ⓑ Ⓒ Ⓓ
75. Ⓐ Ⓑ Ⓒ Ⓓ
76. Ⓐ Ⓑ Ⓒ Ⓓ
77. Ⓐ Ⓑ Ⓒ Ⓓ
78. Ⓐ Ⓑ Ⓒ Ⓓ
79. Ⓐ Ⓑ Ⓒ Ⓓ
80. Ⓐ Ⓑ Ⓒ Ⓓ
81. Ⓐ Ⓑ Ⓒ Ⓓ
82. Ⓐ Ⓑ Ⓒ Ⓓ
83. Ⓐ Ⓑ Ⓒ Ⓓ
84. Ⓐ Ⓑ Ⓒ Ⓓ
85. Ⓐ Ⓑ Ⓒ Ⓓ
86. Ⓐ Ⓑ Ⓒ Ⓓ
87. Ⓐ Ⓑ Ⓒ Ⓓ
88. Ⓐ Ⓑ Ⓒ Ⓓ

89. Ⓐ Ⓑ Ⓒ Ⓓ
90. Ⓐ Ⓑ Ⓒ Ⓓ
91. Ⓐ Ⓑ Ⓒ Ⓓ
92. Ⓐ Ⓑ Ⓒ Ⓓ
93. Ⓐ Ⓑ Ⓒ Ⓓ
94. Ⓐ Ⓑ Ⓒ Ⓓ
95. Ⓐ Ⓑ Ⓒ Ⓓ
96. Ⓐ Ⓑ Ⓒ Ⓓ
97. Ⓐ Ⓑ Ⓒ Ⓓ
98. Ⓐ Ⓑ Ⓒ Ⓓ
99. Ⓐ Ⓑ Ⓒ Ⓓ
100. Ⓐ Ⓑ Ⓒ Ⓓ
101. Ⓐ Ⓑ Ⓒ Ⓓ
102. Ⓐ Ⓑ Ⓒ Ⓓ
103. Ⓐ Ⓑ Ⓒ Ⓓ
104. Ⓐ Ⓑ Ⓒ Ⓓ
105. Ⓐ Ⓑ Ⓒ Ⓓ
106. Ⓐ Ⓑ Ⓒ Ⓓ
107. Ⓐ Ⓑ Ⓒ Ⓓ
108. Ⓐ Ⓑ Ⓒ Ⓓ
109. Ⓐ Ⓑ Ⓒ Ⓓ
110. Ⓐ Ⓑ Ⓒ Ⓓ
111. Ⓐ Ⓑ Ⓒ Ⓓ
112. Ⓐ Ⓑ Ⓒ Ⓓ
113. Ⓐ Ⓑ Ⓒ Ⓓ
114. Ⓐ Ⓑ Ⓒ Ⓓ
115. Ⓐ Ⓑ Ⓒ Ⓓ
116. Ⓐ Ⓑ Ⓒ Ⓓ
117. Ⓐ Ⓑ Ⓒ Ⓓ
118. Ⓐ Ⓑ Ⓒ Ⓓ

119. Ⓐ Ⓑ Ⓒ Ⓓ
120. Ⓐ Ⓑ Ⓒ Ⓓ
121. Ⓐ Ⓑ Ⓒ Ⓓ
122. Ⓐ Ⓑ Ⓒ Ⓓ
123. Ⓐ Ⓑ Ⓒ Ⓓ
124. Ⓐ Ⓑ Ⓒ Ⓓ
125. Ⓐ Ⓑ Ⓒ Ⓓ
126. Ⓐ Ⓑ Ⓒ Ⓓ
127. Ⓐ Ⓑ Ⓒ Ⓓ
128. Ⓐ Ⓑ Ⓒ Ⓓ
129. Ⓐ Ⓑ Ⓒ Ⓓ
130. Ⓐ Ⓑ Ⓒ Ⓓ
131. Ⓐ Ⓑ Ⓒ Ⓓ
132. Ⓐ Ⓑ Ⓒ Ⓓ
133. Ⓐ Ⓑ Ⓒ Ⓓ
134. Ⓐ Ⓑ Ⓒ Ⓓ
135. Ⓐ Ⓑ Ⓒ Ⓓ
136. Ⓐ Ⓑ Ⓒ Ⓓ
137. Ⓐ Ⓑ Ⓒ Ⓓ
138. Ⓐ Ⓑ Ⓒ Ⓓ
139. Ⓐ Ⓑ Ⓒ Ⓓ
140. Ⓐ Ⓑ Ⓒ Ⓓ
141. Ⓐ Ⓑ Ⓒ Ⓓ
142. Ⓐ Ⓑ Ⓒ Ⓓ

WRITING SAMPLE
Use separate ruled sheets of paper.

BIOLOGICAL SCIENCES

143. Ⓐ Ⓑ Ⓒ Ⓓ
144. Ⓐ Ⓑ Ⓒ Ⓓ
145. Ⓐ Ⓑ Ⓒ Ⓓ
146. Ⓐ Ⓑ Ⓒ Ⓓ
147. Ⓐ Ⓑ Ⓒ Ⓓ
148. Ⓐ Ⓑ Ⓒ Ⓓ
149. Ⓐ Ⓑ Ⓒ Ⓓ
150. Ⓐ Ⓑ Ⓒ Ⓓ
151. Ⓐ Ⓑ Ⓒ Ⓓ
152. Ⓐ Ⓑ Ⓒ Ⓓ
153. Ⓐ Ⓑ Ⓒ Ⓓ
154. Ⓐ Ⓑ Ⓒ Ⓓ
155. Ⓐ Ⓑ Ⓒ Ⓓ
156. Ⓐ Ⓑ Ⓒ Ⓓ
157. Ⓐ Ⓑ Ⓒ Ⓓ
158. Ⓐ Ⓑ Ⓒ Ⓓ
159. Ⓐ Ⓑ Ⓒ Ⓓ
160. Ⓐ Ⓑ Ⓒ Ⓓ
161. Ⓐ Ⓑ Ⓒ Ⓓ
162. Ⓐ Ⓑ Ⓒ Ⓓ
163. Ⓐ Ⓑ Ⓒ Ⓓ
164. Ⓐ Ⓑ Ⓒ Ⓓ
165. Ⓐ Ⓑ Ⓒ Ⓓ
166. Ⓐ Ⓑ Ⓒ Ⓓ
167. Ⓐ Ⓑ Ⓒ Ⓓ

168. Ⓐ Ⓑ Ⓒ Ⓓ
169. Ⓐ Ⓑ Ⓒ Ⓓ
170. Ⓐ Ⓑ Ⓒ Ⓓ
171. Ⓐ Ⓑ Ⓒ Ⓓ
172. Ⓐ Ⓑ Ⓒ Ⓓ
173. Ⓐ Ⓑ Ⓒ Ⓓ
174. Ⓐ Ⓑ Ⓒ Ⓓ
175. Ⓐ Ⓑ Ⓒ Ⓓ
176. Ⓐ Ⓑ Ⓒ Ⓓ
177. Ⓐ Ⓑ Ⓒ Ⓓ
178. Ⓐ Ⓑ Ⓒ Ⓓ
179. Ⓐ Ⓑ Ⓒ Ⓓ
180. Ⓐ Ⓑ Ⓒ Ⓓ
181. Ⓐ Ⓑ Ⓒ Ⓓ
182. Ⓐ Ⓑ Ⓒ Ⓓ
183. Ⓐ Ⓑ Ⓒ Ⓓ
184. Ⓐ Ⓑ Ⓒ Ⓓ
185. Ⓐ Ⓑ Ⓒ Ⓓ
186. Ⓐ Ⓑ Ⓒ Ⓓ
187. Ⓐ Ⓑ Ⓒ Ⓓ
188. Ⓐ Ⓑ Ⓒ Ⓓ
189. Ⓐ Ⓑ Ⓒ Ⓓ
190. Ⓐ Ⓑ Ⓒ Ⓓ
191. Ⓐ Ⓑ Ⓒ Ⓓ
192. Ⓐ Ⓑ Ⓒ Ⓓ
193. Ⓐ Ⓑ Ⓒ Ⓓ

194. Ⓐ Ⓑ Ⓒ Ⓓ
195. Ⓐ Ⓑ Ⓒ Ⓓ
196. Ⓐ Ⓑ Ⓒ Ⓓ
197. Ⓐ Ⓑ Ⓒ Ⓓ
198. Ⓐ Ⓑ Ⓒ Ⓓ
199. Ⓐ Ⓑ Ⓒ Ⓓ
200. Ⓐ Ⓑ Ⓒ Ⓓ
201. Ⓐ Ⓑ Ⓒ Ⓓ
202. Ⓐ Ⓑ Ⓒ Ⓓ
203. Ⓐ Ⓑ Ⓒ Ⓓ
204. Ⓐ Ⓑ Ⓒ Ⓓ
205. Ⓐ Ⓑ Ⓒ Ⓓ
206. Ⓐ Ⓑ Ⓒ Ⓓ
207. Ⓐ Ⓑ Ⓒ Ⓓ
208. Ⓐ Ⓑ Ⓒ Ⓓ
209. Ⓐ Ⓑ Ⓒ Ⓓ
210. Ⓐ Ⓑ Ⓒ Ⓓ
211. Ⓐ Ⓑ Ⓒ Ⓓ
212. Ⓐ Ⓑ Ⓒ Ⓓ
213. Ⓐ Ⓑ Ⓒ Ⓓ
214. Ⓐ Ⓑ Ⓒ Ⓓ
215. Ⓐ Ⓑ Ⓒ Ⓓ
216. Ⓐ Ⓑ Ⓒ Ⓓ
217. Ⓐ Ⓑ Ⓒ Ⓓ
218. Ⓐ Ⓑ Ⓒ Ⓓ
219. Ⓐ Ⓑ Ⓒ Ⓓ

The MCAT
Model Examination D

VERBAL REASONING

9 PASSAGES
65 QUESTIONS
85 MINUTES

DIRECTIONS: The questions are based on the accompanying passages. Read each passage carefully, then answer the following questions. Consider only the material within the passage. For each question, select the ONE BEST ANSWER and indicate your selection by marking the corresponding letter on the Answer Form.

Passage I (Questions 1–7)

In the fall of 1990, a vigorous debate broke out at the University of Texas at Austin, a debate that turned into a heated national conversation on the purpose of the writing classroom and, to some extent, the purpose of liberal education. Among composition specialists the debate delineated two separate ways of thinking about freshman composition and the field of composition studies.

The debate focused on a proposed curriculum for the freshman composition program at the University of Texas, English 306, a curriculum which required students to produce approximately 3,900 words of writing and taught students to conduct and sustain rhetorical inquiry into a single topic. Some of the goals of the curriculum were to introduce undergraduates to the intellectual demands of college through the teaching of skills such as analysis, research, and synthesis, to create an intimate, participatory classroom experience for the students whose freshman schedules are often otherwise confined to huge lecture halls, and to help the new graduate student teachers focus on the teaching of writing by creating a bridge between skills learned in the study of literature and the teaching of freshman composition. All seemingly laudable, standard goals for freshman composition. The problem, the reason for the violent debate, was the topic chosen for the class: difference, specifically difference related to legal opinions given in court cases involving issues such as race, gender, bilingualism, and sexual orientation. The debate that followed the submission and ultimate rejection of the program in many ways disregarded the course itself; the discussion became a forum for stating the purpose of composition and liberal education.

One group, that I will call the traditionalists, view the writing classroom as the place to focus on process, a place where students write, primarily, personal essays

to engage in the writing process. The other group, the radical pedagogists, believe that the purpose of the writing classroom is to engage the student as critical thinker, often defined as one who rethinks cultural assumptions and becomes committed to social change. There are varying views among radical pedagogists of the ways and means of teaching critical thinking. . .

. . . The traditionalist point of view is, relatively speaking, fairly new. It arose in the past 25 years or so, in tandem with the advent of composition studies as a legitimate academic discipline. The traditionalist approach focuses on process, and states that a primary way to engage the student is to have the student determine essay topics. As Richard Graves says, "the first lesson in teaching composition is that the writer must find his or her own subject." This student-centered approach assumes that the student will not only be more invested in the essay if the idea originates with her, but that the student learns that she has a wealth of information inside her, information that once organized not only reflects her knowledge base but proves interesting to others. This new knowledge engages the student in her own writing, making it a forum for her voice, thus giving her a sense of legitimacy to her own experiences and reflections. Although aware of the powerful effects of writing on the student as thinker, the primary concern for the traditionalists is the student as writer, as they seek to engage the students in the process and act of writing.

The radical pedagogists are more concerned with the student as thinker and want to use the mind power generated in the writing process to foster social change. Patricia Bizzell states that "we rhetoricians like to see ourselves as social reformers, if not revolutionaries.". . . This concern with social and political change is prevalent among the radial pedagogists. Sharon Crowley states that "freshman composition can be radicalized in the service of social justice" and commends

Adapted from a paper by Abby Arnold, "Empowerment Pedagogy and the Writing Classroom," English 636, VCU, 1996 and used with permission of the author.

writers who "would put literacy to work with the specific goal of effecting social change." There is little mention among these highly political pedagogists of the student as writer, or of developing writing skills in a student for the sake of individual education.

Donald Lazere, a committed leftist educator and radical pedagogist, offers an alternative to both schools of composition theory. He sees student empowerment and social change as coming through the student's learning to write, thus learning to access and manipulate the dialogue of mainstream culture. He criticizes both the "process" contention that skills are less important than the act of writing and the "radical" determination to focus on critical thinking at the expense of writing instruction. He states that "the lack of basic skills and factual knowledge is an obstacle to autonomous critical thinking" and that "a sophisticated level of literacy is virtually necessary, or at least highly advantageous, for effective opposition to the dominant culture in today's society."

Although committed to his view of social change, Lazere is also committed to the growth of the student. He recognizes the coercive nature of some radical pedagogy, the kind of belief in one's agenda which led Sharon Crowley to state that composition teachers "must give up our traditional subscription to liberal tolerance if we are to bring about social change through [our students.]" Lazere believes that to force any ideology on students "is only to replace the coercion . . . in mainstream education with coercion into accord with an opposing ideology."

1. Which of the following was **not** a stated goal of the freshman curriculum at the University of Texas when the debate over English 306 broke out?

   A. to create a smaller, more intimate classroom experience than freshmen typically have
   B. to help new graduate student teachers focus on the teaching of writing
   C. to teach freshmen how to bring about social change through their writing
   D. to introduce freshmen to the intellectual demands of college by teaching various skills

2. Of the two main groups in opposition with each other in the University of Texas debate, which of the following groups have as a goal to use of writing and the teaching of writing to bring about social change?

   A. the traditionalists
   B. the pragmatists
   C. the radical pedagogists
   D. the purists

3. According to the passage, Donald Lazere could best be characterized as

   A. a leftist educator.
   B. a person who would disagree with the methods proposed by Sharon Crowley.
   C. a radical pedagogist.
   D. all of the above.

4. The proposed topic for English 306 was to include

   A. a study of world literature.
   B. an examination of the relationship between writing for the mass media and writing for scholarly journals.
   C. a study of legal opinions from court cases involving, among other things, sexual orientation.
   D. an analysis of fiction and creative nonfiction.

5. Based on the quotations attributed to Sharon Crowley in the passage, we can deduce that she belongs to the group referred to as

   A. the traditionalists.
   B. the radical pedgaogists.
   C. the free thinkers.
   D. the grammar advocates.

6. Though the University of Texas debate originated as a response to a proposed course in the curriculum, it evolved into something larger. Which of the following best describes what the debate became?

   A. a referendum on the role of the teaching of literature in composition classes
   B. an examination of the positive and negative factors in using graduate teaching assistants in the freshman classroom
   C. a forum on the teaching of grammar and usage in freshman composition classes
   D. a forum for stating the purpose of composition and liberal education

7. The proposed curriculum, which involved English 306, was ultimately

   A. defeated.
   B. passed by a slim majority.
   C. deferred for a year.
   D. approved, but only for one year.

Passage II (Questions 8–15)

To establish a prima facie case of sex discrimination in compensation, an employee must present data that compare her salary to that of male coworkers doing the same job under the same circumstances. The standard or test that has emerged from case law is called the equal pay for equal work standard. Not to be confused with the idea that one must hold a job identical to that of someone else, that standard is built on a concept that evaluates jobs within a context of substantial equivalency. The issue to probe thus becomes: Is complainant's job equal in effort and responsibility to that of a male counterpart? A corollary question also is asked. Do the two incumbents in these jobs (the male and the female) possess comparable skills?

On March 11, 1974, the Secretary of Labor took action against Columbia University and its president, seeking to enjoin the University from discriminating against its female custodial workers (classified as light cleaners). Alleging a violation of the Equal Pay Act on the basis of sex, the evidence showed that female light cleaners were paid a lower hourly rate than male heavy cleaners. At trial, the court came to the conclusion that the jobs of light cleaners and heavy cleaners were different. And, because the job of heavy cleaners involved greater effort than that of light cleaners, the plaintiff had failed to sustain the burden of establishing the idea of equal work within the meaning of the Act.

On appeal, the Second Circuit Court of Appeals focused its attention on the "equal effort" criteria in connection with the workers' primary duties. The Court stated:

> The concept of "effort" in the act is straightforward. It calls for a direct comparison of the amount of physical exertion required by the jobs; there is no factor added to compensate for physiological differences between men and women. Based on our careful review of the record before us we cannot say that the district court was clearly erroneous in making this direct comparison and the finding as a fact that heavy cleaning involves "greater effort."

The court also noted that the differences between the heavy cleaner and light cleaner jobs were known by the employees. Furthermore, no heavy cleaner job had ever been denied to a woman. In fact, in 1972, Columbia opened a heavy cleaner category to women, and seven light cleaners were accepted into on-the-job training for that position. However, after seven weeks, four of the seven workers transferred back to light cleaning.

Adapted from Richard S. Vacca: "Sex Discrimination in Public School Employment." In S. B. Thomas, N. H. Cambron-McCabe, and M. M. McCarthy, Eds., *Education and the Law*, New York: Institute for School Law and Finance, 1983.

In conclusion, the circuit court held that based on the evidence of the understanding and experience of the individuals most closely involved, together with the undisputed fact that heavy cleaning called for greater effort, there was no valid claim of unequal pay for substantial equivalent work within the meaning of the Equal Pay Act.

A new and more controversial standard in sex discrimination cases involves the notion of comparable worth. Under the theory of comparable worth, one must look beyond the equal pay for equal work criterion. In such cases, the female plaintiff argues the intrinsic worth, or the intrinsic difficulty of her job, as compared to other jobs in the same organization. Such an argument thus carries the complaint beyond the confines of an equal wage matter and places it under the broader umbrella protection of Title VII.

The judiciary has not yet endorsed the notion of comparable worth, but the Supreme Court has ruled that Title VII provides a remedy for sex discrimination in compensation beyond that covered by the Equal Pay Act. The matter arose in Washington County, Oregon, when four women guards in the female section of the county jail alleged that they were paid unequal wages for work substantially equal to that performed by male guards. In their complaint, the women guards charged that because of intentional discrimination, the county set the pay scale of female guards (but not male guards) "at a level lower than that warranted by its own survey of outside markets and the worth of the jobs."

After an adverse decision at trial, the female guards appealed to the Eighth Circuit Court of Appeals. The appellate court reversed the trial court and held that petitioners were not precluded from suing under Title VII, solely because their jobs were not substantially equal to higher-paying jobs held by male employees. The Supreme Court agreed and ruled in County of *Washington v. Gunther* that the wage differentials were based on intentional sex discrimination even though female guards did not actually perform work equal to that of male guards. Although not adopting the controversial concept of comparable worth, the Court left the door open for a comparable worth argument to be raised in future litigation.

It is significant to note that Justice Rehnquist for the four dissenters in *Gunther* strongly stated that this decision could spell the nullification of the Equal Pay Act if future plaintiffs are allowed to substitute the comparable worth standard for that of the equal pay for equal work standard. He asserted that the majority's opinion must be read narrowly ("the opinion does not endorse the so-called 'comparable worth' theory): though the Court does not indicate how a plaintiff might establish a prima facie case under Title VII, the Court does suggest that allegations of unequal pay for unequal, but comparable, work will not state a claim on which relief may be granted."

Others would argue that the Supreme Court's decision in *Gunther* establishes a possibility for plaintiffs in future cases to be given the opportunity to produce evidence showing a Title VII violation based on a comparable worth, rather than on an equal work basis. For example, female teachers might argue that over the years the historical pattern and practice in public school systems have inflated the value and salaries of certain jobs simply because they were held by men, while depressing the value and salaries of other jobs because they were held by women, even though each of the jobs is of comparable worth to the school system.

8. When one investigates an equal pay issue, attention must be given to:

    I.   equal worth.
    II. equal effort.
    III. equal length of employment.
    IV. equal responsibility.

    A. I, II, and III   **C.** II and IV
    B. I and III   **D.** I, II, III, and IV

9. From information provided in the passage, which of the following conclusions is one justified in drawing?

    A. Identical jobs should receive equal reimbursement.
    B. Substantial equivalency is at the bottom of the issue.
    C. The question also to be asked is whether the concerned possess equal levels of education.
    D. Effort, attitude, drive, and determination are important considerations in equal pay for equal work cases.

10. In sex discrimination cases the courts:

    I.   have considered the fact that women bear children.
    II. have decided that maternity leave is a constitutional right.
    III. have allowed the notion of physical and physiological differences.
    IV. view the Equal Pay Act and the Title VII laws as equal in impact.

    A. I, II, and III
    B. I and III
    C. II and IV
    D. neither I, II, III, nor IV

11. The Columbia University case illustrates:

    A. that on-the-job training is essential in avoiding problems.
    B. the haphazard approach used by the Department of Labor in filing suit.
    C. that employees are not always aware of differences in their jobs.
    D. the well-defined limits of the Equal Pay Act in regard to the equal effort interpretation.

12. Which of the following statement(s) is/are *supported by* the passage?

    I.   Comparable worth is a complex issue.
    II. In comparable worth issues one must probe well beyond the equal pay for equal work issues.
    III. The Supreme Court considers Title VII as a remedy for sex discrimination.
    IV. The judiciary has endorsed Title VII.

    A. I, II, and III   **C.** II and IV
    B. I and III   **D.** I, II, III, and IV

13. In the Oregon case:

    I.   the first trial ended with a ruling for the county.
    II. the first trial resulted in no definitive decision.
    III. the appellate court did not preclude a suit based on job unequality.
    IV. the Supreme court adopted the concept of comparable worth.

    A. I, II, and III   **C.** II and IV
    B. I and III   **D.** I, II, III, and IV

14. The passage substantiates which of the following observations?

    I.   There were four dissenters to the Supreme Court decision.
    II. Concern was voiced about the future effectiveness of the Equal Pay Act.
    III. It is anticipated that litigation might substitute the principle of comparable worth for the argument equal pay and equal work.
    IV. The majority opinion clearly defined the limits of the decision in the *County of Washington v. Gunther* case.

    A. I, II, and III   **C.** IV only
    B. I and III   **D.** I, II, III, and IV

15. The main theme of this passage can be considered to be:

A. Equal Pay Act v. Title VII.
B. comparable worth.
C. sex discrimination.
D. judiciary policy making.

Passage III (Questions 16–24)

There have been two controversies over Eoanthopus, and it is the first of them that has incongruous mandible for its theme. The question at issue was whether this specimen represents a single creature or two different ones. Scientist made reconstructions reconciling jaw and skull; however, one group described the jaw as an ape's separately from the skull that was assigned to Homo sapiens. The finder's argument ran as follows: All of the remains were found very close together. The lower jaw and brain case were both of a similar brown color and apparently in the same state of fossilization. The jaw, even though ape-like, did have human features, particularly in the teeth. The molar teeth had apparently been worn to a flatness never seen in apes, and only expected if the jaw had belonged to a type of human being. The roots of the teeth seen radiologically also resembled human teeth. The appearance of this ape-like man at the beginning of the Ice Age was just what many authorities expected to find. Shortly thereafter, a canine tooth, ape-like, but worn in a way never found in modern apes, was found. This was strong support for the missing link interpretation and man's ape-like ancestry. Questions remained concerning how anatomically the jaw could have worked as part of a human skull, and a wear of the teeth.

Three years later, about two miles away from the first site, pieces of a thick braincase and a molar tooth (both similar to the first find) were unearthed. The climate was ripe for the view that the human ancestor would show a combination of ape and man. However, as more human fossils were found in other parts of the world, this particular specimen differed from all in regard to skull characteristics. Their braincases were far more ape-like and their jaws less so, and a consistent line of evolution was found. Restorations of the cranium resulted in the revisions of brain volume, but in the end the controversial specimen had a brain of modern size to go with its modern skull.

If the remains were old, they would be accepted even though odd and isolated. When the fluorine method was applied, it was found that neither jawbone nor braincase contained more than small traces of fluorine meaning that the specimen did not date before the Ice Age. The speci-

men was now believed to be 50,000 and not 500,000 years old, making it an evolutionary absurdity with no known ancestor or descendants. An explanation was to suppose that a piece of modern ape jaw had been deliberately placed with an ancient braincase and both suitably stained. Another fluorine analysis placed the braincase as ancient, but the jaw and teeth in modern times. In fact, chemical analysis showed that the jaw and teeth contained the same amount of nitrogen and organic carbon as modern specimens, the calvarium, however, much less. Ruling out that the organic matter was not gelatin or glue with which the specimen had been impregnated as a means of hardening was accomplished with electron microscopy because the jaw showed preserved fibers of organic tissue and the calvarium laced this feature. Besides this, it was established that the jaw had been colored artificially with iron to match the calvarium.

The first specimen was apparently made up by placement of an artificially abraded molar tooth of an orangutan with a piece of thick frontal bone; the last fragment found duplicated the thinnest part of the first skull. Chromium detected in the jaw indicates that a dichromate solution was used in an attempt to assist the oxidation of iron salts used to stain these specimens.

16. The skull was classified to belong to:

I. a vertebrate.
II. a mammal.
III. a man.
IV. an ape.

A. I, II, and III
B. I and III
C. II and IV
D. I, II, III, and IV

17. This passage was probably written by:

A. a historian.
B. an anthropologist.
C. a sociologist.
D. an archeologist.

18. From the passage one could surmise that fluorine:

A. was obtained from drinking water.
B. was absorbed from the soil.
C. becomes more concentrated.
D. is a by-product of the decay process.

19. If the jawbone was modern, its fluorine content in relation to the braincase would have been:

A. the same.
B. more.
C. less.
D. not important in the solution.

From H. R. Seibel, "The Piltdown Hoax," *Bioscope*, 1962.

20. The analysis of iron was used to establish:

    A. a color comparison.
    B. the organic matrix pattern.
    C. the age of the specimens.
    D. none of the above.

21. The piece of fossil found last was:

    A. not unusual in size.
    B. thick.
    C. thin.
    D. none of the above.

22. With age, iron salts:

    A. are reduced.
    B. are halogenated.
    C. deteriorate.
    D. are oxidized.

23. Chromium:

    A. is naturally found in bones.
    B. is absorbed from the surrounding areas by a specimen.
    C. is used as a parameter in testing fossils.
    D. none of the above.

24. The passage mainly deals with:

    A. the development of experimental methods of studying fossils.
    B. the verification of the missing link.
    C. a valuable fossil find.
    D. a brilliantly devised falsification.

Passage IV (Questions 25–32)

Many who have seen photographs of Zelda Sayre Fitzgerald note that no two images of her resemble each other. She had many different, unforgettable faces, among them the polished and strikingly beautiful one which appeared on the cover of *Hearst's International* magazine in the early 1920s and which she referred to as her Elizabeth Arden face. But the different faces of Zelda, as the Fitzgeralds' friend Sara Murphy observed shortly after Zelda's first mental breakdown, had much less to do with subtle changes in makeup or lighting than with inner complexity and mystery that no one, not even her husband Scott, ever touched. There have been many constructions of Zelda Fitzgerald, all hinting at the complexity that Sara Murphy noted. But, not surprisingly, the various constructions like the various photographs of Zelda's face rarely resemble each other.

From the actual Zelda Sayre of Montgomery,

Alabama, Scott Fitzgerald constructed a fairy princess, hidden away in a tower to be rescued from her provincial surroundings and taken by him into the more sophisticated world of Princeton and New York. She had been born July 24, 1900, the sixth child of Alabama Judge Anthony Sayre and his wife Minnie, who named Zelda after a gypsy queen in a novel she had read and who spoiled her from the beginning, nursing her, some say, until she was 4 years old. By the time Fitzgerald arrived at Fort Sheridan, near Montgomery, in his tailored Brooks Brothers uniform Zelda was, at 18, thought of as an original, a daring local beauty who was known not only in Montgomery but in most college towns in Alabama. She became not only Scott's idealized version of the Southern Belle but also the incarnation of all that was desirable in woman. He went back to New York from Montgomery after the war was over, finished the novel that was to become *This Side of Paradise*, sent for Zelda, and married her in the rectory of St. Patrick's Cathedral.

The process of Scott's invention and reinvention of Zelda, which had already begun with his creation of the heroine of "The Ice Palace," set in a small southern town, would be repeated numerous times in the next two decades, among other places in Gloria in *The Beautiful and Damned* and in Daisy in *The Great Gatsby*. His two final fictional recreations of Zelda in fiction, as Nicole Diver in *Tender Is the Night* and as Ailie Calhoun in "The Last of the Belles," remain strong at the end, though the hero has lost the ability to sustain a romantic vision of her. Fitzgerald constructed and reconstructed Zelda for as long as he had the emotional vitality to do so. But after Zelda's mental collapse, precipitated in part by her obsessive pursuit of ballet—in effect her obsessive pursuit of an artistic identity of her own that she could have separate from Scott's imagined version of her—Scott began his descent into alcoholism. He left his capacity for hope, he said, on the road leading away from Zelda's sanitarium.

Nancy Milford, Zelda's first major biographer, constructs a Zelda shaped in large part by Scott's exploitation of her, by his appropriation of her image and even of the prose from her diaries for the purpose of enhancing his own literary reputation. There was no room for two artists in the Fitzgerald household, as Milford's description of the bitter conflict that surrounded the publication of Zelda's 1932 novel *Save Me the Waltz* demonstrates. She was, as Scott reminded her, a third-rate talent. But his assault on Zelda's self-esteem is only part of Milford's picture of a self divided by internal forces beyond her control. Her entrapment in a world with little understanding or appreciation of her predica-

Adapted from "Zelda," VCU, 1995 and used with permission of Dr. Bryant Mangum.

ment makes Milford's Zelda a symbol for our time, her death in 1948 by fire while locked away in the upper reaches of a mental institution dramatically underscoring the powerlessness of her plight. Sara Mayfield's competing portrait of Zelda, who was Mayfield's girlhood friend, depicts a southern belle whose major misfortune was her loss of the traditions of the genteel South at the hands of Scott, who took Zelda from her home and set in motion the tragedy of two "exiles from paradise." These are only two of many recreations of Zelda.

The actual Zelda Sayre Fitzgerald is fragmented in the many constructions of her life that we have. Once, in an attempt to establish the historical truth about Zelda's role in Scott's life and his role in hers, someone asked Scott for his analysis. He replied that if one asked Zelda's friends, they would say that his drinking drove her to insanity. His friends would say that her insanity drove him to drink. But the truth, he noted, is that "liquor on my mouth is sweet to her and I cherish her wildest hallucinations." And here we are back where we began. Historically, Scott did cherish, celebrate, and enshrine as art Zelda's wildest hallucinations, particularly during the decade of the Roaring Twenties, which marked the high point of their lives together. After the stock market crash of 1929 and Zelda's first mental collapse which shortly followed it, Scott went through the motions of supporting her, among other things by paying her hospital bills, until his death in 1940.

But, in effect, Scott left Zelda in the mid-1930s to herself and to the biographers, poets, and playwrights who continue to create versions of her from the known facts of her life, from the gallery of her paintings, from her scrapbooks, from her published and unpublished novels, stories, essays, and letters—and from their own imaginations.

25. According to the passage, Zelda Fitzgerald rarely looked the same in any two of the many pictures taken of her. Sara Murphy attributed this to

A. Zelda's inner complexity.
B. the unpredictable quality of photographic equipment in the 1920s and 1930s, during which most of the photographs were taken.
C. Zelda's careful use of makeup.
D. Zelda's insistence that photographers take her picture from unusual angles.

26. Zelda Fitzgerald's first major biographer, according to the passage, was

A. Sara Mayfield.
B. Sara Murphy.
C. Arthur Mizener.
D. Nancy Milford.

27. One could deduce from the passage that Zelda Fitzgerald's husband, F. Scott Fitzgerald,

A. married Zelda on the rebound from his first love, Ginevra King.
B. had known Zelda all of his life and became romantically interested in her only after he had gone off to college.
C. met her when he was stationed near her home in Alabama during the war.
D. agreed to marry Zelda only if she would not pursue her career as a ballet dancer.

28. Minnie Sayre, Zelda's mother, the passage states, named her daughter after

A. a gypsy queen in a novel she was reading.
B. a distant relative who had agreed to remember Zelda in her will.
C. her maternal grandmother.
D. a character in a popular radio drama of the time.

29. The passage would support the following conclusion:

A. Insanity ran in Zelda's family according to family medical records.
B. Zelda was exploited by Scott, but she also suffered from internal conflicts probably not attributable to her husband, according to a major biographer.
C. Zelda was unpopular in her hometown of Montgomery, Alabama, one of her high school friends maintained.
D. Zelda had always wanted to marry a popular author, she told her brother many years after her marriage to Scott.

30. According to the passage, when asked about his role in Zelda's life and her role in his, Scott made an observation that revealed his own belief about their relationship:

A. Their mutual friends were better qualified to comment on this than he was.
B. They were mutually destructive of each other.
C. Zelda was to blame for driving him to drink.
D. His drinking was responsible for driving her to insanity.

31. In which of the following works by F. Scott Fitzgerald, according to the passage, was his wife not the model for a main character in the work?

A. *This Side of Paradise.*
B. "The Last of the Belles"
C. *Tender Is the Night*
D. *The Last Tycoon*

32. The passage asserts that Zelda's death occurred

A. while she was at work on her novel, *Save Me the Waltz.*
B. when she attempted to drive a car down an embankment in the south of France.
C. while she was locked away during a fire in a mental institution.
D. as a result of diving into a dark stairwell.

Passage V (Questions 33–38)

"In this way you shall set the fiftieth year apart and proclaim freedom to all the inhabitants of the land." In this way the ancient writer of *Leviticus* had God speak through Moses for the purpose of commemorating the entrance of the people of Israel into the "Promised Land." This is not the oldest reference to the celebration of an "anniversary," but it does show that celebrating anniversaries is a very old practice, and it also illustrates the role of round numbers in such celebrations.

Thus, the institution's celebration of its one hundred fiftieth year of existence adheres to a very old tradition. We celebrate birthdays and wedding anniversaries annually, whereas we usually commemorate the formation of institutions, businesses, churches, nations and schools on the round-numbered years. (Even with birthdays and weddings we call special attention to the "big" years—tenth, twenty-fifth, fiftieth, and so on.) That we do so, may have something to do with the fact that our numbering is on the base ten system, and the round numbers are those that finish the pattern. Although that explains why we pick the round numbers for our large celebrations, it does not explain why we think it important to celebrate such occasions. A brief discussion of why we *do* observe anniversaries is also an argument for why we *should* do so.

Perhaps the most obvious reason for celebrating the birth of an institution or the commemoration of some dramatic event is our belief that there was a good in it worth perpetuating. Thus, John Adams said of the 1776 Resolution of Independence:

I am apt to believe that it will be celebrated by succeeding generations as the great anniversary festival. It ought to be commemorated as the day of deliverance, by solemn acts of devotion to God Almighty. It ought to be solemnized with pomp and parade, with shows, games, sports, guns, bells, bonfires, and illuminations, from one end of this continent to the other, from this time forward for evermore.

Quite obviously, Adams believed that the launching of a free and independent nation was an act of such worth as to warrant regular celebration. It might be noted in passing that the inauguration of a new enterprise is always an act of hope. It is only at some future time, when folk have seen how an organization, institution, or nation has turned out—when growth and achievement became history—that there can be a confident celebration of the founding day.

But there is also an almost contradictory reason for anniversary celebrations. Instead of perpetuating ancient values they are often viewed as the occasion for a new beginning. As James Russell Lowell wrote, "New occasions teach new duties; time makes ancient good uncouth." So, anniversaries offer the opportunity to reflect on the path traveled, where a people are, where they wish to go next, and what's the best way to get there.

Anniversaries are also a time to honor the people who started the enterprise. Even if it is a romantic conception, we usually think of these pioneers as the hardier sort, whose lives and efforts are worthy of emulation.

Perhaps there is in anniversary celebrations something of an attempt to recapture or to *capture* the drama and emotion of the founding days. Nostalgia, even if it is variously felt, seems to be pleasant to the human spirit. Even if it is tinged with sadness, it is still treasured. Just call to mind (if you can) the lyrics of "Love's Old Sweet Song."

We must confess that part of the motivation for celebrating anniversaries is just plain, human pride. It doesn't matter whether one was among the founding party or joined the institution much later. If the organization has had a long, distinctive history, one may say, "I helped to put that together" or "That eminent institution values me enough to make me a part of it." The power of human pride cannot be underestimated as the motor of an institutional machine.

And we cannot ignore the commercial motivation behind anniversary celebrations. It is not just business organizations that stress, "One Hundred and Fifty Years of Faithful Service to the Community." Organizations of all varieties—churches, clubs, social and humane societies, *and* schools—use anniversaries to emphasize their legitimacy, durability, and trustworthiness and use the occasion to appeal for continued—and expanded—patronage by the public. All of these motivations are *implicit* in the celebration. There is real value in making them *explicit*. To be consciously aware of *why* we're celebrating would make the occasion more meaningful and enjoyable.

From Dr. William E. Blake, Jr., VCU's Sesquicentennial Celebration, 1989.

33. Which of the following statements are *neither supported nor contradicted by* the passage?

A. After 50 years, the Jews celebrated their leaving Egypt.
B. God spoke to Moses to initiate the celebration.
C. Most celebrations are joyous events.
D. Celebrations are a part of civilizations.

34. Which of the following statements is/are *supported by* the passage?

    I. There is a logical reason for celebrating.
    II. Round-numbered year festivities are usually special.
    III. Our mathematical system depends on round numbers that enhance remembering events.
    IV. Independence Day should be observed for always.

A. I, II, and III   C. II and IV
B. I and III   D. IV only

35. The passage either asserts or implies that:

A. Founding Day is an act of hope.
B. history will be the determining factor.
C. a celebration is a renewal.
D. all of the above are valid.

36. In the course of providing historical precedents for celebrations of various kinds, the author reveals his or her personal attitudes related to celebrations in general. Which of the following views of the author emerge from the passage?

A. Nostalgia is good for humankind.
B. Pioneers are usually worthy of emulating.
C. People need a time to reflect.
D. All of the above are viewed positively by the author.

37. The author believes:

A. that a sense of being a part of history is productive.
B. entrepreneurship is part and parcel of a festival.
C. justification for existence is a motive for anniversary celebrations.
D. all of the above statements.

38. The passage could properly be titled:

A. Our One Hundred Fiftieth-Year Celebration.
B. Why We Celebrate.
C. Founding Day.
D. A History of Anniversary Celebrations.

Passage VI (Questions 39–44)

Myths and fairy tales are most often told and remembered as plots (who did what to whom and what happened). But they actually endure in our continuing imaginations because of the "character" of the characters involved. If you place Oedipus into Daedalus's story, or Narcissus into Odysseus's story, you won't have the same story. Cinderella wouldn't do what Red Riding Hood does, nor would Jack-in-the-Beanstalk do what Hansel does. The character doesn't merely *follow* a plot line—the plot happens *because* of the particular human weaknesses and strengths of the particular character.

Underlying all these characters, of course, are larger issues, such as greed and selfishness, pride, acceptance of fate, compassion, cleverness, and risk. But what distinguishes one character from another are the choices, actions, and consequences of those choices peculiar to the individual character. When a teenager (like Theseus) is faced with a dilemma of State (his country must pay human sacrifice tribute in the form of seven youths and seven maidens to a more powerful country), there are a number of choices or decisions he can make. He can ignore the whole problem (it's not his fault, after all); he can take personal responsibility for solving the problem, either because he wants to be a Big Hero or because (as son of the King) he must learn to face problems if he expects to inherit the throne; or he might simply be in a boastful or adventuresome mood when the idea crosses his mind. Once Theseus commits himself to the task (destroying the Minotaur, symbol of the opposing country's power), there are further choices: He can take all the credit but allow his underlings to do all the hard work; he can sacrifice himself on a seemingly impossible task (finding and destroying the Minotaur in its Labyrinth); or he can take advantage of a girl's love for him (agreeing to take Ariadne away with him if she gives him the secret of the Labyrinth). And once he's solved the primary problem of the Minotaur, there are even more choices: does he really want to take Ariadne back with him as he promised? Should he take time out to change the color of his ship's sails (as he promised his father) when he's being pursued by an angry enemy? Because he doesn't change the sails, he directly causes his father's suicide; because he chooses to leave Ariadne behind, he indirectly sets up an even more tragic chain of events in his own life that won't become apparent for a number of years. The series of choices and consequent actions that Theseus takes thus becomes the plot we know, only after we look back on it.

Young people still face seemingly impossible tasks today. These might involve the State (expose corruption, act on one's conscience, protest the military draft), or they might involve other people and relationships

Adapted from Sally V. Doud, "Essay Test Introduction," VCU, Spring 1990.

(whether to live up to an agreement made under different circumstances, such as an engagement, marriage, contract, job, project). People still have to decide whether to try and save a sinking ship, or whether to catch the first lifeboat; whether to admit a harsh truth or to avoid it (lie, exaggerate, use diplomacy, pass blame, run away). Can or should one be loyal to a person or way of life one no longer cares about? What are the risks and benefits of any decision? Does it still "pay" to be a hero, or do other occupations seem more lucrative? Is the difference between a hero and a fool merely success? Should you get involved with someone else's problem or shrug it off? Should you take a stance or merely cast your eyes to heaven and wait for divine intervention and fate? Also, it isn't always easy to separate personal ego or animal needs from more "noble" desires to bring about social or human justice, and often the two run along together for a considerable distance before they part ways. These are matters for contemporary characters in contemporary stories, but these are the same matters Theseus dealt with. We still have our Minotaurs, escape ships, labyrinths, tasks, Ariadnes, and Theseuses, though the forms are different each time. That's why myth and fairy tales (based on folktales or myths) are called Universal.

39. The most appropriate title for this essay would be:

   A. The Role of Fate in Contemporary Life.
   B. Red Riding Hood and Theseus: Two Versions of the Same Character.
   C. Universal Aspects of Everyday Experience.
   D. Myth is Dead.

40. According to the author of the passage:

   A. people today do not face impossible tasks as did the characters in the Greek myths.
   B. the outcomes of fairy tales and myths are rarely determined by choices the characters have made.
   C. myths and fairy tales are universal because the choices that are faced by characters in them are similar to the ones faced by people of all times.
   D. there are fewer choices for heroes today than there were for the heroes of Greek myths.

41. One might infer from this passage that:

   A. Theseus is responsible for the death of his father.
   B. one should not sacrifice himself to a seemingly impossible task.
   C. Theseus should not be blamed for the suicide of his father.

   D. in making decisions, individuals should wait for divine intervention.

42. According to the author of the passage:

   A. plots proceed as a pattern of cause and effect events.
   B. plots are always the same from one story to the next.
   C. plots are merely an accumulated series of events.
   D. plots are the most important part of any story.

43. The most important part of the passage is:

   A. that we not forget the story of Theseus and his adventures surrounding the Labyrinth.
   B. stories change, but the realm of human choices remains the same.
   C. universality deals with language.
   D. we are always punished for our misdoing.

44. According to the passage, the primary problem facing Theseus is:

   A. how he can reward Ariadne for giving him the secret of the Labyrinth.
   B. the killing of the Minotaur.
   C. the changing of his ship's sails so as to inform his father of his fate.
   D. how he will rid himself of guilt after he has killed the Minotaur.

Passage VII (Questions 45–50)

Caricature is a device satirists commonly use in their work. Why is it so common? Caricatures grab readers' or viewers' attention; moreover, they are funny. Caricatures distort reality and that distortion is often hilarious. An audience that will appreciate the caricature recognizes the incongruity between the real object and the satirist's portrayal of it. They also understand why the satirist is attacking this object. In effect, the appreciative audience says, "Of course, this is all out of proportion. But, you know, he's got a point there. This person (place, thing) really does have a weak spot." Meanwhile, as they muse on the message, they are reacting to the incongruities, the exaggeration, with anything from a wry smile to convulsive laughter.

What exactly is a caricature? I would define it as a pictorial (drawing, painting, sculpture, collage, mask, dramatization) or verbal (poem, essay, descriptive sketch in fiction or nonfiction) exaggeration of an object (person, place, thing, situation, organization). The distortion must be based on a fact about the object, for example, bushy eyebrows. The artist or writer just stretches that fact all out of shape; the politician's eyebrows are not *that* bushy. He plays with his object as if it were a glob of silly putty or bread dough. He kneads it, rolls it up, flattens it, stretches it out, shapes it any way to suit his fancy. He must not go so far as to make the object completely unrecognizable, but he has a lot of room to play with his object.

One thing that happens when an object becomes so pliable in the hands of an artist or writer is that the object instantly plummets in value. It becomes ridiculous, at least to some extent, and not as important as it had been. Often the satirist's purpose is to show that the object, because of people's vanity or hypocrisy, is considered more valuable than it really is. By doing a caricature of it, he deflates its value. Furthermore, the artist or writer shows that he has control over the object, at least temporarily. He is exerting his power by the way he portrays the object. It's as if he's saying, "Ah ha! You thought you were so important. But look at you now, the way *I've* made you. I'm calling the shots now . . . ." Needless to say, the people being caricatured rarely think kindly about the creators of the satire—not only do the caricatures deflate their importance, but also the caricatures show that the people who are being satirized don't have control over their image.

It's important to note that one of the effects of caricature is to dehumanize the person being caricatured. This dehumanization is even there in the language of how we discuss satire: the word "object." As the audience, we often enjoy seeing a vaunted person being devalued by caricature and agree that the devaluation is often deserved. But does the means justify the end? Caricatures certainly work, creators and audience have a lot of fun while criticizing the object. However, a side effect is that caricatures serve as one out of many ways we tend in our society to dehumanize each other. Rarely does the creator or the audience notice this; we're caught up in the laughter and disregard any objections to a caricature by saying, "It's just a joke. Don't you have a sense of humor? He (object of caricature) deserved it anyway." Yes, it's just a joke. But also, yes, it makes it easier for us to view people as objects to be manipulated, vilified, destroyed. Think back to the caricatures we did of the Japanese in World War II. It is much easier it work up enthusiasm for killing people when they are depicted as hideous monsters. Hitler readily used caricature to depict Jews as less-than-human animals.

Exaggeration, playing the extremes against each other, distortion—these are all elements of caricature. Caricatures are a quite effective means for satire—creators enjoy creating them, audiences respond eagerly to them, they make their point. However, they are not innocuous little creatures; they can be used to stereotype and dehumanize people. Also, as we use them casually day after day, we sometimes don't even notice anymore that they are caricatures. The cartoon character becomes the norm. Wiley the Coyote makes falling off cliffs, holding an exploding piece of dynamite, or being crushed with huge stones seem like normal, everyday events; he is just a little frazzled after each episode. Numbed day after day with caricatures, might we begin to think of life as a cartoon?

45. Which of the following statements about caricatures is NOT *supported by* the passage?

A. Caricatures do not have to be pictures.
B. People who are satirized often lose the public's respect.
C. People who are satirized often deserve the ridicule.
D. Caricatures can be based on falsehoods.

46. According to the passage, people laugh at caricatures because:

A. bushy eyebrows and other such facial quirks are naturally funny.
B. we laugh at people who are vain and hypocritical.
C. we recognize the incongruities between the object and the caricature of it.
D. the people who create caricatures have a good sense of humor.

47. Which of the following statements best sums up the author's opinion of caricatures?

A. Caricatures are hilarious.
B. Caricatures reveal the hypocrisies of our society.
C. Caricatures have insidious effects.
D. People who do not appreciate caricatures have no sense of humor.

48. According to the passage, caricatures are effective forms of satire because:

I. ridicule devalues an object.
II. caricatures appeal to many kinds of audiences.
III. the satirist controls his object's public image.

A. I and II.   C. I and III
B. II and III   D. I, II, and III

Adapted from Rebecca Dale, "Caricature," VCU, Spring 1989.

49. According to the passage, caricatures can be dangerous because:

    A. people satiated with exaggeration may not recognize the norm.
    B. a person who is satirized may not deserve the ridicule.
    C. caricatures divert our attention from real problems.
    D. caricatures give satirists too much power over society.

50. Of the following titles, which is most appropriate for the passage?

    A. The Cruel Art of Caricature
    B. Caricature and Understatement
    C. Caricature: Exaggeration as a Satirist's Tool
    D. Cartoon Art

Passage VIII (Questions 51–59)

On a physiological level, aggression is a neurochemical impulse, causing tension that necessitates a physical release. According to the evolutionist position, aggression as instinct can be traced from some of the earliest primitive animal forms from which we humans draw a common ancestor, and must therefore, by reason of evolution as well as observed behavioral patterns, be attributable to man. If conflict is the father of all things, it may be the activating force behind all human behavior (love as well as hate), and its ritual forms of appeasement and redirected activity provide a basis for culture.

In order that aggression be considered an element of man's genetic inheritance, some explanation must be offered for its existence in his past. Ethologists maintain that aggression in earliest man, as in all of the lower animals, had a distinct survival advantage, most commonly linked to the defense of territory. "What directly threatens the existence of an animal species," says Konrad Lorenz, "is never the 'eating enemy' but competition" within the species. In this sense, intraspecies aggression provides for the even distribution of a particular species over an inhabitable area; a form of population control as well as quality control. The stronger animal will control the more advantageous territory and subsequently corner the hardier breeding population. Man's traditional attachment to his land is seen as a modern refinement of his territoriality; most human conflicts can be traced back to dispute over land itself or to his sense of independence concerning his property.

According to Robert Ardrey, the defense of the territory holds animals together in breeding pairs or larger groups; but the most powerful defense is offered by the pair, thereby encouraging bonding, to even further selective advantage. Territoriality is also psychological, providing the three basic animal needs: security, identity, and stimulation. The first two are self-explanatory; with the third we are more concerned, for stimulation—by other animals of one's kind—is accomplished through aggression. This may take the form of *inward antagonism*, bickering among one's closest neighbors, which serves no apparent purpose except perhaps sheer stimulation; yet this is considered responsible for socialization. The growth of population into congested cities instead of more evenly spacing out has even been interpreted in this context to be a reaction of man's aggressive needs rather than a practical understanding of cooperation.

Stimulation through aggression can also take the form of *outward antagonism*, the defense of a species group of its territory against outsiders; uniting its members in a common cause and often considered the basis for the human Nation.

Another important aspect of aggression, says Lorenz, is its role in securing the personal bond. "The danger in aggression is its spontaneity . . ." therefore, ". . . aggression of animals toward their own kind is held in check by inhibiting mechanisms" such as ritualization of fighting, appeasement gestures, and redirected activity. As each relationship between two members of the species must be individually negotiated, this consititutes the beginnings of personality. Various forms of greetings as well as many human emotional expressions, such as laughter, are considered ceremonies of redirected activity or appeasement; Lorenz notes that everyone is aware of how laughter tends to create a bond.

Lionel Tiger provides an example of aggression's role in establishing order and custom within a human society: competition between several age groups of males (for females, for prestige) is often responsible for rigid initiatory tradition, along with other political measures prohibitive to one group while enhancing the changes of a second.

The human being who voluntarily places himself within the power of the law embodies the theory of inhibiting mechanisms. Members of the Cheyenne tribe who broke the law during a hunt willingly submitted to the authority of the Shield Soldiers, a gesture of ritual appeasement. In turn, the Shield Soldiers rendered only token punishment, and that on the property of the offenders, acknowledging the appeasement gesture by a redirected activity.

The theory of innate aggression carried to its ultimate climax presents us with the uncomforting image of man with "killer instincts." Although Ardrey points out that territoriality is defensive, that early man hunted because he was hungry, still others point to cannibalism as human acts of aggression as well as a cultural phenomenon.

Adapted from Sally V. Doud, "Aggression and Human Nature," VCU, 1976.

The more dangerously aggressive the particular species is, the firmer is the bond necessary to prevent intraspecies destruction. Here is man's anomaly: he is devoid of the more elaborate safety devices to prevent the abuse of his killing power, because these devices were unnecessary in the harmless protohuman for whom quick and easy killing was impossible. The acquisition of weapons threw off the natural balance, for now he is capable of great destruction without the accompanying mechanics of inhibition; the Cain and Abel, the master of war, the deadly predator who kills for enjoyment.

"It is true," says Morton Hunt, "like other animals, we are impelled to action by hunger, fear, anger, sexual desires . . . but are not directed by instinct to take specific actions in order to satisfy those desires . . . Man may be innately aggressive . . . but he is not programmed . . . the drive can be directed to many different ends." The apparatus with which we are equipped to speak is a product of our evolution, and the particular language is culturally transmitted.

The emphasis then is on interdependence of instinct and culture; no longer is man at the mere beck and call of his instincts, but capable of exercising control over them. His intelligence permits him the conscious choice of goals.

51. The passage suggests that:

A. aggression has not yet been traced to earlier evolutionary forms than man.
B. aggression is a neurochemical impulse.
C. unlike hunger, aggression does not require release.
D. aggression seeks direct expression or appeasement and therefore is not redirected into culture building activities.

52. According to Lorenz, the greatest threat to the survival of an animal species is:

A. what he calls the "eating enemy."
B. natural disaster.
C. various forms of pollution.
D. competition within the species.

53. The passage suggests that of the three basic animal needs, the one that is thought to account for bickering among one's closest neighbors is:

A. identity.   C. stimulation.
B. security.   D. structure.

54. The passage asserts that one of man's greatest anomalies is that:

A. he instinctively pairs with or bonds to another human being, but that he cannot remain monogamous throughout his life cycle.
B. he possesses the "killer instinct" but lacks the internal controls or safety devices that restrict this instinct.
C. he has free access to weapons but lacks the "killer instinct" to take full advantage of them.
D. man is territorial and nomadic at the same time.

55. Morton Hunt, who is quoted in the essay, asserts that:

A. man is innately aggressive, but he is not biologically programmed as to how to direct his aggression.
B. cultural transmission plays only a minor role in determining how aggression is channeled from generation to generation.
C. it is a mistake to think of man as innately aggressive.
D. the existence of anger in man differentiates him from other animals.

56. One might infer from this passage that:

A. the existence of aggression in lower animals is unimportant in the study of aggression in man.
B. aggression plays a very important role in determining the ways in which human beings interact in social groups.
C. humans are not territorial.
D. people live in cities because of innate cooperativeness.

57. The most appropriate title for this essay would be:

A. Lorenz On Aggression.
B. The "Killer Instinct" in Man.
C. Man is Pure Instinct.
D. Aggression as the Basis for Culture.

58. The growth of population into congested cities rather than an even spacing out has been interpreted by the context of Ardery's ideas as:

A. a natural need in man to cooperate.
B. the herding instinct.
C. a need for sharing material goods.
D. a reaction of man's aggressive needs.

59. Members of the Cheyenne tribe who broke the law during a hunt:

A. rebelled against punishment, thus exhibiting aggression.

B. willingly submitted in a gesture of ritual appeasement.

C. insisted that their punishment be on their own land.

D. never broke the same law twice, thus suppressing aggression.

Passage IX (Questions 60–65)

Because the ability to write well is so crucial to success in school, educators are paying more attention to assessments of writing. States have begun requiring students to take minimum competency tests before graduation or before entering high school. Colleges want to limit admissions to students who have shown a certain level of competency in writing. Or they want to place students in an appropriate level of freshman English. How are all these decisions on proficiency, admissions, placement and exemption made? Tests. Because decisions have to be made on large numbers of students, the tests are large scale assessments, tests that *everyone* in the group (school, state, nation) takes.

There are two major types of tests—direct assessments and indirect assessments. Direct assessments are tests that use readers to judge actual samples of students' writing, writing done in timed in-class sessions on a common topic. Indirect assessments are tests that use answers to multiple-choice questions to judge students' knowledge about certain aspects of writing, such as mechanics or grammar.

Statistics show that multiple-choice tests are very reliable, meaning that students' scores are consistent (if Johnny retakes the test, he is likely to receive about the same score), but how valid they are is speculative (validity refers to what extent a test actually tests what it purports to test). Because multiple-choice questions can test only reading and editing skills for the most part, the scores have meaning only about a student's knowledge those areas tested. G. Conlan points out that multiple-choice questions have become more sophisticated recently in the types of knowledge tested and can test such things as principles of organization, logic, ability to shift parts of sentences, and sensitivity to idioms. But still it is someone else's text. Does ability to edit someone else's text necessarily mean ability to *create* texts of one's own?

If we want to measure writing skills, a test that requires a person to write would likely be a more valid test than one that doesn't. However, direct assessment is not proving to be a panacea either. A valid test must necessarily be reliable also, many of the problems with direct assessment testing have to do with reliability. If we change the wording of test topics, the testing conditions, or the readers scoring essays, scores can change dramatically.

Reliability problems are most conspicuous in the scoring process. Here is the main objection to direct assessment—different readers have different reactions to the same essay. How can we determine if an essay has been scored accurately? Reader-response theory has pointed out that readers "recreate" a text when they read it, that interpretation depends on what readers bring to the experience of reading a text as well as what writers put into the text.

Administrators of these tests try to cope with this problem in several ways. One, they develop scoring guides that specify the criteria to be used in evaluating the student papers. Whether they use holistic scoring (scoring an essay as a whole), primary trait scoring (a type of holistic scoring focusing on certain traits found in the particular mode of discourse tested), or analytic scoring (scoring subcategories, such as content, organization, mechanics, and adding the scores up), they all specify in the scoring guides the characteristics of a paper for each score in the scoring range.

Secondly, test administrators train readers with "anchor" papers and trial grading runs. This is sometimes referred to as "calibrating the readers." Readers needs to internalize the criteria in the scoring guide, and by comparing their judgments on an essay to an anchor paper whose score has been predetermined, they can get a feel for how lenient or rigorous the scoring should be. The trial grading runs, where each of the readers grades some sample essays, give additional calibration. After grading the samples, the readers discuss the scores they gave, along with their reasons for assigning those scores. The discussion of discrepancies brings up issues in how to apply the criteria and allow the group to reach greater consensus on what the various scores mean.

Thirdly, each essay is read by two readers, each unaware of the score the other reader has given it. If the scores differ by more than one point, a third reader reads the essay. White considers the practice of multiple readings essential:

> Although there is a constant temptation to reduce the costs by reducing the second reading to samples or by eliminating second readings altogether, such an economy renders the reading unaccountable and unprofessional.

Scores do vary. "Most papers, if rescored by the same readers at the same reading, would probably receive different scores."

These measures in administering tests help increase reliability in scoring essays, but they do not solve the problem. Readers react to the topic and unintentionally may bring some bias to their grading. In cases where readers are aware of their own bias, they even may try to compensate for their bias and be too lenient in grading essays that offend them.

Adapted from Rebecca Dale, "Direct-Indirect Assessment of Writing," Capitol Writing Project, VCU, Summer 1989.

Another problem is reader drift. Readers who are reading hundreds of essays at a time may be more or less lenient at some times than at others. For example, a paper read right after a brilliant one is more likely to receive a lower score than if it's read after an average one. Barritt, Stock, and Clark have raised a provocative question in their study of how expertly trained readers of students' texts can disagree widely in scoring: They found that readers expected to find "average" student papers, and they could agree on scores for papers that met their expectations. But when they read papers that did not fit their expectations of an "average" student, their scores differed widely. S. Freedman had a similar finding in a comparison of student and professional writers: Evaluators gave student work fairly consistent scores, but in scoring the professional essays, "the raters disagreed violently with one another."

60. According to the passage, indirect assessments of writing have been criticized because:

    A.   scores are unreliable.
    B.   only reading and editing skills are tested.
    C.   the tests are biased.
    D.   evaluators cannot agree on the criteria for scoring.

61. Which of the following statements does the passage state or imply is/are true?

    I.   A reliable test is necessarily valid.
    II.   A valid test is necessarily reliable.
    III. A test may be reliable, but not valid.
    IV. A test may be valid, but not reliable.

    A. I and II   **C.** II and III
    B. III and IV   **D.** II only

62. Which of the following statements best sums up the importance of reader-response theory to the problems of evaluating essays on large-scale assessments?

    A.   Scoring guides are necessary to set the criteria by which essays are judged.

    B.   Evaluators are influenced by their own ideas.
    C.   Evaluators need to be calibrated.
    D.   Evaluators give inconsistent scores to professional essays.

63. According to the passage, administrators deal with the reliability problems in scoring direct assessments by all EXCEPT which of the following?

    A.   essays are scored by multiple readers.
    B.   evaluators must use specific criteria in judging essays.
    C.   holistic scoring, primary trait scoring, or analytic scoring is used.
    D.   evaluators are trained with "anchor papers."

64. According to the passage, which of the following affects the reliability of scores on essays?

    A.   Multiple readings mean that scores will likely differ.
    B.   Evaluators may not agree on which criteria are the most important.
    C.   An average paper read after an outstanding one may receive a lower score than if it's read after another average one.
    D.   Trial grading runs do not give sufficient calibration.

65. Which statement probably best sums up the author's evaluation of the ways to test writing in large-scale assessments?

    A.   Indirect assessments are better than direct assessments because of the reliability problems involved in direct assessments.
    B.   Direct assessments are better than indirect assessments because they test a student's ability to create a text.
    C.   Evaluators of essays in direct assessments need to be carefully trained.
    D.   Both indirect assessments and direct assessments have only limited value.

PHYSICAL SCIENCES

10 PROBLEM SETS OF 5–10 QUESTIONS EACH
15 PROBLEMS FOLLOWED BY A SINGLE QUESTION
77 QUESTIONS
100 MINUTES

DIRECTIONS: The following questions or incomplete statements are in groups. Preceding each series of questions or statements is a paragraph or a short explanatory statement, a formula or set of formulas, or a definition. Read the written material and then answer the questions or complete the statements. Select the ONE BEST ANSWER for each question and indicate your selection by marking the corresponding letter of your choice on the Answer Form. Eliminate those alternatives you know to be incorrect and then select an answer from among the remaining alternatives. A periodic table is provided (see p. 583). You may consult it whenever you wish to do so.

Passage I (Questions 66–70)

In a physics class, an experimental motion experiment is devised to allow the study of the motion of a number of objects under a variety of conditions. One part involves projecting identical steel or wooden balls at a variety of initial angles and speeds, starting at various heights above the floor. Equipment, such as protractors and photogate timers, is available so the angles and speeds are known. Rectangular metal blocks of various masses can be slid across horizontal surfaces and also down inclined planes. The surfaces vary from essentially frictionless to quite rough surfaces. The balls can be rolled down the inclined planes also. The masses of each object are measured in advance and the velocities can be measured at any point of the motion with the photogate timers.

66. One of the identical balls is dropped from the edge of a lab table 1.1 m high at the same instant another one is projected horizontally with an initial velocity of 2 m/sec. If there is no air resistance, what are the times for the two balls, respectively, to strike the floor?

   A. 0.11 sec, 0.11 sec
   B. 0.47 sec, 0.47 sec
   C. 0.47 sec, 0.95 sec
   D. 1.2 sec, 2.3 sec

67. One ball is projected horizontally with an initial horizontal velocity of 10 m/sec while the second is projected at an angle of 30° *above* the horizontal with the same initial speed. Both balls strike a vertical wall that is exactly 10 m away. How long does it take each ball, respectively, to hit the wall?

   A. 0.87 sec, 1.5 sec   C. 1 sec, 1 sec
   B. 1 sec, 0.87 sec   D. 1 sec, 1.5 sec

68. A rectangular block of mass 1 kg and one of mass 3 kg are projected across a rough surface with the same starting speed of 4 m/sec. The coefficient of friction is 0.4. How far do the blocks slide, respectively?

   A. 2 m, 2 m   C. 4 m, 4 m
   B. 3 m, 2 m   D. 6 m, 2 m

69. One of the balls is released from rest at the top of an inclined plane 0.5 m high and rolls down without slipping. At the same instant a rectangular block is released and slides down a frictionless plane which is also 0.5 m high. Which of the two objects has the greater speed at the bottom of the inclines?

   A. The ball.
   B. The block.
   C. Both have the same speed.
   D. The question cannot be answered because there is not enough information given.

70. A wooden ball of mass 0.4 kg is dropped down a circular stairwell. It is observed to reach a terminal velocity of 35 m/sec and continues falling at that speed. What is the force of air friction acting on the ball?

   A. 3.9 N   C. 14 N
   B. 7.8 N   D. 28 N

Passage II (Questions 71–76)

Most of the students in an introductory physics class are in premedicine, so the instructor devises a lab in which all the topics are related to the human body. Each student's blood pressure, temperature, weight, height, metabolic rate, pulmonary function, and so on can be measured with reasonable accuracy. A lab handout supplies the following information:

1 kg is equivalent to 2.2 pounds
1 kcal = 4186 joules
Average aortic pressure = 100 mm Hg
1×10^5 N/m^2 = 750 mm Hg
Density of blood = 1050 kg/m^3
Energy of oxidation of fats and oils = 9.5 kcal/gram = 39,700 joules/gram
Oxygen consumption in humans releases about 20,000 joules/liter O^2 (consumed)
1 watt = 1 joule/sec

71. A student with a basal metabolic rate of 100 W exercises vigorously for 10 minutes, during which time his metabolic rate rises to an average of 670 W. What is the approximate number of liters of oxygen that the student consumes during the exercise period?

    A. 9 L   C. 40 L
    B. 20 L   D. 210 L

72. The above student wants to lose 0.52 kg of fat by exercising. Since the average rate of energy expended above that required for ordinary metabolism is 570 W, for how many hours will the student have to exercise?

    A. 3 hr   C. 10 hr
    B. 4 hr   D. 14 hr

73. A student weighs 135 pounds. What is her mass in kilograms and her weight in newtons?

    A. 61.4 kg and 601 N
    B. 42.3 kg and 520 N
    C. 56.5 kg and 554 N
    D. 49.0 kg and 480 N

74. The metabolism for a woman in the class is about 2000 kcal/day. If she has a food intake of 2900 kcal/day for four weeks, what mass of fat, corresponding to the excess intake, might accumulate?

    A. 854 g   C. 1244 g
    B. 2653 g   D. 1995 g

75. What is the gauge pressure in the foot artery, which is 1.35 m below the aorta?

    A. 120 mm Hg   C. 405 mm Hg
    B. 205 mm Hg   D. 660 mm Hg

76. You consume only about 25% of the oxygen that you take into your lungs. If you work for 6 hours at a metabolic rate of 300 W, how many total *liters of oxygen* do you inhale? (The volume of air will be 5 times larger, since O^2 is 20% of the atmosphere).

    A. 900 L   C. 650 L
    B. 1300 L   D. 2800 L

Passage III (Questions 77–81)

A set of experiments in the physics lab is designed to develop understanding of simple electrical circuit principles for direct current circuits. The student is given a variety of batteries, resistors, and DC meters; and is directed to wire series and parallel combinations of resistors and batteries making measurements of the currents and voltage drops using the ammeters and voltmeters. The student calculates expected current and voltage values using Ohm's law and Kirchhoff's circuit rules and then checks the results with the meters.

77. A student connects a 6-volt battery and a 12-volt battery in series and then connects this combination across a 10-ohm resistor. What is the current in the resistor?

    A. 0.8 A   C. 1.8 A
    B. 0.9 A   D. 3.6 A

78. Resistors of 4 ohms and 8 ohms are connected in series. A battery of 6 volts is connected across the series combination. How much power, in watts, is consumed in the 8-ohm resistor?

    A. 0.67 W   C. 12 W
    B. 2 W   D. 24 W

79. Two 4-ohm resistors are connected in series and this pair is connected in parallel with an 8-ohm resistor. A 12-volt battery is connected across the ends of this parallel set. What power, in watts, is consumed in the 8-ohm resistor in this case?

    A. 0.9 W   C. 4.4 W
    B. 2.0 W   D. 18 W

80. A 6-volt battery is connected across a 2-ohm resistor. What is the heat energy dissipated in the resistor in 5 minutes?

A. 430 joules   C. 4300 joules
B. 560 joules   D. 5400 joules

81. A 12-volt battery is connected across a 4-ohm resistor and the heat energy dissipated in the resistor in 10 minutes is used to heat 2 kg of water (which is thermally insulated so that no heat escapes). The initial temperature of the water is 20°C and the specific heat of the water is 4184 joule/kg-°C. What is the final temperature of the water at the end of the 10 minutes of heating?

A. 22.6°C   C. 34.2°C
B. 28.4°C   D. 56.4°C

Passage IV (Questions 82–87)

A set of experiments to study all aspects of sound waves is devised. Several identical audio oscillators with loudspeakers can be used for experiments in audible sound at any frequency between 25 Hz and 40,000 Hz. An old ultrasound (US) unit (an "A scan" unit) is available to study the propagation of ultrasound waves. The unit has a US transducer that transmits a pulse of US and then "rests" and acts as a receiver of the US echo. The transmitted signal and echo are observed on an oscilloscope. The time for the echo to return can be read from the horizontal scope face. Since the returned signals are quite weak, the US unit has the ability to highly amplify the echo. The student can study the conditions of waves in pipes closed on one end or open on both ends. The audio units can be mounted on carts to study the Doppler effect. The waves from the oscillator and US unit are sent through air, water, and aluminum. The speed of sound in these materials is measured by determining the time for the echo to return from a surface a known distance from the transducer. Some of the results are:

Apparatus	Material	Speed of sound	Frequencies
Audio oscillator	Air	340 m/sec	50 Hz, 1000 Hz
	Water	1440 m/sec	50 Hz, 1000 Hz
	Aluminum	5100 m/sec	50 Hz, 1000 Hz
US unit	Air	340 m/sec	2.5 MHz (megahertz)
	Water	1440	2.5 MHz
	Aluminum	5100	2.5 MHz

82. What are the respective wavelengths of the 50 Hz and 2.5 MHz waves in water?

A. 29 m and 13.6 m
B. 29 m and 1.4 cm
C. 136 m and 1.4 cm
D. 29 m and 0.58 mm

83. The audio system is used to send a sound wave from a small speaker into a 25-cm long cylindrical tube which is open on both ends. Both open ends must be antinodes for a standing wave. As the frequency is slowly increased, a louder resonant fundamental is heard. What is the frequency of this fundamental?

A. 340 Hz   C. 170 Hz
B. 680 Hz   D. 1020 Hz

84. At higher frequencies, resonant overtones are created in the open-ended pipe. What are the frequencies of the first and second overtones that are heard?

A. 1360 and 2720 Hz
B. 1360 and 2040 Hz
C. 2720 and 3400 Hz
D. 2720 and 4210 Hz

85. The US transducer at 2.5 MHz is placed just below the surface in a water tank and pointed straight down at a horizontal wooden surface. A reflected echo from the surface is detected after 0.35 milliseconds. How far is the wooden surface from the transducer?

A. 0.82 m   C. 1.1 m
B. 0.34 m   D. 0.25 m

86. The audio system is mounted on a cart and is pulled *toward* a student at 20 m/sec while emitting a 1000 Hz signal. What frequency will be heard by the student?

A. 1063 Hz   C. 1000 Hz
B. 2126 Hz   D. 944 Hz

87. It is a general property of waves that the energy transported by a wave is proportional to the square of the amplitude and the square of the frequency.

$$(E = CA^2f^2)$$

Suppose the 50 Hz and 1000 Hz sound waves have the same amplitude. What is the ratio of the energy in the 1000 Hz wave to the energy of the 50 Hz wave?

A. 400   C. 200
B. 20   D. 2000

Questions 88–95 are independent of any passages and of each other.

88. The naturally occurring radioactive decay series known as the Actinium series begins with the long-lived isotope $_{92}U^{235}$. It decays by a series of alpha (α) and beta (β) decays as follows: $\alpha, \beta, \alpha, \alpha, \beta, \alpha, \alpha, \beta, \alpha, \alpha, \beta$. What isotope is the final result of this series?

   A. $_{88}Ra^{208}$ C. $_{88}Ra^{220}$

   B. $_{82}Pb^{210}$ D. $_{82}Pb^{207}$

89. A positive ion has a horizontal velocity due north. It enters a region where a magnetic field points vertically upward. What is the direction of the force on the positive ion?

   A. vertically down
   B. west, horizontal
   C. east, horizontal
   D. vertically up

90. The absolute temperature of an ideal gas increases by 50% at constant volume. What happens to the absolute pressure of the gas?

   A. The pressure doubles.
   B. The pressure increases by 50%.
   C. The pressure increases by 150%.
   D. The pressure decreases by 50%.

91. A constant force F acts on a mass m which can move without friction. The mass is at rest at the origin of coordinates ($x = 0$) at time $t = 0$. Which graph correctly shows the velocity of the mass as a function of time?

A.

B.

C.

D.

92. What are the highest and lowest values of resistance that one can construct using three 3-ohm resistors?

   A. 12 ohms and 0.33 ohms
   B. 9 ohms and 0.33 ohms

   C. 9 ohms and 1 ohm
   D. 12 ohms and 0.67 ohms

93. A hiker with backpack has a mass of 130 kg. If she hikes up a hill 45 m high, how much mechanical work is done?

   A. 57,300 joules   C. 15,800 joules
   B. 45,400 joules   D. 72,100 joules

94. A net force of 6 N acts on a mass of 3 kg, accelerating it from rest. If the force acts over a distance of 4 m, what is the final speed of the mass?

   A. 4.0 m/sec   C. 5.1 m/sec
   B. 3.6 m/sec   D. 2.8 m/sec

95. A homeowner working in a crawl space touches a "hot" 120 V source. A current of 120 milliamperes passes through his heart and initiates a dangerous ventricular fibrillation. What is the body resistance in ohms?

   A. 400 ohms   C. 1400 ohms
   B. 1000 ohms   D. 800 ohms

Passage V (Questions 96–105)

Students are given a variety of lenses and optics equipment, such as lens holders, lighted object sources, optical benches, meter sticks and tapes, image screens, and several examples of commercial optical equipment, such as microscopes and telescopes. They are to work in an open-ended optics lab in order to learn the general principles of lenses and the optical devices that can be constructed using lenses.

96. A student is given a short focal length converging lens and long focal length converging lens. One lens is placed in a holder. A lighted object is place 18 cm in front of the lens and it is found that a clear image can be focused on a screen placed 36 cm behind the lens. What is the focal length of this lens?

   A. 8 cm   C. 27 cm
   B. 12 cm   D. 46 cm

97. What magnification is produced by the above lens when the object is 18 cm in front of the lens and the image is 36 cm behind the lens?

   A. $2\times$ C. $4\times$
   B. $3\times$ D. $6\times$

98. A lighted object is placed 6 cm in front of the second lens, which has a focal length of +24 cm. Where is the image and which kind of image is it?

   A. 8 cm in front of the lens; a virtual image
   B. 8 cm behind the lens; a real image
   C. 16 cm in front of the lens; a real image
   D. 16 cm behind the lens; a virtual image

99. The 24 cm focal length lens is used as the objective of a simple refracting telescope and a third converging lens of focal length +8 cm is used as the eyepiece. What is the magnification of this simple refractor?

   A. 0.6 ×   **C.** 4 ×
   B. 3 ×   **D.** 6 ×

100. A commercial microscope is examined by the student. The objective is marked 20 × and the eyepiece is marked 10 ×. What power objective should replace the above objective so that the microscope's magnification will be 400 ×?,

   A. 5 ×   **C.** 40 ×
   B. 10 ×   **D.** 100 ×

101. A lighted object is placed 24 cm in front of a +12 cm focal length lens. The image formed by this lens is the object for a second lens of +24 cm focal length. The second lens is placed 72 cm behind the first lens. Where is the final image with respect to the second lens?

   A. 24 cm in front of #2
   B. 24 cm behind #2
   C. 36 cm in front of #2
   D. 48 cm behind #2

102. A lens of local length +24 cm is used to view an object placed 12 cm in front of the lens. The object is 5 cm tall. How tall is the image?

   A. 2.5 cm   **C.** 7.5 cm
   B. 3.3 cm   **D.** 10 cm

103. A diverging lens of focal length −24 cm is now used with the object 12 cm in front of the lens. How tall is the image if the object is 5 cm tall?

   A. 2.5 cm   **C.** 8 cm
   B. 3.3 cm   **D.** 10 cm

104. A nearsighted student cannot see objects clearly unless they are as close as 80 cm (his "far-point"). The image that he sees through his new contact

lens is a virtual image because he looks through the lens to see the image. What focal length lenses does he need in order to see very distant objects, such as the stars?

   A. −20 cm   **C.** −80 cm
   B. −30 cm   **D.** −40 cm

105. A student uses a lens marked "- 4 D," where *D* stands for diopters. What is the focal length of this lens in cm?

   A. −0.04 cm   **C.** −4 cm
   B. −0.25 cm   **D.** −25 cm

Passage VI (Questions 106–110)

Phases include solid, liquid, and gas. Many materials can exist in any of these depending upon conditions. There is, however, usually a gain or loss of heat in the transition.

106. A mechanical refrigerator is cooled by:

   A. conversion of a liquid to a gas.
   B. conversion of a solid to a liquid.
   C. conversion of a solid to a gas.
   D. conversion of a gas to a solid.

107. The freezing point of a crystalline solid is:

   A. several °C lower than the melting point.
   B. equal to the melting point.
   C. several °C higher than the melting point.
   D. not directly related to the melting point.

108. Transition of a material directly from solid to gas:

   A. is not known.
   B. is known as evaporation.
   C. is known as expiration.
   D. is known as sublimation.

109. Boiling point of a pure liquid is:

   A. usually increased by increased pressure.
   B. not usually affected by changes in pressure.
   C. usually decreased by increased pressure.
   D. affected by pressure but in a fairly unpredictable direction.

110. Conversion of oxygen from a gas to a liquid is possible only below −118°C, no matter what pressure is imposed. This temperature is known as the:

A. boiling point.
B. critical temperature.
C. condensation temperature.
D. Clausius temperature.

Passage VII (Questions 111–115)

An enzyme is a special kind of biological catalyst. In many ways it can be considered much as other catalysts.

A series of experiments gave results on the velocity (V) of an enzyme reaction (i.e., rate of formation of products) while keeping the enzyme concentration constant but varying substrate (S). The results are graphed as below:

111. Point A is an area where the reaction is _____ order with respect to the substrate.

A. zero   C. second
B. first   D. third

112. Point B is in an area where the reaction is _____ order with respect to the substrate.

A. zero   C. second
B. first   D. third

113. The substrate concentration of point C is:

A. zero.
B. the maximum soluble.
C. infinite.

D. the minimum amount that will give a measurable product.

114. The reciprocal of the ordinate at point C is:

A. the minimum velocity at minimum substrate.
B. the minimum velocity.
C. the minimum velocity at maximum substrate.
D. zero velocity.

115. Considering the two graphs, maximum velocity would be shown (or could be readily computed from):

A. point B.   C. point E.
B. point C.   D. point B or point C.

Passage VIII (Questions 116–120)

By varying the temperature and pressure for Substance X, the following phase diagram is obtained. It indicates the phase(s) that will be found at a variety of temperatures and pressures.

116. Liquid, solid, and gas may be found in equilibrium at the temperature and pressure indicated by:

A. point 1.   C. point 3.
B. point 2.   D. point 4.

117. Starting at a temperature and pressure indicated by point 4 and heating the material without change of pressure, one would reach a phase change at:

A. point 6.   C. point 8.
B. point 7.   D. point 9.

118. Starting at a temperature and pressure indicated by point 10 and increasing the pressure as much as possible without changing temperature, one would:

A. pass through the point where gas, liquid, and solid are in equilibrium.
B. reach a point where solid is in equilibrium with gas.

C. reach a point where solid is in equilibrium with liquid.

D. note no phase change.

119. The critical temperature is indicated at:

A. point 1.   C. point 3.

B. point 2.   D. point 4.

120. The temperature at point 7, at the indicated pressure, is called the:

A. freezing temperature.

B. sublimation temperature.

C. boiling temperature.

D. allotropic temperature.

Passage IX (Questions 121–125)

A newly discovered reaction is being studied. It is concluded that the reaction consists of

$$2A + 3B \leftrightharpoons 3C + 2D$$

(The letters A, B, C, and D represent hypothetical compounds.)

121. The equilibrium constant as written may be calculated as:

A. $\dfrac{[C]^3 [D]^2}{[A]^2 [B]^3}$ C. $\dfrac{[A]^2 [B]^3}{[C]^3 [D]^2}$

B. $\dfrac{3[C]\, 2[D]}{2[A]\, 3[B]}$ D. $\dfrac{[C]\, [D]}{[A]\, [B]}$

122. If the equilibrium constant is 0.001:

A. reaction to the right will be favored.

B. reaction to the left will be favored.

C. the reaction rate is fast.

D. the reaction rate is slow.

123. If *A*, *B*, and *D* are gases and *C* is a solid, the reaction will:

A. be improved toward the right with increased pressure.

B. be improved toward the left with increased pressure.

C. be unaffected by increased pressure.

D. not proceed in either direction in the presence of increased pressure.

124. At standard temperature and pressure, the volume represented by 3 moles of C is about:

A. 22 liters.

B. 45 liters.

C. 67 liters.

D. more than 80 liters.

125. A small equilibrium constant is indicative of:

A. a fast reaction rate.

B. a slow reaction rate.

C. no reaction.

D. none of the above.

Passage X (Questions 126–135)

A liquid is isolated, containing 5.9% hydrogen and 94.1% oxygen by mass. The elements are 50% hydrogen and 50% oxygen by volume. The molecular weight is determined to be 34.0. In a decomposition reaction this liquid produces water, oxygen, and no other products.

126. The empirical formula is:

A. HO.   C. H_3O_3.

B. H_2O_2.   D. H_3O_4.

127. The molecular formula is:

A. HO.   C. H_3O_3.

B. H_2O_2.   D. H_3O_4.

128. The balanced equation for the decomposition indicates that one mole of the liquid will produce _____ moles of oxygen.

A. 0.25   C. 1.0

B. 0.50   D. 2.0

129. The balanced equation for the decomposition indicates that one mole of the liquid will produce _____ moles of water.

A. 0.25   C. 1.0

B. 0.50   D. 2.0

130. The balanced equation for the decomposition of the liquid indicates the formation of _____ liters of oxygen at S.T.P. from one mole of the liquid.

A. 1.12   C. 11.2

B. 2.24   D. 22.4

131. The balanced equation for the decomposition of the liquid indicates the formation of _____ g of water from 34 g of the liquid.

A. 16   C. 30
B. 18   D. 32

132. For an equilibrium reaction at 25°C, the decomposition we have been considering would be _____ by an increase in pressure.

A. favored
B. unaffected
C. adversely affected
D. affected, but in an unpredictable direction

133. For an equilibrium reaction at 25°C, the decomposition would be _____ by an increase in oxygen without an increase in pressure.

A. favored
B. unaffected
C. adversely affected
D. affected, but in an unpredictable direction

134. In the above question, the equilibrium constant would be:

A. increased.
B. unaffected.
C. decreased.
D. affected, but in an unpredictable direction.

135. The order of the reaction, from information given above, will be definitely

A. zero.   C. second.
B. first.   D. unpredictable.

Questions 136-142 are independent of any passages and of each other.

136. Catalysts:

A. are changed and consumed during a reaction.
B. have virtually no effect on the overall rate of the reaction.
C. are changed but not consumed during a reaction.
D. speed up the rate of the reaction.

137. If solution A is less concentrated in dissolved particle content than solution B, then solution B is said to be:

A. hypertonic.   C. isoosmotic.
B. hypotonic.   D. isotonic.

138. Compared to one mole of oxygen, how many more molecules do two moles of carbon dioxide contain?

A. 25×10^6 C. 6.02×10^{23}
B. 12.04×10^{46} D. 12.04×10^{23}

139. Which one of the following acids does not commonly form acid salts?

A. $HC_2H_3O_2$ C. H_2CO_3
B. H_2SO_4 D. H_3PO_4

140. Which of the statements listed below is false?

A. An aqueous solution in which $[H^+] > 1 \times 10^{-7}$ is said to be acidic.
B. Ions are atoms or groups of atoms that have lost or gained one or more electrons.
C. HCl is a Brønsted acid because it furnishes H^+ ion in solution.
D. NaOH is called a base because it furnishes Na^+ ions in solution.

141. In the decomposition of $KClO_3$ to generate oxygen gas, MnO_2 is added in order to:

A. increase the volume of oxygen obtained from the $KClO_3$.
B. produce oxygen of higher purity.
C. reduce the temperature at which decomposition of $KClO_3$ takes place.
D. increase the temperature at which decomposition of $KClO_3$ takes place.

142. The name applied to a substance such as MnO_2 used in the reaction above is a (an):

A. enzyme.
B. catalyst.
C. isotope.
D. free radical scavenger.

WRITING SAMPLE

2 ESSAYS
60 MINUTES (30 MINUTES/TOPIC)

DIRECTIONS: Your response must be a unified organized essay; it should contain fully developed, logically constructed paragraphs. Remember quality is more important than length. Before you begin writing, make sure you have read the item carefully and understand what is being asked. Write as legibly as possible. Because your essays will be scored as first-draft compositions, you may cross out and make corrections on your response booklet as necessary. It is not necessary to recopy your essay.

Part 1

Consider this statement:

A wise man sees as much as he ought, not as much as he can.

Montaigne

Write a unified essay in which you perform the following tasks. Explain what the above quotation means. Describe a specific situation in which a wise person sees as much as he can, not as much as he ought. Discuss what you think determines the limits that should and should not be placed on vision.

Part 2

Consider this statement:

There is properly no history; only biography

Emerson

Write a unified essay in which you perform the following tasks. Explain what you think the above statement means. Describe a specific situation in which there would, in fact, be history, whether or not there were biography. Discuss what you think determines the relationship between history and biography.

BIOLOGICAL SCIENCES

10 PROBLEM SETS OF 5–10 QUESTIONS EACH
15 PROBLEMS FOLLOWED BY A SINGLE QUESTION
77 QUESTIONS
100 MINUTES

DIRECTIONS: The following questions or incomplete statements are in groups. Preceding each series of questions or statements is a paragraph or a short explanatory statement, a formula or set of formulas, or a definition. Read the written material and then answer the questions or complete the statements. Select the ONE BEST ANSWER for each question and indicate your selection by marking the corresponding letter of your choice on the Answer Form. Eliminate those alternatives you know to be incorrect and then select an answer from among the remaining alternatives.

Passage I (Questions 143–148)

The diagram illustrates a typical neuron, the basic unit of the nervous system, located in a spinal (dorsal root) ganglion. Neurons connect with each other and in that manner an impulse is conducted and transmitted throughout the body. Two types of cell processes are indicated.

143. An impulse on the skin will be picked up by:

A.	4.	**C.**	7.
B.	6.	**D.**	10.

144. The genetic material of the cell is located in:

A.	2.	**C.**	5.
B.	3.	**D.**	7.

145. Protein synthesis is carried out under the direction of:

A.	3 in 5.	**C.**	2 in 5.
B.	2 in 3.	**D.**	2 in 7.

A person has been in an accident and the physician is conducting a neurological examination. Sensation is lost over several fingers and the examiner fears that a nerve has been cut. Note the cut indication on the diagram preceeding question 143.

146. Which process would completely degenerate?

A.	11	**C.**	10a
B.	8	**D.**	10b

147. Retrograde degeneration would be visible in:

A.	2.	**C.**	6.
B.	3.	**D.**	10b.

148. The impulse in the neuron is normally conducted in which direction?

A.	9	**C.**	Neither 9 nor 1
B.	1	**D.**	Both 9 and 1

Passage II (Questions 149–154)

The purpose of these experiments is to illustrate the action of both active and passive driving forces on the absorption of solutions of hemoglobin, Ringer's solution, $MgSO_4$, xylose, and glucose from the lumen of the small intestines *in vivo*.

Fluid can be absorbed from the small intestine even when the luminal solution is isotonic Ringer's. The absence of a net passive driving force for water uptake between lumen and blood indicates that active processes are involved. The active transport is *not* on the water itself but rather on sodium chloride. Active sodium transport from the epithelial cells renders the intercellular spaces sufficiently hypertonic to create osmotic driving forces for water movement out of the lumen.

Glucose is transported from the lumen by means of a specific carrier. The carrier has a site for the sugar and for sodium. It is the sodium gradient across the apical cell membrane that provides the energy for glucose entry. The sodium gradient is maintained by the active extrusion of sodium from the cells. The carrier shows typical saturation kinetics. In the case of glucose, the Km for absorption is 2mM, when sodium levels are 145mM. By contrast, the pentose, xylose, is far less effective as a substrate for this carrier. At the same level of Na, its Km is about 100 mM.

Ions such as Mg^{2+} and SO^{2-}_4, which are poorly absorbed, behave toward the intestinal epithelium almost as if it were a semipermeable membrane. Thus, passive osmotic forces play a predominant role in determining the magnitude and direction of fluid movement. A similar statement can be made about intact proteins such as hemoglobin. These are ordinarily impermeable solutes.

By measuring the changes in fluid volume due to the presence of the test substances and by chemically analyzing for changes in the glucose, xylose, and hemoglobin concentration, data on how the *in vivo* intestine treats each substance will be obtained.

Experiment

In two rats, three successive 10 cm segments of intestine are tied off. Injected into the segments of rat one from proximal to distal were solutions of hemoglobin, Ringer's, and $MgSO_4$.

Injected into the segments of rat two from proximal to distal were solutions of xylose, Ringer's, and glucose. After one hour whatever fluid was present in the respective segments was withdrawn, and volumes recorded. Analysis for solutes present were conducted and percentage of absorption and recovery recorded.

149. From the "absorption from the intestine laboratory: when equal volumes of 100 mM of D-glucose or D-xylose are added in isotonic Ringer's solutions to isolated intestinal segments, the following would be expected (Km, glucose 2mM, xylose 100 mM).

   A. Equal volumes would be absorbed in a one-hour incubation.
   B. A greater volume absorbed from the xylose segment than for glucose.
   C. A greater volume absorbed from the glucose segment than for xylose.
   D. No volume change for either.

150. When 1 ml of a 1.8% solution of D-glucose was added to an intestinal segment in isotonic Ringer's solution and the total glucose analyzed at one hour, it was found that 1.8 mg was recovered. What percent of the D-glucose injected was absorbed or metabolized?

   A. 1.8%   C. 10%
   B. 1%   D. 90%

151. For the "absorption from the intestine laboratory," when a hemoglobin solution in water was injected into the isolated small intestine, at the end of one hour:

   A. more hemoglobin would be recovered than injected because proteins are secreted into the intestine.
   B. less hemoglobin was recovered because intact proteins are normally absorbed.
   C. less hemoglobin was recovered because bleeding into the intestine would normally occur.
   D. less hemoglobin was recovered because some hemoglobin was adsorbed on the surface of the mucosal lumen.

152. For the "absorption from the intestine laboratory," for injection of D-glucose in isotonic Ringer's solution, inhibition of glucose transport would occur when:

   I. D-galactose was also added to the segment.
   II. sodium ion was replaced by a large cation.
   III. when L-glucose replaced D-glucose.
   IV. when an uncoupler of ATP synthesis (dinitrophenol) was added.

   A. I, II, and III   C. II and IV
   B. I and III   D. All are correct

153. For the "absorption from the intestine laboratory," when 25% $MgSO_4$ was injected into the isolated small intestine, the expected change was:

   A. an increase in volume.
   B. a decrease in volume.
   C. no change in volume.

154. For the "absorption from the intestine laboratory," when a hemoglobin solution in water was injected into the isolated small intestine, the expected change was:

   A. an increase in volume.
   B. a decrease in volume.
   C. no change in volume.

Passage III (Questions 155–161)

The schema of thyroxine formation is outlined below:

155. Chemically, thyroid hormones are:

A. iodotyrosines.   C. iodides.

B. iodothyronines.   D. iodines.

156. In proceeding from compound 3 to compound 4, the amino acid tyrosine is:

A. oxidized.   C. iodinated.

B. reduced.   D. synthesized.

157. During transport thyroid hormones are inactive because they are:

A. in the form of thyroglobutin.

B. free hormones.

C. protein-bound.

D. on red blood cells.

158. Untreated goiter is associated with:

A. hyperthyroidism.

B. hypothyroidism.

C. euthyroidism.

D. A, B, and C.

159. TSH:

A. is made up of two peptide chains (alpha and beta).

B. is released by the hypothalamus.

C. binds tightly to thyroid binding globulin (TBG).

D. secretion decreases upon exposure to the cold.

160. Involved in the regulation of the synthesis of thyroid hormone are

A. availability of iodide ions.

B. TSH.

C. negative feedback of circulating T_3 and T_4 at the level of the anterior pituitary (by down regulation of TRH receptors).

D. all of the above.

161. Which of the following describes the metabolic effect of thyroid hormone?

A. decreased myocardial beta adrenergic receptors

B. decreased BMR

C. increased oxygen consumption

D. increased plasma cholesterol

Passage IV (Question 162–166)

The following graph illustrates several phenomena that develop while a muscle is being repetitively stimulated:

162. In the diagram above, region 1 represents:

A. summation.

B. complete or fused tetanus.

C. repeated identical twitches.

D. hyperpolarization.

163. What is the most likely cause of the event in region 3?

A. consumption of ATP stored in the muscle

B. loss of myosin from the muscle

C. gradual failure to transmit the stimulus to the contraction apparatus

D. loss of elasticity within the muscle

164. What is the major difference between regions 1 and 2?

A. Elastic elements have become fully stretched in region 1, but not in region 2.

B. Elastic elements have become fully stretched in region 2, but not in region 1.

C. The stimulus strength is greater in region 2.

D. The stimulus strength is greater in region 1.

165. In the diagram, region 2 represents:

    A. incomplete tetanus.
    B. muscle fatigue.
    C. relaxation.
    D. an absolute refractory period.

166. If a muscle is stimulated to contract, allowed to develop force, but not allowed to shorten, then the contraction is called:

    A. spasmodic.   **C.** tetanic.
    B. isotonic.   **D.** isometric.

Passage V (Questions 167–171)

Epilepsy affects approximately one in 200 people or about 1.2 million persons in the United States alone. Despite pharmacologic treatment, 25% of patients continue to have intermittent seizures, and one-quarter million persons have seizures more frequently than once per month. A form of continuous or recurrent seizures persisting for over 30 minutes is operationally defined as *Status Epilepticus* (SE). SE is associated with an exceptionally high mortality rate of 25%. The incidence of SE is about 250 cases per million population annually.

Seizures are broadly classified as general or partial depending on whether they arise from the entire brain simultaneously or just from a restricted region respectively. They are subclassified on the basis of the presence or absence of associated convulsive activity.

Because of the significance of epilepsy as a public health issue and present inadequacies in drug therapy, better pharmacologic strategies for the treatment of epilepsy are currently being sought. Toward this end, a number of animal models have been developed that can predict the success of new and potentially useful anticonvulsant compounds. These predictions are based on the correlation between the recognized clinical success in treating certain classes of seizures with present anticonvulsants and the degree of efficacy (effectiveness) of these same medications against seizures generated in each of the different animal models.

Class	Generalized			Partial
Subclass	Absence	Tonic-Clonic	Myoclonic	Complex
Convulsive?	No	Yes	Yes	Usually
Animal Model	GABA challenge	Electroshock	Audiogenic mouse	Kindling
First choice	ESM	PHT	VPA	CBZ
Second choice	VPA	VPA	PB	PHT
Third choice				VPA

Abbreviations: CBZ—carbamazepine, ESM—ethosuximide, GABA—gamma amino butyric acid, PB—phenobarbital, PHT—phenytoin, VPA—valproic acid.

167. AntiEpp is a new compound that has shown promise in animal seizure models. It is found to have greatest efficacy in the electroshock model and has slightly less efficacy in the kindling model. This predicts that it might be very good in treating ___i___ seizures and acceptable for treating ___ii___ seizures.

	i	ii
A.	generalized convulsive	partial complex
B.	tonic-clonic	no other
C.	tonic-clonic	partial complex
D.	audiogenic mouse	electroshock

168. New compounds are often tested because of chemical similarity to conventional agents. In drug testing, Compound X was found to be effective against the model of absence seizures. It was ineffective in all animal models of other seizure types. Which agent is Compound X probably most similar to?

    A. carbamazepine
    B. ethosuximide
    C. valproic acid
    D. not enough information is available to answer the question

169. The 1990 population of New York City is about 7 million persons. How many persons are statistically likely to suffer from epilepsy?

    A. 3,500 persons   **C.** 35,000 persons
    B. 1,750 persons   **D.** 17,500 persons

170. A patient is found to have been seizing for over an hour. Electrical activity from her brain recorded on an electroencephalogram reveals that the abnormal activity is localized only to a restricted region. The best description of her condition is:

    A. status epilepticus.
    B. generalized status epilepticus.
    C. partial status epilepticus.
    D. partial complex seizure.

171. From information provided in the reading passage, please indicate the approximate number of patients with epilepsy who continue to have seizures at least once per month despite pharmacologic (drug) therapy.

    A. 30,000   **C.** 1/4 million
    B. 300,000   **D.** 250,000

Passage VI (Questions 172–179)

Using a syringe containing heparin, 50 milliliters of blood were drawn from a healthy male volunteer. Following centrifugation, the "buffy coat" was removed and a lymphocyte-rich cell population was obtained by sedimentation through 2% Dextran. After washing in 0.9% saline, the lymphocytes were placed in cell culture tubes at a concentration of 5×10^6 cells/ml cell culture medium/tube. To one-half of the tubes was added 5 μg of phytohemagglutinin, a substance which causes lymphocytes to undergo mitosis. The other half of the tubes received no phytohemagglutinin. Radioactive tracers for RNA, DNA, and protein synthesis were then added to all tubes and aliquots removed at selected intervals. The following data were obtained:

172. The purpose of this experiment was to:

A. determine the role of heparin in blood clotting.
B. determine the sequence of events in cells stimulated to undergo mitosis, and to compare these data to those gathered from unstimulated cells.
C. isolate a pure population of lymphocytes.
D. determine the lifespan of lymphocytes.

173. From these data it can be seen that increased:

A. RNA synthesis precedes increased protein synthesis.
B. DNA synthesis precedes increased protein synthesis.
C. protein synthesis precedes increased RNA synthesis.
D. DNA synthesis precedes increased RNA synthesis.

174. It may also be assumed that:

A. DNA synthesis is dependent on previous RNA synthesis.
B. protein synthesis is dependent on previous DNA synthesis.
C. RNA synthesis is dependent on previous protein synthesis.
D. unstimulated lymphocytes synthesize RNA, DNA, and protein at a low rate.

175. The smallest unit possessing the capability to maintain life and to reproduce is:

A. an organ. C. DNA.
B. a cell. D. RNA.

176. Normally, a complete set of chromosomes ($2n$) is passed on to each daughter cell as a result of:

A. reduction division.
B. mitotic cell division.
C. meiotic cell division.
D. nondisjunction.

177. Messenger RNA receives its instructions from:

A. ribosomes.
B. endoplasmic reticulum.
C DNA in the nucleus.
D. cytoplasm.

178. During which phase of the mitotic cycle do the two chromatids split apart and start migration toward the poles of the spindle?

A. prophase C. anaphase
B. metaphase D. telophase

179. During metaphase of mitosis:

A. there is a dissolution of the chromosomal material.
B. the centrioles with asters are at the opposite poles.
C. the cell membrane starts to reappear.
D. the nuclear membrane disappears.

Passage VII (Questions 180–189)

The liver from a rat was gently homogenized in buffered sucrose solution using a Dounce homogenizer (which does not break most membranous organelles in cells). The homogenate was layered over a sucrose gradient and centrifuged for four hours at 100,000 xg. The sucrose gradient was then collected as a series of fractions. Each fraction was analyzed for DNA concentration, RNA concentration, cytochrome oxidase activity, acid phosphatase activity, and cytochrome P-450 concentration. Concentrations and enzyme activities are given as relative values, with the fraction giving the highest value for each component being shown as 100 and all other values for that component being scaled relative to the highest value.

180. Which fraction contains most of the nuclei from the hepatocytes?

   A. fraction 1   **C.** fraction 3
   B. fraction 2   **D.** fraction 4

181. Which fraction contains most of the mitochondria from the hepatocytes?

   A. fraction 1   **C.** fraction 3
   B. fraction 2   **D.** fraction 4

182. Which fraction contains most of the rough endoplasmic reticulum from the hepatocytes?

   A. fraction 1   **C.** fraction 3
   B. fraction 2   **D.** fraction 4

183. Which fraction contains most of the lysosomes from the hepatocytes?

   A. fraction 1   **C.** fraction 3
   B. fraction 2   **D.** fraction 4

184. Which fraction contains most of the smooth endoplasmic reticulum from the hepatocytes?

   A. fraction 1   **C.** fraction 3
   B. fraction 2   **D.** fraction 4

185. Which fraction contains most of the Krebs Cycle enzymes from the hepatocytes?

   A. fraction 1   **C.** fraction 3
   B. fraction 2   **D.** fraction 4

186. Which fraction should contain most of the newly synthesized plasma proteins from the hepatocytes?

   A. fraction 1   **C.** fraction 3
   B. fraction 2   **D.** fraction 4

187. Which fraction should appear much larger when isolated from pancreatic exocrine cells than when isolated from hepatocytes? Assume that the assays used in the experiment shown here are used to quantitate the fractions.

   A. fraction 1   **C.** fraction 3
   B. fraction 2   **D.** fraction 4

188. Which fraction should appear much larger when isolated from monocytes or connective tissue macrophages than when isolated from hepatocytes? Assume that the assays used in the experiment shown here are used to quantitate the fractions.

A. fraction 1   **C.** fraction 3
B. fraction 2   **D.** fraction 4

189. Which fraction should appear much larger when isolated from proximal convoluted tubule cells from the kidney than when isolated from hepatocytes? Assume that the assays used in the experiment shown here are used to quantitate the fractions.

A. fraction 1   **C.** fraction 3
B. fraction 2   **D.** fraction 4

Passage VIII (Questions 190–194)

The citric acid cycle (Krebs cycle, tricarboxylic cycle) is the final metabolic pathway for glucose, many amino acids, and fatty acids. The enzymes for the pathway are located in the inner mitochondrial membrane. The electrons from the oxidation of these metabolic fuels are conserved in the formation of reducing equivalents, such as NADH or $FADH_2$ for eventual reoxidation in the respiratory assembly to generate ATP by oxidative phosphorylation. Whereas glucose and fatty acids produce acetyl CoA for oxidation to recover the bond energy and produce CO_2, some amino acids have different routes of catabolism including acetyl CoA, other metabolites of the pathway, and pyruvate formation. The citric acid cycle can accept metabolites at places other than acetyl CoA and is able to supply metabolites for biosynthesis such as in the synthesis of porphyrins or amino acids. However, net glucose cannot be synthesized from acetyl CoA entering the cycle. The reactions have many similarities such as hydration—dehydration or oxidation, particularly of secondary alcohols to ketone. For every mole of acetyl CoA entering the cycle and condensing with oxaloacetate, 12 moles of ATP and two moles of CO_2 are formed and a mole of oxaloacetate is recovered. The rate of the cycle is controlled by energy levels of the cell at specific enzymatic points including the formation of citric acid and the formation of α-ketoglutarate.

190. For one mole of acetyl CoA entering the Krebs (TCA) cycle (coupled to oxidative phosphorylation):

A. one mole of carbon dioxide and 38 ATP are formed.
B. two moles of carbon dioxide and 38 ATP are formed.
C. two moles of carbon dioxide and 24 ATP are formed.
D. two moles of carbon dioxide and 12 ATP are formed.

191. All of the following are similar pairs of types of reactions starting with pyruvate EXCEPT:

A. isocitrate to oxalosuccinate; malate to oxaloacetate.
B. alpha ketoglutarate to succinyl CoA; acetyl CoA to pyruvate.
C. cis-aconitase to isocitrate; fumarate to malate.
D. pyruvate to acetyl CoA; alpha ketoglutarate to succinyl CoA.

192. The citric acid cycle provides biosynthetic intermediates (net) for the following EXCEPT:

A. acetyl CoA to oxaloacetate.
B. acetyl CoA to malonyl CoA.
C. succinyl CoA to porphyrins.
D. oxaloacetate to aspartate.

193. All of the following are metabolic functions or possible interactions of the tricarboxylic acid cycle EXCEPT:

A. decreased activity when ATP levels are high.
B. control of glycolysis.
C. accepting acetyl CoA from fatty acids, glucose, and some amino acids.
D. net synthesis of glucose occurs from acetyl CoA.

194. All of the following are correct about the citric acid cycle EXCEPT:

A. active in the mature red blood cell in humans.
B. occurs in the mitochondria.
C. provides about 24 ATP/moles of glucose (coupled to ox-phos).
D. when acetyl CoA amount increases it may increase gluconeogenesis from other carbon atoms.

Passage IX (Questions 195–199)

The carbon atom can have four different substituted groups. Because these molecules are not flat, but occupy a three-dimensional shape, they become chiral (handedness, like your right and left hand). The basal molecule that originally all other molecules were compared to was D(+) glyceraldehyde. It has a mirror image L(-) glyceraldehyde with the same chemical and physical properties (with special exceptions) but different biological properties. The D isomer has the OH group on the right side, whereas the L isomer has the OH on the left side. These are enantiomers. The next higher homolog of this aldotriose is an aldotetrose. The family of the aldosugars for trioses and tetroses is shown below. Note that the D tetroses (erythrose and threose) are not entiomers (not mirror images) but are diastereoisomers with different chemical, physical, and biological properties. These D tetroses are also epimers, because they differ only by the configuration around a single carbon atom. The stability of certain stereoforms has allowed them to predominate in nature (D-glucose, for example). The specificity of enzymes allows them to recognize three dimensional stereodifferences. For example, D-glucose and an epimer at the C4 carbon D-galactose. The translation of amino acids in proteins in humans is for the L-form.

195. Amino acids found in humans are usually:

    A. optically inactive.
    B. of the L-series.
    C. of the D-series.
    D. a racemic mixture.

196. Carbohydrates in humans (glucose, galactose, fructose, mannose, for example) are usually:

    A. optically inactive.
    B. of the L-series.
    C. of the D-series.
    D. a racemic mixture.

197. D-glucose and L-galactose are:

    A. epimers.   C. enantiomers.
    B. diastereomers.   D. A and B.

198. Epimers of D-glucose include:

    A. D-galactose.   C. D-fructose.
    B. D-mannose.   D. A and B.

199. D-glucose (assume no cyclic structure) has the OH group at _____ carbon as its D indicator.

    A. 1   C. 3
    B. 2   D. 5

Passage X (Questions 200–204)

The mature human red blood cell is unique in that it has no nucleus and no mitochondria, and has a finite lifetime of 120 days. Its main function is as a carrier of hemoglobin. In fact, the signal for its death is triggered by the loss of hemoglobin function. The red blood cell metabolizes glucose by two pathways with glucose-6-

phosphate as the branch point. One direction is the glycolytic pathway to provide energy through substrate level phosphorylation and to produce pyruvate. In order to maintain the glycolytic pathway, the pyruvate is reduced enzymatically using L-lactic dehydrogenase and the coenzyme NADH. The oxidized coenzyme NAD⁺ is then used as an electron acceptor in oxidation of 3-phosphoglyceraldehyde in the glycolytic pathway. Lactate leaves the red blood cell and is reoxidized in the liver to pyruvate, which has many fates in metabolism. The second direction for glucose-6-phosphate in metabolism is in the hexose monophosphate pathway (pentose pathway). This pathway produces special reducing equivalents (NADPH) that are used to maintain the red cell membrane, the ferrous ion and molecules, that are the cells reservoir of -SH groups (glutathione). Drug metabolism frequently requires NADPH so that a deficit in the first enzyme directing this pathway (glucose-6-phosphate dehydrogenase) results in a premature hemolysis of the red blood cell.

200. The end product(s) of catabolism of glucose in the red blood cell by the glycolytic pathway is/are:

A. glucose-6-phosphate.
B. carbon dioxide.
C. acetyl CoA.
D. pyruvate and lactate.

201. The first step in the metabolism of glucose:

A. occurs in the cytoplasm.
B. requires ATP.
C. produces glucose-6-phosphate.
D. all are correct.

202. ATP producing steps in glycolysis include:

A. glucose to glucose-6-phosphate.
B. phosphoenol pyruvate to pyruvate.
C. 1,3 bis phosphoglycerate to 3-phosphoglycerate.
D. B and C.

203. A genetic defect in the red blood cell enzyme glucose-6-phosphate dehydrogenase will result in all of the following EXCEPT:

A. decrease in the formation of NADPH.
B. increase in the hemolysis of red blood cells.
C. failure to reduce pyruvate to lactate.
D. A and B are correct.

204. Glycolysis and the hexose monophosphate shunt:

A. have no common places of interaction.
B. only interface through glucose-6-phosphate.
C. both produce CO_2 in the red blood cell.
D. interact through common intermediates, such as glyceraldehyde-3-phosphate.

DIRECTIONS: Read each passage carefully, study each table, chart, or formula, then answer the question following it. Eliminate those choices that you think to be incorrect and mark the letter of your choice on the answer sheet.

Effect of Various Treatments on Organ Weights

| Treatments | No. of Animals | Body Weight Grams | Organ Weight (mg/100 g Body Weight) | | |
			Organ 1	Organ 2	Organ 3
Control	8	70	1509 ± 34	223 ± 20	22 ± 0.8
Drug A	8	66	1044 ± 30	87 ± 14	23 ± 1.0
Drug B	8	73	1432 ± 51	224 ± 24	26 ± 0.9
Drug A + B	8	71	1586 ± 68	208 ± 28	25 ± 1.2
Drug C	8	73	1393 ± 80	146 ± 19	31 ± 2.0
Drug B + C	8	65	954 ± 50	61 ± 3	26 ± 2.0

205. The following statements are related to the table above. Based on the information given, select the statement *contradicted by* the information in the table.

A. Causal evaluation of the results leads one to believe that treatment resulted in significant effects.
B. Drugs B and C seem to have acted in an additive manner.
C. The experimenters should have paid closer attention to body weights.
D. Drug C affects all parameters under investigation.

Diet	Losing Weight	Mortality
Balanced Diet	4%	2%
Diet A	90%	74%
Diet A + Vitamin C	84%	72%
Diet A + Vitamin B	4%	2%
Diet A + Vitamin A	88%	76%

Groups of 50 mice were fed the diets listed in the table, and the percentage losing more than 10% of their initial body weight and the percentage mortality after 30 days were recorded.

206. The best conclusion to be drawn from this study is that

    A. diet A is a good reducing diet.
    B. diet A lacks B vitamins.
    C. vitamin C is not necessary for life.
    D. vitamin A is necessary for life.

The epiphyseal cartilage plate is very sensitive to somatotrophin (growth hormone) and, therefore, can be used as an assay for this compound. Species variations exist and other hormones such as estrogen, thyroxine, and several antibiotics also have an effect upon cartilage growth. The assay must be carried out on hypophysectomized animals.

The following experiments were conducted as can be seen from the table:

Test Groups	No. of Animals	Cartilage Growth in μ	
		1 Injection Daily	2 Injections/Day (1/2 amount each time)
Control (normal) (saline)	20 (10/injecting group)	100	100
Hyphophysectomized (saline)	20	60	60
Hypox + 100 mg STH	20	150	160
Hypox + 300 mg STH	20	180	195
Stressed normal animals (saline)	20	175	190
Hypox + stressed (saline)	20	50	50
Stressed normal + 100 mg STH	20	200	210
Hypox, stressed + 100 mg STH	20	110	120

207. The reason the assay must be carried out on hypophysectomized rats is:

    A. just to add another sophisticated method to the experiment.
    B. because the pituitary produces its own growth hormone and it might interfere with the assay.
    C. to study the pituitary composition of growth hormone.
    D. to obtain the animals' own growth hormone.

The following experimental protocol was carried out. Bean seeds were picked for their uniformity and 20 were planted/pot. One hundred percent germination was observed; and when the seedlings were nine days old, the seedlings of uniform growth were selected for treatment with X rays. Four hundred r units/minute were applied at a distance of 30 cm from the object. Seedlings were exposed up to 60 minutes with up to 24,000 r. After exposure, seedlings were placed in a greenhouse and kept at uniform light, temperature, and moisture conditions. Seedlings were measured as indicated in the table.

Code

	I		II
1	From ground to cotyledon (a mark was made on the seedling near the ground with india ink)	A	0 minutes—control
		B	7.5 minutes—3,000 r
		C	15 minutes—6,000 r
		D	30 minutes—12,000 r
		E	60 minutes—24,000 r
2	Cotyledon to 1st node		
3	Petiole length of 1st leaf		
4	Midrib of 1st leaf		
5	From 1st node to tip of the plant (when included)		

EXPERIMENTAL RESULTS

10 Days

	A	B	C	D	E
1	6.20	6.58	7.30	5.45	4.43
2	2.17	2.16	2.30	1.15	.76
3	.87	1.11	1.10	0.65	.53
4	3.00	3.23	3.02	2.03	1.86
5					

17 Days

	A	B	C	D	E
1	7.08	6.73	8.00	6.99	5.82
2	8.06	7.11	5.36	2.50	1.63
3	4.12	4.50	4.15	2.13	1.70
4	5.44	5.27	5.68	5.33	4.97
5					

33 Days

	A	B	C	D	E
1	7.21	6.73	8.00	7.00	6.05
2	8.07	7.11	5.48	2.65	1.65
3	4.33	4.61	4.86	2.30	1.90
4	5.50	5.50	6.13	5.91	5.25
5	12.56	11.38	5.27		

208. The purpose of this experiment was:

    A. to observe the germination rate.
    B. to check for uniform growth rate.
    C. test output and scatter of the X ray machine.
    D. observe X ray effect on growth.

Both sexes carry a complete complement of sex-linked genes. A female, however, with the XX arrangement will only exhibit a recessive gene if she has received it from both parents (a rare event if we are dealing with an uncommon gene of the population); while in the male with the XY arrangement the recessive gene cannot be masked since there is no partner X chromosome and, therefore, a larger number of recessive genes are expressed (examples are hemophilia and color blindness). A man receives his X chromosome from his mother and passes it on to his daughters, not his sons. His daughters in this respect are the carriers of his sex-linked traits and their sons will be the affected ones. Let us illustrate with an example. The normal czarina of Russia produced sons suffering from hemophilia, a disease that is caused by a sex-linked recessive gene, h. The more dominant gene, H, produces normal blood clotting. Genotypically, these women must have carried Hh (X_H and X_h). A daughter, depending on the father ($X_H Y$ or $X_h Y$), could have carried $X_H X_h$ or $X_H X_H$, while a son could have been born either with an $X_H Y$ or an $X_h Y$ (hemophilic) chromosomal complement.

209. The following statements are related to the information presented above. Select the statement *supported by* the information given.

    A. A cattle breeder has in a herd a dominant Y-linked trait. A calf sired by a bull carrying this trait is born. The chances of the inheritance of the trait are 50%.
    B. A female calf was born; the chances of exhibiting the trait are zero.
    C. If the sex in the above cross is known, there is no doubt about whether a calf has the trait.
    D. All of the above.

Melanoma tumors were implanted into three strains of mice. Experiments were then performed to determine the types and amounts of host serum antibodies produced against the lipid components of the virus contained in the melanoma cells. The results are summarized in the table below.

		Antilipid Antibody	
Host	Ag A Phenotype	Day 40 Post Implant	Day 60 Post Implant
Strain 1	3/3	4.5 ± 0.3	6.3 ± 1.7
Strain 2	1/3	3.4 ± 0.4	5.5 ± 1.3
Strain 3	1/1	1.3 ± 0.1	1.3 ± 0.3

210. The following statements are related to the information presented above. Select the statement *supported by* the information given.

    A. Strain 1 produced less antilipid antibody at both time periods measured than the other two hosts.
    B. On the basis of this information, Strain 1 animals are less resistant to melanoma type cancers than either Strain 2 or 3 animals.
    C. All three hosts produced more antibody at 60 days than they did at 40 days.
    D. An Ag A phenotype containing three seems to be related to higher antibody production.

During wound healing, proliferation of cells in epithelial tissues, connective tissues, and vascular tissues occurs in order to fill in and resurface the defect caused by necrotic (dead) tissue. In experimental studies of the cellular kinetics of wound healing, it is often necessary to assess the amount of proliferation in various cell populations. Because cells replicate DNA within 8 to 12 hours before dividing, determination of the frequency of DNA synthesis at a particular time among cells in a population is a good index of the rate of cell division. DNA synthesis can be determined by tagging replicating DNA with radioactive thymidine. By the procedure of autoradiography, the nuclei of cells which have incorporated radioactive thymidine can be identified on histological sections. The percentage of cells labeled with radioactive thymidine is called the labeling index.

The following table includes data on the labeling index of endothelial cells which form the lining of blood vessels.

^{3}H-THYMIDINE INDEX IN WOUND HEALING

Wound Age	Amount of Epidermal Resurfacing	Endothelial Labeling Index
1 day	0%	3.5%
2 days	0%	13.3%
3 days	0–5%	10.5%
6 days	60–70%	5.6%
10 days	90–100%	2.5%

211. The following statements are related to the information presented. Select the statement *not supported by* the information given.

A. The ^{3}H-thymidine labeling index, and hence the amount of endothelial prolifetation, increased before epidermal resurfacing had become evident.

B. The endothelial labeling index, after 2 days, decreased both with advancing wound age and with advancing surface coverage.

C. The increased endothelial proliferation at 2 and 3 days led to the formation of new blood vessels, which then induced epidermal resurfacing.

D. Endothelial proliferation ceases when the wounds are 90–100% resurfaced with epidermis.

Androgen compounds are responsible for maintaining the secondary sex organs and characteristics of organisms. An endocrinology class was divided into 4 groups to conduct a blind experiment and at the end was asked to compare results. Each group received a compound and injected a similar amount. The experimental protocol in male animals was: 1) Unoperated control animals; 2) Unoperated control animals receiving vehicle only; 3) Bilaterally castrated (testes removed) animals; and 4) Bilaterally castrated animals receiving unknown. The results were summarized in table form.

Experimental Groups	Prostate Weight-mg Student Groups				Seminal Vesicle Weight-mg Student Groups			
	1	2	3	4	1	2	3	4
Unoperated Control	33	31	29	34	68	65	63	67
Unoperated Control and Vehicle	31	32	30	31	69	70	65	64
Bilaterally Castrated	10	9	7	8	12	14	10	15
Bilaterally Castrated and Unknown	37	33	28	31	70	64	61	59

212. The following statements are related to the information presented above. Select the statement *supported by* the information given.

A. The prostate gland is more sensitive than the seminal vesicle to a lack of androgens.

B. These experiments were properly controlled.

C. The results obtained are probably not statistically significant.

D. Bilateral castration removes a major source of sex hormones.

Gerbils were used for this experiment. One group served as a control; one group was thyroidectomized and maintained on 1% calcium gluconate since the parathyroids were probably removed also; one group received daily injections of thyroxin; and one group that was thyroidectomized and maintained as described above also received daily injections, of thytoxin. Oxygen was measured in a standard manner. The following were the results.

Groups	Initial Body Weight gm	Final Body Weight gm	Thyroid Gland Weight mg	Liter of O_2 Consumed hour/ meter^2
Normal	143	150	5.0	1.54
Hypothyroid	160	174	0.0	0.16
Hyperthyroid	123	120	8.0	7.33
Hypothyroid + thyroxin	164	158	4.9	1.23

213. The following statements are based on the information presented above. Select the statement(s) *consistent with* the information given.

A. The quantity of heat liberated by an organism as calculated on the basis of respiratory exchange is decreased by deficiencies and elevated by excesses of the active thyroid principle.

B. After total thyroidectomy, the basal metabolic rate falls to 10% of its normal value.

C. Hypothyroid animals probably exhibited sluggishness.

D. All of the above.

A manufacturer is testing a newly designed line of autoclaves that will be marketed. Calibration of timers and temperature controls is critical to insure destruction of bacteria.

214. Bacteria Z will grow following exposure to temperature below 160°C. Which autoclave will fail to inactivate bacteria Z?

A. autoclave 1.
B. autoclave 1 and 2.
C. autoclave 2 and 3.
D. autoclave 3.

The pineal complex is implicated in the modulation of reproductive functions of the golden hamster. Surgical removal of the eyes produced atrophy of the testes and seminal vesicle within four to six weeks, and simultaneous pinealectomy prevented the atrophy. In the following experiment the drug MTPH was injected subcutaneously daily for 30 days to learn if there was an enhancement of atrophy. The results are summarized below.

Organ Weight
(mg/100g body weight)

Treatment	Number of Hamsters Treated	Testes	Seminal Vesicles
Untreated Control	6	2884	722
Blinding	6	1695[a]	396[a]
Pinealectomy	6	2600	544
Blinding, Pinealectomy	6	2580	577
MTPH, No Surgery	6	3069	699
MTPH, Blinding	6	1419[a]	398[a]
MTPH, Pinealectomy	6	2875	591
MTPH, Blinding, Pinealectomy	6	2635	577

[a]$(P < 0.05)$

215. The following statements are related to the information presented above. Select the statement *supported by* the information given.

A. Drug MTPH increased the testicular atrophy in blinded hamsters when compared with blinded hamsters not receiving MTPH.
B. Drug MTPH increased the seminal vesicle atrophy in blinded hamsters when compared with blinded hamsters not receiving MTPH.
C. Drug MTPH had no effect on atrophy, either testicular or seminal vesicles.
D. Drug MTPH, when administered without surgery, would affect reproductive organ weight.

216. In the reaction sequence used in breakdown of glycogen in the liver or muscle—glycogen → glucose-1-phosphate → glucose-6-phosphate → glucose—the first step is:

A. catalyzed by phosphorylase.
B. catalyzed by pepsin.
C. catalyzed by pancreatic amylase.
D. nonenzymatic.

217. A metabolic process that produces energy to convert ADP + phosphate into ATP is the:

A. production of fructose and glucose from sucrose.
B. production of fatty acids and glycerol from triglycerides.
C. production of CO_2 and water from fatty acids.
D. production of steroids from acetate.

218. A negative iodoform test (i.e., no yellow precipitate) will be the result when NAOH + I_2 is reacted with:

A. $CH_3-CH-CH_3$
         |
        OH

B. $CH_3-C-CH_2-CH_3$
         ||
        OH

C. $\emptyset-\overset{\overset{O}{||}}{C}-CH_3$

D. $CH_3-CH_2-CH_2-\overset{\overset{H}{|}}{C}=O$

Phenylamine is cooled to 0°C and treated with HCl and $NaNO_2$. After a few minutes of reaction time cuprous bromide is added, and the solution is heated.

219. The final product would primarily be a (an):

A. azo dye.
B. organometallic compound.
C. monosubstituted benzene containing no metal.
D. disubstituted benzene.

Model Examination D Answer Key

Verbal Reasoning

1.	C	14.	A	27.	C	40.	C	53.	C
2.	C	15.	C	28.	A	41.	A	54.	B
3.	D	16.	A	29.	B	42.	A	55.	A
4.	C	17.	D	30.	B	43.	B	56.	B
5.	B	18.	B	31.	D	44.	B	57.	D
6.	D	19.	C	32.	C	45.	D	58.	D
7.	D	20.	D	33.	C	46.	C	59.	B
8.	C	21.	C	34.	C	47.	C	60.	B
9.	B	22.	D	35.	D	48.	C	61.	C
10.	D	23.	D	36.	D	49.	A	62.	B
11.	D	24.	D	37.	D	50.	B	63.	C
12.	A	25.	A	38.	B	51.	B	64.	C
13.	B	26.	D	39.	C	52.	D	65.	D

Physical Sciences

66.	B	82.	D	98.	A	113.	C	128.	B
67.	D	83.	B	99.	B	114.	B	129.	C
68.	A	84.	B	100.	C	115.	D	130.	C
69.	B	85.	D	101.	D	116.	B	131.	B
70.	A	86.	A	102.	D	117.	B	132.	C
71.	B	87.	A	103.	B	118.	D	133.	C
72.	C	88.	D	104.	C	119.	A	134.	B
73.	A	89.	C	105.	D	120.	C	135.	D
74.	B	90.	B	106.	A	121.	A	136.	D
75.	B	91.	A	107.	B	122.	B	137.	A
76.	B	92.	C	108.	D	123.	A	138.	C
77.	C	93.	A	109.	A	124.	C	139.	A
78.	B	94.	A	110.	B	125.	D	140.	D
79.	D	95.	B	111.	B	126.	A	141.	C
80.	D	96.	B	112.	A	127.	B	142.	B
81.	A	97.	A						

Biological Sciences

143.	A	159.	A	175.	B	190.	D	205.	C
144.	A	160.	D	176.	B	191.	B	206.	B
145.	C	161.	C	177.	C	192.	A	207.	B
146.	D	162.	A	178.	C	193.	D	208.	D
147.	A	163.	C	179.	B	194.	A	209.	D
148.	B	164.	B	180.	D	195.	B	210.	D
149.	C	165.	A	181.	C	196.	C	211.	D
150.	D	166.	D	182.	A	197.	B	212.	D
151.	D	167.	C	183.	B	198.	D	213.	D
152.	D	168.	B	184.	A	199.	D	214.	A
153.	A	169.	C	185.	C	200.	D	215.	A
154.	B	170.	C	186.	A	201.	D	216.	A
155.	B	171.	B	187.	A	202.	D	217.	C
156.	C	172.	B	188.	B	203.	C	218.	D
157.	C	173.	A	189.	C	204.	D	219.	C
158.	D	174.	D						

Explanation of Answers for Model Examination D

VERBAL REASONING

1 **C.** The author characterizes the goals for freshman composition at the University of Texas as "standard" (three of them are listed in **A, B,** and **D**) and enumerates them in paragraph two. The goal not listed is **C**, the goal of teaching freshmen to bring about social change, an objective of the radical pedagogists.

2. **C.** See the explanation of question 1 (above). Bringing about social change is the goal of the radical pedagogists, according to paragraph five.

3. **D.** In paragraph six, Lazere is described as a "leftist educator and radical pedagogist" (**A** and **C**); in paragraph seven the passage clearly suggests that he would be in disagreement with the methods proposed by Sharon Crowley because they would force ideology on the student. The correct answer, therefore, would be **D**, all of the above.

4. **C.** The course, described in paragraph two, would examine the subject of "difference, specifically difference related to legal opinions given in court cases involving issues such as race, gender, bilingualism, and sexual orientation." Answer **C** partially describes the content of the course and is the correct response.

5. **B.** One can easily infer from the statements attributed to her in the passage that Crowley fits the definition for a radical pedagogist given in paragraph three. Among other things, she asserts that composition teachers "must give up our traditional subscription to liberal tolerance if we are to bring about social change through [our students]" (see paragraph seven).

6. **D.** Though **A, B,** and **C** are certainly logical areas for study in establishing a curriculum, they were not the endpoints for discussion sparked by the University of Texas debate. As the passage states in paragraph two, "the discussion became a forum for stating the purpose of composition and liberal education," the answer provided by **D**.

7. **D.** Early in the passage (in paragraph two), the author observes that the "debate that followed the submission and ultimate rejection of the program in many ways disregarded the course itself," a statement that provides the only evidence in the passage of the outcome of the specific curriculum proposal.

8. **C.** Paragraph one makes it clear that the investigator must focus on the question: "is complainant's job equal in effort and responsibility to that of a male counterpart?" Paragraph seven indicates that the judiciary has not yet endorsed the notion of comparable worth, and the length of employment is not addressed in the reading passage.

9. **B.** Paragraph one makes the point that identical jobs are not necessary because the standard is built on the concept that jobs must be evaluated within a context of substantial equivalency. None of the other statements is supported.

10. **D.** Statements **A** and **B** are not discussed in the passage. Paragraph three contradicts statement **C**, whereas paragraph five implies that Title VII encompasses very broad aspects and reaches beyond the confines of equal wage matters.

11. **D.** Although we might assume that the program of on-the-job training was a positive factor, the law does not address the issue. We could argue that the Department of Labor acted irresponsibly; however, we have no data to substantiate our claim. In the Columbia case, employees were aware of the differences in their positions. Paragraph five supports statement **D** because the court took into consideration the fact that heavy cleaning called for greater effort.

12. **A.** Paragraphs six and seven support statements I, II, and III; however, paragraph seven makes it clear that although the Supreme Court has ruled that Title VII provides a remedy for sex discrimination, the judiciary has not yet endorsed the notion of comparable worth.

13. **B.** Paragraph eight mentions the adverse decision the female guards received during the initial

trial, and statement I is supported. It also makes it clear that the appellate court reversed the trial court and held that one could sue even though jobs were not substantially equal; statement III is supported. The paragraph also states that although the Supreme Court did not adopt the concept of comparable worth, it left the door open for further litigation.

14. **A.** Paragraphs nine and ten clearly substantiate statements I, II, and III. Paragraph nine also indicates that the Supreme Court did not indicate how a plaintiff might establish a prima facie case under Title VII, and so statement IV is not supported.

15. **C.** It should be clear to the reader that the issue under consideration is sex discrimination and its resolution.

16. **A.** Paragraph one assigns the skull to Homo sapiens. Man is a vertebrate (subphylum); a mammal (class); Homo is the genus and sapiens is denoted as the species.

17. **D.** Because we are dealing with a fossil, the best answer is an archeologist.

18. **B.** The specimen was found in soil. The fluorine method of dating fossils was developed in 1949 and is based on the fact that buried bones absorb fluorine from the soil, and the amount increases with time.

19. **C.** The older a fossil is, the more fluorine would have been present. A modern jawbone would, on testing, yield a lesser amount of fluorine in comparison to an ancient cranium.

20. **D.** Iron in this case was used to artificially color the mandible to match the cranium.

21. **C.** The last fragment was quite thin; in reality it was chosen by the perpetrator of the hoax (Piltdown Hoax) to duplicate the thinnest part of the first skull.

22. **D.** The passage points out that iron salts are oxidized.

23. **D.** The chromium detected in the jawbone indicates that a dichromate solution was at first used by the forger in an attempt to assist the oxidation of iron salts used to stain the specimens.

24. **D.** There were developments of several methods to study fossils in the 50 years it took to resolve this matter. Although one of the theories proposed was that the missing link was found, the investigation centered on solving the disparity of evidence between the cranium and the jaw. This was a brilliantly devised falsification and no one to date knows for sure who the culprit was.

25. **A.** There is no evidence in the passage that Sara Murphy believed anything other than **A,** Zelda's inner complexity, caused her to appear different in the various photographs that were taken of her. Murphy's observation is cited in paragraph one.

26. **D.** In paragraph four, the author characterizes Nancy Milford as Zelda's first major biographer. Sara Mayfield was Zelda's girlhood friend, and she wrote a biography after Milford had published hers. The passage does not provide that information, however. Arthur Mizener was Scott Fitzgerald's first major biographer, and Sara Murphy was a close friend of the Fitzgeralds. But again, the passage does not provide this information. **A, B,** and **C,** therefore, are incorrect answers.

27. **C.** Paragraph two indicates that Fitzgerald was stationed at Fort Sheridan, near Zelda's hometown of Montgomery, and that he returned to New York after the war was over.

28. **A.** In paragraph two, the author tells of Zelda's, mother naming her after a gypsy queen in a novel she was reading, and goes on to add details that suggest Zelda's mother spoiled her daughter.

29. **B.** Biographically there may be evidence to support the assertion that insanity ran in Zelda's family (**A**), but the passage does not supply such information. **C** and **D** present details that are not factual and do not appear in the passage. Milford's biography, according to paragraph four, presents a picture of Zelda as one who was exploited by her husband, but who also had conflicts not related to his treatment of her, the answer provided by **B.**

30. **B.** While Zelda's friends, according to Scott, would have blamed her insanity on his drinking (**D**), and his friends would have blamed her insanity for his drinking (**C**), neither would have been correct: "liquor on my mouth is sweet to her and I cherish her wildest hallucinations," he said, clearly characterizing their relationship to each other as mutually self-destructive. The correct

answer, therefore, is **B**. Obviously he did not consider their friends as the best judges, the incorrect answer suggested in **A**. See paragraph five.

31. **D.**   Paragraph three provides the works by Scott in which Zelda is the model for the heroine. The novel not listed in the passage is *The Last Tycoon* (D), which was in fact—though the passage does not say so—the only Fitzgerald novel for which Zelda was not the model for the main character.

32. **C.**   Paragraph four in the passage notes the historical fact that Zelda died in 1948 while confined to a mental institution.

33. **C.**   Paragraph one indicates that the fiftieth anniversary in the "Promised Land" was celebrated. Also found in paragraph one is the fact that the writer of *Leviticus* had God speak to Moses; there is no evidence in the passage that God ever spoke to Moses. The passage does point out that celebrating is an old practice of mankind, however; there is no comment anywhere to make the reader assume that most celebrations are joyous events.

34. **C.**   Statements II and IV are supported by the passage. Paragraph two points out that even with birthdays we call special attention to the "big" years, and the quotation from John Adams leaves no doubt that our Independence Day celebration should be carried out "from this time forward for everyone."

35. **D.**   Paragraph three mentions that the inauguration of a new enterprise is always an act of hope and when achievement is history a confident celebration is appropriate. Paragraph four mentions that a celebration is often viewed as the occasion for a new beginning.

36. **D.**   Paragraph five indicates that nostalgia, although differently felt, is good for the human spirit. In paragraph four we are told that we usually think that the lives of pioneers are worth emulating and that anniversaries offer us an opportunity to reflect.

37. **D.**   Paragraphs seven and eight mention the facts that human pride is a motor of an institutional machine, that we use anniversaries to emphasize legitimacy, and that one cannot ignore the commercial motivation behind celebrations.

38. **B.**   The author did use the one hundred fiftieth anniversary of an institution to essentially write a treatise on why we need the act of regular celebrations.

39. **C.**   The story cites universal experiences both in myth and in everyday life.

40. **C.**   The passage focuses on choice, which, because it is human, is universal.

41. **A.**   Because changing or not changing the sail was Theseus's choice, the death of his father resulting from that choice was clearly his responsibility.

42. **A.**   The plot itself is a series of choices, one following the other.

43. **B.**   The author shows how choices in a myth can be the same choices that anyone can face at any time.

44. **B.**   The passage is concerned with the ways in which a character's actions determine his destiny and how major choices lead to other important choices. In Theseus's case, the primary problem is how he will kill the Minotaur.

45. **D.**   All the other statements are supported by the passage. It is stated in the passage that caricatures must be based on *fact*.

46. **C.**   Statements **A**, **B**, and **D** may be true, but they are not stated in the passage. Statement **C** is cited as a cause of laughter.

47. **C.**   Although the author states **A** and **B**, they are not the main point. The passage is set up to lead toward statement **C**. Statement **D** is dismissed in the passage.

48. **C.**   Statements I and III are stated in the passage to show how caricatures work. Statement II may be true, but it does not indicate why caricatures are effective.

49. **A.**   The passage does not deal with the possible objections to caricatures stated in **B**, **C**, and **D**. However, **A** is cited as a danger.

50. **B.**   The entire essay deals with the ways in which satirists use exaggeration as a means of communicating their ideas.

51. **B.** The first sentence of the passage identifies aggression as a neurochemical impulse. **A, C,** and **D** are contradicted in paragraph one.

52. **D.** **B** and **C** are not dealt with in the passage. Lorenz points out specifically that it is *not* the eating enemy, but competition within the species, that poses the greatest threat to an animal species.

53. **C.** According to the passage, there seems to be no other reason for this bickering among one's own, other than the need for stimulation. **A** and **B** are mentioned as the other two basic needs; **D,** structure, is not listed as a need.

54. **B.** The passage identifies the invention of weapons as important in throwing off the natural balance precisely because man possesses the killer instinct without the internal controls or safety devices to limit his use of this instinct.

55. **A.** Hunt's point that man is aggressive without having been programmed as to how he might channel the aggression is a major point on which the author of this passage relies in emphasizing the interdependence of instinct and culture in man's development.

56. **B.** The passage cites a number of ways, many of them perhaps surprising, in which activities of humans can be traced to innate aggression.

57. **D.** Although the essay addresses **A** and **B** specifically, the essay goes far beyond both of these. **D** incorporates both the cultural and the instinctual. The essay addresses the interdependence of the two.

58. **D.** Though one might think, the essay asserts, that people are congested in cities because they like to cooperate, it actually is due to aggressive needs.

59. **B.** The passage states this specifically, and adds that the Shield Soldiers to whom they submitted rendered only token punishment, thus acknowledging the appeasement gesture.

60. **B.** Indirect assessment scores are reliable, so **A** is incorrect. The tests may be biased, but that issue is not addressed in the passage, so **C** is incorrect. **D** is not addressed.

61. **C.** Statement I is contradicted in the passage. Statement II is stated directly. Indirect assessments are an example of a reliable test that is not necessarily valid, so statement III is also correct. Statement IV cannot be true if statement II is true.

62. **B.** Statements **A, C,** and **D** are correct, but they do not deal with the idea in reader response theory that readers bring their own experiences to the reading of a text.

63. **C.** It is the use of a scoring guide, not the particular kind of scoring guide (holistic, primary trait, analytic), that helps increase reliability.

64. **C.** Multiple readings increase the reliability of scores, so **A** is incorrect. **B** and **D** are not addressed in the passage.

65. **D.** The author points out problems with both kinds of testing and does not choose one type as better than the other. The author may agree with **C,** but that is not an evaluation.

PHYSICAL SCIENCES

66. **B.** In the absence of air resistance, both balls have the same vertical acceleration, $g = 9.8$ m/sec^2. Because they start from rest at the same height, they will fall equal distances in equal times as shown by the equation $y = 1/2\ gt^2$.

67. **D.** The horizontal velocity of the second ball is $(10\ \text{m/sec})\ (\text{COS } 30°) = 8.7$ m/sec, so it takes it more than 1 s to reach the wall.

68. **A.** The easier way to solve this problem is to equate the work done against friction to the loss of kinetic energy of the masses, i.e.: $F_f\ x = 1/2\ mv^2$, where $F_f = \mu\ N = \mu\ mg$ where N is the "normal" force (equal to the weight in this case). Solving for $x = v^2/(2\ \mu\ g) = 2$ m for *both* bodies. An alternative solution is to calculate the frictional force and the deceleration. One can then use the equations for uniformly accelerated motion to find the distance. The methods are completely equivalent.

69. **B.** It is possible to calculate the velocities exactly. The initial gravitational potential energy of the block and the ball are converted entirely into kinetic energy at the bottom of the incline. However, part of the kinetic energy of the ball is in the form of rotational kinetic energy about the ball's center of mass. Therefore, at the bottom of the incline, the velocity of the ball's center of mass is less than the linear velocity of the sliding block's center of mass. Understanding this con-

cept, the question can be answered without calculating the velocities. One can do the actual calculations as follows:

$$\text{Ball: } mgh = 1/2 \, mv^2 + 1/2 \, I \, \omega^2$$

where I is the moment of inertia (of a sphere) and ω is the angular velocity. Substituting $I = 2/5 \, mr^2$ and $v = r\omega$, one can solve for v.

$$\text{Ball: } v = \sqrt{(10\text{-}7)gh} = 2.646 \text{ m/sec.}$$

For the block,
$$\text{Block: } mgh = 1/2 \, mv^2 \text{ and } V = \sqrt{2gh}$$
$$= 3.13 \text{ m/sec.}$$

70. **A.** At the terminal velocity (regardless of the actual terminal velocity), the upward frictional force of air resistance is equal to the weight. $F_f - mg = 0$, because the acceleration is zero.

$$F_f = 0.4 \times 9.8 = 3.92 \text{ N.}$$

71. **B.** Power is the "rate of doing work;" 1 watt = 1 joule/sec. This student is using 670 joules each second. In 10 minutes the total energy expended is 402,000 J. The amount of O^2 consumed is 402,000 joules × 1 L/20,000 joules = 20 L.

72. **C.** The desired loss of 0.52 kg of fat requires an energy expenditure of 0.52 kg × 1000 g/kg × 39,700 joule/g = 20,644,000 joules. Since 570 W = 570 joule/sec, the time required is $t = 20,644,000$ joule/570 joule/sec or $t = 36,218$ sec = 10 hr.

73. **A.** This is a conversion problem: 135 lb/2.2 kg/lb = 61.4 kg. Then $W = mg = 61.4 \times 9.8 = 601$ N.

74. **B.** The excess intake per day is 900 kcal. In four weeks the excess will be 900 × 28 = 25,200 kcal. From the energy oxidation value for fats, 25,200 kcal/9.5 kcal/g = 2653 grams.

75. **B.** The gauge pressure in the foot is higher than at the level of the aorta. (This is the reason blood pressure is taken with the cuff on the upper arm at the level of the aorta.) The 1.35 m height difference causes "added pressure," $P' = dgy$, where d is the density of the blood. Thus:

$$P' = 1050 \text{ kg/m}^3 \times 9.8 \text{ m/sec}^2 \times 1.35 \text{ m}$$
$$= 13,900 \text{ N/m}^2$$

Converting P' to mm Hg gives 13,900 N/m² × 750 mm Hg/1 × 10⁵ N/m² = 105 mm Hg. Since this *adds* to the aortic pressure of 100 mm Hg, the gauge pressure in the foot will be 205 mm Hg.

76. **B.** A metabolic rate of 300 W for 6 hours is a total energy expenditure of 300 joules/sec × 6 hours × 3600 sec/hr = 6,480,000 joules. The O^2 consumed is 6,480,000 joules/20,000 joules/L = 324 L. The O^2 actually inhaled is 324 L/0.25 = 1300 L.

77. **C.** The voltages of batteries connected in series add. The 6- and 12-volt batteries in series are equivalent to an 18-volt battery. Applying Ohm's law, $V = IR$, to the equivalent circuit; the current through the resistor is:

$$I = V/R = 18 \text{ volts/10 ohm} = 1.8 \text{ A.}$$

78. **B.** The expression for the equivalent resistance of resistors connected in series is: $R_s = R_1 + R_2 + \ldots = 4 + 8 = 12$ ohms. We can find the current in this circuit using Ohm's law: $I = V/R_s = 6/12 = 0.5$ A. The power consumed in the 8-ohm resistor is then found from $P = I^2R = (0.5)^2 \times 8 = 2$ watts. There is additional power consumed in the 4-ohm resistor, of course.

79. **D.** Although this question could be answered in the same manner as the preceding question, one would have to find the individual current through the 8-ohm resistor. It is easier and simpler to note that the full 12 volts is applied across the terminals of the 8-ohm resistor. The power consumed can be found using the expression: $P = IV = (V/R)V = V^2/R$ where we have applied Ohm's law, $V = IR$ to the 8-ohm resistor. Then: $P = (12)^2/8 = 18$ watts.

80. **D.** We can find the power from the given information: $P = V^2/R = 18$ W. Power is the "time rate of doing work": (1 W = 1 J/s) $P = E/t$ so that $E = Pt$ where t is the time in seconds. Thus: $E = 18$ joules/s × 300 s = 5400 joules.

81. **A.** ($t_i = 20°C$) This heat is generated electrically in the resistor, $H = E = Pt = (V^2/R)t$. Then $m \, C_w \, (t_f - t_i) = (V^2/R)t$. We can solve this expression for t_f, the only unknown. $t_f = 22.6°C$.

82. **D.** The velocity of any wave is equal to the product of its frequency and wavelength, $v = f\lambda$. The data shows that $v = 1440$ m/s for all frequencies, indicating that the wave velocity is independent of the frequency. Thus, $\lambda = v/f = 1440/50 = 29$ m for the 50 Hz audible wave and $\lambda = 1440/2.5 \times 10^6$ Hz = 0.58 mm for the 2.5 MHz (US) wave.

83. **B.**

The sketch shows the node-antinode (N-A) pattern for the fundamental (lowest) frequency of standing waves. Each node-to-antinode distance is always a quarter-wavelength. There are two quarter-wavelengths in the pipe length, $L = 0.25$ m. Thus, $\lambda = 0.5$ m. Also, $v = 340$ m/sec in air, so $f = v/\lambda = 340/0.5 = 680$ Hz.

84. **B** For these standing waves the overtones are integer multiples of the fundamental:

$$f_2 = 2f = 2 \times 680 = 1360 \text{ Hz}$$
$$f_3 = 3f = 3 \times 680 = 2040 \text{ Hz}$$

85. **D.** The US wave travels down and back to the wooden surface a distance of $2d$. Since velocity equals distance/time, $v = 2d/t$, so:

$$d = vt/2 = \frac{1440 \text{ m/sec} \times 0.35 \times 10^{-3} \text{ sec}}{2} =$$
$$1.44 \times 0.35/2 = 0.25 \text{ m}$$

86. **A.** Since the source is moving ($v_s = 20$ m/sec) toward the student, she will hear a higher frequency according to the Doppler effect. The most general form for sound waves of the Doppler formula is:

$$f' = f(v \pm v_o)/(v \mp v_s)$$

where f' is the shifted frequency, f is the frequency of the source, v is the speed of sound, v_o is the speed of the observer, and v_s is the speed of the source. Here $v_o = 0$. (One uses the upper signs for "approach" as in this case.) Thus:

$$f' = 1000(340)/(340 - 20) = 1063 \text{ Hz}$$

87. **A.** Since C and A will be the same, we can simply take the ratio of the two expressions for the energy. The C and A will cancel:

$$E_{1000}/E_{50} = \frac{CA^2(1000)^2}{CA^2(50)^2} = (1000/50)^2 = 400$$

88. **D.** $_{92}U^{235}$ has $z = 92$, the charge number (number of protons) while $A = 235$ is the mass number, or number of nucleons (i.e., protons + neutrons). The emission of each alpha, α, comprised of He^4 nuclei, reduces the charge by 2 and reduces the mass by 4. Each beta, β, decay involves the emission of a negative electron from the nucleus. The nuclear charge increases by 1 unit but the mass number is unchanged, since the mass of the electron is negligible.

The net change in z is $-14 + 4 = -10$, so the new $z = 82$.

The net change in A is $-7 \times 4 = -28$, so the new $A = 207$.

89. **C.** We use the right-hand rule to find the direction of the force. The force (F) is perpendicular to the plane of the velocity (v) vector and the magnetic field vector, B, and points in the direction that a right-hand screw would advance if one turned the velocity vector toward the B field vector. If one turns the horizontal north velocity vector toward the upward vertical B vector, the result shows that a right-hand screw turned that way would advance toward the east.

90. **B.** The Ideal Gas Law is usually written $P_1V_1/T_1 = P_2V_2/T_2$. Since the volume is constant, $P_1V_1/T_1 = P_2V_2/T_2 = \text{constant}$, so the pressure is directly proportional to the absolute temperature. The pressure increases by exactly the same factor as the temperature, namely 50%.

91. **A.** Newton's Second law states that if the force is constant, the acceleration is constant, $F = ma$. The slope of the velocity versus time graph is the acceleration. The slope is positive, sloping upward, since the velocity will increase. The correct graph is **A**.

92. **C.** There 3-ohm resistors in series will equal a 9-ohm resistor and is the highest possible value. Three 3-ohm resistors in parallel are equivalent to a 1-ohm resistor. Although there are six other possible combinations of the three resistors, no combination will equal more than 9 ohms or less than 1 ohm.

93. **A.** The mechanical work done equals the gain in gravitational potential energy. So $W = mgh = 130 \text{ kg} \times 9.8 \text{ m/sec}^2 \times 45 \text{ m} = 57,300$ joules.

94. **A.** Newton's Second Law will give the acceleration: $F = ma$, so $a = F/m = 67 \text{ N}/3 \text{ kg} = 2 \text{ m/sec}^2$. The equation for constant acceleration (when the

initial velocity is zero) yields $v^2 = 2as = 2 \times 2$ m/sec$^2 \times 4$ m $= 16$ m^2/sec^2. Then $v = 4.0$ m/sec. An alternate solution is to equate the work done by the net force to the gain in kinetic energy: $Fs = 1/2\ mv^2 - 0$, yielding the same result.

95. **B.** As in an electrical circuit, Ohm's Law will apply: $V = IR$. Here $I = 120$ mA $= 0.120$ A. then $R = V/I = 120$ V/0.120 A $= 1000$ ohms.

96. **B.** $f, p,$ and q are all positive because the light rays do travel from the object toward the lens and from the lens toward the image point.

$$1/f = 1/18 + 1/36; f = 12\ cm.$$

97. **A.** The linear magnification is the negative ratio of the image distance to the object distance. $M = -q/p = -36/18 = -2$. The minus sign indicates that the image is inverted and it is 2 times the size of the object. (If q were negative as it might be for a virtual image the magnification would be positive, $-(-q/p)$, which would indicate that the image was upright and not inverted with respect to the object.)

98. **A.** The object is placed inside the focal length (closer to the lens than the focal length). This is the way that one uses a magnifying glass. The image is virtual as shown by the negative image distance; it is upright and it is magnified.

$$1/q = 1/f - 1/p = 1/24 - 1/6$$

and $q = -8$ cm. The image is on the same side of the lens as the object (in "front") and can only be seen by looking through the lens at the image.

99. **B.** The magnification of a simple refracting telescope is known as the angular magnification and is given by the ratio of the focal length of the objective to the focal length of the eyepiece:

$$M = f_o/f_e = 3\ X.$$

100. **C.** For a microscope, the magnification is the product of the magnification of the objective and the magnification of the eyepiece. $M = M_o M_e$

$$M_o = M/M_e = 400/10 = 40\times.$$

101. **D.** This problem is solved by two successive applications of the thin lens formula. One must calculate the object distance for lens #2.
Lens #1: $1/q_1 = 1/f_1 - 1/p_1$; $q_1 = 24$ cm (behind #1). For lens #2, $p_2 = 72$ cm $- 24$ m $= 48$ cm (in front of #2). Then $1/q_2 = 1/f_2\ 1/p_2 = 1/24 - 1/48$, and thus $q_2 = +48$ cm (behind #2) The final image is real.

102. **D.** The magnification is the ratio of the image distance, q, to the object distance, p, for a thin lens. ($m = -q/p$). In order to find the image distance, q, we use the thin lens formula:

$1/f = 1/p + 1/q,\ 1/q = 1/f - 1/p$ or $1/q = 1/24 - 1/12 = -1/24$. Then $q = 24$ cm and the magnification is:

$$m = -\left(\frac{-24}{12}\right) = +2.$$

The image is twice as large as the object, or 10 cm tall. (The plus sign means that this virtual image is upright.)

103. **B.** This problem is done exactly as in the explanation for question 102. This time the focal length $f = -24$ cm so that the image distance is found to be: $1/q = -1/24 - 1/12$ or $q = -8$ cm. The magnification is then equal to: $m = -(-8)/12 = +0.67$ and the image is only 3.3 cm tall. (This image is upright as shown by the plus sign for the magnification. A diverging lens always produces an upright image.)

104. **C.** The very distant objects, such as stars, are effectively an infinite distance away. The thin lens formula, $1/f = 1/p + 1/q$, then yields the result that the image distance is the same as the focal length because $1/p$ is equal to zero for $p =$ infinity. The image must appear at the actual far-point of the eye, that is, at -80 cm (for the virtual image) and thus the required focal length is also -80 cm.

105. **D.** The power in diopters is equal to the reciprocal of the focal length in *meters*. Thus: $P = 1/f$. Then $f = 1/P = -1/4$ meter $= -0.25$ m or $f = -25$ cm.

106. **A.** The coolant is compressed to form a liquid and becomes warm. The heat is dissipated by a fan. Then the pressure is released from the liquid, allowing its conversion to a gas. This conversion requires heat, the heat of vaporization. It draws heat from surrounding materials.

107. **B.** The transition temperature from solid to liquid should be the same without regard to the direction from which it is approached.

108. **D.** Sublimation is the process of a solid becoming a gas without an intervening liquid.

109. **A.** Increased pressure increases the boiling point.

110. **B.** The critical temperature is the highest temperature at which a gas may be condensed by imposition of high pressure.

111. **B.** Velocity varies in linear fashion with variation of substrate in the area of point A. In this area, the reaction is first order with respect to substrate.

112. **A.** In the area where point B is located, there is no significant change in velocity with a change in substrate. This is zero order with respect to substrate.

113. **C.** At point C the reciprocal substrate concentration is zero, and the substrate concentration would be infinite. Obviously this point cannot be determined by laboratory measurement but must be extrapolated from other data.

114. **B.** The ordinate is reciprocal velocity, and the reciprocal of reciprocal velocity is velocity. Because this extrapolated point corresponds to the reciprocal of infinite substrate, it also will correspond to the reciprocal of maximum velocity.

115. **D.** Point B represents essentially maximum velocity and point C represents the reciprocal of maximum velocity. The zero order portion of the first graph (encompassing point B) does show some change, and it is somewhat difficult to ascertain at what point maximum velocity has been attained.

116. **B.** The three phases will exist together only at the triple point, point 2.

117. **B.** To raise the temperature without changing the pressure, one would proceed on a horizontal line to the right. Such a line intersects the phase transition line for liquid/gas at point 7.

118. **D.** Proceeding vertically toward the top of the diagram, no phase transition from the existing solid phase is indicated.

119. **A.** No liquid can exist above point 1, regardless of the pressure.

120. **C.** The transition from liquid to gas indicates the boiling temperature at the indicated pressure.

121. **A.** This is the definition of equilibrium constant. Note that the coefficients in the reaction equation become exponents in the equilibrium equation.

122. **B.** When the resultants on the right are written in the numerator, a small number such as this indicates that the reaction as written will be favored to go toward the left.

123. **A.** Five moles of gas are being converted to two moles of gas. Increased pressure will improve reaction toward the right, thus relieving the pressure (Principle of LeChatelier).

124. **C.** At STP, a mole of any gas occupies 22.4 liters. Three moles times 22.4 liters equals 67.2 liters.

125. **D.** Equilibrium constant indicates the concentrations at equilibrium. It does not deal with the rate in reaching equilibrium.

126. **A.** Knowing the atomic weight of hydrogen as 1.0 and oxygen at 16.0, the simplest proportions are one H and one O. Thus, the empirical formula is HO.

127. **B.** The empirical formula has only a molecular weight of 17.0. Because the true molecular weight is determined as 34.0, the molecular formula must be a multiple, in this case H_2O_2.

128. **B.** $H_2O_2 \rightleftharpoons H_2O + O_2$ (unbalanced)
Note that we have two hydrogen atoms on each side. However, we have two oxygen atoms on the left side and three on the right. We may try to balance by multiplying H_2O and H_2O_2 by two. We now have

$$2\,H_2O_2 \rightleftharpoons 2\,H_2O + O_2$$

and find that this is balanced. As written, one mole of H_2O_2 will produce only 0.5 mole of O_2.

129. **C.** The balanced equation indicates two moles of H_2O_2 will produce two moles of H_2O or one mole of H_2O_2 will produce one mole of H_2O.

130. **C.** As noted above, one mole of H_2O_2 will produce 0.5 mole of O_2. Because one mole of any gas occupies a volume of 22.4 liters at S.T.P., 0.5 mole will occupy 11.2 liters.

131. **B.**
$$\begin{array}{ccc} 34 & & x \\ 2\,H_2O_2 & \rightleftharpoons & 2\,H_2O + O_2 \\ 68 & & 36 \end{array}$$
$$\frac{34}{68} = \frac{x}{36}$$
$$x = \frac{(36)(34)}{68} = 18.$$

132. **C.** The LeChatelier principle indicates that if a system in equilibrium experiences a change in conditions, chemical reaction will occur to shift the equilibrium and reduce the effect of the changed conditions. Even if reactants and products are all in the gaseous state, there are two moles on the left side and three moles on the right side. Increased pressure would be expected to shift an equilibrium to the left.

133. **C.** If an equilibrium exists, there is an equilibrium constant. Addition of one or more products without changing conditions otherwise will not change the equilibrium constant, but the concentrations of reactants and other products must adjust to maintain the equilibrium constant.

134. **B.** See above. The equilibrium constant would not be affected.

135. **D.** Although it is expected that this would be a first order reaction (rate = k $[H_2O_2]$) it cannot be predicted with certainty. The order of the reaction must be determined on the basis of experimental evidence.

136. **D.** A catalyst is defined as a substance that increases the velocity of a chemical reaction. They are not consumed.

137. **A.** *Hypertonic*: the solution has a higher osmotic pressure than the solution with which it is compared. There is a higher concentration of solute and a lower concentration of solvent. *Hypotonic:* a lower concentration of solute and a higher concentration of solvent are present. *Isotonic:* both solutions have the same osmotic pressure.

138. **C.** One mole of any compound contains 6.02×10^{23} molecules. Two moles of carbon dioxide would contain one mole of molecules more than that contained by one mole of oxygen.

139. **A.** Acid salts are formed by di- and tribasic acids. For example, H_2CO_3 can form the acid salt ($NaHCO_3$) known as sodium hydrogen carbonate or sodium bicarbonate.

140. **D.** NaOH may be called a base because it produces OH^- ions, but it is more properly called a base because it consumes H^+ ions.

141. **C.** The thermal decomposition of $KClO_3$ to produce oxygen will occur if the temperature is sufficiently high. The addition of a catalyst MnO_2 will decrease the activation energy and increase the rate at a lower temperature.

142. **B.** See explanation for question 141.

WRITING SAMPLE

Part 1, Essay

The definition of a wise person generated by this quote hinges on the interpretation of the words "ought" and "can." These words, however, as well as "see," remain ambiguous out of context, thus permitting opposing definitions of a "wise man." If "ought" is taken as a limitation of "can," that is if the wise individual sees only what he should or is obliged to see, then the quote takes on overtones of pragmatism. The wise person, or person who would be happy, does not see further than he ought. He sees less than he "can" or could. To see all he is capable of seeing would be unwise, perhaps because seeing all would be painful or would necessitate prying. He could find out more but sees only that which is his business. The wise individual limits even his perception to avoid painful realities. On first reading, the quote seems to imply some such limited wisdom, perhaps because the shades of meaning in "ought" and "can" have changed over time. Repulsed by the definition of wisdom generated by this interpretation, one might be driven to reverse the relative magnitude of the terms "ought" and "can." What a wise person ought to see is more than what he can see. He must go beyond what is obvious or visible. The implication here is that the wise individual looks beyond or below the surface of perceptible reality. "See" begins to take on shades of meaning akin to "understand" or "infer" beyond superficial perception. The obligation implied by "ought" becomes an obligation to extend rather than an obligation to limit. This second wise person, to be wise, must either dig for more information (things he "ought" to see) or use intuition to understand more than he can see. Without further information on the context of the quote, two possible and opposing wise people remain.

Situations in which the pragmatic position does not apply can be found in psychology. If one believes that unconscious urges or forgotten traumas can have harmful effects on the individual, the wise individual might be advised to "see" more than he "can." A person might, for example, have difficulty relating to authority figures who, judging by what he "can" see, restrict him unfairly. If he can "dig down" to or be made to see oedipal impulses underlying the perception of oppression, he may become better able to respond to authority in a prudent, less self-defeating manner. Seeing only what one ought may also have parallels in jurisprudence, where a judge sometimes suppresses information. A decision reached based on the visible, limited facts may then be different (not to mention wrong) from a conclusion based on what one ought to have seen beyond what could be seen. This analogy, if true, argues that if one only attends to what he can see he may be misled. The other wise person, the one who sees more than he "can," may have a less assailable position. Perhaps, the pragmatic wise person is the best example of a situation in which limited wisdom is advisable. It is arguable that seeing too much is painful and potentially harmful. One might travel to study different cultures only to be more and more sickened by the pain and misery he finds everywhere. One could argue, I suppose, that he would have been wiser, that is happier, less potentially misanthropic, had he limited his vision.

In my mind there are no conditions under which vision or perception or understanding should be limited, if wisdom is the goal. According to the pragmatic reading of the quote, seeing all one can is a mistake, but I would argue limited wisdom is self-contradictory. The truly wise individual is one who sees not only all he "can," but what he "ought" as well. In other words, his vision intuits or infers beyond the visible. The wise person and the happy person may inhabit mutually exclusive positions due to the potential pain involved in seeing too far into oneself or others. However, pleasure and the avoidance of pain should not be used as conditions for defining wisdom.

Part 1
Explanation of First Response: 5

The paper focuses on the statement and addresses the three writing tasks. The most difficult task in writing this essay is the first: explaining what Montaigne's quotation actually means. This essay confronts the difficulty squarely, making it clear that one's interpretation of the quotation depends very much on the meanings of the word "ought" and "can." The irony is that "ought" in one sense could be considered a weaker word than "can"; but in another it is stronger. The essay suggests that one must conclude that two entirely different wise individuals emerge from the quotation, depending on the way in which "ought" is defined. Paragraph two then, moves to the task of providing specific situations in which the two different wise persons see as much as they ought and then as much as they should. The example taken from the psychology of unconscious motivation is appropriate and the analogy using judge and jury is particularly imaginative. Finally the essay confronts the ambiguities and paradoxes raised when one considers Montaigne's quotation by taking the stand that a wise individual never limits his vision. And ultimately, the essay concludes, wisdom should not be defined in terms simply of pleasure or the avoidance of pain.

This essay provides a sensitive insight into a difficult quotation. The introduction is tightly reasoned; the writing is clear. Paragraph two brings the essay down into the realm of the concrete in its use of unconscious motives and of the judge-jury examples. Because the subject is so highly philosophical, this essay would be strengthened by the use of more concrete details, both in paragraphs one and two. The final paragraph, in which the essay winds down nicely, would especially benefit from a well-chosen concrete illustration. The addition of such specific details would elevate the rating of this essay rating from 5 to 6.

Part 2, Essay

History exists, according to Emerson, only as a document tracing the events of individuals. Without people, there can be no history. Therefore, history is not a recording of events, but of the individuals who participated in them. The history of the Cathedral at Chartres does not concern itself primarily with the building, not its stones, it ironworks, its bells. The history of the Cathedral at Chartres focuses on the people who designed and built it, who worshipped and died in it, who tended their flocks in its walls. It is their history, and the history of these individuals is biography.

If it is true that by definition history is necessarily biography, then the events must take second place to the individuals. After all, biography is typically a document showing how the events have shaped the individual. Is history about the individual? It is not. True, history without the human element is dead, but history enjoys a longer continuum than the life of those it influences, and those influenced by it. History is about eras, thoughts, and ages. The Age of Reason is neither a biography of Rousseau, nor a story with those who believed the tenets as the main characters. It is about the events that took place during the time. History encompasses wars, art, politics, science, and philosophy. No biography can encompass all this. History is a larger container than just the human beings. It must hold many people, many actions, both intended and accidental. History records mistakes, quirks, even coincidences and accidents. So, the history of the Cathedral at Chartres is not about Abbot Sugar or King Louis, it is larger than that. Like the stones, the cathedral's history is longer than the life of humans, for the stones live longer than an abbot or king. The space is larger than the area taken up by the bodies it encompasses. It holds many ages of humankind, their thoughts, errors, reasons, and hopes. No, history cannot be biography, for biography is only a part of history. There are no biographies of stones and ideas, of errors and wars; there are only biographies of people.

But who shaped and stacked the stones? From whom do the errors, ideas, and reasons come? Though one person cannot live as long as a cathedral, the cathedral is nothing but a pile of stones and shards of glass with humans and their God to give it meaning. Eras are eras of Humankind, and the Age of Reason reflects a change of thinking in the minds of people. For if we think of history as biography, we must think of Humans as opposed to men and women. Emerson believed that humans and nature were inextricably entwined. Humans and their consciousness were part stone, part God, part evil, part time. Though one person's story cannot be history, Humankind's story, or biography, certainly can, and this story is what we call history. History, then, redefines biography. This definition of biography is not about us as the limited creatures we are as individuals so much as it is about the limitless, encompassing Humankind as a unified whole. The stones are part of this and when labeled as Cathedral and joined to religion, the stones become more of Humankind. The history of the stones and of the space are then the history of Humankind and that, true, is biography.

Part 2
Explanation of Second Response: 5

The essay focuses on the topic defined by Emerson's statement and addresses the three writing tasks. Paragraph one explains Emerson's idea that "there is properly no history; only biography" and illustrates the explanation with a concrete reference to the Cathedral at Chartres. The second paragraph explores in detail the other side of the issue, arguing through historical references that there is, indeed, history independent of biography. The final paragraph presents a balanced consideration of the relation between biography and history, concluding finally that the history of Humankind, not of men and women, is biography.

The first section of the essay uses an interesting rhetorical strategy: that of paraphrasing Emerson's statement in such a way that the paraphrases become premises leading to the conclusion that "Therefore, history is not a recording of events, but of the individuals who participated in them." Some will argue that Emerson's statement is not saying "without people, there can be no history" (the essay's second premise), and thus some will question the foundation of the essay from the beginning. A simple qualifier, such as "perhaps," would strengthen the logic. The second paragraph provides an eloquent defense of the idea that there is indeed history that includes more than biography. It does so by extending the example of the Cathedral at Chartres used in paragraph one and by citing various historical eras and ages. The essay's final paragraph brings the point back to Emerson's assertion and balances it by the concept of the history of Humankind, a creative solution to the task of exploring the circumstances that determine the relationship between history and biography.

The writing in this essay is clear, and it flows nicely from sentence to sentence. The essay could use a clear transition leading into paragraph two. This is the paragraph that reverses the position explained in paragraph one, and the reader could use help in getting into that position. The essay is rich in concrete details. Especially effective is the extended reference to the Cathedral at Chartres. If this paper had led the reader more smoothly from one task to the next, and if the logic in the first several sentences were tightened, the paper would receive a rating of 6.

BIOLOGICAL SCIENCES

143–148.   **(143-A) (144-A) (145-C) (146-D) (147-A) (148-B)** Let us identify the components of the neuron numbered: (2) nucleus with nucleolus, containing the genetic material of the cell and directing the synthetic activity of the cell; (3) Golgi apparatus (zone), the packaging and concentrating area of the cell's secretory activity; (4) dendrites; dendrites are the processes that pick up an impulse and carry it towards the cell body; (5) endoplasmic reticulum (rough in this case—ribosomes are attached), the synthetic machinery of the cell (proteins etc.); (6) cell membrane, semipermeable and the protector of the cell from its environment; (7) cytoplasm (specifically the area here is called the axon hillock); (8) myelin sheath (Schwann cell covered by its neurilemma, the insulator of the axon); (1) direction of conduction of an impulse; axon (10a) and (10b) conducts impulses away from the dendrites to the function with the dendrites of another neuron. The junction point is known as the synaptic area; the impulse can cross the synapse only from the axon to the dendrite and no backflow is permitted; (11) terminal branches of the axon. In a lesion (cut) the process distal from the cell body would completely degenerate; retrograde degeneration would be detected in the proximal portion and the cell body, however, the proximal portion has the capacity and will regenerate.

149.   **C.**   Because glucose is absorbed at a faster rate than xylose, due to both passive and active transport, then as the glucose is absorbed, water follows. The transport system for glucose is working maximally as indicated by the initial concentration of glucose being 50 times the apparent Km of transport.

150.   **D.**   A 1.8% solution contains 1.8 g/100 m of solution. This is 1,800 mg/100 ml, which is 18 mg/ml. For the recovery of 1.8 mg, this represents $(1.8/18 \times 100)$ a 10% recovery meaning that 90% has been metabolized or transported out of the lumen of the intestine.

151. **D.** Hemoglobin is a large (64,000 MW) molecule. Because the gut was ligated below the pancreas and proteolytic enzymes present were washed out, no digestion of the protein could occur. Large molecules are not readily transported across cell membranes. Due to the vast surface area of the small intestine with its many microvilli, some of the protein would be adsorbed on this surface and visible through the heme prosthetic group color.

152. **D.** All are correct. I. D-galactose is transported by the same carrier as glucose, therefore, by addition of galactose, a competition for transport between glucose and galactose occurs. II. The transport carrier is sodium ion selective. A larger cation, while having the appropriate charges, does not fit the selective carrier. III. The carrier is specific for the D-glucose; L-glucose would be transported by passive diffusion only. IV. Because the carrier is an energy requiring process, by limiting the supply of ATP, the transport is decreased.

153. **A.** A 25% solution of $MgSO_4$ is hypertonic. Neither Mg nor SO_4 ions are readily transported so the net effect is a water flow into the lumen becoming an isotonic solution.

154. **B.** Hemoglobin is not absorbed and an aqueous solution is not isotonic. Assuming that the hemoglobin is not ionized, a 0.3 M solution would have to have $64,000 \times 0.3$ g/liter. This solution must be hypotonic, which can be only modified by water flow out of the lumen.

155-157. **(155-B) (156-C) (157-C)** The answers can be found in the flow diagram of the question. Thyroid-hormones (T_3 and T_4) are iodothyronines. The union of iodine and tyrosine is called iodination, and the active thyroid principal is protein-bound during transport to the target organs.

158. **D.** Hyperthyriodism, hypothyroidism, and euthyroidism can be associated with goiter. In hyperthyroidism, thyroxin is released into the bloodstream at a rate exceeding needs. BMR accelerates resulting in rapid pulse and respiration, increased appetite with concomitant weight loss, nervousness, and protruding eyes. If not treated, goiter and thyroid exhaustion can occur; treatment involves antithyroid drugs or thyroidectomy. The opposite, hypothyroidism, exhibits a gland that cannot meet secretory demands; the body's metabolic rate is depressed

and symptoms are the reverse of the above cited. When hypothyroidism occurs during childhood, a cretin is the result; mental retardation and stunted growth are features. Treatment requires administration of thyroid hormone. Goiter simply means enlargement of the gland and can be present in the normal (euthyroid) state.

159. **A.** Thyroid stimulating hormone produced by the basophils of the anterior pituitary is a glycoprotein made up of two peptide chains (alpha and beta). Certain regions of the hypothalamus have a neuroendocrine function because neurosecretory cells release hormones that affect anterior pituitary function. TRH secreted by the hypothalamus reaches the pituitary via the hypophyseal-portal circulation and elicits TSH production. Thyroxin binds to TBG. Exposure to cold would elicit a compensatory increase in BMR and, hence, thyroid activity.

160. **D.** Also see explanations for questions 158 and 159. Control of thyroid principal is via the pituitary. TSH stimulates the thyroid to produce thyroxin; its release is related to levels in the bloodstream. Low levels increase TSH and thyroxin release, but as levels rise to normal and above, further production and release of TSH is curtailed and thyroxin production falls. This feedback system maintains balance.

161. **C.** See explanations for questions 158–160.

162. **A.** The effect of repeated close-spaced stimuli is that a summation occurs: each contraction is somewhat larger than the preceding one.

163. **C.** ATP continues to be supplied in adequate amounts, even during the period of loss of contraction ability (fatigue). Some link between the stimulating event and the responding event (sliding of actins over myosins), however, gradually becomes less efficient.

164. **B.** During the summation period each new stimulus arrives before the preceding twitch can reach the relaxation period, and elastic elements in the muscle become stretched without rebounding to their original shape. The muscle eventually reaches a steady state of nearly full contraction (region 2), when all elastic elements are fully stretched.

165. **A.** When a volley of stimuli is applied to a muscle, each succeeding stimulus may arrive before the muscle can completely relax in the

contraction caused by the preceding stimulus. The result is summation, an increased strength of contraction. If the frequency of stimulation is very fast, individual contractions refuse and the muscle smoothly and fully contracts. This is a tetanus.

166. **D.** The word contraction refers to those processes that are manifested externally by either a shortening of a muscle or by tension development in a muscle. If the muscle length is held constant the contraction is referred to as an isometric contraction. In an isometric contraction, the passive tension remains constant with the active tension being added to it to produce the total tension of the muscle. If the muscle shortens during contraction, it is called an isotonic contraction and the total tension remains constant.

167. **C.** The drug most closely resembles PHT (phenytoin) in terms of its high efficacy in the electroshock model of tonic-clonic seizures and its adequate efficacy in the kindling model of partial complex seizures. **A**, though not completely incorrect, is not the best answer. PHT, the drug this experimental agent AntiEpp acts most like, is not effective in the androgenic mouse model of myoclonic seizures, which is also a form of generalized convulsive seizures. **D** is also incorrect for this reason. The better answer is **C**.

168. **B.** Ethosuximide is the only drug that is exclusively effective against the animal model of absence seizures. **A** is incorrect, because carbamazepine has highest efficacy in the kindling model and in partial complex seizures. **C** is incorrect because valproic acid shows some degree of efficacy in all seizure models and the corresponding clinical conditions. Again, Compound X, like ethosuximide, shows efficacy only against the GABA challenge model of absence seizures. Given the premise that investigational compounds are selected in part because of a chemical nature similar to presently used compounds, there is enough information to respond that this agent is "probably most similar" to ethosuximide. So **D** is also incorrect.

169. **C.** It is stated that 1 in 200 persons suffer from epilepsy in the United States and that there are 7 million persons in New York City. Thus, the correct answer can be derived as follows:

$$\frac{1}{200} = \frac{X}{7,000,000} \text{ or rearranging,}$$

$$X = \frac{(7,000,000)(1)}{200} \text{ or } X = 35,000$$

This can be calculated more rapidly in your head realizing that:

$$\frac{1}{200} = \frac{5}{100} = \frac{5}{1,000} = \frac{50}{10,000} = \frac{500}{100,000} =$$

$$\frac{5,000}{1,000,000} \text{ or } \frac{35,000}{7,000,000}$$

A or **D** reflect a mathematical mistake. **B** is the probable number of yearly deaths from status epilepticus.

170. **C.** Status epilepticus is defined in the first paragraph of the passage as a seizure that persists for over 30 minutes. A partial seizure emanates from a restricted region. This woman's seizure is described as having lasted for "over an hour" and was observed on the electroencephalogram as "localized only to a restricted region." Thus, "partial status epilepticus" is the *best* answer. **A**, status epilepticus is correct but does not fully describe the patient's condition. Neither does partial complex seizure **(D)**. Finally, generalized seizures, you are told, arise from the entire brain simultaneously. Again, this woman's seizure is restricted or partial. For this reason, **B** is incorrect.

171. **B.** The reading passage states that there are approximately 1.2 million persons with epilepsy in the United States. It also indicates that 25% of patients with epilepsy continue to have seizures at least once per month. So, the correct answer is generated by taking 25% of 1.2 million, or

$$0.25 \times 1,200,000 = 300,000$$

A, 30,000 represents a mathematical mistake. So does **D**, 250,000. **C**, 1/4 million, is just another way of saying 250,000 and is also incorrect.

172. **B.** It is the purpose of this experiment to determine the sequence of events in cells stimulated to undergo mitosis, and to compare the data to those gathered from unstimulated cells.

173. **A.** Analysis of the graphs clearly shows that RNA synthesis precedes increased protein synthesis; at around 17 hours they are equal and RNA continues to drop, whereas protein synthesis increases.

174. **D.** It is safe to assume that unstimulated lymphocytes synthesize RNA, DNA, and protein at a low rate. One of the premier functions of DNA is the production of RNA; most RNA is produced in the nucleus. DNA determines and acts as a template for RNA synthesis. With the help of a transcription enzyme (RNA polymerase), a complimentary RNA strand is produced; once produced it moves into the cytoplasm.

175. **B.** The cell is the basic unit of structure and function and the basis of all life; all cells come from preexisting cells.

176. **B.** A complete set of chromosomes ($2n$) is passed on to each daughter cell as a result of mitotic cell division. Cells that are produced mitotically are genetically alike.

177. **C.** Messenger RNA (MRNA) from the nucleus brings the coded message for protein synthesis to ribosomes in the cytoplasm.

178. **C.** Mitosis is divided into:

    (1) prophase—chromosomes become distinct and nucleoli disappears centrioles, asters, and spindle appear; nuclear membrane disappears.
    (2) metaphase—chromosomes move to equator of cell.
    (3) anaphase—the two chromatids split apart and start migration toward the poles of the spindle, and the spindle loses its definition.
    (4) telophase—chromosomes lengthen and become less distinct and nucleon reappear.
    (5) interphase—cell growth, protein + DNA synthesis, and chromosomes duplicate.

179. **B.** During metaphase of mitosis, the centrioles with asters are at the opposite poles; the chromosomes move to the equator of the cell. Also see explanation for question 178.

180. **D.** Nuclei have the highest DNA concentration among cellular organelles. The DNA in fraction 3 is in mitochondria.

181. **C.** Cytochrome oxidase is the enzyme complex that transfers electrons from the mitochondrial electron transport chain to oxygen and is therefore located in mitochondria.

182. **A.** Most of the RNA found in a mature cell is ribosomal RNA, and the cytoplasmic ribosomal RNA in a hepatocyte should occur in a mixture of free ribosomes and rough endoplasmic reticulum. Because only one peak of RNA occurred at the top of the gradient, fraction 1 must contain both free and membrane-bound ribosomes and therefore contains the rough endoplasmic reticulum. The RNA in fraction 3 probably represents ribosomes in mitochondria. The RNA in fraction 4 is probably partially assembled ribosomes in the nucleoli in the nuclei.

183. **B.** Acid phosphatase is a lysosomal enzyme and occurred only in fraction 2 among the choices.

184. **A.** Cytochrome P-450 is involved in detoxification reactions in smooth endoplasmic reticulum and only occurred in fraction 1 among the choices.

185. **C.** Krebs cycle enzymes are located in the mitochondria and should therefore occur in the same fractions that contain cytochrome oxidase activity.

186. **A.** Plasma proteins are secreted proteins and therefore should be made on the rough endoplasmic reticulum in fraction 1.

187. **A.** A cell that secretes large amounts of protein (such as a pancreatic exocrine cell) should contain large arrays of rough endoplasmic reticulum, which would increase fraction 1. Secretory granules could increase fraction 2 or fraction 3, but the assays used would not detect pancreatic enzymes or their contribution to a fraction.

188. **B.** Phagocytic cells, such as monocytes or macrophages, contain large numbers of lysosomes that would contribute to the acid phosphatase activity measured in fraction 2.

189. **C.** Proximal convoluted tubule lining cells contain large numbers of mitochondria that supply the large amounts of energy needed to support the active transport used for resorption of solutes from urine. High numbers of mitochondria should increase fraction 3.

190. **D.** Two moles of carbon dioxide formed and 12 ATP formed per mole of acetyl CoA. The reactions produce three moles of NADH and one mole of $FADH_2$. Reoxidation of these coenzymes in the respiratory assembly will produce three ATP/NADH and two ATP/$FADH_2$. The remain-

ing one ATP is a substrate level phosphorylation of GDP to GTP by succinyl CoA. GTP can phosphorylate ADP to ATP.

191. **B.** The reaction acetyl CoA to pyruvate does not occur. This is one of the reasons that we cannot make (net) glucose from acetyl CoA. Choice **D** shows two very similar reactions of oxidative decarboxylation. The same coenzymes, mechanism, and release of CO_2 occur. Choice **A** indicates both oxidations of a secondary alcohol. The product, oxalosuccinate, spontaneously decarboxylates due to the instability of the keto acid formed to yield alpha ketoglutarate. Choice **C** indicates both hydration reactions.

192. **A.** For the citric acid cycle to function, as acetyl CoA is catabolized it reacts with oxaloacetate to form citrate. In specific reactions, CO_2 is lost and oxaloacetate is regenerated. Oxaloacetate may be considered catalytic for the cycle. Oxaloacetate plus acetyl CoA forms 2 CO_2 and oxaloacetate. **B** is a true statement in that the synthesis of fatty acids in the cytoplasm occurs through this step. **C** is also true because the first step in the synthesis of the porphyrin ring (heme) occurs from succinyl CoA. The last two choices are also true because transamination from these keto acids (using some other amino acids as the amino group donor) results in the formation of the specific amino shown.

193. **D.** Net synthesis of glucose does not take place because the reaction pyruvate to acetyl CoA is not reversible under physiological conditions and also because for every acetyl CoA condensing with oxaloacetate, 2 CO_2 is formed. Choice **A** is true because specific enzymes of the pathway are inhibited by high levels of ATP (citrate synthase) or stimulated by low levels of ADP (isocitrate dehydrogenase). Choice **B** is correct. One control of the glycolytic pathway has citrate as a negative effector (phosphofructokinase). Choice **C** is a true statement. The citric acid cycle is the final metabolic pathway for many metabolites.

194. **A.** The red blood cell (mature RBC) does not contain mitochondria where the citric acid cycle takes place; see **B.** Choice **C** is true; for every acetyl CoA (two per glucose mole) 12 ATP are formed. Substrate level phosphorylation (GTP + ADP to ATP + GDP) form one and reoxidation of reducing equivalents in oxidative phosphorylation forms 11 ATP. When acetyl CoA levels are high, several things can happen: (1) the citric

acid cycle may be maximal (depends on ATP needs); (2) fatty acids may be synthesized; (3) ketone bodies may be formed; (4) gluconeogenesis is stimulated because the enzyme pyruvate carboxylase requires high levels to activate it for the synthesis of net oxaloacetate from pyruvate and CO_2. Eventually glucose may be formed anew from the pyruvate (gluconeogenesis).

195. **B.** L-amino acids are those coded for translation into proteins. D-amino acids are rare, although found in some bacteria. All of the amino acids with one exception, glycine, are optically active. This is a physical property that molecules may have when they are chiral.

196. **C.** In contrast to the amino acids, all of the main carbohydrates are of the D configuration. Notable exceptions are some L sugars found in blood group glypoproteins, such as L-fucose.

197. **B.** Diastereomers (diastereo-isomers) are not mirror images (enantiomers) and have different chemical, physical, and biological properties. If the question had asked D-glucose and D-galactose, the answer would be **D.** That is, they are both epimers and diastereomers.

198. **D.** D-galactose is an epimer at C4 of glucose, and D-mannose is an epimer at C2 of glucose. D-fructose is a keto hexose and has similar OH configuration to D-glucose at C atoms 3, 4, 5.

199. **D.** One may compare D-glyceraldehyde to D-glucose. It is as if the three carbon atom difference were by addition to the C-1 of glyceraldehyde.

200. **D.** Pyruvate is formed from the high energy compound phosphoenolpyruvate catalyzed by the enzyme pyruvate kinase. As NADH builds up from an earlier step, the keto acid pyruvate is reduced to the hydroxy-acid lactate. Choice **A** is the first product formed in all cells that metabolize glucose. Carbon dioxide **B** is not produced in the glycolytic pathway. Acetyl CoA **C** is formed in mitochondria from pyruvate by the pyruvate dehydrogenase complex.

201. **D.** The glycolytic pathway takes place in the cytoplasm. The first step, glucose to glucose-6-phosphate, is catalyzed by a kinase and uses ATP to phosphorylate glucose.

202. **D.** Choice **A** requires ATP, whereas **B** and **C** are substrate level phosphorylations (ADP + high energy phosphate to give ATP).

203. **C.** The enzyme glucose-6-phosphate dehydrogenase, the first enzyme in the hexosemonophosphate shunt, catalyzes the oxidation to 6-phosphogluconate and the reduction of $NADP^+$ to NADPH. Red cell lysis occurs for a number of different reasons, including changes in hemoglobin, such as the oxidation of ferrous ion to ferric ion (which does not carry oxygen). Failure to maintain a reduced cell membrane results in a cell that does not fit through capillaries. Pyruvate is reduced to lactate by NADH.

204. **D.** After the formation of pentose phosphate, further catabolism produces common intermediates, such as glyceraldehyde-3-P, and fructose-6-phosphate provide an interchange between these two pathways. Only the hexose monophosphate shunt produces carbon dioxide in the red blood cell. This occurs by oxidation of 6-phosphogluconate to reduce $NADP^+$. The oxidized product is decarboxylated to a pentose phosphate and carbon dioxide. Another name for the hexose monophosphate shunt is the pentose pathway.

205. **C.** Except for statement C, all of the others are supported by the evidence. To infer that the experimenters should have paid closer attention to body weights is not supported because the greatest difference between the six groups (8 animals/group) was 8 grams, organ weights were corrected for body weight, and organ weights/g body weight do not appear to vary with body weight.

206. **B.** This study was designed to determine what vitamins were missing from diet A. The data indicated that diet A lacked the B vitamins. Thiamine (B_1) is essential for the proper functioning of the nervous system; deficiency will result in beriberi. Riboflavin (B_2) converts tryptophan to nicotinic acid; general problems with vision, skin, coordination, and growth can occur. In the experiment, the difference between the percentage losing weight and percentage mortality within each group is best explained by individual variation among mice within each group.

207. **B.** Acidophils (alpha cells) of the pituitary secrete somatotropic hormone (STH, growth hormone), which stimulates generalized body growth. Hypersecretion before ossification is complete results in giantism, whereas thereafter, acromegaly is the consequence. Hyposecretion leads to dwarfism. Our assay had to be conducted on hypophysectomized rats because the pituitary produces growth hormone that might interfere with the assay.

208. **D.** The purpose of this experiment was to observe X ray effect on growth. X rays can be lethal; they are used in combination with chemotherapy to treat certain malignant growths. The table also shows that plants exposed to 24,000 r units exhibit a marked effect; growth from the cotyledon to the first node was greatly decreased. This was the part most affected; the midrib lengths were not affected.

209. **D.** Because the Y-chromosome always passes from father to son, all male offspring (half of the total, on average) have the father's Y-chromosome. If the gene is dominant, all males will exhibit the trait. Female offspring could not, because they get the father's X-chromosome, not the Y.

210. **D.** Melanoma is a malignancy. The data shows that an Ag A phenotype containing three seems to be related to higher antibody production . If one possesses a 1/3 Ag A phenotype, the mouse resulting from a cross of Strain 2 with one of Strain 3 would probably be a better antibody producer than a sibling having a 1/1 Ag A phenotype. Statements A and C are clearly contradicted by the data, whereas statement B is neither contradicted nor supported.

211. **D.** Statement C is neither supported nor contradicted by the data. Statement D is contradicted by the evidence because even after 90–100% resurfacing, an endothelial labeling index of 2.5% is exhibited. Statements A and B are supported by the information presented.

212. **D.** The actions of LH and FSH in the male on the testes are to promote androgen secretion and spermatogenesis. Androgenic actions of testosterone are: (1) maintenance of secondary sex organs; (2) promotion of secondary sex characteristics (size of genitalia, voice, muscle development, and hair distribution); (3) normal development of body growth and psychological balance. The statement (**D**) that bilateral castration removes a major source of sex hormones is clearly the only one supported by the experiment; all others are contradicted.

213. **D.** Thyroid hormone controls the rate of metabolism, growth, maturation, and differentiation of the organism, and it influences nervous

system activity. All the statements are consistent with the information and are true concerning thyroid activity. The quantity of heat liberated is decreased by deficiencies and elevated by excesses of thyroxin; after thyroidectomy the basal metabolic rate drops, and animals probably exhibit sluggishness and slight obesity.

214. **A.** It is obvious that because bacteria Z could grow following exposure to temperatures below 160°C, it cannot be destroyed in autoclave 1.

215. **A.** The testes of blinded hamsters weighed 1695 mg/100 g of body weight if no MTPH was given. Application of MTPH reduced the weight to 1419 mg/100 g, indicating increased atrophy.

216. **A.** Conversion of glycogen to glucose-l-phosphate is catalyzed by the enzyme, phosphorylase. Pancreatic amylase is usually not in contact with glycogen (except dietary glycogen); in any case it would not catalyze the formation of glucose-l-phosphate.

217. **C.** Production of glucose and fructose from sucrose and production of fatty acids and glycerol from triglycerides are both simple hydrolytic reactions in which essentially no energy is gained or lost. Production of steroids from acetate (as is true with most synthetic reactions) requires energy input. Production of CO_2 and water from fatty acids yields large amounts of energy.

218. **D.** A yellow precipitate of iodoform is produced in this reaction with methyl ketones, alcohols that may be oxidized to methyl ketones, or acetaldehyde.

219. **C.** We have described conditions for the formation of a diazonium salt and then replacement of the diazonium salt by Br to produce monobromobenzene. (The replacement is known as the Sandmeyer reaction.) The intermediate diazonium salt is often unstable at room temperature, so a lower temperature is used.

Appendix

LOGARITHMS AND EXPONENTS

Logarithms

The logarithm of any number is the exponent of the power to which 10 must be raised to produce the number. The logarithm X of the number N to the base 10 is the exponent of the power to which 10 must be raised to give N (for example, $\log_{10} N = X$). Logarithms consist of two parts. First, there is the "characteristic," which is determined by the position of the first significant figure of the number in relation to the decimal point. If we count leftwards from the decimal point as positive and rightwards as negative, the characteristic is equal to the count ending at the right of the first significant figure. Thus, the characteristic of the logarithm of 2340 is 3, and of 0.00234 is –3. Second, there is the "mantissa." It is always positive, is found in logarithm tables, and depends only on the sequence of significant figures. Thus, the mantissa for the two numbers is the same, namely 0.3692. The logarithm of a number is the sum of the characteristic and the mantissa. Thus, $\log 2340 = 3.3692$ while $\log 0.00234 = -3 + 0.3692 = -2.6308$.

The logarithms of the whole integers 1 to 10 are given below.

$\log 1.0 = 0.000$	$\log 6.0 = 0.778$
$\log 2.0 = 0.301$	$\log 7.0 = 0.845$
$\log 3.0 = 0.477$	$\log 8.0 = 0.903$
$\log 4.0 = 0.602$	$\log 9.0 = 0.954$
$\log 5.0 = 0.699$	$\log 10.0 = 1.000$

Useful Rules in Handling Logarithms

1. The logarithm of a product is equal to the sum of the logarithms of the factors:

$$\log ab = \log a + \log b$$

(Check this out by solving for $\log 6$, using $\log 2 + \log 3$.)

2. The logarithm of a fraction is equal to the logarithm of the numerator minus the logarithm of the denominator:

$$\log \frac{a}{b} = \log a - \log b$$

Example:

$$\log \frac{10}{2} = \log 10 - \log 2 = \log 5$$

How about $\log 2.5$? The answer from the log tables is 0.398.

3. The logarithm of the reciprocal of a number is the negative logarithm of the number:

$$\log \frac{1}{a} = \log 1 - \log a$$

Since $\log 1 = 0$, then

$$\log \frac{1}{a} = -\log a$$

Equally,

$$\log \frac{1}{2} = -\log 2 = -0.301$$

4. The logarithm of a number raised to a power is the logarithm of the number multiplied by the power:

$$\log a^b = b \log a$$
$$\log 2^2 = 0.603$$

Exponents

It is convenient to express large numbers as 10^x, where x represents the number of places that the decimal must be moved to place it after the first significant figure. This also represents $10 \cdot 10$ for x times. For example, 1,000,000 may be expressed as 1×10^6; 3663 as 3.663×10^3; and so on. To multiply, the exponents are added, but coefficients are multiplied. To divide, the exponents are subtracted, but coefficients are divided.

Multiplying: $(1 \times 10^x) \cdot (1 \times 10^y) = 1 \times 10^{x+y}$

$$(4 \times 10^2) \cdot (2 \times 10^3) = 8 \times 10^5$$

Dividing: $(1 \times 10^x) \div (1 \times 10^y) = 1 \times 10^{x-y}$

$$(4 \times 10^2) \div (2 \times 10^3) = 2 \times 10^{-1}$$

Numbers less than 1 are 10^{-x}. For example, 0.000001 is 1×10^{-6}.

Multiplying: $(1 \times 10^{-x}) \cdot (1 \times 10^{-y}) = 1 \times 10^{-(x+y)}$

$$(4 \times 10^{-2}) \cdot (2 \times 10^{-3}) = 8 \times 10^{-5}$$

A large number multiplied by a small number:

$$(4 \times 10^{-2})(2 \times 10^3) = 8 \times 10^1$$

(Logarithms and Exponents are reproduced through the courtesy of Dr. Richard B. Brandt, Dept. of Biochemistry, MCV, VCU, Richmond, Virginia, 23298.)

Table of Common Logarithms

Numbers	0	1	2	3	4	5	6	7	8	9
10	0000	0043	0086	0128	0170	0212	0253	0294	0334	0374
11	0414	0453	0492	0531	0569	0607	0645	0682	0719	0755
12	0792	0828	0864	0899	0934	0969	1004	1038	1072	1106
13	1139	1173	1206	1239	1271	1303	1335	1367	1399	1430
14	1461	1492	1523	1553	1584	1614	1644	1673	1703	1732
15	1761	1790	1818	1847	1875	1903	1931	1959	1987	2014
16	2041	2068	2095	2122	2148	2175	2201	2227	2253	2279
17	2304	2330	2355	2380	2405	2430	2455	2480	2504	2529
18	2553	2577	2601	2625	2648	2672	2695	2718	2742	2765
19	2788	2810	2833	2856	2878	2900	2923	2945	2967	2989
20	3010	3032	3054	3075	3096	3118	3139	3160	3181	3201
21	3222	3243	3263	3284	3304	3324	3345	3365	3385	3404
22	3424	3444	3464	3483	3502	3522	3541	3560	3579	3598
23	3617	3636	3655	3674	3692	3711	3729	3747	3766	3784
24	3802	3820	3838	3856	3874	3892	3909	3927	3945	3962
25	3979	3997	4014	4031	4048	4065	4082	4099	4116	4133
26	4150	4166	4183	4200	4216	4232	4249	4265	4281	4298
27	4314	4330	4346	4362	4378	4393	4409	4425	4440	4456
28	4472	4487	4502	4518	4533	4548	4564	4579	4594	4609
29	4624	4639	4654	4669	4683	4698	4713	4728	4742	4757
30	4771	4786	4800	4814	4829	4843	4857	4871	4886	4900
31	4914	4928	4942	4955	4969	4983	4997	5011	5024	5038
32	5051	5065	5079	5092	5105	5119	5132	5145	5159	5172
33	5185	5198	5211	5224	5237	5250	5263	5276	5289	5302
34	5315	5328	5340	5353	5366	5378	5391	5403	5416	5428
35	5441	5453	5465	5478	5490	5502	5514	5527	5539	5551
36	5563	5575	5587	5599	5611	5623	5635	5647	5658	5670
37	5682	5694	5705	5717	5729	5740	5752	5763	5775	5786
38	5798	5809	5821	5832	5843	5855	5866	5877	5888	5899
39	5911	5922	5933	5944	5955	5966	5977	5988	5999	6010
40	6021	6031	6042	6053	6064	6075	6085	6096	6107	6117
41	6128	6138	6149	6160	6170	6180	6191	6201	6212	6222
42	6232	6243	6253	6263	6274	6284	6294	6304	6314	6325
43	6335	6345	6355	6365	6375	6385	6395	6405	6415	6425
44	6435	6444	6454	6464	6474	6484	6493	6503	6513	6522
45	6532	6542	6551	6561	6571	6580	6590	6599	6609	6618
46	6628	6637	6646	6656	6665	6675	6684	6693	6702	6712
47	6721	6730	6739	6749	6758	6767	6776	6785	6794	6803
48	6812	6821	6830	6839	6848	6857	6866	6875	6884	6893
49	6902	6911	6920	6928	6937	6946	6955	6964	6972	6981
50	6990	6998	7007	7016	7024	7033	7042	7050	7059	7067
51	7076	7084	7093	7101	7110	7118	7126	7135	7143	7152
52	7160	7168	7177	7185	7193	7202	7210	7218	7226	7235
53	7243	7251	7259	7267	7275	7284	7292	7300	7308	7316
54	7324	7332	7340	7348	7356	7364	7372	7380	7388	7396

Numbers	0	1	2	3	4	5	6	7	8	9
55	7404	7412	7419	7427	7435	7443	7451	7459	7466	7474
56	7482	7490	7497	7505	7513	7520	7528	7536	7543	7551
57	7559	7566	7574	7582	7589	7597	7604	7612	7619	7627
58	7634	7642	7649	7657	7664	7672	7679	7686	7694	7701
59	7709	7716	7723	7731	7738	7745	7752	7760	7767	7774
60	7782	7789	7796	7803	7810	7818	7825	7832	7839	7846
61	7853	7860	7868	7875	7882	7889	7896	7903	7910	7917
62	7924	7931	7938	7945	7952	7959	7966	7937	7980	7987
63	7993	8000	8007	8014	8021	8028	8035	8041	8048	8055
64	8062	8069	8075	8082	8089	8096	8102	8109	8116	8122
65	8129	8136	8142	8149	8156	8162	8169	8176	8182	8189
66	8195	8202	8209	8215	8222	8228	8235	8241	8248	8254
67	8261	8267	8274	8280	8287	8293	8299	8306	8312	8319
68	8325	8331	8338	8344	8351	8357	8363	8370	8376	8382
69	8388	8395	8401	8407	8414	8420	8426	8432	8439	8445
70	8451	8457	8463	8470	8476	8482	8488	8494	8500	8506
71	8513	8519	8525	8531	8537	8543	8549	8555	8561	8567
72	8573	8579	8585	8591	8597	8603	8609	8615	8621	8627
73	8633	8639	8645	8651	8657	8663	8669	8675	8681	8686
74	8692	8698	8704	8710	8716	8722	8727	8733	8739	8745
75	8751	8756	8762	8768	8774	8779	8785	8791	8797	8802
76	8808	8814	8820	8825	8831	8837	8842	8848	8854	8859
77	8865	8871	8876	8882	8887	8893	8899	8904	8910	8915
78	8921	8927	8932	8938	8943	8949	8954	8960	8965	8971
79	8976	8982	8987	8993	8998	9004	9009	9015	9020	9025
80	9031	9036	9042	9047	9053	9058	9063	9069	9074	9079
81	9085	9090	9096	9101	9106	9112	9117	9122	9128	9133
82	9138	9143	9149	9154	9159	9165	9170	9175	9180	9186
83	9191	9196	9201	9206	9212	9217	9222	9227	9232	9238
84	9243	9248	9253	9258	9263	9269	9274	9279	9284	9289
85	9294	9299	9304	9309	9315	9320	9325	9330	9335	9340
86	9345	9350	9355	9360	9365	9370	9375	9380	9385	9390
87	9395	9400	9405	9410	9415	9420	9425	9430	9435	9440
88	9445	9450	9455	9460	9465	9469	9474	9479	9484	9489
89	9494	9499	9504	9509	9513	9518	9523	9528	9533	9538
90	9542	9547	9552	9557	9562	9566	9571	9576	9581	9586
91	9590	9595	9600	9605	9609	9614	9619	9624	9628	9633
92	9638	9643	9647	9652	9657	9661	9666	9671	9675	9680
93	9685	9689	9694	9699	9703	9708	9713	9717	9722	9727
94	9731	9736	9741	9745	9750	9754	9759	9763	9768	9773
95	9777	9782	9786	9791	9795	9800	9805	9809	9814	9818
96	9823	9827	9832	9836	9841	9845	9850	9854	9859	9863
97	9868	9872	9877	9881	9886	9890	9894	9899	9903	9908
98	9912	9917	9921	9926	9930	9934	9939	9943	9948	9952
99	9956	9961	9965	9969	9974	9978	9983	9987	9991	9996

List of Elements with Their Symbols

Element	Symbol	Element	Symbol	Element	Symbol	Element	Symbol	Element	Symbol
Actinium	Ac	Cobalt	Co	Iridium	Ir	Oxygen	O	Sodium	Na
Aluminum	Al	Copper	Cu	Iron	Fe	Palladium	Pd	Strontium	Sr
Americium	Am	Curium	Cm	Krypton	Kr	Phosphorus	P	Sulfur	S
Antimony	Sb	Dysprosium	Dy	Lanthanum	La	Platinum	Pt	Tantalum	Ta
Argon	Ar	Einsteinium	Es	Lawrencium	Lr	Plutonium	Pu	Technetium	Tc
Arsenic	As	Element 106		Lead	Pb	Polonium	Po	Tellurium	Te
Astatine	At	Erbium	Er	Lithium	Li	Potassium	K	Terbium	Tb
Barium	Ba	Europium	Eu	Lutetium	Lu	Praseodymium	Pr	Thallium	Tl
Berkelium	Bk	Fermium	Fm	Magnesium	Mg	Promethium	Pm	Thorium	Th
Beryllium	Be	Fluorine	F	Manganese	Mn	Protactinium	Pa	Thulium	Tm
Bismuth	Bi	Francium	Fr	Mendelevium	Md	Radium	Ra	Tin	Sn
Boron	B	Gadolinium	Gd	Mercury	Hg	Radon	Rn	Titanium	Ti
Bromine	Br	Gallium	Ga	Molybdenum	Mo	Rhenium	Re	Tungsten	W
Cadmium	Cd	Germanium	Ge	Neodymium	Nd	Rhodium	Rh	Uranium	U
Calcium	Ca	Gold	Au	Neon	Ne	Rubidium	Rb	Vanadium	V
Californium	Cf	Hafnium	Hf	Neptunium	Np	Ruthenium	Ru	Xenon	Xe
Carbon	C	Helium	He	Nickel	Ni	Samarium	Sm	Ytterbium	Yb
Cerium	Ce	Holmium	Ho	Niobium	Nb	Scandium	Sc	Yttrium	Y
Cesium	Cs	Hydrogen	H	Nitrogen	N	Selenium	Se	Zinc	Zn
Chlorine	Cl	Indium	In	Nobelium	No	Silicon	Si	Zirconium	Zr
Chromium	Cr	Iodine	I	Osmium	Os	Silver	Ag		

Reference Tables for Chemistry

PHYSICAL CONSTANTS AND CONVERSION FACTORS

Name	Symbol	Value(s)	Units
Angstrom unit	Å	1×10^{-10} m	meter
Avogadro number	N_A	6.02×10^{23} per mol	
Charge of electron	e	1.60×10^{-19} C	coulomb
Electron volt	eV	1.60×10^{-19} J	joule
Speed of light	c	3.00×10^{8} m/s	meters/second
Planck's constant	h	6.63×10^{-34} J · s	joule-second
		1.58×10^{-37} kcal · s	kilocalorie-second
Universal gas constant	R	0.0821 L · atm/mol · K	liter-atmosphere/mole-kelvin
		1.98 cal/mol · K	calories/mole-kelvin
		8.31 J/mol · K	joules/mole-kelvin
Atomic mass unit	μ(amu)	1.66×10^{-24} g	gram
Volume standard, liter	L	1×10^{3} cm^3 = 1 dm^3	cubic centimeters, cubic decimeter
Standard pressure, atmosphere	atm	101.3 kPa	kilopascals
		760 mmHg	millimeters of mercury
		760 torr	torr
Heat equivalent, kilocalorie	kcal	4.18×10^{3} J	joules

Physical Constants for H$_2$O

Molal freezing point depression . . . . 1.86°C
Molal boiling point elevation . . . . 0.52°C
Heat of fusion . . . . 79.72 cal/g
Heat of vaporization . . . . 539.4 cal/g

STANDARD UNITS

Symbol	Name	Quantity
m	meter	length
kg	kilogram	mass
Pa	pascal	pressure
K	kelvin	thermodynamic temperature
mol	mole	amount of substance
J	joule	energy, work
		quantity of heat
sec	second	time
C	coulomb	quantity of electricity
V	volt	electric potential, potential difference
L	liter	volume

Selected Prefixes

Factor	Prefix	Symbol
10^{6}	mega	M
10^{3}	kilo	k
10^{-1}	deci	d
10^{-2}	centi	c
10^{-3}	milli	m
10^{-6}	micro	μ
10^{-9}	nano	n

RELATIVE STRENGTHS OF ACIDS IN AQUEOUS SOLUTION AT 1 atm AND 298 K

Conjugate Pairs	K_a
ACID BASE	
$HI = H^+ + I^-$	very large
$HBr = H^+ + Br^-$	very large
$HCl = H^+ + Cl^-$	very large
$HNO_3 = H^+ + NO_3^-$	very large
$H_2SO_4 = H^+ + HSO_4^-$	large
$H_2O + SO_2 = H^+ + HSO_3^-$	1.5×10^{-2}
$HSO_4^- = H^+ + SO_4^{2-}$	1.2×10^{-2}
$H_3PO_4 = H^+ + H_2PO_4^-$	7.5×10^{-3}
$Fe(H_2O)_6^{3+} = H^+ + Fe(H_2O)_5(OH)^{2+}$	8.9×10^{-4}
$HNO_2 = H^+ + NO_2^-$	4.6×10^{-4}
$HF = H^+ + F^-$	3.5×10^{-4}
$Cr(H_2O)_6^{3+} = H^+ + Cr(H_2O)_5(OH)^{2+}$	1.0×10^{-4}
$CH_3COOH = H^+ + CH_3COO^-$	1.8×10^{-5}
$Al(H_2O)_6^{3+} = H^+ + Al(H_2O)_5(OH)^{2+}$	1.1×10^{-5}
$H_2O + CO_2 = H^+ + HCO_3^-$	4.3×10^{-7}
$HSO_3^- = H^+ + SO_3^{2-}$	1.1×10^{-7}
$H_2S = H^+ + HS^-$	9.5×10^{-8}
$H_2PO_4^- = H^+ + HPO_4^{2-}$	6.2×10^{-8}
$NH_4^+ = H^+ + NH_3$	5.7×10^{-10}
$HCO_3^- = H^+ + CO_3^{2-}$	5.6×10^{-11}
$HPO_4^{2-} = H^+ + PO_4^{3-}$	2.2×10^{-13}
$HS^- = H^+ + S^{2-}$	1.3×10^{-14}
$H_2O = H^+ + OH^-$	1.0×10^{-14}

Note: $H^+ (aq) = H_3O^+$

Sample equation: $HI + H_2O = H_3O^+ + I^-$

CONSTANTS FOR VARIOUS EQUILIBRIA AT 1 atm AND 298 K

$H_2O(\ell) = H^+ (aq) + OH^-(aq)$	$K_w = 1.0 \times 10^{-14}$
$H_2O(\ell) + H_2O(\ell) = H_3O^+(aq) + OH^-(aq)$	$K_w = 1.0 \times 10^{-14}$
$CH_3COO^-(aq) + H_2O(\ell) = CH_3COOH(aq) + OH^-(aq)$	$K_b = 5.6 \times 10^{-10}$
$Na^+F^-(aq) + H_2O(\ell) = Na^+ (OH)^- + HF(aq)$	$K_b = 1.5 \times 10^{-11}$
$NH_3(aq) + H_2O(\ell) = NH_4^+(aq) + OH^-(aq)$	$K_b = 1.8 \times 10^{-5}$
$CO_3^{2-}(aq) + H_2O(\ell) = HCO_3^-(aq) + OH^- (aq)$	$K_b = 1.8 \times 10^{-4}$
$Ag(NH_3)_2^+(aq) = Ag^+(aq) + 2NH_3(aq)$	$K_{eq} = 8.9 \times 10^{-8}$
$N_2(g) + 3H_2(g) = 2NH_3(g)$	$K_{eq} = 6.7 \times 10^5$
$H_2(g) + I_2(g) = 2HI(g)$	$K_{eq} = 3.5 \times 10^{-1}$

Compound	K_{sp}	Compound	Ksp
AgBr	5.0×10^{-13}	Li_2CO_3	2.5×10^{-2}
AgCl	1.8×10^{-10}	$PbCl_2$	1.6×10^{-5}
Ag_2CrO_4	1.1×10^{-12}	$PbCO_3$	7.4×10^{-14}
AgI	8.3×10^{-17}	$PbCrO_4$	2.8×10^{-13}
$BaSO_4$	1.1×10^{-10}	PbI_2	7.1×10^{-9}
$CaSO_4$	9.1×10^{-6}	$ZnCO_3$	1.4×10^{-11}

STANDARD ENERGIES OF FORMATION
OF COMPOUNDS AT 1 atm AND 298 K

Compound	Heat (Enthalpy) of Formation* kcal/mol (ΔH°_f)	Free Energy of Formation* kcal/mol (ΔG°_f)
Aluminum oxide $Al_2O_3(s)$	−400.5	−378.2
Ammonia $NH_3(g)$	−11.0	−3.9
Barium sulfate $BaSo_4(s)$	−352.1	−325.6
Calcium hydroxide $Ca(OH)_2(s)$	−235.7	−214.8
Carbon dioxide $CO_2(g)$	−94.1	−94.3
Carbon monoxide $CO(g)$	−26.4	−32.8
Copper (II) sulfate $CuSO_4(s)$	−184.4	−158.2
Ethane $C_2H_6(g)$	−20.2	−7.9
Ethene (ethylene) $C_2H_4(g)$	12.5	16.3
Ethyne (acetylene) $C_2H_2(g)$	54.2	50.0
Hydrogen fluoride $HF(g)$	−64.8	−65.3
Hydrogen iodide $HI(g)$	6.3	0.4
Iodine chloride $ICl(g)$	4.3	−1.3
Lead (II) oxide $PbO(s)$	−51.5	−45.0
Magnesium oxide $MgO(s)$	−143.8	−136.1
Nitrogen (II) oxide $NO(g)$	21.6	20.7
Nitrogen (IV) oxide $NO_2(g)$	7.9	12.3
Potassium chloride $KCl(s)$	−104.4	−97.8
Sodium chloride $NaCl(s)$	−98.3	−91.8
Sulfur dioxide $SO_2(g)$	−70.9	−71.7
Water $H_2O(g)$	−57.8	−54.6
Water $H_2O(\ell)$	−68.3	−56.7

*Minus sign indicates an exothermic reaction.

Sample equations:

$$2Al(s) + \frac{3}{2} O_2(g) \rightarrow Al_2O_3(s) + 400.5 \text{ kcal}$$

$$2Al(s) + \frac{3}{2} O_2(g) \rightarrow Al_2O_3(s) \quad \Delta H = -400.5 \text{ kcal/mol}$$